T0327616

Equine Pharmacology

Equine Pharmacology

EDITORS

Cynthia Cole DVM, PhD, DACVCP

Director of Research & Development, Mars Veterinary, Portland, Oregon, USA

Bradford Bentz VMD, MS, DACVIM, DACVECC, DABVP (equine)

Equine Medicine and Surgery, Bossier City, Louisiana, USA

Lara Maxwell DVM, PhD, DACVCP

Oklahoma State University, Stillwater, Oklahoma, USA

WILEY Blackwell

Contents

Contributors

Bradford Bentz, VMD, MS, DACVIM, DACVECC, DABVP (equine)
Equine Medicine and Surgery
Bossier City, LA, USA

Jennifer E. Carter, DVM, MANZCVS, DACVAA, CVPP
Lecturer in Veterinary Anaesthesia
Faculty of Veterinary Science
University of Melbourne
Werribee, Australia

Michelle L. Ceresia, PharmD
Associate Professor
MCPHS University
Boston, MA, USA

Cynthia Cole, DVM, PhD, DACVCP
Director of Research & Development
Mars Veterinary
Portland, OR, USA

Tad Coles, DVM
Kansas City, MO, USA

Jennifer Durenburger, DVM, JD
Director of Racing
Massachusetts Gaming Commission
Boston, MA, USA

Amber Labelle, DVM, MS, DACVO
Assistant Professor
Comparative Ophthalmology
Veterinary Teaching Hospital
University of Illinois Urbana-Champaign
Urbana, IL, USA

Randy Lynn, DVM, MS, DACVCP
Greensboro, NC, USA

K. Gary Magdesian, DVM, DACVIM, ACVCP, ACVECC
Henry Endowed Chair in Emergency Medicine
and Critical Care
School of Veterinary Medicine
University of California
Davis, CA, USA

Dianne McFarlane, DVM, PhD, DACVIM, ABVP
Associate Professor/Ricks-Rapp Professor
Oklahoma State University
Stillwater, OK, USA

Lara Maxwell, DVM, PhD, DACVCP
Associate Professor
Oklahoma State University
Stillwater, OK, USA

Melissa R. Mazan, DVM, Diplomate ACVIM
Associate Professor
Department of Clinical Sciences
Cummings School of Veterinary Medicine
Tufts University
North Grafton, MA, USA

Nora Nogradi, DVM, DACVIM
Equine Internal Medicine Specialist
Dubai Equine Hospital
Dubai, United Arab Emirates

Sheilah A. Robertson, BVMS (Hons), PhD, DECVAA, DACVAA, Dip ECAWBM (WSEL)
Specialist in Welfare Science, Ethics and Law, DACAW,
MRCVS
Professor
Department of Large Animal Clinical Sciences
University of Florida College of Veterinary Medicine
Gainesville, FL, USA

L. Chris Sanchez, DVM, PhD, DACVIM
Associate Professor
Department of Large Animal Clinical Sciences
University of Florida College of Veterinary Medicine
Gainesville, FL, USA

Meg Sleeper, VMD, DACVIM (Cardiology)
Associate Professor of Cardiology/Clinician Educator
School of Veterinary Medicine
University of Pennsylvania
Philadelphia, PA, USA

Brett Tennent-Brown, BVSc, MS, DACVIM, DACVECC
The University of Melbourne
Hawthorn, Victoria, Australia

Balazs Toth, DVM, MS, MSc, DACVIM
Section Head
Equine Internal Medicine
Equine Department and Clinic
Szent István University
Dora-Major, Hungary

Scot Waterman, DVM
Animal Welfare and Medical Advisor
Arizona Department of Racing
Tucson, AZ, USA

Preface

The objective of this book is to provide practitioners and veterinary students with a concise and practical guide to equine clinical pharmacology. Although some equine pharmacology texts choose to emphasize complete in-depth reviews of the scientific literature, this approach does not necessarily help the practitioner choose the best therapeutic approach for a specific clinical situation. In contrast, whereas formulary texts are extremely popular for their ease of use and simplicity, there is much more to the successful use of therapeutic medications in horses than simply choosing a dose and dosing frequency. Therefore, we sought authors for this book who are both experts in the specific topic of interest and also had experience or interest in clinical pharmacology. Because we wanted the text to be very practical with a clinical approach, we sought individuals who deal with medication issues on a regular basis, either in their patients in the clinics, in the course of their research, or in many cases a combination of both.

The text is divided into two sections. Section 1 begins with a discussion of some of the important differences between horses and other species in terms of clinical pharmacology. This is an extremely important chapter because many of the therapeutics used in horses have not been well studied and their potential benefits and risks are extrapolated from studies in other species. Practitioners need to be aware of the limitations and caveats of such extrapolations. This section also covers a broad range of clinical pharmacology topics that commonly confront the equine practitioner, including antimicrobials, anesthesia, analgesics, nonsteroidal anti-inflammatory drugs (NSAIDs), and anti-parasiticides. A separate chapter on the clinical pharmacology of foals was included to stress how their unique physiology has ramifications in the use of therapeutics in neonates. Although fluids and electrolytes are not uniformly considered to be within the realm of clinical pharmacology, we included a chapter on this topic because fluids and electrolyte balance are critical components of many therapeutic plans for critically ill horses. Finally, a discussion of drug and medication control programs was included because most equine athletes compete under such regulations, so it is important for practitioners to know where they can get accurate, up-to-date information on those rules. Section 2 takes a systems approach to clinical pharmacology. Often pharmacology is presented by drug classes, but rarely is only a single class of drugs indicated in the treatment of a disease condition. By discussing therapeutic approaches for diseases that affect each organ system, a concise, logical, and comprehensive guide is provided to the practitioner. The systems covered range from the ophthalmic to cardiovascular. Because the same drug may be used in the therapy of several different diseases, therapeutics may appear in multiple chapters. For example, the use of NSAIDs is discussed in a summary chapter in Section 1 but are also included in several chapters in Section 2.

SECTION 1
General Review Section

CHAPTER 1

Horse of a different color: Peculiarities of equine pharmacology

Lara Maxwell

Oklahoma State University, Stillwater, OK, USA

Introduction

Horses are different. Practitioners expect such differences, given the unique anatomy and physiology of the many species encountered within veterinary medicine. Nonetheless, the appropriate use of therapeutic agents can be particularly challenging in the horse. Small animal practitioners have an advantage over other veterinary clinicians when novel therapeutics are investigated for veterinary use, as the pharmacology of investigational drugs is often described in dogs before they are used in people. However, if the dog is the prototypical species of basic pharmacological research, then the horse is just the opposite. The many idiosyncrasies of equine anatomy and physiology can make the behavior of drugs in this species highly unpredictable. Drugs that are well absorbed after oral administration, safe, and efficacious in other species may be poorly absorbed, toxic, or ineffective in horses. This chapter will investigate the sources of some of these pharmacological peculiarities and address strategies for using drugs safely and effectively in horses despite these inherent challenges.

Idiosyncrasies related to route of administration

Enteral absorption

Administration of drugs per os is the most natural route in companion animals. Administering foreign material to the gastrointestinal tract (GIT) is safer than parenteral administration, since the immunological and physical defenses in the GIT are designed to cope with all manner of foreign substances. Particulates, excipients, bacteria, fungi, endotoxins, and other toxins can be devastating if inadvertently administered parenterally, but most of these contaminants will have little impact if inadvertently delivered to the GIT. The cost of a drug formulated for oral administration is often less than its injectable counterpart, because of the stringent requirements needed to prepare safe injectable formulations. In addition, owner and patient compliance is usually better when oral drug administration is employed, especially when the duration of therapy encompasses days, weeks, or even for the remaining life of the patient. For all of these reasons, the oral route of administration is generally preferred in the nonhospitalized equine patient. In counterpoint to all of the advantages of oral drug administration, there are certainly disadvantages that the equine practitioner will recognize. First, getting the drug into the stomach of the horse can be challenging. Some small capsules and powders can be administered as a top-dressing to highly palatable feed. For horses that don't avoid top-dressed drugs and drugs that are palatable, this method of administration probably represents the most effective and convenient method of oral administration. Capsules, tablets, and powders may be hidden in pieces of carrot or apple with space carved or drilled by drug placement. Capsules and powders can also be mixed with applesauce, molasses, or syrup and mixed with feed, bran, or beet pulp. These methods can all be effective but require that the feed bucket be observed after

Equine Pharmacology, First Edition. Edited by Cynthia Cole, Bradford Bentz and Lara Maxwell.
© 2015 John Wiley & Sons, Inc. Published 2015 by John Wiley & Sons, Inc.

administration to confirm that the entire dose was ingested. For unpalatable drugs and horses that avoid top-dressings, a powder can be mixed with applesauce, syrup, or molasses and placed in a syringe. A catheter-tipped syringe can be used for thinner mixtures, or the tip of the syringe can be removed and surfaces sanded smooth for the administration of thicker mixtures. Tablets can be crushed with a mortar and pestle, coffee grinder, or hammer to make a powder for administration. Some tablets and capsules can also be dissolved in a small volume of water. However, not all drugs are soluble and stable in water, so knowledge of the drug's aqueous stability is necessary if the drug does not quickly dissolve and is not immediately administered. Drugs should not be heated to speed solubilization unless aqueous and thermal stability is known, since heating will also speed hydrolysis of an unstable drug. Drugs with beta-lactam rings, including penicillins and cephalosporins, as well as some drugs with ester bonds, such as valacyclovir, have poor aqueous stability (see Chapter 2) [1, 2]. Some tablets and capsules that are insoluble in water will instead dissolve in the acidic pH of lemon juice [3]. The volume of lemon juice should be minimized to limit administration of the acidic solution, and it should be mixed with syrup or feed prior to administration.

Administration of drugs by a nasogastric tube is sometimes employed clinically and is often the route used when the oral absorption of a drug is being investigated. However, nasogastric intubation requires the presence of the veterinarian and is poorly tolerated for chronic dosing regimens. The bioavailability, or the total amount of the drug that reaches systemic circulation, of an orally administered drug is often reported in the initial assessments of a drug's utility in horses. As described in the following text, the knowledge of a drug's oral bioavailability will assist the practitioner with decisions regarding selection of the best available drug for a particular condition, dose modifications, and the likelihood of therapeutic failure with a particular drug. Since bioavailability is often known from studies detailing the drug's pharmacokinetic properties, the presentation of bioavailability after nasogastric administration to a fasted horse represents the best possible bioavailability of that drug in the horse. However, the actual bioavailability in the field, where fasting is difficult and nasogastric administration is seldom used, may be considerably lower than the reported value.

Although we expect that cattle and other ruminants will exhibit unique absorption patterns when drugs are administered per os, we may conversely expect that horses will absorb drugs in a similar manner to other monogastric species. Certainly, this expectation is met for some therapeutics, with drugs such as fluconazole being nearly completely absorbed after oral administration to horses and other species [4]. If the bioavailability is less than 100% but still adequate, an increase in dose can be used to obtain therapeutic results comparable to that of intravenous (IV) administration [5]. However, other drugs, such as acyclovir and azathioprine, are subject to abysmal oral bioavailability in horses [6, 7]. There are numerous pharmacological examples of drugs, such as furosemide, tramadol, metformin, ciprofloxacin, and amoxicillin, that are adequately absorbed after oral administration to other monogastric species but are poorly absorbed in horses, with average bioavailability of less than 10% [8–13]. Such drugs are rarely if ever administered orally to adult horses due to the recognition that their bioavailability is too low to allow a predictable therapeutic effect at doses that are practical to administer.

Parallels may be drawn between ruminants and horses, with ruminants often exhibiting very poor oral absorption of therapeutics due to the propensity of ruminal microbes to cleave xenobiotics to an inactive form and the dilution of drugs by the tremendous volume of the ruminal fluid [14]. Although horses have a monogastric digestive system, the poor bioavailability of some drugs in horses can also be attributed to their herbivorous diet. Whereas horses do not maintain the full complement of cellulolytic gastric bacteria as ruminants, both ruminants and horses do ingest a large volume of herbaceous feed, and horses do maintain some fermentative bacteria as part of the normal stomach flora [15]. Although the effect of the equine gastric flora on drug stability is poorly understood, it has been shown that some drugs, such as ampicillin, will specifically bind to equine ingesta, limiting their bioavailability [16]. Although feeding status also impacts some drug absorption profiles in other species, the presence of feed can be even more important to the absorption of orally administered drugs in horses. For example, the *rate* of flunixin absorption is greatly affected by fasting in horses, with the time of maximal plasma drug concentration occurring much later in fed horses (7 h) than in fasted ones (<1 h) [17]. Interestingly, whereas the *rate* of flunixin absorption was dependent on feeding, the *extent* of absorption was not, so efficacy is probably unaffected. However, a decrease in the maximal plasma drug concentration that occurs with slower absorption can reduce the efficacy of drugs that must reach some threshold concentration to obtain the desired effect, since a slower rate of absorption will produce a lower peak plasma concentration. Alternatively, the presence of feed may affect both the rate and extent of absorption of some drugs, such as moxidectin [18]. It should also be noted that the presence of feed does not affect the absorption of some orally administered drugs. For example, the absorption of orally administered meclofenamic acid is not affected by feeding status [19].

For those drugs that are poorly absorbed after feeding, strategic fasting can increase the peak concentration, the extent of absorption, or both properties. However, fasting can be difficult to implement with a prolonged multiple-dose regimen. Complicating the design of a strategic fasting schedule, the amount of fasting time required to enhance drug absorption in horses is poorly defined, with some studies reporting enhanced absorption with fasting for as little as a few hours before and after oral drug administration and others after fasting overnight [17, 20]. The rate of gastric emptying depends on both diet composition and amount ingested, with large amounts of high-starch feeds taking longer to leave the equine stomach as compared to smaller meals with a lower proportion of starch [21]. Since it takes longer than a few hours of fasting to completely empty the equine stomach, it appears that a reduction of gastric volume, rather than complete gastric emptying, can enhance drug absorption. Such a goal makes pharmacokinetic sense, since dilution of drug by stomach contents will reduce the drug concentration in gastric juice and thereby reduce the concentration gradient between gastric juice and blood, which is the driving force of diffusion into systemic circulation.

Further support for the notion that the herbaceous diet of adult horses is to blame for sporadic poor bioavailability of drugs is found in the adequate oral absorption of some drugs, such as amoxicillin, when administered to foals, despite their poor absorption in adult horses [8, 9, 22]. As a consequence, some drugs that are not clinically useful in adult horses due to poor oral absorption are well absorbed in foals and so can be used in young, prefermentative animals (see Chapter 7).

Even drugs that are adequately absorbed after oral administration to horses may be subject to considerable variability in plasma concentrations due to erratic and unpredictable absorption patterns. Inconsistent therapeutic responses can follow such unpredictable absorption patterns, and the clinical importance of variable bioavailability is often underappreciated. For example, the absorption of metronidazole exhibits oral bioavailability ($74 \pm 18\%$, mean $\pm$ SD) that is fairly typical of a drug with adequate oral absorption in horses. A casual inspection of these values might suggest that there will be little variation in the plasma metronidazole concentrations between different horses, leading to a reliable therapeutic effect. However, a closer inspection of this data shows that the 95% confidence interval for metronidazole bioavailability for the extrapolated population would then be from 52 to 96%. As a consequence of this nearly twofold difference in bioavailability, plasma drug concentrations would also vary by at least twofold between horses at the lower and higher ends of typical bioavailability. The impact of erratic bioavailability on plasma concentrations will be further compounded by variability in other aspects of drug disposition, such as the extent of drug distribution and the rate of drug metabolism. Although pharmacokinetic differences between horses can be important sources of therapeutic failure for a drug administered by any route, interindividual differences are particularly pronounced when drugs are administered orally, as the initial variability in absorption combines with all other sources of variation.

Similarly, intrarectal administration, as is routinely employed for metronidazole administration to horses, may result in even more irregular absorption. For example, the average intrarectal bioavailability for metronidazole in horses is $30 \pm 9\%$, giving a 95% confidence interval of 19–41% or a greater than twofold difference in absorption. For any drug where mean bioavailability is relatively low, perhaps 50% or less, there will be a substantial chance of clinically relevant variability in drug absorption between horses. This variability arises because a relatively small change in drug absorption will have a disproportionately large effect on fluctuation in plasma drug concentrations. As illustrated earlier for intrarectally administered metronidazole, as well as for more poorly absorbed orally administered drugs like digoxin, the range in the bioavailability of such drugs will generally vary by at least twofold [23]. Plasma drug concentrations that are lower or higher than expected can lead to therapy that does not produce the desired effect or, conversely, to drug toxicity. Such pharmacokinetic considerations should therefore be considered in horses that fail to respond to therapy as expected. The solution to such a failure may be to change the dose to the upper or lower end of the range of suggested doses or to switch to an alternate drug that is more reliably absorbed in horses. Drugs with bioavailability less than

10% are rarely useful when orally administered to horses due to low and erratic plasma drug concentrations. The oral administration of ciprofloxacin to horses is such an example, with a reported bioavailability of $7 \pm 5\%$. [13] The associated 95% confidence interval for oral ciprofloxacin bioavailability in horses, therefore, varies almost sevenfold. Such extreme variability typically accompanies the very poor bioavailability of such drugs, as small absolute changes in absorption account for a large change in the overall proportion of drug absorbed. This high variability generally precludes the safe and effective use of drugs with very low bioavailability, since the variability in drug absorption will continue at the higher dose rate. Consequently, even if a higher dose is administered in an attempt to reach targeted plasma concentrations, the resulting highly variable drug plasma concentrations will lead to a similarly unpredictable therapeutic response. Thus, very low bioavailability of drugs is usually an insurmountable obstacle to their clinical utility, necessitating a more reliable route of administration for the drug to be useful.

Formulations that enhance oral bioavailability

Poor bioavailability of some classes of drugs is a problem not only of horses but of other species as well. Therefore, specific drug formulations have been developed to combat poor oral absorption, and horses have benefited from many of these "designer drugs." For example, erythromycin base is rapidly hydrolyzed by the acidic pH of gastric juice, so it is administered in other species as an enteric-coated tablet, where the enteric coating prevents drug dissolution until the tablet reaches the more basic pH of the small intestine [24]. Grinding of the enteric-coated tablet for administration to horses disrupts the enteric coating, so the erythromycin is hydrolyzed in the stomach and subject to poor bioavailability. However, administration of an erythromycin estolate formulation produces much higher plasma erythromycin concentrations as the ester form is much more stable in acidic conditions [25]. As a prodrug, the ester bond must be broken by drug-metabolizing enzymes that are primarily present in enterocytes, the blood, and the liver, as only the liberated ester base will be active. Several other drugs, such as valacyclovir and cefpodoxime proxetil, are also ester prodrugs with enhanced bioavailability of the active drug in horses or foals [26, 27]. However, ester prodrugs are not always advantageous in horses, as is the case with

prednisone, an ester prodrug of prednisolone. Both prednisone and prednisolone are well absorbed after oral administration to people, but prednisone was the first synthetic glucocorticoid developed for use in patients and so was the first synthetic, orally administered glucocorticoid to be widely used [28]. Despite administration of oral prednisone to equine patients for many years, only within the past decade was it reported that horses do not absorb orally administered prednisone well and do not readily convert prednisone to its active form, prednisolone, by the hepatic enzymes that are quite effective in dogs and people [29]. As prednisone is inactive, its administration cannot therefore be expected to produce a therapeutic effect in the horse. This finding shows again how important species-specific differences in drug absorption and metabolism can be. In addition, the dramatic differences between the metabolism of the ester bonds of prednisone and more useful prodrugs, like erythromycin estolate, demonstrate that the activation of prodrugs cannot be assumed in horses, but must be determined individually for each prodrug.

Parenteral routes of administration

Horses with altered perfusion, shock, or colic cannot be expected to absorb orally administered drugs normally, so IV administration should be selected in the physiologically compromised patient. IV administration is also preferred when a rapid onset of action is needed, such as for the administration of anesthetic agents or for assurance that the entire dose reaches the systemic circulation. Some drugs, such as potassium penicillin, must be administered slowly when given IV in order to avoid side effects associated with rapid administration (see Chapter 2). Other drugs, such as phenylbutazone, are irritants and will cause phlebitis and sloughing if any portion of the dose is administered extravascularly (see Chapter 5). Drugs that are known irritants, or those with very high or low pH in solution, should be administered very carefully to avoid extravasation and the possible sequelae of clostridial myositis [30]. Most irritants can only be administered topically or IV via a large vessel; the intramuscular (IM) and subcutaneous (SC) routes should be avoided to prevent tissue damage [31].

IM administration is generally preferred over IV administration if an owner must administer therapeutics, as personnel with insufficient training are at an increased risk of inadvertent intracarotid administration when attempting to use the jugular vein. Intracarotid administration is associated with severe effects on the central nervous system (CNS), such as seizure, and so IV administration should be used judiciously. IM drug administration can be preferred to the oral route for some drugs with low oral bioavailability, such as penicillin G. Some drugs are subject to higher bioavailability when administered IM rather than orally, but without prior pharmacokinetic study, the clinician cannot predict whether the IM route will provide faster or better absorption than the oral route. One of the most important advantages of the IM route of administration as compared to IV or oral routes is that depot drug formulations can be administered IM for a prolonged effect. The extended effect of depot formulations can be ascribed to "flip-flop" kinetics, where drug absorption from the site of administration is the rate-limiting step of disposition and is much slower than the rate of drug elimination. Consequently, the slow absorption rate instead appears to be the rate of drug disappearance from the plasma, and the drug's effect can persist much longer than if the same dose was administered IV. However, the drug effect will only occur for as long as the drug concentration is able to remain at effective plasma concentrations, since depot formulations produce lower peak drug concentrations than do equivalent doses of the nondepot formulations. Penicillin benzathine formulations are an example of a depot formulation for which the resulting low plasma concentrations may reduce drug efficacy (see Chapter 2). Depot formulations also include corticosteroids, such as methylprednisolone acetate, which are most often used in joints for a prolonged anti-inflammatory effect, and several important antibacterial agents, such as procaine penicillin G and ceftiofur crystalline free acid (see Chapters 2 and 13). The neck, semitendinosus/semimembranosus muscle (buttocks), and, occasionally, the pectoral muscles are the sites most often used for IM administration. Injections may be rotated between sites when drugs, such as procaine penicillin G, are given more frequently. For drugs given infrequently, such as ceftiofur crystalline free acid, clinicians should select the site for which pharmacokinetic or efficacy data is available, since the site of administration can affect drug absorption [32]. Side effects specific to the IM route of administration are infrequent but can occur and, on rare occasion, are life threatening. Localized reactions can range from stiffness and swelling to bacterial abscessation and clostridial myositis. Because the rump or gluteal muscles are poorly drained in the event of abscess formations, this site is seldom used unless rotation between multiple IM sites is needed [33]. Administration of drugs into the buttocks has the advantage of injecting into a large, well-vascularized muscle mass, which can decrease the chance of tissue reactions and infection [30]. Clostridial myositis has followed the administration of a variety of drugs and vaccines IM but is most closely linked with the IM administration of flunixin meglumine, so it is most judicious to avoid IM administration of flunixin and other nonsteroidal anti-inflammatory drugs (NSAIDs) and use oral or IV routes instead [30]. Inadvertent administration of procaine penicillin G into the vasculature supplying muscle can result in CNS signs ranging from excitement to seizure, probably due to the rapid delivery of high concentrations of procaine to the CNS (see Chapter 2). For this reason, the IM injection site should be checked for inadvertent intravascular placement prior to injection.

Drug interactions

Over several decades, equine practice has become increasingly sophisticated in its use of therapeutic agents. There has been an exponential increase in studies investigating the therapeutic potential of novel agents, and new drugs have been specifically developed for use in horses. With the availability of new therapeutic options and treatment modalities, equine patients are increasingly likely to be exposed to multiple drug regimens or the inadvertent combination of several drugs to treat concurrent diseases. Drug combinations can be advantageous, detrimental, or neutral, with no net effect on efficacy or toxicity. Although some combinations are specifically chosen for their advantageous properties, most combinations that the clinician encounters are not adequately characterized to allow better than empirical predictions of their effects. With little information available regarding drug interactions in horses and the increasing use of "polypharmacy" in veterinary medicine, clinicians must be alert to potential interactions when administering multiple drugs to a patient. With clinical experience of common drug combinations, as well as knowledge of a drug's mechanism of action and pharmacokinetic properties, the clinician can assess the odds of a drug interaction and identify the most likely side effects.

Pharmacodynamic drug interactions

Drug–drug interactions can be either pharmacodynamic or pharmacokinetic in nature. Pharmacodynamic interactions occur when one drug increases or decreases the effect of another. Synergistic and potentiated combinations can be therapeutically beneficial and are most commonly selected for the use of antimicrobial, anesthetic, and analgesic agents. For example, the combination of penicillin with gentamicin produces a synergistic antibacterial effect (see Chapter 2). In addition, the anesthetic effects of isoflurane are potentiated by the addition of ketamine and lidocaine (see Chapter 3). Similarly, the use of multimodal analgesia can reduce the doses of each individual drug, thus decreasing the potential for adverse effects while still providing effective pain relief (see Chapter 4). On the other hand, drug combinations can instead be detrimental. Chloramphenicol coadministered with enrofloxacin can produce an antagonistic effect that impedes bacterial killing (see Chapter 2). The simultaneous administration of multiple drugs with similar mechanisms of action can enhance toxicity, as in the combination of firocoxib and phenylbutazone (see Chapters 5 and 13).

Pharmacokinetic drug interactions

Pharmacological compounds are xenobiotics, originating outside the body. As such, one can conceptualize drug metabolism as the body's attempt to render such substances inactive and more readily excreted. Whereas some drugs, such as gentamicin and penicillin, are primarily excreted intact into the urine, many other drugs are too highly protein bound or too lipophilic to be efficiently excreted into the urine. Biotransformation either activates or inactivates such drugs but will generally make them more polar, so that the resulting metabolite will be more readily excreted. Metabolism can also conjugate a bulky, highly charged moiety to the backbone of the drug, allowing biliary and/or renal excretion of the resulting metabolite. Although there are multiple sites, including the liver, blood, enterocytes, and lung, in the body where metabolizing enzymes are located, the liver metabolizes the majority of therapeutic substances. Both cytosolic and membrane-bound enzymes, such as cytochrome P450 enzymes, perform similar functions in the metabolism of xenobiotics. Surveys of drugs approved for use in people reveal that the majority of approved therapeutics are metabolized by P450 enzymes [34]. Due to wide interspecies variability, cytochrome P450 density

and activity require direct study for each substrate in each species, with horses expressing high metabolizing activity for some drugs but low activity for others [35]. Since metabolites might be active or inactive, P450 metabolism is often responsible for drug–drug interactions due to induction or inhibition of their activity, with increased metabolism to active metabolites being an important source of drug toxicity. Phenobarbital induction of P450 enzymes is a well-recognized interaction that speeds the metabolism of phenobarbital itself but also increases the metabolism of other therapeutic drugs (see Chapter 12). Since the method of enzyme induction involves upregulation of expression and requires synthesis of new enzyme, induction is a relatively slow process, requiring days to weeks for the full effect to be realized. Conversely, inhibitors of P450 enzymes, such as ketoconazole, can immediately inhibit the metabolism of numerous other drugs (see Chapter 2). Other interactions involve more subtle competition for metabolism when two drugs are metabolized by the same P450 isoform. Cytochrome P450 isoforms are the expression of related metabolizing enzymes that differ with respect to their xenobiotic specificity and tissue location. P450 isoforms are divided into families, such as CYP1A, CYP3A, CYP2D, and CYP3C, by genotypic homology. The CYP3A family, specifically the CYP3A4 isoform, metabolizes the majority of therapeutics in people. Unfortunately, the CYP isoforms, their metabolizing specificity, and products are species specific, although CYP families are conserved between mammals. As a consequence, drug–drug interactions noted in one species, such as in humans, do not definitively indicate the likelihood of interactions in other species, such as in horses [36]. Such interactions are well recognized in people, where the individual hepatic P450 isoforms have been cloned, expressed in recombinant systems, and are routinely used to test all new therapeutics for interactions against a panel of substrates [37]. Even though the dog may be considered the model species of pharmacology and recombinant canine P450 isoforms are commercially available, recognition of drug–drug interactions is poorly understood even in this species [38]. Nonetheless, clinically relevant interactions, such as the inhibition of ketamine metabolism by concurrent medetomidine administration, have been noted in dogs [39]. However, if pharmacokinetic drug–drug interactions are poorly understood in dogs, then their recognition in horses is nearly in its infancy. Some equine P450 isoforms have been sequenced and expressed in recombinant systems, but are not yet commercially available for routine testing [40, 41]. Therapeutics that are used in horses and have been found to present clinically relevant pharmacokinetic interactions in other species include the P450 inducers phenobarbital and rifampin and the inhibitors ketoconazole, itraconazole, cimetidine, and erythromycin (Table 1.1). Some of these drugs have been used in combination (e.g., rifampin with erythromycin in foals with *Rhodococcus equi* pneumonia) in horses with apparent efficacy and safety. However, dramatic interactions have also been reported, such as a 90% decrease in the oral bioavailability of clarithromycin when rifampin was coadministered to foals for several weeks [42]. Interestingly, this decrease in clarithromycin bioavailability by rifampin coadministration appears to be due to both the well-recognized P450-inducing effects by rifampin and a decrease in unknown intestinal transporters [43]. Conversely, ivermectin increased the bioavailability of cetirizine when ivermectin was administered 12 h prior to cetirizine but not when administered 1.5 h before [44]. On the other hand, a known inhibitor of P450 enzymes in people, cimetidine, failed to decrease the metabolism of coadministered phenylbutazone in horses [45]. Furosemide has been well recognized for its propensity to decrease the urine concentrations of drugs of regulatory interest, but the diuretic actions of furosemide are also blunted by the coadministration of NSAIDs [46]. Where novel or poorly studied combinations are used, clinicians should be alert to potential interactions when administering multiple drugs to a patient. Particular vigilance is warranted in drugs that are known inhibitors or inducers of P450 enzymes in other species, even though species-specific differences may preclude such interactions (Table 1.1).

Species-specific difference in hepatic metabolizing enzymes not only results in unique drug–drug interaction but can also result in metabolites that are unique to a particular species. As these unique metabolites can either be active or inactive, differences in drug activity between species can occasionally be explained by differences in drug metabolites. In equine pharmacology, however, the identity of drug metabolites can be particularly important when identifying whether prohibited drugs have been administered to horses where forensic testing of plasma or urine is employed (see Chapter 9). Specific analysis of postrace or show samples may include testing for both the restricted parent drug and its metabolite, as the existence of the metabolite corroborates a positive finding since it suggests metabolism of the parent drug by the body, as opposed to contamination of the sample with the parent drug alone. The metabolic pathways of many illicit and prohibited drugs are well understood in people, due to the forensic testing routinely employed by high-stakes athletic competitions. In order for such metabolite testing to be accurate in equine competitions, the metabolic patterns of the restricted drug within horses must be similarly elucidated, since the existence of a particular major metabolite in human beings does not mean that the same metabolic pathways will predominate in horses. Some drugs for which oxidative or phase I metabolism produces unique major metabolites in horses include fentanyl, ractopamine, and nimesulide [57–59]. Synthetic or phase II metabolites may also differ between horses and other species, with glucuronyltransferase being the major high-capacity conjugative enzyme system, often producing glucuronidated metabolites that are similar to those found in people and dogs [60]. In the forensic setting, equine urine is routinely incubated with glucuronidase in order to liberate the conjugated metabolite from the parent drug or oxidative metabolite for identification. Although the glucuronidated metabolite can also be directly measured, cleavage of the glucuronide moiety simplifies analysis and so is routinely employed [61].

Veterinary compounding pharmacies

Introduction

The ethics, safety, and liability of prescribing drugs prepared by compounding pharmacies are issues that face all facets of veterinary practice. However, in 2009, the shocking deaths of 21 polo ponies that received an IV administered, compounded vitamin supplement illustrated the worst of the compounding industry woes, where a seemingly small measurement error can have disastrous consequences for all involved [62]. Veterinarians are faced daily with the therapeutic challenge of treating species and conditions for which no approved drug exists. Other challenges include the differing needs of patients that have species-specific requirements, as well as individual needs for palatability and formulation. Some of these needs can be met by extralabel drug use under the regulations of the Animal Medicinal Drug Use Clarification Act (AMDUCA) of 1994 [63]. However, extralabel drug use is insufficient if

Table 1.1 Pharmacokinetic and pharmacodynamic drug interactions in horses

Drug	Effect	Drugs affected	Possible effect	Evidence
P450 enzyme inducers/increased elimination rate				
Phenobarbital	Increases its own metabolism by autoinduction	Phenobarbital	Decreased efficacy	*In vivo* [47]
Phenylbutazone	Decreased elimination half-life and distribution of coadministered drug	Gentamicin	Decreased efficacy	*In vivo* [48]
Rifampin	Increases clearance of coadministered drug	Phenylbutazone, clarithromycin	Decreased efficacy	*In vivo* [42, 49]
Rifampin	Decreased bioavailability of coadministered drug	Clarithromycin	Decreased efficacy	*In vivo* [42, 43]
P450 enzyme or efflux pump inhibitors				
Chloramphenicol	Decreases clearance of coadministered drug	Thiamylal, phenylbutazone	Increased activity and toxicity	*In vivo* [49]
Ivermectin	Increased bioavailability of select drugs	Cetirizine	Increased activity and toxicity	*In vivo* [44]
Ketoconazole	Decreases clearance of coadministered drug	Ketamine	Increased activity and toxicity	*In vitro* [50]
Methadone	Decreased metabolism of coadministered drug	Ketamine	Increased activity and toxicity	*In vitro* [51]
Quinidine	Decreases clearance of coadministered drug	Digoxin	Increased activity and toxicity	*In vivo* [52]
Xylazine	Decreased metabolism of coadministered drug	Ketamine	Increased activity and toxicity	*In vitro* [51]
Pharmacodynamic/miscellaneous				
Furosemide	Dilution of urine by diuresis	Clenbuterol, phenylbutazone, flunixin, fentanyl, and others	Decreased urine drug concentrations	*In vivo* [46, 53, 54]
Ketamine	Increases effectiveness of other anesthetics	Halothane	Increased activity and toxicity	*In vivo* [55]
NSAIDs	Decrease diuretic effects	Furosemide	Decreased activity	*In vivo* [46, 56]

a drug is no longer available as either a human or veterinary formulation, if the palatability of a formulation is poor, or if a formulation needs to be a different strength than the approved product. Under these circumstances, compounded drugs are often used. Drug compounding can be described as a change in the dosage form of a drug from that of the approved product. Although provisions for compounding are included under AMDUCA, much of the regular practice of compounding stands outside of clear regulatory guidelines. In the wake of considerable regulatory confusion and disturbing accounts of therapeutic failure with compounded products, veterinarians, pharmacists, and regulators are revisiting the role of compounding pharmacies in veterinary practice.

What are the rules?

There are several laws and regulations to consider in the legality of drug compounding. First, the federal government was given regulatory authority over drugs by the Pure Food and Drugs along with the Food, Drug, and Cosmetic Acts of 1906 and 1938. However, regulations that specifically covered drug compounding took longer. Human compounding was addressed by the Food and Drug Administration (FDA) Modernization Act in 1997, but veterinary use was ignored. Like extralabel drug use, veterinary use of compounding was included in the AMDUCA of 1994. This act laid the provisions for both extralabel drug use and for drug compounding, resulting in some confusion among veterinary practitioners about which regulations cover which specific practice. Given these combinations of provisions, FDA guidelines for drug compounding include [64].

1 A valid veterinarian–client–patient relationship (VCPR) must exist.

2 The health of an animal must be threatened or suffering or death may result from failure to treat.

3 There must be no FDA-approved commercially available animal or human drug that, when used as labeled or in an extralabel fashion in its available dosage form and concentration, will appropriately treat the patient.

4 The product must be made from an FDA-approved commercially available animal or human drug.

5 The product must be compounded by a licensed veterinarian or a licensed pharmacist on the order of a veterinarian within the practice of veterinary medicine.

6 The compounded product must be safe and effective.

7 The amount of product compounded must be commensurate with the need of the animal identified in the VCPR-based prescription.

8 For animals produced for human consumption, the veterinarian must establish an extended withdrawal interval for the compounded product and ensure food safety. Compounding is not permitted if it results in violative food residue or any residue that may present a risk to public health.

9 No drug may be compounded for food animals from drugs listed on the prohibited list.

10 Veterinarians must comply with all aspects of the federal extralabel drug use regulations including record-keeping and labeling requirements.

11 All relevant state laws relating to compounding must be followed.

Suggestions issued by the AVMA for compounding provisions include (https://www.avma.org/KB/Resources/Reference/Pages/Compounding.aspx):

1 The decision to use a compounded drug should be veterinarian (not pharmacist) driven, based on a VCPR. Whenever possible, the veterinarian should make that decision utilizing evidence-based medicine.

2 Compounding must be implemented in compliance with the AMDUCA and the FDA Compliance Policy Guide (CPG) 608.400 titled Compounding of Drugs for Use in Animals. Use of compounded drugs in

food animals is accompanied by food safety concerns that preclude their use unless information exists to assure avoidance of illegal tissue residues.

3 The use of a compounded drug should be limited to:
   (a) Those drugs for which both safety and efficacy have been demonstrated in the compounded form in the target species
   (b) Disease conditions for which response to therapy or drug concentration can be monitored
   (c) Those individual patients for which no other method or route of drug delivery is practical

4 Use of a compounded drug should be accompanied by the same precautions followed when using an approved drug, including counseling of the client regarding potential adverse reactions and attention to the potential for unintended human or animal exposure to the drug.

A quick review of these requirements reveals several areas where common compounding practices may deviate from federal regulations. First, the need for a valid VCPR dictates that compounding cannot occur independent of the needs of a specific patient. As a consequence, the practice of stocking compounded drugs before the need for these drugs arises would be in violation of the first and seventh requirements. This presents a problem for veterinary practices that routinely need compounded products on an emergency basis, without the luxury of time required to fill a prescription and obtain the final compounded product. The 2004 FDA CPG, last issued in 2003, attempts to clarify some of the confusion arising from existing compounding regulations with regard to obtaining compounded product without a VCPR and to resale of a compounded product. The CPG states that FDA regulatory enforcement may be undertaken under the condition of "compounding of drugs in anticipation of receiving prescriptions, except in very limited quantities in relation to the amounts of drugs compounded after receiving prescriptions issued within the confines of a valid VCPR." The CPG further opposes third-party (e.g., veterinarian) sale of drugs compounded by a pharmacy. State pharmacy regulations also apply and may differ somewhat, with some allowing a practitioner to stock and sell a small supply of compounded medications sufficient for an anticipated patient need until the compounded prescription can be filled. Taken together, these statements suggest that practitioners may keep a very limited supply of routinely needed medications on hand to administer or dispense while a compounded prescription is concurrently filled. However, the practice of purchasing large amounts of compounded medications in the absence of a specific patient in need of that compounded product and especially of reselling such products is clearly discouraged by the FDA CPG and by most state pharmacy regulations.

The third requirement of drug compounding—that no FDA-approved veterinary or human drug currently exists that can meet the needs of the patient—is clearly counter to common practice. A perusal of current catalogs of compounding pharmacies shows many products and formulations that are substituted for approved drugs. The practice of substituting compounded drugs for approved drugs may be necessary in a few special circumstances, such as when the concentration of the approved drug is inappropriate for an individual patient or when palatability of the approved product is an issue for a particular patient. However, substitution of compounded products for approved products is often performed in an effort to reduce costs of drug therapy. A price reducing intention is clearly counter to FDA guidance and can expose patients to unnecessary risk, as some of these substitute products are prepared from drug stocks of unknown purity and potency. This raises the most contentious issue currently surrounding the practice of veterinary compounding: the use of bulk drugs to prepare the compounded product. Bulk drug is a compound in its raw, often powdered, form that is ordered directly from a chemical or pharmaceutical manufacturer. Some drugs, such as cisapride and some antidotes, are not currently manufactured as approved drugs and so can only be prepared from bulk ingredients [65]. Other compounded drugs may be prepared from bulk supplies in order to meet a specific concentration need. However, the majority of drugs compounded from bulk chemicals have the appearance of being cost-saving measures.

In order to put the use of bulk chemicals into perspective, let's compare the manufacture of approved drugs with that of bulk drugs used in compounding. Pharmaceutical companies will use bulk drugs as one step of the manufacturing process. However, pharmaceutical companies are also subject to strict oversight and regulations, such as Good Manufacturing Practice, that are designed to establish and maintain the purity, potency, stability, and sterility (if applicable) of the final manufactured product. Compounding pharmacies are bound to no such manufacturing regulations, with the result that the patient, client, and veterinarian are left to trust completely that a compounding pharmacy can reliably ascertain whether the drug source, preparation steps, product stability, and sterility all meet high standards. Several independent studies of compounded

pharmaceutical products have demonstrated that compounded drugs often fail to meet such standards [66–69]. While bulk drug may be certified by the US Pharmacopeia (USP) to be of high purity, the use of many USP drugs will result in final compounded product that is at least as expensive as the FDA-approved product. Therefore, many bulk drugs are instead obtained from uncertain and questionable sources where certificates of analysis are not performed by independent testing. Given the not-too-distant melamine scare in pet foods, independent testing for purity and potency has become a matter of great concern when using drugs of unknown origin. Further, the use of bulk drugs introduces an extra preparation step that a pharmacy technician must undertake, which can increase the chance of formulation errors. The 2009 deaths of 21 polo ponies that received a compounded vitamin supplement was apparently due to just such a formulation error, which can all too easily happen without sufficient oversight and redundancy in the formulating process. Similarly, the well-publicized outbreak of fungal meningitis in people treated with a supposedly sterile compounded formulation of methylprednisolone acetate illustrated the disastrous consequences of microbial contamination of injectable drugs [70].

Can self-regulation be enough?

There is clearly a need for compounding of selected veterinary products, and compounding pharmacies fill an important role in veterinary practice. Compounding pharmacies have themselves recognized the challenges that face their industry and have formed several organizations that seek to maintain and improve the practice of compounding. The International Academy of Compounding Pharmacists (IACP) was founded in 1991 and has become the main trade group and advocate of compounding pharmacies [71]. Although IACP is probably most visible as an advocacy and lobbying group, they are also one of the founders of a more recent organization, the Pharmacy Compounding Accreditation Board (PCAB), established in 2004. In an attempt to facilitate voluntary regulation of compounding pharmacies, PCAB has established ethical, record-keeping, and practice standards that all pharmacies are required to meet before being accredited. Participation in PCAB is voluntary, however, so its ability to standardize compounding practices is still being explored. In the meantime, legislative action resulting from the fungal meningitis outbreak mentioned earlier is unlikely to substantially affect veterinary compounding practices at this time [72].

What the veterinarian can do

In addition to looking for PCAB accreditation, the following are some commonsense guidelines that can help veterinarians to select high-quality compounding pharmacies:

1 Are they ethical?
   (a) Do they sell compounded versions of marketed, approved drugs?
   (b) Do they sell without a veterinary–client–patient relationship?
   (c) Do they offer financial incentives to physicians to buy their product?
2 Is there a licensed pharmacist on-site?
   (a) Is the pharmacist trained in veterinary pharmacology and physiology?
   (b) Do they have additional compounding training? Membership in
      (i) International Academy of Compounding Pharmacists
      (ii) Professional Compounding Centers of America
      (iii) PCAB Accreditation
3 Where are the bulk chemicals coming from?
   (a) Is the supplier FDA licensed and/or registered?
   (b) Do the bulk drugs come with a certificate of analysis?
   (c) How is quality control testing performed on the bulk chemical?
4 What quality testing is being done on end product?
   (a) Are there records of adverse reactions?
   (b) Were any trials done on the products?
   (c) Were these trials done by a disinterested, masked third party?
   (d) Any information on bioavailability? Shelf life? Strength?
5 How are sterile drugs formulated?
   (a) Is there a laminar flow hood?
   (b) Is sterility of the product checked?
6 Is there appropriate product labeling?
   (a) Preparation date
   (b) Expiration date: Is there one and has it been verified by testing?
   (c) Storage advice
   (d) Proper directions for use labels

References

1 Granero, G.E. & Amidon, G.L. (2006) Stability of valacyclovir: Implications for its oral bioavailability. *International Journal of Pharmaceutics*, **317**, 14–18.

2 Yamana, T. & Tsuji, A. (1976) Comparative stability of cephalosporins in aqueous solution: Kinetics and mechanisms of degradation. *Journal of Pharmaceutical Science*, **65**, 1563–1574.

3 Carmichael, R.J., Whitfield, C. & Maxwell, L.K. (2013) Pharmacokinetics of ganciclovir and valganciclovir in the adult horse. *Journal of Veterinary Pharmacology and Therapeutics*, **36**, 441–449.

4 Latimer, F.G., Colitz, C.M.H., Campbell, N.B. & Papich, M.G. (2001) Pharmacokinetics of fluconazole following intravenous and oral administration and body fluid concentrations of fluconazole following repeated oral dosing in horses. *American Journal of Veterinary Research*, **62**, 1606–1611.

5 Cornelisse, C.J., Robinson, N.E., Berney, C.E., Kobe, C.A., Boruta, D.T. & Derksen, F.J. (2004) Efficacy of oral and intravenous dexamethasone in horses with recurrent airway obstruction. *Equine Veterinary Journal*, **36**, 426–430.

6 Bentz, B.G., Maxwell, L.K., Erkert, R.S. *et al.* (2006) Pharmacokinetics of acyclovir after single intravenous and oral administration to adult horses. *Journal of Veterinary Internal Medicine*, **20**, 589–594.

7 Liska, D.A., Akucewich, L.H., Marsella, R., Maxwell, L.K., Barbara, J.E. & Cole, C.A. (2006) Pharmacokinetics of pentoxifylline and its 5-hydroxyhexyl metabolite after oral and intravenous administration of pentoxifylline to healthy adult horses. *American Journal of Veterinary Research*, **67**, 1621–1627.

8 Ensink, J.M., Klein, W.R., Mevius, D.J., Klarenbeek, A. & Vulto, A.G. (1992) Bioavailability of oral penicillins in the horse: A comparison of pivampicillin and amoxicillin. *Journal of Veterinary Pharmacology and Therapeutics*, **15**, 221–230.

9 Wilson, W.D., Spensley, M.S., Baggot, J.D. & Hietala, S.K. (1988) Pharmacokinetics and estimated bioavailability of amoxicillin in mares after intravenous, intramuscular, and oral administration. *American Journal of Veterinary Research*, **49**, 1688–1694.

10 Johansson, A.M., Gardner, S.Y., Levine, J.F. *et al.* (2004) Pharmacokinetics and pharmacodynamics of furosemide after oral administration to horses. *Journal of Veterinary Internal Medicine*, **18**, 739–743.

11 Shilo, Y., Britzi, M., Eytan, B., Lifschitz, T., Soback, S. & Steinman, A. (2008) Pharmacokinetics of tramadol in horses after intravenous, intramuscular and oral administration. *Journal of Veterinary Pharmacology and Therapeutics*, **31**, 60–65.

12 Hustace, J.L., Firshman, A.M. & Mata, J.E. (2009) Pharmacokinetics and bioavailability of metformin in horses. *American Journal of Veterinary Research*, **70**, 665–668.

13 Dowling, P.M., Wilson, R.C., Tyler, J.W. & Duran, S.H. (1995) Pharmacokinetics of ciprofloxacin in ponies. *Journal of Veterinary Pharmacology and Therapeutics*, **18**, 7–12.

14 Vynckier, L.J. & Debackere, M. (1993) Plasma ronidazole concentrations in sheep after intravenous, oral, intraruminal and intraabomasal administration. *Journal of Veterinary Pharmacology and Therapeutics*, **16**, 70–78.

15 de Fombelle, A., Varloud, M., Goachet, A. *et al.* (2003) Characterization of the microbial and biochemical profile of the different segments of the digestive tract in horses fed two distinct diets. *Animal Science*, **77**, 293–304.

16 McKellar, Q.A. & Horspool, L.J. (1995) Stability of penicillin G, ampicillin, amikacin and oxytetracycline and their interactions with food in in vitro simulated equine gastrointestinal contents. *Research in Veterinary Science*, **58**, 227–231.

17 Welsh, J.C., Lees, P., Stodulski, G., Cambridge, H. & Foster, A.P. (1992) Influence of feeding schedule on the absorption of orally administered flunixin in the horse. *Equine Veterinary Journal Supplement*, **24**, 62–65.

18 Alvinerie, M., Sutra, J.F., Cabezas, I., Rubilar, L. & Perez, R. (2000) Enhanced plasma availability of moxidectin in fasted horses. *Journal of Equine Veterinary Science*, **20**, 575–578.

19 Snow, D.H., Baxter, P. & Whiting, B. (1981) The pharmacokinetics of meclofenamic acid in the horse. *Journal of Veterinary Pharmacology and Therapeutics*, **4**, 147–156.

20 Maitho, T.E., Lees, P. & Taylor, J.B. (1986) Absorption and pharmacokinetics of phenylbutazone in Welsh Mountain ponies. *Journal of Veterinary Pharmacology and Therapeutics*, **9**, 26–39.

21 Metayer, N., Lhote, M., Bahr, A. *et al.* (2004) Meal size and starch content affect gastric emptying in horses. *Equine Veterinary Journal*, **36**, 436–440.

22 Baggot, J.D., Love, D.N., Stewart, J. & Raus, J. (1988) Bioavailability and disposition kinetics of amoxicillin in neonatal foals. *Equine Veterinary Journal*, **20**, 125–127.

23 Sweeney, R.W., Reef, V.B. & Reimer, J.M. (1993) Pharmacokinetics of digoxin administered to horses with congestive heart failure. *American Journal of Veterinary Research*, **54**, 1108–1111.

24 Periti, P., Mazzei, T., Mini, E. & Novelli, A. (1989) Clinical pharmacokinetic properties of the macrolide antibiotics. Effects of age and various pathophysiological states (Part I). *Clinical Pharmacokinetics*, **16**, 193–214.

25 Prescott, J.F., Hoover, D.J. & Dohoo, I.R. (1983) Pharmacokinetics of erythromycin in foals and in adult. *Journal of Veterinary Pharmacology and Therapeutics*, **6**, 67–73.

26 Maxwell, L.K., Bentz, B.G., Bourne, D.W. & Erkert, R.S. (2008) Pharmacokinetics of valacyclovir in the adult horse. *Journal of Veterinary Pharmacology and Therapeutics*, **31**, 312–320.

27 Carrillo, N.A., Giguere, S., Gronwall, R.R., Brown, M.P., Merritt, K.A. & O'Kelley, J.J. (2005) Disposition of orally administered cefpodoxime proxetil in foals and adult horses and minimum inhibitory concentration of the drug against common bacterial pathogens of horses. *American Journal of Veterinary Research*, **66**, 30–35.

28 Patrick, G. (2001) *History of Cortisone and Related Compounds*. *eLS*: John Wiley & Sons, Ltd, New York.

29 Peroni, D.L., Stanley, S., Kollias-Baker, C. & Robinson, N.E. (2002) Prednisone per os is likely to have limited efficacy in horses. *Equine Veterinary Journal*, **34**, 283–287.

30 Peek, S.F., Semrad, S.D. & Perkins, G.A. (2003) Clostridial myonecrosis in horses (37 cases 1985–2000). *Equine Veterinary Journal*, **35**, 86–92.

31 Toutain, P.L., Lassourd, V., Costes, G. *et al.* (1995) A non-invasive and quantitative method for the study of tissue injury caused by intramuscular injection of drugs in horses. *Journal of Veterinary Pharmacology and Therapeutics*, **18**, 226–235.

32 Firth, E.C., Nouws, J.F., Driessens, F., Schmaetz, P., Peperkamp, K. & Klein, W.R. (1986) Effect of the injection site on the pharmacokinetics of procaine penicillin G in horses. *American Journal of Veterinary Research*, **47**, 2380–2384.

33 Thiemann, A. (2003) Treatment of a deep injection abscess using sterile maggots in a donkey: A case report. http://www.worldwidewounds.com/2003/november/Thiemann/Donkey-Maggot-therapy.html [accessed on July 18, 2014].

34 Jones, B.C., Middleton, D.S. & Youdim, K. (2009) Cytochrome P450 metabolism and inhibition: Analysis for drug discovery. *Progress in Medicinal Chemistry*, **47**, 239–263.

35 Nebbia, C., Dacasto, M., Rossetto Giaccherino, A., Giuliano Albo, A. & Carletti, M. (2003) Comparative expression of liver cytochrome P450-dependent monooxygenases in the horse and in other agricultural and laboratory species. *Veterinary Journal*, **165**, 53–64.

36 Tobin, T., Blake, J.W. & Valentine, R. (1977) Drug interactions in the horse: Effects of chloramphenicol, quinidine, and oxyphenbutazone on phenylbutazone metabolism. *American Journal of Veterinary Research*, **38**, 123–127.

37 Bjornsson, T.D., Callaghan, J.T., Einolf, H.J. *et al.* (2003) The conduct of in vitro and in vivo drug-drug interaction studies: A Pharmaceutical Research and Manufacturers of America (PhRMA) perspective. *Drug Metabolism and Disposition*, **31**, 815–832.

38 Trepanier, L.A. (2006) Cytochrome P450 and its role in veterinary drug interactions. *Veterinary Clinics of North America-Small Animal Practice*, **36**, 975–985.

39 Baratta, M.T., Zaya, M.J., White, J.A. & Locuson, C.W. (2010) Canine CYP2B11 metabolizes and is inhibited by anesthetic agents often co-administered in dogs. *Journal of Veterinary Pharmacology and Therapeutics*, **33**, 50–55.

40 Knych, H.K., McKemie, D.S. & Stanley, S.D. (2010) Molecular cloning, expression, and initial characterization of members of the CYP3A family in horses. *Drug Metabolism and Disposition*, **38**, 1820–1827.

41 Peters, L.M., Demmel, S., Pusch, G. *et al.* (2013) Equine cytochrome P450 2B6—genomic identification, expression and functional characterization with ketamine. *Toxicology and Applied Pharmacology*, **266**, 101–108.

42 Peters, J., Block, W., Oswald, S. *et al.* (2011) Oral absorption of clarithromycin is nearly abolished by chronic comedication of rifampicin in foals. *Drug Metabolism and Disposition*, **39**, 1643–1649.

43 Peters, J., Eggers, K., Oswald, S. *et al.* (2012) Clarithromycin is absorbed by an intestinal uptake mechanism that is sensitive to major inhibition by rifampicin: Results of a short-term drug interaction study in foals. *Drug Metabolism and Disposition*, **40**, 522–528.

44 Olsen, L., Ingvast-Larsson, C., Bondesson, U., Broström, H., Tjälve, H. & Larsson, P. (2007) Cetirizine in horses:

Pharmacokinetics and effect of ivermectin pretreatment. *Journal of Veterinary Pharmacology and Therapeutics*, **30**, 194–200.

45 Sams, R.A., Gerken, D.F., Dyke, T.M., Reed, S.M. & Ashcraft, S.M. (1997) Pharmacokinetics of intravenous and intragastric cimetidine in horses. I. Effects of intravenous cimetidine on pharmacokinetics of intravenous phenylbutazone. *Journal of Veterinary Pharmacology and Therapeutics*, **20**, 355–361.

46 Soma, L.R. & Uboh, C.E. (1998) Review of furosemide in horse racing: Its effects and regulation. *Journal of Veterinary Pharmacology and Therapeutics*, **21**, 228–240.

47 Knox, D.A., Ravis, W.R., Pedersoli, W.M. *et al.* (1992) Pharmacokinetics of phenobarbital in horses after single and repeated oral administration of the drug. *American Journal of Veterinary Research*, **53**, 706–710.

48 Whittem, T., Firth, E.C., Hodge, H. & Turner, K. (1996) Pharmacokinetic interactions between repeated dose phenylbutazone and gentamicin in the horse. *Journal of Veterinary Pharmacology and Therapeutics*, **19**, 454–459.

49 Burrows, G.E., MacAllister, C.G., Tripp, P. & Black, J. (1989) Interactions between chloramphenicol, acepromazine, phenylbutazone, rifampin and thiamylal in the horse. *Equine Veterinary Journal*, **21**, 34–38.

50 Mossner, L.D., Schmitz, A., Theurillat, R., Thormann, W. & Mevissen, M. (2011) Inhibition of cytochrome P450 enzymes involved in ketamine metabolism by use of liver microsomes and specific cytochrome P450 enzymes from horses, dogs, and humans. *American Journal of Veterinary Research*, **72**, 1505–1513.

51 Capponi, L., Schmitz, A., Thormann, W., Theurillat, R. & Mevissen, M. (2009) In vitro evaluation of differences in phase 1 metabolism of ketamine and other analgesics among humans, horses, and dogs. *American Journal of Veterinary Research*, **70**, 777–786.

52 Parraga, M.E., Kittleson, M.D. & Drake, C.M. (1995) Quinidine administration increases steady state serum digoxin concentration in horses. *Equine Veterinary Journal Supplement*, **27**, 114–119.

53 Roberts, B.L., Blake, J.W. & Tobin, T. (1976) Drug interactions in the horse: Effect of furosemide on plasma and urinary levels of phenylbutazone. *Research Communications in Chemical Pathology and Pharmacology*, **15**, 257–265.

54 Stevenson, A.J., Weber, M.P., Todi, F. *et al.* (1990) The influence of furosemide on plasma elimination and urinary excretion of drugs in standardbred horses. *Journal of Veterinary Pharmacology and Therapeutics*, **13**, 93–104.

55 Muir, W.W., 3rd & Sams, R. (1992) Effects of ketamine infusion on halothane minimal alveolar concentration in horses. *American Journal of Veterinary Research*, **53**, 1802–1806.

56 Hinchcliff, K.W., McKeever, K.H., Muir, W.W., 3rd & Sams, R.A. (1995) Pharmacologic interaction of furosemide and phenylbutazone in horses. *American Journal of Veterinary Research*, **56**, 1206–1212.

57 Frincke, J.M. & Henderson, G.L. (1980) The major metabolite of fentanyl in the horse. *Drug Metabolism and Disposition*, **8**, 425–427.

58 Sarkar, P., McIntosh, J.M., Leavitt, R. & Gouthro, H. (1997) A unique metabolite of nimesulide. *Journal of Analytical Toxicology*, **21**, 197–202.

59 Lehner, A.F., Hughes, C.G., Harkins, J.D. *et al.* (2004) Detection and confirmation of ractopamine and its metabolites in horse urine after Paylean administration. *Journal of Analytical Toxicology*, **28**, 226–238.

60 Krishnaswamy, S., Duan, S.X., Von Moltke, L.L. *et al.* (2003) Serotonin (5-hydroxytryptamine) glucuronidation in vitro: Assay development, human liver microsome activities and species differences. *Xenobiotica*, **33**, 169–180.

61 Kioussi, M.K., Lyris, E.M., Angelis, Y.S., Tsivou, M., Koupparis, M.A. & Georgakopoulos, C.G. (2013) A generic screening methodology for horse doping control by LC–TOF-MS, GC–HRMS and GC–MS. *Journal of Chromatography B*, **941**, 69–80.

62 Desta, B., Maldonado, G., Reid, H. *et al.* (2011) Acute selenium toxicosis in polo ponies. *Journal of Veterinary Diagnostic Investigation*, **23**, 623–628.

63 US Food and Drug Administration (FDA) (1994) Animal Medicinal Drug Use Clarification Act of 1994 (AMDUCA). http://www.fda.gov/AnimalVeterinary/Guidance ComplianceEnforcement/ActsRulesRegulations/ ucm085377.htm [accessed on July 18, 2014].

64 US Food and Drug Administration (FDA) (2003) CPG Sec. 608.400 Compounding of Drugs for Use in Animals. http://www.fda.gov/iceci/compliancemanuals/compliancepoli-cyguidancemanual/ucm074656.htm [accessed on July 18, 2014].

65 Post, L.O. & Keller, W.C. (2000) Current status of food animal antidotes. *Veterinary Clinics of North America. Food Animal Practice*, **16**, 445–453, vi.

66 Davis, J.L., Kirk, L.M., Davidson, G.S. & Papich, M.G. (2009) Effects of compounding and storage conditions on stability of pergolide mesylate. *Journal of the American Veterinary Medical Association*, **234**, 385–389.

67 Boothe, D.M. (2006) Veterinary compounding in small animals: A clinical pharmacologist's perspective. *Veterinary Clinics of North America. Small Animal Practice*, **36**, 1129–1173, viii.

68 Lust, E. (2004) Compounding for animal patients: Contemporary issues. *Journal of the American Pharmacists Association*, **44**, 375–384; quiz 384–386.

69 Papich, M.G. (2005) Drug compounding for veterinary patients. *AAPS Journal*, **7**, E281–E287.

70 Centers for Disease Control and Prevention (CDC) (2012) Multistate outbreak of fungal infection associated with injection of methylprednisolone acetate solution from a single compounding pharmacy—United States, 2012. *Morbidity and Mortality Weekly Report*, **61**, 839–842.

71 Clark, A. (2005) Battles over compounding from bulk drugs move forward. *Journal of the American Veterinary Medical Association*, **227**, 9–10.

72 Hinkley, K.N. (2013) Compounding interest: A tragedy caused by contaminated steroids turned the spotlight on compounding pharmacies. *State Legislatures*, **39**, 22–23.

CHAPTER 2

Basics of antimicrobial therapy for the horse

Cynthia Cole
Mars Veterinary, Portland, OR, USA

Historical perspective

Bacteria were first observed by the Dutch naturalist Antoni van Leeuwenhoek with the aid of a simple microscope of his own construction. He reported his discovery to the Royal Society of London in 1683, but the science of bacteriology was not firmly established until the middle of the 19th century. For nearly 200 years, it was believed that bacteria were produced by spontaneous generation. The fundamental fact that bacteria, like all living organisms, arise only from other similar organisms was not established until 1860 by the French scientist Louis Pasteur. Pasteur and another scientist, Joubert, published the first account of antimicrobial activity when they reported that common microorganisms could inhibit the growth of anthrax bacilli in urine in 1877. In 1928, Alexander Fleming observed that mold in one of his *Staphylococcus* cultures had caused bacteria in the vicinity to lyse. He later observed that broth from cultures of that mold could inhibit growth of a number of different bacterial species. As the mold belonged to the genus *Penicillium*, Fleming named the antibacterial substance penicillin. Modern era antimicrobial therapy dates back only to 1936 with the introduction of sulfanilamide. Penicillin came into clinical use in 1941, and streptomycin, chloramphenicol, and chlortetracycline were introduced toward the end or soon after the end of WWII. One of the biggest challenges for modern medical research is to address the increasing prevalence of antimicrobial resistance. Equine medicine is no exception, and clinicians need to recognize the risks associated with the indiscriminate use of antimicrobials. Appropriate selection, dosing, and duration of therapy, along with appropriate infection control procedures, are essential to maintain the efficacy of antimicrobials currently available to the equine practitioner.

The bacterial cell wall

The bacterial cell wall is a unique structure that surrounds the cell membrane. Although not present in every bacterial species, the cell wall is very important as a cellular component. Structurally, the wall is necessary for maintaining the cell's characteristic shape, the rigid wall compensating for the flexibility of the phospholipid membrane. It also helps counter the effects of osmotic pressure that develops when the intracellular osmolarity is greater than the extracellular osmolarity. In addition, the cell wall also provides attachment sites for bacteriophages and a rigid platform for surface appendages, such as flagella, fimbriae, and pili, all of which emanate from the wall and extend beyond it.

The cell walls of all bacteria are not identical. In fact, cell wall composition is one of the most important factors in bacterial species analysis and differentiation. For example, through a process invented by Hans Christian Gram now commonly referred to as Gram staining, bacteria can be divided into two major classifications. Gram-positive bacteria have thick cell walls containing large amounts of peptidoglycan that bind crystal violet stain, turning the bacteria a blue/purple color after exposure. In contrast, Gram-negative bacteria have cell walls that contain much less proteoglycan, and therefore, the crystal violet stain is easily removed. The Gram-negative bacteria are then stained a red/pink color by a safranin stain in a second counterstaining process.

Equine Pharmacology, First Edition. Edited by Cynthia Cole, Bradford Bentz and Lara Maxwell.
© 2015 John Wiley & Sons, Inc. Published 2015 by John Wiley & Sons, Inc.

Gram-negative bacteria also have two unique regions that surround the plasma membrane: the periplasmic space and the lipopolysaccharide (LPS) layer. The periplasmic space separates the plasma membrane from the peptidoglycan layer. The LPS layer is located adjacent to the exterior peptidoglycan layer. It has a phospholipid bilayer construction similar to that of the cell membrane and is attached to the peptidoglycan layer by lipoproteins. The lipid portion of LPS contains Lipid A, which is responsible for most of the pathogenic effects associated with Gram-negative bacteria. Polysaccharides, which extend out from the bilayer, also contribute to the toxicity. The LPS, lipoproteins, and the associated polysaccharides together form what is known as the outer membrane.

Antimicrobials versus antibiotics

An antimicrobial is any substance (natural, semisynthetic, or synthetic) that kills or inhibits the growth of a microorganism, but causes little or no host damage [1]. In contrast, an antibiotic is a substance produced by a microorganism that, at low concentrations, inhibits or kills other microorganisms. Although these terms are often used interchangeably, they are technically different.

Isolate

A bacterial isolate commonly refers to an individual bacterial strain cultured or isolated from infectious material taken from a patient.

Aerobes and anaerobes

Bacteria differ in their need and tolerance for oxygen. Obligate aerobes are organisms that are dependent upon the presence of oxygen for their metabolism. In contrast, obligate anaerobes cannot survive in oxygen-rich environments, while facultative anaerobes are able to exist with or without oxygen. Many yeasts; enteric bacteria, such as the Gram-negative *E. coli*; and skin-dwelling Gram-positive bacteria, such as *Staphylococcus* spp., are facultative anaerobes. Microaerophile bacteria require oxygen but at a lower concentration than that found in the atmosphere. Finally, aerotolerant anaerobes are not

affected by oxygen; although they cannot utilize it, they are not harmed by it either. For example, *Lactobacillus* spp. are part of the normal gut flora and are aerotolerant microorganisms.

When obtaining a sample for culture or selecting an antimicrobial for treatment, it is important for clinicians to consider the environment from which the bacteria have been isolated. For example, although oxygen concentrations are relatively high in normal lung parenchyma, in the presence of pneumonia with inflammatory exudates, necrotic tissue, and lung consolidation, oxygen may be very low in the tissues, allowing for the growth of obligate anaerobic organisms. Samples for anaerobic cultures must obviously be handled in a manner to minimize exposure to oxygen. Because effectively culturing anaerobic bacteria is notoriously difficult, treatment for these agents is often based on the suspicion of their presence rather than their confirmation.

Empirical versus culture and sensitivity-guided treatment

A medical treatment not derived from the scientific method, but from observation, survey, or common use, is referred to as empirical therapy. In the case of a serious life-threatening infection or in cases of therapeutic failure, "best practice" considerations dictate that a culture should be used to identify the infectious agent and determine the sensitivity of that isolate to representative antimicrobials. An empirical approach to therapy is often used initially, pending the results of culture and sensitivity (C&S) testing or in cases where clinical acumen suggests that a definitive diagnosis is not required for effective treatment.

Spectrum approach for empirical therapy

The term "spectrum of activity" is often used to describe the general activity of an antimicrobial against various microorganisms. A narrow spectrum implies activity against some limited subset of bacteria, such as only Gram-positive aerobes, while broad spectrum usually implies activity against a wide range of bacteria, for example, both Gram-negative and Gram-positive aerobes, as well as some anaerobes. Practitioners should bear in mind, however, that the spectrum of activity of an antimicrobial is a relative classification, and the efficacy against any specific bacterial isolate is never guaranteed.

Antimicrobial pharmacodynamics

Some antimicrobial agents do not kill bacteria at typical therapeutic concentrations, but only inhibit their replication. These agents are often classified as having "bacteriostatic" activity, and their ultimate efficacy depends upon the host's immune system to kill the microbe. In contrast, an antimicrobial with "bactericidal" activity can kill the microbe (Table 2.1) if certain conditions are met. Generally, the antimicrobial concentration must exceed some threshold and be maintained for some minimal period of time in order for bactericidal activity to occur. If those conditions are not met, even agents generally considered bactericidal, such as aminoglycosides and beta-lactams, may only be bacteriostatic. For some antimicrobials, the difference between bactericidal and bacteriostatic activity depends on the pathogen involved and the concentration of the drug that can be achieved in the tissue of interest. General pharmacological principles stipulate that in cases of serious or life-threatening infections or in individuals without competent immune systems, bactericidal agents are preferred. However, there may be clinical situations where this dogma is not followed and practitioners need to consider the entire clinical presentation when choosing the appropriate antimicrobial regimen.

In vitro sensitivity testing

When treating a microbial infection, it is obviously important to select an antimicrobial that is likely to be effective against the causative agent. Although empiric

therapy is commonly practiced, identifying the specific pathogens present by culturing them *in vitro* is often preferred, particularly if the infection is serious. In addition, isolation of the causative agent allows the *in vitro* susceptibility of that isolate to representative antimicrobial agents to be determined. Although there are numerous approaches, the two most common tests used in veterinary medicine to determine antimicrobial activity *in vitro* are the broth microdilution and the disk diffusion methods.

For the broth microdilution method, microtiter plates containing nutrient broth supplemented with decreasing concentrations of the antimicrobials are inoculated with a standard number of the cultured organisms. The lowest concentration at which there is no visible growth of the bacteria is referred to as the minimum inhibitory concentration (MIC) for that specific antimicrobial. The MIC is a measurement of the susceptibility of the isolate to the antimicrobial; the lower the MIC, the more susceptible the isolate. For the disk diffusion method (also known as the Kirby–Bauer test), isolates from an initial culture are plated on an agar surface of standardized growth media, and filter disks, impregnated with antimicrobials, are applied. During incubation, the antimicrobial diffuses out of the disk and into the agar. If the microbe is sensitive to the antimicrobial, it will not grow in agar in which inhibitory concentrations of the antimicrobial are present. This inhibition of growth produces a clear ring around the disk. The larger the diameter of the ring, the more effective the antimicrobial is against that isolate. It is extremely important that the testing follow standardized protocols as variations in the process, such as the thickness of the agar, the number of microbes plated, etc., can significantly alter the results. Under standard conditions, there is an inverse linear relationship between the diameter of the zone of inhibition of growth and the MIC. Although standard disk diffusion assays cannot accurately determine the MIC, newer variations of the method can provide MIC data, although their use in equine medicine has not been extensive.

Although *in vitro* sensitivity testing can provide clinically valuable information, it does not always accurately predict the outcome of antimicrobial therapy *in vivo*. By itself, *in vitro* testing indicates that if a particular concentration of the antimicrobial agent can be achieved at the site of an infection, bacteria may be inhibited. It does not tell the clinician whether typical dosing regimens are likely to produce that target concentration at

Table 2.1 General PD classification of common antimicrobials.

Bactericidal	Bacteriostatic
Fluoroquinolones	Chloramphenicol
Aminoglycosides	Macrolides
Beta-lactams	Tetracyclines
Potentiated sulfonamides	Sulfonamides

the site of the infection, nor whether conditions at the site of infection, such as a particularly low pH or the presence of inflammatory debris, will decrease the activity of the antimicrobial. Therefore, *in vitro* MIC testing alone is of little utility until combined with *in vivo* testing of drug concentrations that can be achieved from specific dosing regimens and the outcomes associated with the treatment of veterinary species. As a consequence, current emphasis in antimicrobial clinical research has been to derive MIC breakpoints, also referred to as clinical or pharmacokinetic/pharmacodynamic (PK/PD) breakpoints. These breakpoints are discriminating concentrations of an antimicrobial used in the interpretation of the results of susceptibility testing to provide predictive value as to the probable outcome of therapy. Three criteria are used to determine breakpoints: (i) MIC data from populations of bacteria collected in the field or in clinical efficacy studies, (ii) PK/PD properties of the antimicrobial, and (iii) clinical efficacy of the drug during clinical field trials at the standard dose [2]. While the classification of an isolate as susceptible, intermediate, or resistant to a particular antimicrobial has not changed from traditional interpretations, the reliability of that determination is greater using MIC breakpoints. In the USA, the Clinical Laboratory Standards Institute is the group responsible for setting standards for antimicrobial testing and classification and also determines breakpoints. The major limitation to the use of MIC breakpoints for the equine practitioner is that they have been set for only a few antimicrobials, such as ceftiofur, gentamicin, and ampicillin. In some cases where equine-specific breakpoints do not exist, data from other species, including human values, may be substituted. The clinician needs to be aware, however, that these values may not accurately predict the efficacy of these antimicrobials against equine pathogens due to differences in the PK and PD characteristics of the antimicrobials in the horse, as well as resistance patterns among equine pathogens.

Other parameters of bacterial susceptibility are also used in some scenarios. For example, an MIC_{90}, the concentration that will inhibit 90% of the isolates in a given population, is derived from pooled quantitative susceptibility data for individual isolates. The minimum bactericidal concentration (MBC) is the lowest drug concentration that kills 99.9% of a particular bacterial isolate *in vitro*. To determine the MBC, aliquots of microtiter wells used for MIC determinations are diluted

and recultured without any additional antimicrobials. If growth occurs, then the isolate was only inhibited, not killed. The lowest concentration of an antimicrobial from which no growth occurs is considered the MBC. If the ratio of the MBC to the MIC is small (<4–6), it is likely that the antibiotic will be bactericidal (i.e., it is possible to produce bactericidal concentrations *in vivo*). If the ratio is high, it may not be possible to achieve bactericidal serum or tissue concentrations without producing signs of toxicity or requiring larger doses of drugs than can be practically administered. Because it is time consuming and cumbersome to conduct MBC testing, it is not commonly determined in commercial laboratories.

Postantibiotic effect (PAE)

Following exposure to some antimicrobials, the growth rate of bacteria may remain suppressed even after concentrations of the drug have decreased below the MIC. This effect is due to antimicrobial-induced damage to the bacteria, which may increase the sensitivity of the bacteria to host defenses. The postantibiotic effect (PAE) varies with the antimicrobial and the bacterial pathogen but can partially explain why some effective antimicrobial regimens allow the plasma drug concentrations to drop below the MIC for some portion of the dosing interval.

Patterns of microbial killing

For some antimicrobials, their efficacy correlates directly to the intensity of the exposure; once the MIC is exceeded, their rate of killing increases with the concentration. This pattern of killing is termed "concentration-dependent". Within this group, there are subgroups for which specific PK parameters are the best predictors of efficacy. For example, for aminoglycosides, efficacy correlates most closely with the maximum serum concentration, or Cmax. For other agents, such as fluoroquinolones, the total drug exposure, defined by the area under the plasma concentration versus time curve or simply the area under the curve (AUC), is a better correlate of efficacy. Finally, there are some antimicrobials, such as metronidazole and the azalide azithromycin, for which both parameters correlate fairly well with efficacy. Ratios of drug kinetic parameters, such as the Cmax:MIC or AUC:MIC (sometimes ambiguously expressed as AUIC), are often used to predict efficacy for agents exhibiting concentration-dependent killing.

The second pattern described for antimicrobial efficacy is termed "time-dependent" killing. For agents in this class, it is the duration of exposure of the microbe to the antimicrobial at concentrations above the MIC that is the critical parameter. Agents that exhibit time-dependent killing include beta-lactams, macrolides, glycopeptides, tetracyclines, sulfonamides, trimethoprim, and chloramphenicol. For antimicrobials within this group that do not exhibit a prolonged PAE (i.e., beta-lactams and vancomycin), efficacy can be maximized by maintaining serum concentrations above MIC for as much of the dosing interval as possible [3]. For antimicrobials within this group that do exhibit a prolonged PAE (i.e., macrolides, tetracycline, and clindamycin), efficacy is best correlated to the dosing regimens that maximize the AUC.

The aforementioned PK/PD classifications can be overly simplistic and are not without some controversy. In addition, implementation of appropriate dosing regiments by the practitioner in the field is sometimes problematic. Nevertheless, the practitioner can benefit from understanding the general concepts of the various PK/PD groups. For example, for an antimicrobial drug that exhibits concentration-dependent killing, such as an aminoglycoside, administering a single large dose once a day is likely to be more efficacious than administering one-third of that dose every 8 h, as was recommended in older dosing protocols. In contrast, for a beta-lactam that exhibits time-dependent killing with a brief PAE, smaller doses administered more frequently would be a better approach. Unfortunately, unless the PK of the antimicrobial are well described, altering the dose and dosing interval to manipulate the AUC can be difficult. In addition, the safety of the antimicrobial being administered must also be considered when using alternative dosing strategies.

Susceptibility, sensitivity, and resistance

Susceptibility refers to the presence of targets of the antimicrobial activity within a genre or species of bacteria. For example, E. coli organisms, as a species, are generally susceptible to gentamicin. In contrast, sensitivity refers to a particular isolate of a given bacterial species and indicates whether an antimicrobial is likely to be effective against that isolate. For example, a specific E. coli isolate could be sensitive or resistant to gentamicin, depending on the MIC determined for that isolate. Resistance to an antimicrobial or class of antimicrobials can be divided into two categories: constitutive and acquired. "Constitutive resistance" indicates that the bacterial species does not possess the target of antimicrobial action or that it possesses some intrinsic protection from the antimicrobial. In other words, bacteria that are constitutively resistant to an antimicrobial are not susceptible to it. In contrast, it is possible for bacteria that were susceptible to an antimicrobial to obtain or develop a mechanism that allows them to become resistant; this change over time is termed "acquired resistance." This resistance can occur by point mutation in the bacteria's own genome, or the bacteria can acquire exogenous DNA by one of three different mechanisms. Conjugation, in which plasmids containing antimicrobial resistance genes are transported across an intercellular bridge, is most common in Gram-negative bacteria. Transduction involves transfer of resistance genes by bacteriophages, and it is most common in Gram-positive bacteria. Finally, transformation involves incorporation of free DNA carrying resistance genes from the environment. Depending on the mechanism of the resistance, it may be relative, where the resistance can be overcome by increased exposure to the antimicrobial, or absolute, when it cannot be overcome by increasing drug exposure.

Mechanisms of resistance

There are numerous mechanisms by which bacteria can resist the effects of an antimicrobial, and some isolates may possess multiple mechanisms. Resistance mechanisms can loosely be classified into four different categories. Inactivation of the antimicrobial drug, for example, the degradation of penicillins and cephalosporins by beta-lactamase enzymes, is one of the most common mechanisms. Another mechanism is a reduction in the intracellular accumulation of the antimicrobial. For example, membrane-associated efflux pumps remove tetracyclines from the bacterial cell, preventing intracellular accumulation. Bacteria may also develop modifications of the antimicrobial target site, resulting in a decrease in efficacy of the antimicrobial. For example, structural changes in bacterial DNA gyrase and topoisomerase decrease the binding affinity of fluoroquinolones to those enzymes, which decreases efficacy. Finally, bacteria may develop alternative metabolic pathways that bypass the antimicrobial-produced blockage. For example, potentiated sulfonamides block several enzymes necessary for the production of folic acid, but resistant bacteria produce folic acid by alternative pathways, counteracting the antimicrobial activity.

Antimicrobial drug interactions

Antimicrobials may interact with one another in three ways. Some effects may simply be additive, where the action of the combination of two products is equal to the sum of the actions of each component. Combinations of agents may also have synergistic effects, where the action of the combination is significantly greater than the sum of the actions of each component. For example, the mechanism of action of beta-lactam antimicrobials compromises the integrity of the bacterial cell wall, and those compromised sites facilitate entry of aminoglycosides; thus, their interaction is synergistic. Some interactions are antagonistic, however, where the efficacy of the combination is significantly less than the sum of the two combined when used individually. For example, bacteriostatic antimicrobials often decrease the growth rate of bacteria; this can decrease the efficacy of bactericidal drugs, which are most effective in rapidly dividing cells. For this reason, combinations of bacteriostatic and bactericidal antimicrobials are best avoided unless the efficacy of that combination has been specifically studied.

Antimicrobials used in equine medicine

Beta-lactams
Chemistry
All antimicrobials in this class, which include the penicillins, cephalosporins, carbapenems, and monobactams, have four-member beta-lactam rings that are responsible for both their activity and instability. Hydrolysis of the ring structure is the primary cause of drug inactivation. Bacterial-produced beta-lactamases act by this mechanism, but the ring can also be hydrolyzed in an acid environment and by drug–drug interactions.

Substitutions on the ring structure are responsible for characteristic class differences, such as in susceptibility to beta-lactamases, enhanced antimicrobial activity, and/or altered PK characteristics among the different classes of beta-lactams.

Mechanism of action
The beta-lactams interfere with the production and integrity of bacterial cell walls by binding irreversibly to integral components of the wall referred to as penicillin-binding proteins (PBPs). The binding of the beta-lactam ring to the transpeptidase enzyme, the most critical PBP, prevents it from catalyzing cross-linking among the peptidoglycan strands. It has been proposed that this impairment of cell wall formation compromises the integrity of the wall, leading to cell lysis. Due to this mechanism of action, beta-lactams are much more effective against actively dividing cells that have a higher rate of cell wall synthesis than quiescent cells. The beta-lactam mechanism of action also results in a slower rate of killing as compared to some other bactericidal drugs. In some Gram-positive cocci, very high concentrations of beta-lactams are associated with reduced efficacy. It has been proposed that at concentrations far above those associated with maximum killing, beta-lactams interfere with cell growth by binding to bacterial proteins other than the PBP targets. As previously described under antagonist drug combinations, a decrease in the rate of cell division can result in a decrease in efficacy.

Differences in the spectrums of activity of beta-lactams are the result of differences in their binding affinities for PBPs, as well as their susceptibility to enzymatic degradation. Gram-negative bacteria are inherently less sensitive to beta-lactams because they possess (i) an outer cell membrane that inhibits penetration of beta-lactams, (ii) less peptidoglycan in their cell walls, and (iii) potent beta-lactamases that hydrolyze the beta-lactam structure. Nevertheless, many new generations of beta-lactams overcome these traditional limitations and can be extremely effective against Gram-negative microbes.

Beta-lactams exhibit a time-dependent killing profile and have a very brief PAE. Therefore, it is recommended that they be administered in a manner to maintain concentrations above the MIC for at least 40% of the dosing interval for infections caused by Gram-positive microbes and for at least 80% of the dosing interval for infections caused by Gram-negative microbes [3]. The exception to this rule may be the carbapenems, which may be effective if concentrations exceed the MIC for only 30% of the dosing interval, due to their high degree of efficacy. Overdosing should be avoided because of the previously discussed paradoxical response on bacterial killing associated with very high concentrations.

Pharmacokinetics

Following intravenous (IV) administration, most beta-lactams display a rapid distribution. Most are also well and rapidly absorbed following intramuscular (IM) or subcutaneous (SC) administration. Some of the third-generation cephalosporins, however, have much slower absorption rates, and there are also formulations of other beta-lactams that exhibit slow-release characteristics. Absorption following oral administration is highly variable and depends on the subclass. Beta-lactams are hydrophilic weak acids, and as such, most distribute throughout the body in the extracellular fluid but do not cross biological membranes or enter mammalian cells. In addition, most beta-lactams are eliminated from the body primarily by the kidneys, often as unchanged parent compounds. Notable exceptions for this generalization are nafcillin, ceftriaxone, and cefoperazone, although these antimicrobials are not typically used in equine medicine. Elimination of most beta-lactams is generally rapid with terminal elimination half-lives in the range of 1–2 h. This rapid elimination can limit the usefulness of beta-lactams in field situations; however, some of the cephalosporins have prolonged elimination rates, and as mentioned previously, slow-release formulations have also been developed.

Mechanisms of resistance

There are three common mechanisms of resistance to beta-lactams. First, as previously described, some bacteria produce beta-lactamases that hydrolyze the beta-lactam ring, inactivating the drug. Currently, almost 200 unique beta-lactamases have been identified, and they vary in a myriad of ways. For example, some are constitutively produced, while others are induced, and some are encoded for on plasmids and others on chromosomes. Some enzymes are specific for penicillin and are referred to as penicillinases, while others are active only against cephalosporins and so they are referred to as cephalosporinases. Finally, some beta-lactamases have activity against both the penicillins and cephalosporins. Resistance to beta-lactams in Gram-positive bacteria is primarily mediated through

production of beta-lactamases. The development of compounds that inhibit beta-lactamases, such as clavulanic acid and sulbactam, has dramatically improved the efficacy of beta-lactams against beta-lactamase-producing bacteria, particularly the Gram-negative agents.

The second most common mechanism of resistance is alteration of the outer cell membrane, limiting penetration by the beta-lactam. For example, the outer cell membrane layer of LPS found in Gram-negative bacteria decreases the penetration of beta-lactams, making Gram-negatives intrinsically less sensitive than Gram-positive bacteria. However, aqueous channels in the outer membrane formed by proteins called porins can be penetrated by small hydrophilic agents, such as ampicillin and amoxicillin, which explains their increased activity against Gram-negative bacteria over larger molecules, such as penicillin G. Highly resistant microbes, such as *Pseudomonas aeruginosa*, lack porins, preventing penetration by even small hydrophilic molecules.

The third common mechanism of resistance involves changes in the structure of PBPs that decrease the binding affinity of beta-lactams. Methicillin-resistant *Staphylococcus* organisms are commonly produced by this mechanism. Other mechanisms, such as energy-dependent efflux pumps that prevent the beta-lactam agent from accessing the site of action, have also been described.

Drug interactions

Beta-lactams are considered to act synergistically with aminoglycosides. It is proposed that the disruption of the cell wall by the beta-lactams enhances the penetration of the aminoglycosides. Also, as previously described, beta-lactamase inhibitors and beta-lactams have synergistic effects against beta-lactamase-producing bacteria.

Penicillins

Penicillins are generally divided into four classes: natural penicillins, aminopenicillins, antistaphylococcal penicillins, and extended-spectrum penicillins.

Natural penicillins

Natural penicillins are produced by mold cultures followed by extraction and purification. Today, only penicillin G is used clinically in veterinary medicine. It has excellent activity against most Gram-positive aerobic and Gram-positive and Gram-negative anaerobic organisms, except the Gram-negative anaerobe *Bacteroides fragilis*, which is often resistant.

Penicillin G is only used parenterally, because of its instability in acid environments. Penicillin is commercially available, formulated with benzathine and procaine (SC and IM administration only) and as potassium and sodium (IV administration) salt preparations. Penicillin potassium and sodium salts are manufactured as dry crystalline formulations that are quite stable; however, once dissolved for administration, they have a short shelf life. Penicillin G, unlike many antimicrobials, is still measured in units rather than weight. One international unit (IU) is the amount of activity in 0.6 µg of the pure crystalline standard salt of penicillin G. Thus, 1 mg of pure penicillin G contains 1667 IU. Penicillin G is dosed by IU per unit of body weight (bwt), while the dose of other beta-lactams is expressed in milligrams per unit of bwt.

In horses, penicillin is active against streptococcal infections, such as *Streptococcus equi* subsp. *equi*, which causes strangles, and *S. equi* subsp. *zooepidemicus*, which is often associated with infections of the respiratory tract, including pneumonia. In addition, it can be effective against nonpenicillinase-producing *Staphylococci* spp. and against infections caused by anaerobic microbes including *Fusobacterium*, *Peptococcus*, *Clostridium*, and some *Bacteroides* strains, but usually not *B. fragilis*. A few Gram-negative agents, such as *Haemophilus* and *Pasteurella* spp., are often sensitive. Penicillin is also active against spirochetes including *Leptospira* and *Borrelia burgdorferi*. *Pseudomonas* spp., most *Enterobacteriaceae*, and penicillinase-producing *Staphylococcus* spp. are consistently resistant to penicillin G.

Slow- or immediate-release formulations of penicillin G are available for parenteral administration in horses. Penicillin G procaine, which is a poorly soluble salt suspended in an aqueous vehicle, is administered IM or occasionally SC, every 12–24 h most commonly at a dose of 22 000–25 000 IU/kg of bwt. At this dosage, the slow-release formulation produces serum penicillin concentrations adequate for most organisms considered sensitive to penicillin. It should be noted that labels on over-the-counter preparations of penicillin G procaine recommend a dose of 3000 IU/lb bwt, although the efficacy of this very low dose is not supported by the scientific literature. There is also another formulation of penicillin available over the counter, which is a combination of benzathine penicillin and procaine penicillin G that produces very low serum concentrations. It is efficacious against only the most sensitive organisms, and therefore, its use should be avoided. Practitioners

need to be aware, however, that in most states clients can obtain and administer these over-the-counter preparations to their horse without veterinary consult.

The sodium or potassium salts of penicillin G are immediate-release crystalline formulations and are generally administered IV at a dosage of 10 000–40 000 IU/kg bwt every 6 h. The results of one study indicated that the potassium salt formulation administered IM to horses produced serum concentrations of penicillin comparable to procaine penicillin [4]. This mode of administration for the potassium salt formulation, however, has not been widely adopted, perhaps because the unexpected study findings have not been confirmed. IV administration should be slow, particularly when administering the potassium salt formulation, to avoid the negative effects of high serum potassium concentrations on cardiac function. The potassium formulation is most commonly used in equine practice, but there is no pharmacological basis for this preference over the sodium formulation.

The rate and extent of absorption of penicillin G depends on the route and location of the injection [5]. Absorption is generally more rapid following IM administration than SC. In addition, there is evidence that injections in the neck are absorbed more rapidly and to a greater extent than those in the gluteals. Whether this difference is clinically significant has not been evaluated. In addition, injections in the neck can be associated with complications, such as pain and swelling, which can interfere with the horse's willingness to eat. In clinical practice, procaine penicillin injections are often rotated between the neck and hindlimbs and on occasion other sites, such as the pectorals.

As a weak organic acid (pK_a 2.7), penicillin G is primarily ionized in plasma, with a relatively small apparent volume of distribution (0.2–0.3 l/kg) and short elimination half-life. Because penicillin G is ionized and hydrophilic at physiological pH, it does not readily cross biological membranes. Inflammation may increase membrane penetration, but the extent is variable and clinically significant concentrations cannot be reliably expected. As with most beta-lactams, penicillin G is eliminated primarily by the kidneys. Decreased renal function will slow elimination, but as penicillin G has a wide safety margin, dosages are rarely adjusted in patients with mild renal disease.

Although common in humans, anaphylactic reactions in horses are unusual, but they can occur. Cross-sensitization with other penicillins, such as ampicillin, should be expected, but not necessarily with cephalosporins. Immunological studies have demonstrated that approximately 20% of humans allergic to penicillins also react to cephalosporins; however, the observed clinical frequency is more on the order of 1%. Nevertheless, practitioners should take care when administering cephalosporins to horses that have a history of penicillin reactions. Although rare, severe immune-mediated hemolytic anemia with icterus has been reported in horses following penicillin administration.

The primary safety concern with the administration of penicillin to horses derives from the procaine component of procaine penicillin G. A local anesthetic, procaine also has stimulatory effects on the CNS. CNS excitation is thought to be the result of an initial blockade of inhibitory pathways in the cerebral cortex by the local anesthetic. The blockade of inhibitory pathways allows facilitatory neurons to function in an unopposed fashion, which results in an increase in excitatory activity leading to convulsions. An increase in the dose of local anesthetic leads to an inhibition of activity of both inhibitory and facilitatory circuits, resulting in a generalized state of CNS depression. Therefore, if procaine penicillin is inadvertently administered IV or if absorption is very rapid following IM administration, the observed effects can vary from mild excitation to seizures and collapse. Because high serum potassium concentrations can have negative effects on cardiac function, potassium penicillin should be administered slow IV.

Antistaphylococcal or beta-lactamase-resistant penicillins

This group, also referred to as the beta-lactamase-stable penicillins, includes dicloxacillin, cloxacillin, oxacillin, nafcillin, and methicillin. As the name implies, this group is used primarily against beta-lactamase-producing *Staphylococcus* spp., infections that are not particularly common in horses. In addition, although they maintain good to excellent activity against other Gram-positive organisms, cost and formulation issues limit their use in the horse for other susceptible infections. Methicillin, which was first approved in 1959 in England to treat penicillin-resistant *Staphylococcus aureus* infections in humans, has historically been considered the prototypical antimicrobial in this group. The first *S. aureus* isolate resistant to methicillin was reported in 1961, and the term methicillin-resistant *S. aureus* spp. (MRSA) was

adopted soon after. Resistance to methicillin is indicative of resistance across the entire class, including all the penicillins (the natural penicillins, aminopenicillins, and the extended-spectrum penicillins) as well as the cephalosporins. Strains susceptible to these antimicrobials are referred to as methicillin-sensitive *S. aureus* or MSSA. MRSA are of increasing concern in human and veterinary medicine, because the rates of MRSA infections have been on the rise in both man and animals and because these resistant microbes can cause infections in multiple species. Resistance is mediated by the mecA gene that codes for a PBP that does not bind any of the beta-lactams. These microbes are not necessarily more pathogenic than nonresistant strains, and often, individuals, human and animals, colonized by these bacteria do not show signs of infection. Nevertheless, they are pathogens, and when an opportunity presents itself, such as a wound or injury, the bacteria can cause serious infections. In addition, individuals colonized by the bacteria may spread them. This is of particular concern in hospital settings where immunocompromised individuals and those with wounds or surgical sites are particularly at risk. Other methicillin-resistant Staphylococcal species, such as *Staphylococcus pseudintermedius*, have also been described.

Oxacillin has been recommended for the treatment of MSSA infections in horses and administered at a dosage of 25 mg/kg bwt, IV, every 6 h, and IM, every 8–12 h, for susceptible infections.

Semisynthetic aminopenicillins

This group contains amoxicillin, ampicillin, and other related esters, although only ampicillin is used with any frequency in equine medicine. Their small size and the addition of an amino group to the beta-lactam ring allow aminopenicillins to penetrate the outer layer of Gram-negative bacteria better than penicillin G, and therefore, they have improved activity against these microbes, which include *E. coli*, *Salmonella*, *Pasteurella*, and some *Proteus* and *Klebsiella* spp. In contrast, *Serratia*, *Enterobacter*, and *Pseudomonas* spp. are generally not sensitive to the aminopenicillins. Their activity against Gram-positive aerobes and anaerobes is similar to penicillin. Because aminopenicillins are still susceptible to beta-lactamases, inhibitors, such as clavulanic acid and sulbactam, have been added to some formulations, although these are rarely used in equine medicine.

Sodium ampicillin is most commonly administered IV at a dosage of 10–20 mg/kg bwt every 6–8 h. It can also be administered IM at 10–22 mg/kg bwt every 8–12 h. It is often used for treatment of respiratory and other susceptible infections and can be used in place of penicillin or when a broader spectrum of activity is desired, such as prophylactically perioperatively.

Ampicillin trihydrate is administered to adult horses IM at a dosage 20 mg/kg every 12–24 h. Oral preparations are not absorbed sufficiently in adult horses to be useful, but have sufficient bioavailability in foals to be efficacious. In foals, a dosage of 13–20 mg/kg bwt, orally, every 8–12 h has been recommended.

Amoxicillin trihydrate has been recommended for administration to foals at a dosage of 13–20 mg/kg bwt, orally, every 8–12 h.

Similar to penicillins, ampicillin and amoxicillin have wide safety margins in the horse. Anaphylactic reactions are possible but rare. Broad-spectrum antibiotics, like ampicillin and amoxicillin, are thought to increase the risk of colitis in horses by altering the balance in gastrointestinal (GI) flora. Because it is only administered parenterally and is primarily eliminated by tubular secretion in the urine, however, the risk of antibiotic-associated colitis following ampicillin administration to horses is considered minimal.

Extended-spectrum penicillins (antipseudomonal penicillins)

The major advantage of antimicrobials in this class, which include carbenicillin and ticarcillin, is their activity against *Pseudomonas*, *Proteus*, and other Gram-negative agents resistant to other penicillins. Most *Klebsiella*, *Citrobacter*, and *Serratia* are resistant, as are all *Enterobacter*. These antimicrobials are also susceptible to beta-lactamases, and so they are often administered with an inhibitor agent, such as clavulanic acid. They are active against Gram-positive aerobic and anaerobic bacteria, but are not more efficacious against these agents than penicillin or the aminopenicillins, except for *Bacteroides fragilis* for which they do have improved activity. A relatively new subgroup of ureidopenicillins, which includes azlocillin, mezlocillin, and piperacillin, have increased activity against some microbes including *Klebsiella* and *B. fragilis*, but they have not been extensively studied in the horse.

Ticarcillin was approved in the USA for treatment of uterine infections in mares caused by beta-hemolytic streptococci, but the veterinary formulation is no longer marketed. The kinetics of ticarcillin have been studied in the horse [6, 7]. IV doses of 44 and 60 mg/kg of bwt were characterized by rapid elimination with a half-life of approximately 1 h. Following IM administration at a dosage of 44 mg/kg bwt, ticarcillin had bioavailability of approximately 65%, but it was poorly absorbed following intrauterine administration. There are no reports of its use in clinical cases. Given the expense of the human formulations and the lack of evidence in clinical cases, it cannot be recommended for use in adult horses unless C&S results indicate that the use of other antimicrobials is unlikely to be successful. In foals, a combined dosage of ticarcillin 50 mg/kg bwt and clavulanic acid 1.67 mg/kg has been recommended for IV administration every 6 h [8, 9]. IM administration was reported to be painful in foals and was not recommended.

Cephalosporins

Cephalosporins have a six-membered dihydrothiazine ring attached to the beta-lactam ring, which has the effect of making them more resistant to beta-lactamases than the penicillins. They do, however, share many properties with the penicillins in that they commonly have short elimination half-lives and wide margins of safety and are most commonly excreted primarily by the kidney. They are generally divided in four generations. Although these divisions are primarily based on their chronological development, some generalities regarding their activity can be made.

Cephalosporins are generally considered very safe, but hypersensitivity and anaphylactic reactions have been reported. Cross-sensitivity with penicillins can occur, but not always. Increased bleeding times can also occur, although these are rarely clinically significant. In horses, cephalosporins have been associated with the development of colitis even when administered parenterally. Although most of these agents are eliminated in the urine, some portion of the dose must be excreted in the bile to an extent sufficient to alter GI flora. Anecdotal reports indicate that colitis is more likely to develop in stressed horses, particularly racing horses, but there is no objective data to support this observation.

<u>First Generation.</u> As a class, their activity is similar to the aminopenicillins (i.e., good Gram-positive and some Gram-negative activity). They have some activity against anaerobes, and they are effective against many *Staph* spp., because they are more resistant to beta-lactamases than the aminopenicillins.

Cephalothin in one study was administered to horses at a dosage of 11 mg/kg bwt IV and IM [10]. The bioavailability of cephalothin given IM ranged from 38.3 to 93.1% and averaged 65.0 ± 20.5%. Cephalothin has been recommended to be administered to horses at dosages of 20–30 mg/kg bwt, IV, every 6 h and 20 mg/kg bwt, IM, every 8 h [11].

Cephapirin PK have been determined in adult horses and foals in several studies [12–15]. In both adults and foals, it is recommended to be administered at dosages of 20 mg/kg bwt, IV and IM, every 6 and 8 h, respectively [11].

Cephalexin can be administered to adult horses and foals at a dosage of 10 mg/kg bwt, IV, every 6 h [11, 16]. In foals, cephalexin can also be administered orally at a dosage of 30 mg/kg bwt every 6 h. Oral administration of cephalexin to adult horses, however, cannot be recommended at this time because the bioavailability is extremely low at approximately 5% and the effect of chronic daily dosing on GI flora has not been determined. In ponies, cephalexin administered at a dosage of 7 mg/kg bwt, IM, was well absorbed and tolerated, but this mode of administration should be used cautiously because in other species, it is generally associated with pain and muscle damage [17].

Cefadroxil was administered in one study to adult horses at a dosage of 25 mg/kg IV, and it was well tolerated and produced serum concentrations likely to be effective against sensitive Gram-positive infections [18]. In that same study, however, the oral bioavailability of cefadroxil administered at that same dose to adult horses was too low to be determined. Therefore, oral administration of cefadroxil to adult horses cannot be recommended. In contrast, bioavailability of orally administered cefadroxil was high (≈99.6%) in foals 0.5 month of age administered 10 mg/kg bwt. Cefadroxil has been recommended to be administered to foals less than 5 months of age orally at a dose of 20–40 mg/kg bwt every 8–12 h [11, 19].

Second Generation. As a class, their activity against Gram-positives is similar to aminopenicillins and first-generation cephalosporins, but they have increased activity against many Gram-negative pathogens, and some are effective for infections caused by *Enterobacter*, *Klebsiella*, *Proteus*, and *Serratia* spp.

Cefoxitin has less activity against Gram-positive aerobes than most first-generation cephalosporins, but it does have significant activity against Gram-negative aerobes that are often resistant to first-generation agents including *E. coli*, *Klebsiella*, and *Proteus* spp. It also has excellent activity against Gram-negative anaerobes including *B. fragilis*. It is recommended to be administered to horses at a dosage of 20 mg/kg IV or IM, every 6 h although laminitis has been reported associated with its administration.

Third Generation. As a class, these agents have more activity against Gram-negative aerobes and less activity against *Staph* spp. and Gram-positive aerobes than the second-generation cephalosporins. Their efficacy against anaerobes is variable with some having excellent activity and others negligible.

Ceftiofur is approved for use in horses in the USA for the treatment of *S. equi* subsp. *zooepidemicus*. In general, however, ceftiofur has good activity against Gram-positive aerobes, such as *Corynebacterium* spp., and some Gram-negative aerobes, including *Pasteurella* and *Actinomyces* spp. Some *E. coli* and *Salmonella* spp. are sensitive, but the MICs for these agents are often several fold higher than more sensitive microbes. In a similar manner, the sensitivity of anaerobic organisms to ceftiofur is variable. It has good activity against many anaerobes, but *B. fragilis* is often resistant. In addition, some *Staph* spp. may be sensitive, but C&S testing should be used as a guide as many are not. *Pseudomonas* spp. are also usually resistant.

There are currently two formulations of ceftiofur available. Per the label recommendations, the sodium salt formulation (Naxcel®, Zoetis Animal Health, Florham Park, NJ) is reconstituted with sterile water and administered IM at a dosage of 2.2–4.4 mg/kg bwt once a day. Reports in the literature indicate that IV and SC routes of administration at the same dose rate produce serum concentrations similar to those achieved following IM administration and are acceptable alternative dosing regimens. In neonatal foals, much higher dosages (5–10 mg/kg bwt, IV or SC, every 6–12 h) of Naxcel have been used to achieve serum concentrations likely to be effective against bacteria commonly associated with sepsis in foals, such as Gram-negative enteric organisms. These higher doses should not be administered to adult horses and older foals due to the risk of colitis. The crystalline-free acid formulation (Excede®, Zoetis Animal Health, Florham, NJ) is suspended in a caprylic/capric triglyceride and cottonseed oil mixture that slowly releases the ceftiofur into the circulation. This latter formulation exhibits what is termed "flip-flop" kinetics, where the rate of release of the drug from the formulation is responsible for the apparent drug elimination rate. Per the label recommendations, Excede should be administered twice, IM, at a dosage of

6.6 mg/kg bwt, 4 days apart. If required, additional treatments can be administered at the same dose every 4–7 days depending on the sensitivity of the pathogen. Although the label of Excede indicates that up to 20 ml can be administered at one injection site, the dose can be split into two separate injections sites to decrease irritation without significantly changing the PK. In neonatal foals, the results of one study support the administration of Excede at a dosage of 6.6 mg/kg, SC, every 72 h [20].

Cefoperazone, which has good activity against *Pseudomonas* spp., has been evaluated in one kinetic study in horses [21]. Following IV administration, it is rapidly eliminated, and therefore, the recommended dose of 30 mg/kg bwt should be administered every 6–8 h to maintain adequate serum concentrations. Cefoperazone, unlike many cephalosporins, has been shown in many species to be eliminated by hepatic metabolism. Although its primary route of elimination has not been determined in the horse, if it is similar to other species, this would raise concerns about a risk of antibiotic-associated colitis, even though no adverse effects were reported in the study. Nevertheless, it should be used very cautiously and only when C&S results indicate that other antimicrobials with more well-described safety and efficacy profiles in the horse are unlikely to be successful.

Cefpodoxime, in the form of the ester cefpodoxime proxetil, is approved in the USA for use in dogs (Simplicef, Zoetis Animal Health, Florham Park, NJ). Based on the results of one study, cefpodoxime is recommended to be administered orally to foals at a dose of 10 mg/kg bwt every 6–8 h for treatment of infections with *E. coli* and *Salmonella* organisms [22]. For more sensitive microbes, such as *Streptococcus* and *Pasteurella* spp., the same dose can be administered every 12 h. Cefpodoxime is not effective against *Pseudomonas*, *Enterococcus*, and *Rhodococcus* spp. It should not be administered to adult horses due to the risk of disruption of the GI flora and production of antibiotic-associated colitis [22].

Fourth Generation. As a class, their spectrum of activity is similar to third-generation cephalosporins, but because they are more resistant to beta-lactamases, they have extremely broad spectrums of activity, which include *Pseudomonas* spp. and cephalosporin-resistant nosocomial bacteria, such as *Citrobacter* and *Enterobacter* spp. They are not, however, effective against MRSA or resistant strains of *Enterococcus faecium*. One particular advantage of this class is that they produce a rapid kill of

bacteria, which is less likely to result in the release of endotoxin when treating Gram-negative sepsis.

Cefepime, like most fourth-generation cephalosporins, has good activity against many aerobic Gram-positive and Gram-negative bacteria and is resistant to many beta-lactamase enzymes. It has variable activity against anaerobic organisms, and it is not effective against MRSA or enterococci. Cefepime has been evaluated in foals and adult horses, but its efficacy in clinical cases has not been determined [23, 24]. A dose of 2.2 mg/kg administered IM or IV was associated with the occurrence of colic in a significant number of the adult horses studied. Therefore, based on these results, cefepime administration cannot be recommended in adult horses. In foals, a dosage of 11 mg/kg administered IV every 8 h is recommended [23]. Cefepime has a large volume of distribution including crossing the blood–brain barrier, so it can be used for meningitis.

Cefquinome, although not approved in the USA, is available in the UK. In adults horses, it is administered at a dosage of 1 mg/kg bwt, IV, once a day for the treatment of respiratory tract infections. In foals, the same dose is administered every 12 h for the treatment of septicemia caused by susceptible microbes.

Carbapenems: Imipenem–cilastin

The carbapenems are very similar in structure to the penicillins, but the sulfur atom in the five-member ring attached to the beta-lactam ring has been replaced with a carbon atom, and an unsaturation has been introduced, which renders the structure highly resistant to beta-lactamases. They have excellent activity against a wide range of Gram-positive and Gram-negative bacteria, including species resistant to many other antimicrobials, such as *B. fragilis* and *P. aeruginosa*. Resistance has been reported, however, so C&S testing should be conducted. In addition, this class is considered the last resort for humans with multidrug-resistant infections, and as such, its use in veterinary medicine is extremely controversial. Imipenem is the only member of this class that has been studied in the horse.

Imipenem, when administered alone, is rapidly degraded by the renal enzyme dehydropeptidase 1, and therefore, it is always coadministered with the enzyme inhibitor cilastatin. Imipenem is not absorbed following oral administration and is most commonly administered IV, because IM administration is painful. It has a rapid and widespread distribution to extracellular fluid following IV administration, but it does not readily cross biological membranes. It is eliminated almost entirely by the kidney. In the adult horse, it is recommended to be administered IV, slowly over 20–30 min, at a dosage of 10–20 mg/kg bwt every 6–8 h [25]. In foals, a lower dose of 5 mg/kg administered by the same regimen used in adult horses has been recommended, although the adult dose has been used in foals by some clinicians. In humans, the most common side effects are GI disturbances, and seizures have been reported. Imipenem was well tolerated in the limited number of horses studied.

Beta-lactamase inhibitors

These agents bind to beta-lactamase enzymes and inhibit their activity. These are most effective against plasmid-encoded beta-lactamases and are clinically inactive against chromosomal beta-lactamases induced in Gram-negative bacilli, such as *Enterobacter* and *Acinetobacter*. Clavulanic acid is the most common of these inhibitors, others include sulbactam and tazobactam.

Aminoglycosides
Chemistry

The aminoglycoside antibiotics include gentamicin and amikacin, which are commonly used in equine medicine, as well as dihydrostreptomycin, streptomycin, kanamycin, tobramycin, and neomycin that are either rarely used or used for topical and/or ophthalmic applications only. Aminoglycosides are large polycations that are highly charged at physiological pH. To a large extent, their chemical structure dictates their PK characteristics, which are shared by all members of the group. For example, they are not absorbed following oral administration, they do not cross biological membranes to any clinically significant degree, and they are all excreted fairly rapidly by the kidney primarily as unchanged molecules.

Mechanism of action

Aminoglycosides act by inhibiting protein synthesis in bacterial cells. They bind to one or more receptor proteins on the 30S ribosome, interfering with mRNA translation and resulting in formation of aberrant proteins. As these proteins are inserted into the cell membrane, they alter permeability and increase aminoglycoside transport. Aminoglycosides also act through other mechanisms including inducing the breakdown of RNA, altering DNA metabolism, and damaging cell membranes. Their penetration of the bacteria involves

passive and active transport. First, aminoglycosides passively diffuse through the outer membranes of Gram-negative bacteria passing through aqueous channels formed by porin proteins. Once in the periplasmic space, however, the aminoglycosides are transported into the cell by oxygen-requiring drug transport proteins. Because this second process requires oxygen, obligate anaerobes and facultative anaerobes (under anaerobic conditions) are resistant to aminoglycosides. In addition, the transportation can be inhibited by divalent cations, such as calcium and magnesium, hyperosmolarity, and a reduction in pH. Thus, the antimicrobial activity of aminoglycosides is reduced in environments with these characteristics, such as hyperosmolar acidic urine.

Aminoglycosides are bactericidal and their effect is concentration dependent. Therefore, as previously discussed, maximizing the Cmax:MIC and AUC:MIC ratios is the best predictor of bactericidal success. For aminoglycosides, a Cmax:MIC ratio of 10 has been recommended [26]. The clinical translation for this is that high peak serum concentrations, particularly initially, will maximize bacterial killing and accordingly should improve clinical outcomes. The duration of the PAE of aminoglycosides also increases with the concentration of the antibiotic.

Spectrum of activity

Aminoglycosides have good activity against most aerobic, Gram-negative bacteria, including *E. coli*, *Klebsiella*, *Pseudomonas*, *Proteus*, and *Serratia* spp. Some of these microbes are facultative anaerobes, so depending on the nature of the infection, the isolates may appear sensitive in an aerobic culture environment, but in the anaerobic *in vivo* environment, they prove to be resistant. They are also active against a few Gram-positive aerobes, most notably *Staphylococcus* spp. The efficacy of aminoglycosides against enterococci and streptococci is significantly improved when they are combined with agents that inhibit cell wall synthesis, such as beta-lactam agents. *Mycoplasma* spp. and spirochetes may also be sensitive, but *Salmonella* and *Brucella* spp. are often resistant to aminoglycosides.

Pharmacokinetics and therapeutic drug monitoring

The aminoglycosides, highly polar and cationic, are not absorbed from a normal GI tract. Therefore, they are either applied topically or administered parenterally. If given orally, the goal is to depopulate the GI tract of unwanted bacteria. Nevertheless, care should be used when administering aminoglycosides to neonates or adults with enteritis as absorption can be greater in these individuals than expected due to ulceration and inflammation in the gut. Absorption following IM and SC administration is usually good at 65–90% bioavailability, but the injections are painful. The apparent volumes of distributions (V_d) for most aminoglycosides are relatively small in the adult horse, less than 0.2 l/kg. In foals, however, V_d are larger, at approximately 0.34 l/kg, because a higher percentage of their bwt is extracellular water. The plasma elimination half-lives of aminoglycosides in horses are relatively short (1–2 h), and they are not highly protein bound (<20%). Because of their polycationic nature, aminoglycosides do not readily cross membranes, and so their concentrations in the CSF, prostrate, and respiratory secretions are low. They do, however, reach clinically significant concentrations in synovial, perilymph, pleural, peritoneal, and pericardial fluids.

Aminoglycosides are eliminated primarily by glomerular filtration as unmetabolized parent molecules, but the rate of elimination is highly variable among horses. Many physiologic (age, weight, etc.) and pathologic (dehydration, decreased renal function, etc.) processes may affect their clearance. Because of the high degree of variation in their elimination rates, and because they have a narrow therapeutic range, therapeutic drug monitoring (TDM) is undertaken with this class of antibiotics, but its use in equine medicine is not common. Briefly, serum aminoglycoside concentrations are determined on plasma samples collected after dosing (5–10 min after IV administration and 30–60 min after SC or IM administration) and then at least 8 h after dosing. The elimination half-life can then be calculated and the dosing regimen altered if serum concentrations are outside of the desired therapeutic range. Actual or predicted trough concentrations should be less than 2 μg/ml for gentamicin and less than 6 μg/ml for amikacin [27].

Toxicity

The aminoglycosides are nephrotoxic and ototoxic because both organs have very high concentrations of phospholipids in their cellular matrixes relative to other tissues [28]. Cationic aminoglycosides are attracted to the anionic membrane phospholipids and accumulate in high concentrations accordingly in these tissues.

Renal toxicity

Mild and reversible renal impairment is commonly observed during prolonged aminoglycoside therapy. The initial signs are only observed in the urine and include excretion of renal tubular brush border enzymes, decreased urine concentration, mild proteinuria, and hyaline and granular casts. Eventually, however, increases in plasma creatinine and blood urea nitrogen are observed. Aminoglycosides are freely filtered from the blood by the glomerulus into the renal tubule. There, the cationic molecules bind to anionic phospholipids on the proximal tubular cells. After binding, the drugs are internalized by pinocytosis and are eventually stored in lysosomes. Intracellular concentrations in these renal cells can be 50× those in serum. The more cationic charges on the molecule, the more the drug will accumulate, which is why neomycin is more toxic than gentamicin. The exact mechanism by which accumulation causes damage is not known. It has been proposed that with sufficient accumulation lysosomes rupture, releasing enzymes, phospholipids, and aminoglycosides into the cytosol, which causes organelle dysfunction and eventually cell death. Increases in urine lysosomal enzymes (gamma-glutamyl transferase (GGT)) are an indication of proximal tubule cell necrosis. Mitochondria, the glomerulus, and cellular plasma membranes are also likely targets of toxicity. A number of factors are associated with an increased risk of the development of nephrotoxicity, which include prolonged therapy (i.e., >7 days), metabolic acidosis and electrolyte disturbances, volume depletion, concurrent nephrotoxic drug therapy, preexisting renal disease, and elevated trough plasma concentrations.

Although TDM in an effort to prevent toxicity is the best approach, it may not always be available, practical, or affordable. In other species, increases in urine GGT and the GGT–urine creatinine ratio are early indicators of renal toxicity, but they have not proven to be as reliable in the horse. An elevation in the urine protein concentration has been suggested, but not evaluated, as a reliable parameter to monitor in the horse. The least sensitive parameters are blood urea nitrogen and creatinine, as they do not increase until renal damage is well established.

There are several approaches to decreasing accumulation of aminoglycosides in the renal tubules. First, minimizing trough concentrations by extending the dosing interval enhances back diffusion of the aminoglycosides into the tubular filtrate. Second, because the interaction between the cationic drugs and the anionic membrane phospholipids is saturable and competitively inhibited by divalent cations, such as magnesium and calcium, diets high in calcium and administration of calcium containing IV fluids can theoretically decrease accumulation. Finally, high-protein diets may also decrease the renal accumulation of aminoglycosides because they increase the glomerular filtration rate and renal blood flow.

Ototoxicity

In a mechanism similar to that observed in the kidney, progressive accumulation of aminoglycosides occurs in the perilymph and endolymph during periods of high serum concentrations. Also as in the kidney, back diffusion, in this case into the bloodstream, is slow but is enhanced by low trough concentrations. The biochemical mechanism of ototoxicity is not well understood, but histologically, it is associated with progressive degeneration of the sensory hair cells in the cochlea and vestibular labyrinth. Although it may be reversible in the early stages, it is often irreversible by the time it is diagnosed. While dogs tend to present with auditory signs and cats with vestibular signs, preferential organ toxicity in the horse has not been determined. Ototoxicity is generally observed after signs of renal toxicity are well established, unless administration has been into the ear itself.

Neuromuscular blockade

Acute neuromuscular blockade accompanied by apnea has rarely been reported associated with aminoglycoside administration. In humans, its occurrence is most commonly associated with intrapleural and intraperitoneal instillation of large doses of aminoglycosides, but it has been reported following other modes of administration. In addition, most incidents occur with concurrent administration of anesthetic or neuromuscular blocking agents. Aminoglycosides appear to inhibit prejunctional release of acetylcholine while reducing postsynaptic activity. As with other forms of toxicity, calcium antagonizes the effect, and IV administration of calcium containing fluids, either calcium chloride at 10–20 mg/kg bwt or calcium gluconate at 30–60 mg/kg bwt, is the preferred treatment [27]. Neostigmine at 100–200 µg/kg bwt IV will also assist with reversal of the dyspnea, and edrophonium at 0.5 mg/kg bwt IV will assist with reversal of the neuromuscular blockade.

Avoiding administration of aminoglycosides to horses under general anesthesia is recommended, if possible. However, given the growing use of regional limb perfusion with aminoglycosides, awareness of this rare, but serious, toxicity and its treatment is important.

Mechanisms of resistance

Anaerobes do not have the oxygen-dependent mechanisms required to transport aminoglycosides into the bacterial cell, and therefore, they are inherently resistant. Some resistant organisms have altered membrane transport structures, which prevent penetration of the aminoglycoside; others produce enzymes that can inactivate the drug or altered ribosomal proteins that have little affinity for the antimicrobial. Amikacin is the least sensitive to enzymatic degradation.

Gentamicin is the most commonly used aminoglycoside in equine medicine. Organisms with MIC ≤ 4 µg/ml are considered sensitive, and those with MICs ≥ 16 µg/ml are considered resistant [27]. Organisms commonly found to be resistant would include anaerobes, many Gram-positive aerobes, and some *Pseudomonas* spp. In the USA, it is approved for intrauterine administration to mares with endometritis at a dosage of 2.5 gm of gentamicin administered in 250 ml of saline, daily for 3–5 days. Much more commonly, however, it is administered IV or IM for severe Gram-negative infections at dosages of 4.4–6.6 mg/kg bwt once a day [29]. In foals less than 12 weeks of age, a dose of 12–14 mg/kg bwt once a day is recommended [28]. Older foals can be administered the adult dose. Gentamicin is also used for regional limb perfusion (IV or intraosseous) and impregnated in polymethylmethacrylate (PMMA) beads to provide high local concentrations but less systemic exposure.

Amikacin possesses the broadest spectrum of the aminoglycosides, because it is the most resistant to enzymatic inactivation. Organisms with MIC ≤ 16 µg/ml are considered sensitive, and those with MICs ≥ 64 µg/ml are considered resistant [27]. Organisms commonly found to be resistant would include anaerobes, streptococci, and some *Pseudomonas* spp. Because of its stability, it often has activity against bacteria resistant to gentamicin including *Pseudomonas* and *Klebsiella* spp., and its use is best reserved for those resistant infections. It is approved in the USA for intrauterine administration to mares with bacterial endometritis. For this purpose, a dose of 2 g in 200 ml of saline, administered as an intrauterine infusion once a day for 3–5 days, is commonly recommended. Amikacin is commonly used in foals with septicemia or pneumonia at a dose of 20–25 mg/kg bwt, IV, once day [30]. Expense generally limits the use of amikacin in adult horses, but it has been studied at a dose of 10 mg/kg, which produced serum concentrations likely to be effective against sensitive organisms [31]. Like gentamicin, amikacin is also used in regional limb perfusions and impregnated in PMMA beads. In addition, it is often used concurrently with corticosteroids or chondroprotective agents, such as polysulfated glycosaminoglycans or hyaluronic acid in intra-articular administrations.

Neomycin, **streptomycin**, and **dihydrostreptomycin** are older agents that are fairly toxic. They are rarely used except in topical preparations.

Kanamycin has a limited spectrum of activity and is one of the more toxic aminoglycosides, so it is rarely used in equine medicine.

Tobramycin has been proposed to be particularly effective against *Pseudomonas* spp. It is very expensive and its use is generally limited to topical treatment of *Pseudomonas*-infected corneal ulcers.

Chloramphenicol
Spectrum of activity
Chloramphenicol has broad-spectrum activity against Gram-positive and some Gram-negative aerobes, many anaerobes, and rickettsial and chlamydial organisms. Resistance is common, however, so use of chloramphenicol should be supported by the results of C&S testing. In addition, human toxicity concerns and its questionable bioavailability limit its usefulness in equine medicine.

Mechanism of action
Chloramphenicol, which is considered bacteriostatic, acts by binding to the 50S ribosomal subunit and inhibiting peptidyl transferase, which ultimately inhibits protein synthesis. Chloramphenicol also inhibits protein synthesis in mammalian bone marrow cells in a dose-dependent manner [27].

Mechanisms of resistance
The most common mechanism of resistance involves plasmid-mediated production of enzymes that acetylate the hydroxyl groups on the chloramphenicol molecule, which prevents it from binding to the 50S ribosome.

Other mechanisms of resistance include decreased bacterial cell wall permeability, alteration of the structure of the 50S ribosomal subunit, and inactivation by nitroreductases [32].

Formulations
Chloramphenicol base is very bitter, and therefore, a palmitate ester was developed to try to improve palatability. Following oral administration, it is hydrolyzed in the small intestine to the freebase form. Chloramphenicol succinate, formulated for parenteral administration, is hydrolyzed in the blood to release the active parent molecule. Formulations for topical and ophthalmic administration have also been developed. Many of these formulations may not be readily available, however.

Pharmacokinetics
When chloramphenicol is administered IV to adult horses, serum concentrations decline rapidly with an elimination half-life of less than 1 h. Part of this rapid decline is due to its widespread distribution throughout the body, with a volume of distribution greater than 1 l/kg bwt. This large distribution is consistent with its unionized state at physiological pH, low protein binding, and high degree of lipophilicity, and because of these characteristics, chloramphenicol can reach therapeutic concentrations in many secluded sites, such as the CNS and ocular tissue. It also readily crosses the placenta, which can cause toxicity to the fetus, because they are deficient in hepatic glucuronyl transferase activity. Despite its rapid and widespread distribution, clinically significant serum concentrations in tissues are maintained for only brief periods of time, because of its rapid elimination. For example, when mares were administered chloramphenicol sodium succinate IV at a dose of 25 mg/kg bwt, synovial and peritoneal concentrations peaked at 3–4 µg/ml 30 min after administration and were below the limit of detection of the assay 2.5 h later [33]. To maintain serum concentrations in the clinically significant range, horses in a different study were administered 22 mg/kg bwt, IV, every 4 h for 3 days [34]. Following oral administration of chloramphenicol to adult horses at a dose of 50 mg/kg bwt every 6 h by gastric gavage, the bioavailability was only 40% on day 1 and it decreased to 21% after 5 days of dosing [35]. Based on these studies, it is difficult to recommend this use of chloramphenicol; nevertheless, it is used and anecdotal reports are favorable.

In foals, the elimination rate of chloramphenicol was age related. For example, the elimination half-life of chloramphenicol administered at a dose rate 25 mg/kg to foals 1 day of age was over 5 h, but it decreased to approximately 30 min when the foals were 14 days of age [36]. The bioavailability also seems to be increased in foals with one study finding a bioavailability of over 83% in foals less than 10 days of age [37].

Drug interactions and toxicity

One of the most significant issues surrounding the use of chloramphenicol by equine practitioners is the rare, but well documented, occurrence of bone marrow toxicity in humans associated with exposure to chloramphenicol. Most commonly, chloramphenicol causes dose-related and reversible anemia by inhibition of protein synthesis. However, it is also associated with a dose-independent and irreversible bone marrow aplasia, pancytopenia. While most of the cases of aplastic anemia occurred in humans actually treated with chloramphenicol, they have also been reported from contact exposure including just handling the drug. Therefore, veterinarians, technicians, and owners should wear gloves and face masks to prevent exposure. Reversible dose-dependent anemia has also rarely been reported in small domestic animals. Although anemia has not been reported in the horse, there is no reason to think it could not occur with prolonged treatment or administration of high dosages.

Chloramphenicol should not be administered concurrently with many other antibiotics, because antagonistic effects have been documented. For example, chloramphenicol decreases the efficacy of fluoroquinolones, because it inhibits production of autolysins that induce cell lysis after fluoroquinolones interfere with DNA gyrase function. Other antibiotic combinations that should be avoided because of possible antagonist interactions include penicillin G, aminoglycosides, macrolides, and tetracyclines. Chloramphenicol is also an inhibitor of hepatic microsomal activity, so the clearance of other drugs metabolized by the liver (i.e., most barbiturates) may decrease.

Chloramphenicol, as previously described, is rapidly eliminated following IV administration in the horse. When this rapid elimination is combined with its PD characteristics of bacteriostatic killing with a time-dependent mechanism of effect, it is evident that maintaining clinically significant serum concentrations will require frequent dosing. Oral administration has been used clinically, but given the poor and progressively declining bioavailability demonstrated in one study of repeated dosings, it is difficult to recommend that route of administration. In addition, the human risk associated with exposure should always be considered, even if the true incidence of toxicity is extremely rare. Despite all of these caveats, chloramphenicol is used in equine practice and clinical anecdotes abound regarding its efficacy. An oral dose of 25–50 mg/kg administered every 6–8 h has been used in clinical practice. Although the PK of IM administration of chloramphenicol has not been characterized in the horse, the sodium succinate formulation has been administered in clinical practice at a dose of 30–50 mg/kg every 6 h.

Florfenicol is a fluorinated derivative of chloramphenicol. It is approved for use in cattle, swine, and fish and has been studied in a number of different species. The one published study in the horse, however, indicated that it consistently caused loose manure and elevated bilirubin, even after just one dose, raising the concern that it might cause enteritis, and therefore, its use cannot be recommended [38].

Lincosamides: Lincomycin and clindamycin

Lincosamides are a group of monoglycoside antibiotics containing an amino acid-like side chain. There are two members of this group: lincomycin and clindamycin. Both of these agents have been implicated in the development of colitis in horses and other hindgut fermenters, such as rabbits. Neither agent should be used in either adult horses or foals.

Tetracyclines

The tetracyclines are a group of four-ringed amphoteric antibiotics with broad-spectrum activity. Resistance to agents in this class is widespread, however, and often limits their usefulness. The class includes tetracycline, chlortetracycline, minocycline, oxytetracycline, and doxycycline, but only tetracycline and the latter two antimicrobials are used with any frequency in equine medicine.

Spectrum of activity

Tetracyclines have broad-spectrum activity against Gram-positive and Gram-negative aerobes, anaerobes, spirochetes, neorickettsia, and anaplasma organisms. Their activity against *Staphylococcus* spp. is limited, and they are not effective against *Enterococci* spp., *E. coli*, *Klebsiella*, *Proteus*, or *Pseudomonas* spp. While doxycycline and minocycline appear more active *in vitro*, *in vivo* differences in activity between the various tetracyclines are more likely the result of differences in absorption, distribution, and/or excretion rather than absolute activity.

Mechanism of action

These agents act by binding reversibly to the 30S ribosomal subunit inhibiting protein synthesis. They are considered bacteriostatic, but at high concentrations, they may be bactericidal against particularly sensitive microbes.

Mechanisms of resistance

Over 30 different genes providing resistance to tetracyclines have been identified, and most commonly, these genes are located on mobile elements including plasmids, transposons, and integrons. The most common resistance genes encode for energy-dependent membrane-spanning transporter pumps that actively excrete the drug from the bacterial cell. Other resistance genes encode for proteins that interfere with the binding of tetracycline to the ribosomes. Resistance to one tetracycline will generally provide resistance to others in the class. It is important to note that resistance to tetracyclines is rare among *Neorickettsia* and *Anaplasma* spp., organisms of particular interest to equine practitioners.

Pharmacokinetics

In horses, doxycycline is not particularly well absorbed following oral administration, but it does have good tissue penetration [39]. It is highly protein bound in the plasma and has a relatively slow rate of elimination. IV administration of doxycycline to horses results in cardiovascular collapse and death regardless of how slowly it is administered. Most tetracyclines are eliminated unchanged both in the bile by hepatic mechanisms and in the urine, although minocycline (and probably doxycycline) is primarily eliminated in the bile. Enterohepatic cycling, the reabsorption of drugs eliminated in the bile, can occur.

Drug interactions and toxicity

IV administration of oxytetracycline must be slow to avoid collapse. Although calcium chelation is suspected, the exact mechanism of the effect is not known; nevertheless, it is repeatable, predictable, and best avoided. Doxycycline cannot be administered IV, because it causes

cardiovascular collapse and death, regardless of the speed of administration. The mechanism for this reaction is not well understood, but does not seem to be related to changes in serum calcium concentrations. Allergic reactions and anaphylactic reactions to tetracyclines have been reported in many species, though rarely in the horse. In other species, tetracyclines have been reported to cause renal and hepatic damage. Although this has not been reported in the horse, the potential for this adverse reaction should be considered. In all species, tetracyclines are incorporated into forming bone and teeth and can cause discoloration in young animals. Phototoxicity, particularly associated with doxycycline, is common in humans and presumably can occur in animals with exposed nonpigmented skin. Oxytetracycline administration has been associated with alteration in normal intestinal microflora, resulting in potentially fatal enterocolitis. It appears that doxycycline is associated with a lower risk of antimicrobial-associated colitis. Some practitioners totally avoid the use of tetracyclines in horses with the exception of treating *Anaplasma* and *Neorickettsia*, while others report positive effects and few adverse reactions.

Oxytetracycline is the drug of choice to treat Potomac horse fever, which is caused by *Neorickettsia risticii* (formerly *Ehrlichia risticii*), and equine ehrlichiosis, caused by *Anaplasma phagocytophilum* (formerly *Ehrlichia equi*). Oxytetracycline should be administered IV slowly at a dose of 5.0–6.6 mg/kg every 12–24 h for 5 days. IM administration is not recommended, because achievable serum concentrations are unlikely to be effective against most pathogens, and it is associated with severe tissue irritation. Depending on the severity of the disease, some practitioners switch to oral doxycycline after a week of oxytetracycline treatment. This therapeutic regimen (IV oxytetracycline followed by oral doxycycline) has also been used to treat *Lawsonia intracellularis*. Oxytetracycline may also be effective against *Corynebacterium equi*, *S. equi*, and *Actinobacillus* spp., although in most cases there are better therapeutic options available.

Tetracycline has been recommended for treatment of Lyme disease caused by the spirochete *B. burgdorferi*. During an acute presentation of the disease associated with limb stiffness, edema, and fever, tetracycline can be administered at a dose of 6.6 mg/kg bwt, IV, every 24 h. After a week and depending on the clinical response, many clinicians will switch to oral doxycycline as described earlier.

Doxycycline, as discussed earlier under oxytetracycline, has been used in horses for the treatment of diseases caused by *Neorickettsia* and *Anaplasma* spp. It has also been recommended for treatment of chronic Lyme disease, caused by *B. burgdorferi*, and leptospirosis. The optimal dose of doxycycline is controversial. A dosage of 10 mg/kg administered, orally, every 12 h has been recommended in foals, but serum concentrations produced by this regimen in adult horses were very low. Therefore, a dosage of 20 mg/kg, orally, every 24 h in adult horses has been recommended for sensitive organisms with MIC ≤ 0.25 µg/ml, and the same dose administered every 12 hours has been recommended for organisms with MIC of 0.5–1.0 µg/ml [39]. It was also suggested that the presence of ingesta may decrease absorption of doxycycline; therefore, in an ideal treatment situation, food would be withheld for 8 h before dosing and for 2 h after dosing.

Non-antimicrobial uses of tetracyclines

Oxytetracycline has been administered IV at high doses (50–70 mg/kg bwt) every 48 h to newborn foals for the treatment of contracted tendons. The mechanism of action has not been determined, but calcium chelation has been proposed. Although no evidence exists in the literature to support its use for this purpose, anecdotal reports abound. One study examining the PK of these doses in 4- and 5-day-old foals found no adverse effects.

Tetracyclines, particularly doxycycline, have been shown to have anti-inflammatory properties. In humans, they are used as adjunct therapies for arthritis and autoimmune diseases. Doxycycline was shown to improve the outcomes of dogs with a surgically induced model of arthritis, but it has not been studied in horses. It has been proposed that some of the response observed while treating chronic Lyme disease is due more to the anti-inflammatory effects of these agents rather than their antimicrobial activity.

Fluoroquinolones

The quinolones are a group of synthetic antimicrobials that were first introduced in the 1960s. The fluorinated quinolones include enrofloxacin, which is the most commonly used quinolone in veterinary medicine, and ciprofloxacin, danofloxacin, difloxacin, sarafloxacin, norfloxacin, orbifloxacin, and marbofloxacin. To date, none have been approved in the USA for use in the horse, but some are used quite commonly in an extralabel manner.

Spectrum of activity

The fluoroquinolones have broad-spectrum activity against most aerobic Gram-negative bacteria (particularly *Enterobacteriaceae* spp.) and some Gram-positive, as well as *Mycoplasma*, *Chlamydia*, and *Rickettsia* spp. *Pseudomonas* spp. are often susceptible but may require higher doses. As a class, fluoroquinolones are usually active against *Staphylococcus* spp. but have variable activity against *Enterococcus* and *Streptococcus* spp. Except for some of the newest agents, which have not been studied in the horse, they are not effective against MRSA or anaerobes.

Mechanism of action

DNA in bacterial cells exists in supercoiled structures. DNA gyrase enables the formation of these space-saving structures by producing single-stranded nicks in the DNA, allowing it to coil upon itself and then resealing it. Fluoroquinolones bind to the DNA–DNA–enzyme complex and prevent resealing of the DNA strand. The result is in an abnormal spatial configuration of the DNA, which in turn leads to its degradation by bacterial autolysins. A secondary target is topoisomerase IV, an enzyme that regulates relaxation and unlinking of the DNA. In Gram-positive bacteria, topoisomerase IV is likely the primary target, while in Gram-negative bacteria, it is the inhibition of DNA gyrase that is primarily responsible for the antimicrobial activity of fluoroquinolones.

Fluoroquinolones are bactericidal and their effect is concentration dependent. As discussed previously, maximizing the AUC_{24}:MIC ratio is the best predictor of bactericidal success for fluoroquinolones. Ideally, an AUC_{24}:MIC ratio greater than 100 should be achieved [26]. An alternative goal is to achieve a peak serum concentration of 10× the MIC value for the microbe of interest. Because fluoroquinolones are considered to have a wide margin of safety in adult horses, TDM is not commonly used. Therefore, the ratios and peak serum concentrations are theoretical goals based on PK parameters determined in previously published studies. The PAE of fluoroquinolones is significant and increases with the concentration of the antimicrobial.

Mechanisms of resistance

There are at least three mechanisms of resistance to fluoroquinolones that are currently mediated by chromosomal mutations. Alterations of the DNA gyrase, which decrease the binding of the fluoroquinolone to the enzyme, are the most common form and produce high level resistance. Decreased bacterial cell permeability, by decreasing cell wall porin size, for example, also occurs. Finally, some mutations encode for energy-dependent pumps that export the drug out of the cell. Because these efflux membrane pumps may also be active against other antimicrobials, they can confer cross-resistance. Resistance mediated by chromosomal elements is extremely stable and is not eliminated when the selective drug pressure is removed. Plasmid-mediated resistance genes, which are inherently less stable, have been reported for fluoroquinolones, but their clinical significance is unclear.

Pharmacokinetics

In adult horses, the oral bioavailability of enrofloxacin, by far the most common fluoroquinolone used in this species, is 50–60%. In contrast, in ponies, the bioavailability of ciprofloxacin was only 6%. Although *in vivo* a significant proportion of the absorbed enrofloxacin is metabolized to ciprofloxacin, the two cannot be dosed interchangeably. Fluoroquinolones are generally lipid soluble and distribute well, including into the CSF and milk. In addition, they tend to accumulate in inflammatory cells, which may contribute to their higher concentrations in areas of infection/inflammation. Enrofloxacin is excreted unchanged in the urine by glomerular filtration and active tubular secretion, but ciprofloxacin is eliminated through both renal elimination and hepatic metabolism.

Drug interactions and toxicity

Chronic administration of high doses of enrofloxacin has been shown to produce articular cartilage damage in foals. The exact time frame of vulnerability, however, is not known, and fluoroquinolones have been used in older foals when other therapeutic options were minimal. Nevertheless, this class of antimicrobials should be avoided whenever possible in foals and pregnant mares. High doses can also produce arthropathies in adults. Colitis has been reported, but the risk is considered low to moderate. Transient neurological signs have been associated with bolus IV injections, although generally at doses higher than those used clinically. Nevertheless, slow IV injections or diluting the dose in normal saline is recommended.

In other species, adverse events have been reported that have not been observed in the horse at clinically relevant doses. For example, acute blindness has been reported in cats, but not in horses. In humans, tendonitis and spontaneous tendon rupture have been associated with fluoroquinolone therapy. Tendonitis and cellulitis of the plantar ligament were observed in some horses treated with high dosages of enrofloxacin for extended periods of time (15–25 mg/kg bwt, IV, daily for 21 d). Quinolones inhibit the metabolism of some drugs, which may increase the elimination times for these other agents. For example, in humans, theophylline toxicity has been reported in individuals concurrently administered with ciprofloxacin. The clinical importance of this in horses has not been determined, but clinicians should be cognizant of the possibility when administering other drugs concurrently with fluoroquinolones.

Enrofloxacin is commonly used in horses at a dosage of 7.5 mg/kg bwt, every 24 h, either orally or IV. The cattle product (Baytril 100®, Bayer Animal Health, Shawnee, KS) is used for IV administration and can also be used for oral administration. The small animal unflavored tablet formulation, however, has better bioavailability. Although the kinetics of **marbofloxacin** and **orbifloxacin** have not been studied as extensively as enrofloxacin, they have been described and their safety assessed, preliminarily. Marbofloxacin is recommended to be administered orally at a dose of 2.0 mg/kg bwt once a day, and orbifloxacin orally at a dose of 5.0–7.5 mg/kg bwt once a day.

Ciprofloxacin should not be used in horses. The bioavailability of orally administered ciprofloxacin is very low, and numerous adverse events including mild to severe colitis, endotoxemia, and laminitis occurred following oral and IV administration to horses [40].

Macrolides

Structurally, macrolides are many-membered lactone rings with sugar moieties attached. Erythromycin, which is naturally occurring, and azithromycin and clarithromycin, which are erythromycin derivatives, are the only macrolides used with any frequency in equine medicine.

Spectrum of activity

For equine medicine, the spectrum of activity of macrolides is primarily aerobic Gram-positive bacteria, including *Campylobacter jejuni*, *Staphylococcus*, *Streptococcus* spp., and a few Gram-negative bacteria, such as *Pasteurella* spp. They have very little activity against anaerobic organisms. In horses, they are used most commonly against the intracellular pathogens *Rhodococcus equi* and *L. intracellularis*.

Mechanism of action

Macrolides bind reversibly to the 50S ribosomal subunit and are generally considered bacteriostatic agents, although at high concentrations they may be bactericidal. The newer agents, azithromycin and clarithromycin, concentrate in phagocytic cells to a very large degree, which enhances their efficacy.

Mechanisms of resistance

There are three common mechanisms of resistance to macrolides: (i) active efflux of the drug from the cell by membrane pumps; (ii) inducible or constitutive production of an enzyme that modifies the ribosomal protein, resulting in a decrease in the binding of the macrolide; and (iii) esterase-mediated hydrolysis of the macrolide.

Pharmacokinetics

The macrolides used in equine medicine are almost exclusively administered orally. They are generally well absorbed, but some are inactivated by low gastric pH. Specific formulations of erythromycin, such as enteric-coated and ester derivatives, have been developed to decrease acid inactivation of the molecule. Clarithromycin and azithromycin are significantly more acid stable than erythromycin.

Macrolides have a wide distribution and a tendency to concentrate in cells. Erythromycin, for example, diffuses readily into intracellular fluids, and clinically significant concentrations can be achieved throughout the body except in the brain and the CSF. After oral administration of clarithromycin, it is rapidly absorbed and undergoes significant first-pass metabolism to an active metabolite, 14-hydroxyclarithromycin. Both the parent and metabolite distribute widely throughout the body and achieve high intracellular concentrations. Azithromycin also has extensive tissue distribution, and it accumulates within cells, including phagocytes, to a very large degree. The extensive accumulation of azithromycin, and to a somewhat lesser degree clarithromycin, in cells results in very slow elimination rates, allowing for long dosing intervals.

Drug interactions and toxicity

Erythromycin, like many macrolides, is eliminated as metabolites and unchanged parent molecules in the bile and may undergo enterohepatic cycling. It is this metabolic characteristic that raises concerns in adult horses. As much of the eliminated drug is active, the risk of antibiotic-associated colitis is significant. Therefore, erythromycin should be used in adult horses with extreme caution. The metabolic pathways for elimination of clarithromycin and azithromycin have not been elucidated in the horse, but in humans and other species, both are primarily eliminated in the bile. In one published study, mild decreases in appetite and alterations in fecal consistency were observed when azithromycin was administered orally at a dose of 10 mg/kg bwt daily for 5 days [41].

In foals, erythromycin appears to interfere with normal thermoregulatory responses. Hyperthermia and heat stroke can occur in foals turned out on moderately warm days while undergoing treatment with erythromycin. It is unclear whether clarithromycin and azithromycin share this adverse effect with erythromycin, but foals treated with these agents should be monitored closely.

Erythromycin and clarithromycin can also impair metabolism of other drugs by liver cytochrome P-450 enzymes. Therefore, concurrent administration of these macrolides and drugs, such as theophylline, midazolam, ranitidine, and chloramphenicol, which are primarily eliminated by the liver, should be avoided. Azithromycin does not appear to share this effect, but because the use of this agent has not been fully characterized in equines, caution should still be used.

Erythromycin is used in foals in combination with rifampin to treat *R. equi* infections, although its use has been largely supplanted by clarithromycin and to a lesser extent azithromycin. For the treatment of *R. equi* in foals, erythromycin is administered orally at a dose of 25 mg/kg bwt every 6–8 h along with rifampin, which is administered orally at a dose of 5 mg/kg bwt every 12 h. In foals, erythromycin has been recommended for the treatment of *L. intracellularis*, a Gram-negative bacillus that causes proliferative enteropathy. Oral dose of 25 mg/kg bwt every 8–12 h has been recommended, often in combination with rifampin (5–10 mg/kg bwt, orally, every 12–24 h). Treatment should be continued for 3–4 weeks. Erythromycin in combination with rifampin at the same dosage previously described has also been used for the treatment of colitis caused by *N. risticii*, although IV oxytetracycline and oral doxycycline are more commonly used for this indication. Because rifampin can decrease the bioavailability of macrolides when they are coadministered, dosing of each agent should be separated temporally as much as possible.

Azithromycin and **clarithromycin** are used primarily in foals in combination with rifampin for treatment of *R. equi*. Of the two, there is some evidence that clarithromycin is more efficacious for that disease [42]. In foals, azithromycin is administered orally at a dosage of 10 mg/kg bwt every 24 h, and clarithromycin is administered orally at a dosage of 7.5 mg/kg bwt every 12 h. Concurrent therapy with rifampin (5–10 mg/kg bwt, orally, every 12–24 h) is recommended. As mentioned previously, dosing of each agent should be separated temporally as much as possible. Clarithromycin has also been used for the treatment of *L. intracellularis* in foals at a dosage of 7.5 mg/kg bwt, orally, every 12 h.

There are numerous new macrolides that have been approved for use in food animal species in recent years, but only a few have been studied in horses, and all to a very limited degree. **Tilmicosin** should not be used in horses because of poor bioavailability when administered orally and safety concerns following parenteral administration. **Tulathromycin** has been studied in foals, but the primary pathogen of interest, *R. equi*, is inherently resistant to it. The PK of **gamithromycin** in foals has been evaluated in one study and the results were favorable. A single IM dose of 6.6 mg/kg bwt maintained pulmonary epithelial lining fluid and phagocytic cell concentrations likely to be effective against *S. equi* subsp. *zooepidemicus* and *R. equi*, respectively, for 7 days [43]. Nevertheless, safety and clinical efficacy studies are lacking at this point in time, so its use cannot be recommended.

Non-antimicrobial effects of macrolides

Some of the macrolides have been shown to have immunomodulatory effects apart from their antimicrobial activity. For example, in the respiratory tract, erythromycin, clarithromycin, and azithromycin have all been shown to inhibit chemotaxis and infiltration of neutrophils in the airways, resulting in a decrease in mucus production. In addition, macrolides inhibit production of many proinflammatory mediators. Although many of the studies demonstrating these events were conducted *in vitro* or in humans or laboratory animals, the anti-inflammatory effects of erythromycin have been documented in foals [44].

In addition to anti-inflammatory effects, macrolides within the 14-member ring group, including erythromycin

and clarithromycin, have been shown to have prokinetic effects within the GI tract. These effects are mediated by the macrolides binding to the motilin receptor and have been demonstrated in horses. The clinical applicability of these effects, however, has not been determined.

Polypeptide antibiotics

The polypeptide antibiotics used commonly in equine medicine are vancomycin, polymyxin, and bacitracin.

Vancomycin
Spectrum of activity

The tricyclic glycopeptide vancomycin is a large molecule with a molecular weight of approximately 1500 Da. It is highly effective against aerobic Gram-positive cocci, including MRSA and *S. pseudintermedius* organisms, and beta-lactam-resistant enterococci (*E. faecium* and *Enterococcus faecalis*). In addition, it is active against Gram-positive anaerobic bacteria, including *Clostridium* spp., but most Gram-negative bacteria are inherently resistant.

Mechanism of action

Vancomycin inhibits bacterial cell wall formation by interfering with the synthesis of long polymers of *N*-acetylmuramic acid and *N*-acetylglucosamine, which form the backbone strands of the bacterial cell wall, and preventing the backbone polymers that do form from cross-linking with each other. It is bactericidal and its activity is generally considered to be time-dependent. There is some evidence, however, that its efficacy also correlates to parameters typically associated with concentration-dependent killing including Cmax:MIC and AUC:MIC ratios.

Mechanisms of resistance

Resistance to vancomycin, due to plasmid-mediated changes in cell wall permeability and decreased binding of the drug to target molecules, is increasing particularly in *E. faecium* isolates. The VanA gene has been well characterized and confers resistance to all glycopeptides. Other resistant genes, VanB and VanC, have also been described. Resistant MRSA isolates have also been recognized with increasing frequency in recent years.

Pharmacokinetics

Because it is not absorbed following oral administration and because extravascular administration is extremely irritating, for systemic therapy, vancomycin must be administered by a slow IV infusion. Its distribution into tissues is limited, although it will cross the blood–brain barrier in the presence of significant inflammation. Vancomycin is eliminated primarily as unchanged parent molecule in the urine, and therefore, if used in patients with compromised renal function, the dose should be decreased. TDM has been advocated in human medicine, where target peak serum concentrations are below 50 µg/ml and trough concentrations are above 5 µg/ml. For the treatment of antibiotic-associated enterocolitis, vancomycin is administered orally.

Drug interactions and toxicity

Renal damage is the most common toxicity observed following vancomycin administration, and it appears to be associated with rapid IV infusion, although the mechanism of toxicity is not well defined. Ototoxicity has also been reported. Coadministration of aminoglycosides with vancomycin, which is not uncommon due to the narrow spectrum of activity of each class, may be synergistic in their effects but also potentiate their toxicity. Rapid infusion in humans also appears to cause histamine release, producing flushing of the skin, pruritus, and tachycardia.

Vancomycin should only be used when the results of C&S testing indicate the presence of a highly resistant organism, such as MRSA or *Enterococcus* spp. A dosage of 7.5–12.5 mg/kg bwt is recommended to be administered slowly IV over the course of 30–60 min every 8 h [45]. Vancomycin has also been administered intraosseously and by regional limb perfusion techniques to treat distal limb infections with resistant organisms [46, 47]. For these administrations, 300 mg of vancomycin was diluted into 60 ml of saline. For the treatment of antibiotic-associated colitis, when a metronidazole-resistant clostridial organism, such as *C. difficile*, is cultured or suspected, vancomycin is administered orally at a dosage of 125 mg (total dose) every 6 h.

The use of vancomycin in horses, and in veterinary species in general, is somewhat controversial. Vancomycin-resistant organisms, specifically resistant *Enterococci* spp., have been identified. In order to slow the rate of their development and given the threat that these microbes pose to human health, some have proposed that vancomycin should not be used in veterinary species. Most veterinary pharmacologist believe, however, that if used judiciously and appropriately the risk to human health

is minimal and the benefit to the individual animal's life can be significant.

Bacitracin inhibits bacterial cell wall synthesis by interfering with the dephosphorylation of a molecule that carries the building blocks of the peptidoglycan bacterial cell wall outside of the inner membrane. It is only effective against Gram-positive bacteria, and it is also highly nephrotoxic, so it is limited to topical use. It is most commonly formulated in a cream or ointment, for topical application to wounds or ophthalmic indications. Often, these formulations include neomycin and polymyxin B to provide broader-spectrum coverage. Oral administration of bacitracin for the treatment of enteric infections is rare in equine medicine, because of the high prevalence of resistance among pathogens, such as *C. difficile*.

Polymyxins are a large group of acetylated decapeptides that interact with phospholipids within the cell membranes, resulting in alterations in the membrane structure and causing an increase in permeability. Although numerous polymyxins have been isolated, only E, which is also known as colistin, and B are still in use clinically.

Spectrum of activity

Polymyxins are rapid-acting bactericidal agents with good activity against many Gram-negative bacteria including *E. coli*, *Salmonella* spp., and *P. aeruginosa*. Only *Serratia*, *Providencia*, and *Proteus* spp. are usually resistant, as well as all Gram-positive microbes. A number of compounds, however, including divalent cations, purulent exudates, and unsaturated fatty acids, can interfere with their activity.

Resistance

Although acquired resistance is rare, it has been reported in *P. aeruginosa*. The mechanism is not well understood.

Pharmacokinetics

When administered orally, polymyxins are not absorbed to any significant degree. Because they are nephrotoxic and neurotoxic and can produce neuromuscular blockade at antimicrobial doses, they are not administered parenterally in equine medicine.

Polymyxins are used quite commonly topically in ointments and creams formulated for the skin, eye, or ear. Occasionally, they are administered orally for the treatment of enteritis caused by *E. coli* or *Salmonella* spp. They must be used with caution for this purpose, however, because if ulceration of the GI tract is significant, absorption will be increased and so with it the risk of systemic toxicity. Rarely, oral administration is also used prior to surgery to decrease bacterial populations in the bowel. A dosage of 10 000 IU/kg bwt every 8 h has been recommended for oral administration.

In horses, formulations of polymyxin B, bacitracin, and neomycin (i.e., triple antibiotic) are commonly used to treat superficial bacterial keratitis.

Polymyxin has also been shown to bind the anionic lipid component of LPS, commonly referred to as endotoxin, rendering it inactive. As this effect is produced at subantimicrobial and, more importantly, subtoxic serum concentrations, polymyxin B has been used clinically to bind endotoxin in horses suffering from Gram-negative sepsis. Several studies have demonstrated its beneficial effects, but it should be used as early in the onset of endotoxemia as possible to maximize the response. A dosage of 6000 units/kg bwt given by slow IV administration every 8 h for the first 24–48 h is commonly recommended for this indication.

Potentiated sulfonamides

The sulfonamides are one of the oldest groups of antimicrobials. Sulfanilamide, an amide of sulfanilic acid, was the first sulfonamide used clinically. Resistance is very widespread, however, and therefore, they are of limited efficacy when used alone as sole antimicrobial agents. When combined with diaminopyrimidines (trimethoprim, pyrimethamine, or ormetoprim), however, their efficacy is increased. These combinations are referred to as potentiated sulfonamides.

Spectrum of activity

The spectrum of potentiated sulfas includes Gram-positive and Gram-negative aerobes and anaerobes. They are also active against *Chlamydia* spp. and protozoa (i.e., toxoplasma and coccidia). Resistance, even to the potentiated agents, however, is common, so C&S testing results should ideally guide their use in critically ill patients or when treating chronic infections. They are generally not useful against *Serratia*, *Pseudomonas*, *Enterococcus*, or *Bacteroides* spp. In general, their activity against anaerobes is less than *in vitro* sensitivity testing would suggest.

Mechanism of action

Sulfonamides are structurally similar to *p*-aminobenzoic acid (PABA) and act as competitive substrates for the dihydropteroate synthetase enzyme. This enzyme normally converts PABA into dihydrofolic acid, which eventually is converted to folic acid, an essential substrate for protein production. An additional block in the folic acid synthesis pathway is provided by the diaminopyrimidines, which prevent the conversion of dihydrofolic acid to tetrahydrofolic acid by dihydrofolate reductase (DHFR). When used alone, sulfonamides are static agents, but the potentiated sulfas are considered bactericidal for nonresistant strains. In the presence of excess amounts of PABA, the sulfonamides may be less effective, so exudates and necrotic tissue should be removed to the extent that is possible in order to enhance efficacy.

Mechanisms of resistance

Chromosomal-mediated resistance mechanisms for sulfonamides result in impaired drug penetration, reduced affinity of the enzyme for the drug substrate, and increased PABA production by the bacterial cell. Plasmid- and integron-mediated resistance mechanisms are much more common and result in altered drug penetration or synthesis of altered dihydropteroate synthetase enzymes. For the diaminopyrimidines, plasmid-encoded production of a DHFR enzyme that is resistant to the drug is the primary resistance mechanism. In addition, excessive production of DHFR and a reduction in the drug's penetration of the cell wall also occur.

Pharmacokinetics

Sulfonamides are weak acids, and as such, when the pH of a biological fluid is less than their pK_a, they will exist predominantly in their nonionized form. Most are rapidly absorbed following oral administration, and as nonionized compounds, they are well, but slowly, distributed throughout the body. Sulfadiazine, but not all other sulfas, can attain therapeutic concentrations in the CSF. The binding of sulfonamides to plasma proteins is extremely variable, ranging from 15 to 90%. Diaminopyrimidines are weak bases, and they distribute well and rapidly throughout the body, including the CSF. Sulfas and diaminopyrimidines are metabolized in the liver, and the parent compound and conjugated metabolites are excreted in the urine and bile.

Drug interactions and toxicity

In small animals and humans, sulfonamides can produce a wide array of adverse reactions in the skin, kidney, liver, and eye; however, these adverse events appear to occur less often in horses. Although rare, sulfonamides can also cause immune-mediated thrombocytopenia and anemia secondary to folate deficiency. In the presence of dehydration or the use of high doses, crystalluria with concurrent renal damage can also occur. Sulfonamides cross the placenta and are teratogenic. Therefore, their use to treat pregnant mares suffering from equine protozoal myeloencephalitis (EPM) is controversial as abortions and fetal defects have been reported even with folate supplementation. Folate and the diaminopyrimidines compete for absorption in the GI tract; therefore, they should be administered at least 2 h apart if folate supplementation is used. Some sulfonamides are highly protein bound and can affect the disposition of other highly protein bound drugs, such as phenylbutazone. Procaine is metabolized to PABA, so it is contraindicated to administer procaine penicillin and sulfas concurrently. As with all orally administered antibiotics in horses, there is an increased risk of colitis and GI disturbances with the administration of potentiated sulfas. The injectable formulations are suspensions and should be given slowly IV. They are also extremely irritating if administered perivascularly. In addition, these formulations should not be administered to horses sedated with alpha-2 agonists, such as xylazine and detomidine, because it appears that the risk of cardiac arrhythmias is increased.

Trimethoprim–sulfadiazine is used commonly in horses for treating acute respiratory tract infections, urinary tract infections, skin wounds, and abscesses. Resistance is common, so C&S testing is warranted in critical infections. The recommended dosage range is wide at 15–30 mg/kg bwt, orally, every 12 h. Some recommend withholding hay for 30 min after dosing. Human formulations of trimethoprim–sulfamethoxazole are often substituted for the veterinary product that contains sulfadiazine.

Pyrimethamine–sulfadiazine has been used for the treatment of EPM caused by *Sarcocystis neurona*. A liquid formulation approved for use in horses in the USA (ReBalance® Antiprotozoal Oral Suspension, PRN Pharmacal, Pensacola, FL) is labeled to be administered at a dosage of 20 mg/kg bwt sulfadiazine and 1 mg/kg pyrimethamine bwt daily or 4 ml of the formulation per 110 lb (50 kg) of bwt once per day. The duration of treatment is dependent upon clinical response, but the usual treatment regimen ranges from 90 to 270 days.

Miscellaneous antibiotics

Rifampin

Rifampin is a semisynthetic member of the rifamycin antibiotic class and is the only class member used in equine medicine. Because resistance develops rapidly, it should always be administered concurrently with other antimicrobials.

Spectrum of activity

Rifampin is primarily effective against Gram-positive aerobes including *Staphylococci* spp., as well as *Mycobacterium*, *Mycoplasma*, *Chlamydia*, and *Neisseria* spp. It is also active against anaerobes including *Clostridium* and *Bacteroides* spp. Many Gram-negative microbes are resistant. Rifampin also has some antifungal and antiviral activity, although it is rarely used for those indications in equine medicine. Depending on the sensitivity of the organism, it can be bactericidal or bacteriostatic in its effects. It concentrates in white blood cells, and so it is effective against intracellular pathogens, such as *R. equi*.

Mechanism of action

Rifampin inhibits the beta subunit of DNA-dependent RNA polymerase, thus suppressing RNA synthesis.

Mechanisms of resistance

Resistance develops rapidly due to changes in the beta subunit of the DNA-dependent RNA polymerase. A single mutation can change the affinity of the drug for the target enzyme, and therefore, it should never be used as a sole therapeutic agent.

Pharmacokinetics

Rifampin is fairly well absorbed following oral administration with bioavailability of 40–70%. It is very lipid soluble and distributes well throughout the body, including the CNS. It concentrates in phagocytes and is effective against intracellular pathogens. Its activity is enhanced in acid environments. Rifampin is extensively metabolized by the liver producing some active metabolites. It is primarily eliminated in the bile, with enterohepatic cycling possible, but some renal elimination also occurs.

Drug interactions and toxicity

Rifampin is a potent inducer of hepatic microsomal enzymes, so chronic therapy will increase its own elimination rate, as well as that of other drugs eliminated by hepatic metabolism, such as chloramphenicol and barbiturates. Occasionally in other species, hepatitis has been observed and rarely thrombocytopenia, anorexia, vomiting, and diarrhea. It is teratogenic in laboratory animals, and so it should not be used in pregnant mares. Clinicians should remember that rifampin stains everything red, including urine, tears, sweat, etc. It is not harmful, but it does stain clothes as well. There is evidence that when rifampin is administered concurrently with macrolides, the bioavailability of the macrolide is decreased. Therefore, temporal separation of the administrations is recommended.

Rifampin is most commonly used in combination with erythromycin, clarithromycin, or azithromycin for the treatment of *R. equi* in foals. It is also used to treat infections with *Staphylococcus* spp. It is administered orally at a dosage of 5–10 mg/kg bwt once a day.

Metronidazole

Although there are numerous members of the nitro-imidazole class of antimicrobials, only metronidazole is used with any frequency in equine medicine. Metronidazole is a weak base that is moderately lipophilic with a small molecular weight, characteristics that enhance its penetration across membranes.

Spectrum of activity

Metronidazole has excellent bactericidal activity against Gram-negative and many Gram-positive anaerobes, including *B. fragilis* (penicillin resistant), *Fusobacterium*, and *Clostridium* spp., but very little activity against aerobes. It also has activity against a number of protozoa including *Tritrichomonas foetus* and *Giardia lamblia*.

Mechanism of action

Bacteria rapidly take up metronidazole and reduce it to cytotoxic short-lived free radicals. These compounds damage DNA and other macromolecules. Aerobic bacteria lack the pathways necessary to reduce the compound and thus are not affected.

Metronidazole resistance

Although not common, resistance among *C. difficile* isolates has been reported, and therefore, C&S testing is warranted when treating enteritis associated with this pathogen [48]. The method of resistance has not been well defined, but it appears to result from decreased cellular activation of the drug.

Pharmacokinetics

Metronidazole is rapidly and generally well absorbed after oral administration with bioavailability reports of 58–91%. It is lipophilic and distributes throughout the body including into bone, abscesses, and the CNS. It is metabolized by the liver with both unchanged drug and metabolites excreted in the bile and urine.

Drug interactions and toxicity

Cimetidine has been reported to decrease the metabolism of metronidazole and may increase serum metronidazole concentrations. Neurotoxicity has been reported to occur with high doses or chronic therapy; signs include ataxia, lethargy, and anorexia.

Metronidazole is administered orally at dosages ranging from 15 to 25 mg/kg bwt every 12 h. Injectable formulations are available, but they are expensive and care must be used when administering them IV because their low pH makes them very irritating if inadvertently administered perivascularly. Metronidazole is commonly administered for the treatment of anaerobic infections in horses, and it is the drug of choice for the treatment of antibiotic-associated colitis in horses. Metronidazole-resistant *C. difficile* organisms have been isolated, however, and in those cases, oral vancomycin is a good secondary choice.

References

1 Giguere, S. (2006) Antimicrobial drug action and interaction: An introduction. In: S. Giguere, J. Prescott, J.D. Baggot *et al.* (eds), *Antimicrobial Therapy In Veterinary Medicine*, 4th edn, pp. 3–10. Blackwell Publishing, Ames.

2 Papich, M.G. (2007) *Susceptibility Testing in Animals—How Breakpoints are Derived and Interpretation of Susceptibility Data.* AAVPT 15th Biennial Symposium, Asilomar Conference Center, Monterey Peninsula, Pacific Grove, CA, May 20–24, 2007.

3 Marilyn Martinez, P.-L.T. & Robert, W. (2006) The pharmacokinetic-pharmacodynamic (PK/PD) relationship of antimicrobial agents. In: S. Giguere, J. Prescott, J.D. Baggot *et al.* (eds), *Antimicrobial Therapy in Veterinary Medicine*, 4th edn, pp. 81–106. Blackwell Publishing, Ames.

4 Uboh, C.E., Soma, L.R., Luo, Y. *et al.* (2000) Pharmacokinetics of penicillin G procaine versus penicillin G potassium and

procaine hydrochloride in horses. *American Journal of Veterinary Research*, **61**, 811–815.

5 Firth, E.C., Nouws, J.F., Driessens, F., Schmaetz, P., Peperkamp, K. & Klein, W.R. (1986) Effect of the injection site on the pharmacokinetics of procaine penicillin G in horses. *American Journal of Veterinary Research*, **47**, 2380–2384.

6 Sweeney, C.R., Soma, L.R., Beech, J., Reef, V. & Simmons, R. (1984) Pharmacokinetics of ticarcillin in the horse after intravenous and intramuscular administration. *American Journal of Veterinary Research*, **45**, 1000–1002.

7 Sweeney, R.W., Beech, J., Simmons, R.D. & Soma, L.R. (1988) Pharmacokinetics of ticarcillin and clavulanic acid given in combination to adult horses by intravenous and intramuscular routes. *Journal of Veterinary Pharmacology and Therapeutics*, **11**, 103–108.

8 Sweeney, R.W., Beech, J. & Simmons, R.D. (1988) Pharmacokinetics of intravenously and intramuscularly administered ticarcillin and clavulanic acid in foals. *American Journal of Veterinary Research*, **49**, 23–26.

9 Wilson, W.D., Spensley, M.S., Baggot, J.D., Hietala, S.K. & Pryor, P. (1991) Pharmacokinetics and bioavailability of ticarcillin and clavulanate in foals after intravenous and intramuscular administration. *Journal of Veterinary Pharmacology and Therapeutics*, **14**, 78–89.

10 Ruoff, W.W., Jr & Sams, R.A. (1985) Pharmacokinetics and bioavailability of cephalothin in horse mares. *American Journal of Veterinary Research*, **46**, 2085–2090.

11 Giguere, S. (2006) Antimicrobial drug use in horses. In: S. Giguere, J. Prescott, J.D. Baggot *et al.* (eds), *Antimicrobial Therapy in Veterinary Medicine*, 4th edn, pp. 449–462. Blackwell Publishing Professional, Ames.

12 Brown, M.P., Gronwall, R., Gossman, T.B. & Houston, A.E. (1987) Pharmacokinetics and serum concentrations of cephapirin in neonatal foals. *American Journal of Veterinary Research*, **48**, 805–806.

13 Brown, M.P., Gronwall, R.R. & Houston, A.E. (1986) Pharmacokinetics and body fluid and endometrial concentrations of cephapirin in mares. *American Journal of Veterinary Research*, **47**, 784–788.

14 el-Komy, A.A. (1995) Disposition kinetics and bioavailability of piperacillin and cephapirin in mares. *Deutsche tierärztliche Wochenschrift*, **102**, 244–248.

15 Short, C.R., Beadle, R.E., Aranas, T., Pawlusiow, J. & Clarke, C.R. (1987) Distribution of cephapirin into a tissue chamber implanted subcutaneously in horses. *Journal of Veterinary Pharmacology and Therapeutics*, **10**, 241–247.

16 Davis, J.L., Salmon, J.H. & Papich, M.G. (2005) Pharmacokinetics and tissue fluid distribution of cephalexin in the horse after oral and i.v. administration. *Journal of Veterinary Pharmacology and Therapeutics*, **28**, 425–431.

17 Lees, P., May, S.A., Hooke, R.E. & Silley, P. (1990) Cephalexin in ponies: A preliminary investigation. *Veterinary Record*, **126**, 635–637.

18 Wilson, W.D., Baggot, J.D., Adamson, P.J., Hirsh, D.C. & Hietala, S.K. (1985) Cefadroxil in the horse: Pharmacokinetics and in vitro antibacterial activity. *Journal of Veterinary Pharmacology and Therapeutics*, **8**, 246–253.

19 Duffee, N.E., Stang, B.E. & Schaeffer, D.J. (1997) The pharmacokinetics of cefadroxil over a range of oral doses and animal ages in the foal. *Journal of Veterinary Pharmacology and Therapeutics*, **20**, 427–433.

20 Hall, T.L., Tell, L.A., Wetzlich, S.E., McCormick, J.D., Fowler, L.W. & Pusterla, N. (2011) Pharmacokinetics of ceftiofur sodium and ceftiofur crystalline free acid in neonatal foals. *Journal of Veterinary Pharmacology and Therapeuticsc*, **34**, 403–409.

21 Soraci, A.L., Mestorino, O.N. & Errecalde, J.O. (1996) Pharmacokinetics of cefoperazone in horses. *Journal of Veterinary Pharmacology and Therapeuticsc*, **19**, 39–43.

22 Carrillo, N.A., Giguere, S., Gronwall, R.R., Brown, M.P., Merritt, K.A. & O'Kelley, J.J. (2005) Disposition of orally administered cefpodoxime proxetil in foals and adult horses and minimum inhibitory concentration of the drug against common bacterial pathogens of horses. *American Journal of Veterinary Research*, **66**, 30–35.

23 Gardner, S.Y. & Papich, M.G. (2001) Comparison of cefepime pharmacokinetics in neonatal foals and adult dogs. *Journal of Veterinary Pharmacology and Therapeuticsc*, **24**, 187–192.

24 Guglick, M.A., MacAllister, C.G., Clarke, C.R., Pollet, R., Hague, C. & Clarke, J.M. (1998) Pharmacokinetics of cefepime and comparison with those of ceftiofur in horses. *American Journal of Veterinary Research*, **59**, 458–463.

25 Orsini, J.A., Moate, P.J., Boston, R.C. *et al.* (2005) Pharmacokinetics of imipenem-cilastatin following intravenous administration in healthy adult horses. *Journal of Veterinary Pharmacology and Therapeuticsc*, **28**, 355–361.

26 McKellar, Q.A., Sanchez Bruni, S.F. & Jones, D.G. (2004) Pharmacokinetic/pharmacodynamic relationships of antimicrobial drugs used in veterinary medicine. *Journal of Veterinary Pharmacology and Therapeuticsc*, **27**, 503–514.

27 Dowling, P. (2006) Aminoglycosides. In: S. Giguere, J. Prescott, J. Baggot *et al.* (eds), *Antimicrobial Therapy in Veterinary Medicine*, pp. 207–230. Blackwell Publishing Professional, Ames.

28 Papich, M.G. & Riviere, J.E. (2009) Aminoglycoside antibiotics. In: J.E. Riviere & M.G. Papich (eds), *Veterinary Pharmacology and Therapeutics*, pp. 915–944. Wiley-Blackwell, Ames.

29 Magdesian, K.G., Hogan, P.M., Cohen, N.D., Brumbaugh, G.W. & Bernard, W.V. (1998) Pharmacokinetics of a high dose of gentamicin administered intravenously or intramuscularly to horses. *Journal of the American Veterinary Medical Association*, **213**, 1007–1011.

30 Magdesian, K.G., Wilson, W.D. & Mihalyi, J. (2004) Pharmacokinetics of a high dose of amikacin administered at extended intervals to neonatal foals. *American Journal of Veterinary Research*, **65**, 473–479.

31 Pinto, N., Schumacher, J., Taintor, J., Degraves, F., Duran, S. & Boothe, D. (2011) Pharmacokinetics of amikacin in plasma and selected body fluids of healthy horses after a single intravenous dose. *Equine Veterinary Journal*, **43**, 112–116.

32 Papich, M.G. & Riviere, J.E. (2009) Chloramphenicol and derivatives, macrolides, lincosamides, and miscellaneous antimicrobials. In: J.E. Riviere & M.G. Papich (eds), *Veterinary Pharmacology and Therapeutics*, pp. 945–982. Wiley-Blackwell, Ames.

33 Brown, M.P., Kelly, R.H., Gronwall, R.R. & Stover, S.M. (1984) Chloramphenicol sodium succinate in the horse: Serum, synovial, peritoneal, and urine concentrations after single-dose intravenous administration. *American Journal of Veterinary Research*, **45**, 578–580.

34 Varma, K.J., Powers, T.E. & Powers, J.D. (1987) Single- and repeat-dose pharmacokinetic studies of chloramphenicol in horses: Values and limitations of pharmacokinetic studies in predicting dosage regimens. *American Journal of Veterinary Research*, **48**, 403–406.

35 Gronwall, R., Brown, M.P., Merritt, A.M. & Stone, H.W. (1986) Body fluid concentrations and pharmacokinetics of chloramphenicol given to mares intravenously or by repeated gavage. *American Journal of Veterinary Research*, **47**, 2591–2595.

36 Adamson, P.J., Wilson, W.D., Baggot, J.D., Hietala, S.K. & Mihalyi, J.E. (1991) Influence of age on the disposition kinetics of chloramphenicol in equine neonates. *American Journal of Veterinary Research*, **52**, 426–431.

37 Brumbaugh, G.W., Martens, R.J., Knight, H.D. & Martin, M.T. (1983) Pharmacokinetics of chloramphenicol in the neonatal horse. *Journal of Veterinary Pharmacology and Therapeuticsc*, **6**, 219–227.

38 McKellar, Q. & Varma, K. (1996) Pharmacokinetics and tolerance of florfenicol in Equidae. *Equine Veterinary Journal*, **28**, 209–213.

39 Davis, J.L., Salmon, J.H. & Papich, M.G. (2006) Pharmacokinetics and tissue distribution of doxycycline after oral administration of single and multiple doses in horses. *American Journal of Veterinary Research*, **67**, 310–316.

40 Yamarik, T.A., Wilson, W.D., Wiebe, V.J., Pusterla, N., Edman, J. & Papich, M.G. (2010) Pharmacokinetics and toxicity of ciprofloxacin in adult horses. *Journal of Veterinary Pharmacology and Therapeuticsc*, **33**, 587–594.

41 Leclere, M., Magdesian, K.G., Cole, C.A. *et al.* (2012) Pharmacokinetics and preliminary safety evaluation of azithromycin in adult horses. *Journal of Veterinary Pharmacology and Therapeuticsc*, **35**, 541–549.

42 Giguere, S., Jacks, S., Roberts, G.D., Hernandez, J., Long, M.T. & Ellis, C. (2004) Retrospective comparison of azithromycin, clarithromycin, and erythromycin for the treatment of foals with Rhodococcus equi pneumonia. *Journal of Veterinary Internal Medicine*, **18**, 568–573.

43 Berghaus, L.J., Giguere, S., Sturgill, T.L., Bade, D., Malinski, T.J. & Huang, R. (2012) Plasma pharmacokinetics, pulmonary distribution, and in vitro activity of gamithromycin in foals. *Journal of Veterinary Pharmacology and Therapeuticsc*, **35**, 59–66.

44 Lakritz, J., Wilson, W.D., Watson, J.L., Hyde, D.M., Mihalyi, J. & Plopper, C.G. (1997) Effect of treatment with erythromycin on bronchoalveolar lavage fluid cell populations in foals. *American Journal of Veterinary Research*, **58**, 56–61.

45 Orsini, J.A., Snooks-Parsons, C., Stine, L. *et al.* (2005) Vancomycin for the treatment of methicillin-resistant staphylococcal and enterococcal infections in 15 horses. *Canadian Journal of Veterinary Research* , **69**, 278–286.

46 Rubio-Martinez, L., Lopez-Sanroman, J., Cruz, A.M., Santos, M. & San Román, F. (2005) Medullary plasma pharmacokinetics of vancomycin after intravenous and intraosseous perfusion of the proximal phalanx in horses. *Veterinary Surgery*, **34**, 618–624.

47 Rubio-Martinez, L.M., Lopez-Sanroman, J., Cruz, A.M., Santos, M., Andrés, M.S. & Román, F.S. (2005) Evaluation of safety and pharmacokinetics of vancomycin after intravenous regional limb perfusion in horses. *American Journal of Veterinary Research*, **66**, 2107–2113.

48 Magdesian, K.G., Dujowich, M., Madigan, J.E., Hansen, L.M., Hirsh, D.C. & Jang, S.S. (2006) Molecular characterization of Clostridium difficile isolates from horses in an intensive care unit and association of disease severity with strain type. *Journal of the American Veterinary Medical Association*, **228**, 751–755.

CHAPTER 3

Anesthesia and sedation in the field

Jennifer E. Carter

Faculty of Veterinary Science, University of Melbourne, Werribee, Australia

The principles of general anesthesia in the horse do not differ significantly from those of other species. The primary goals include muscle relaxation, unconsciousness, and analgesia. This is typically best accomplished by using a balanced anesthesia regimen that includes premedication, induction, maintenance, and additional analgesics. There are, however, significant differences between equine and small animal anesthesia that warrant review.

Equine anesthesia requires medications with a high degree of predictable activity in order to minimize risks to the horse and its handlers. In addition, equine practice often mandates techniques and procedures that are adaptable to a field situation in which inhalant anesthesia is impossible. Field anesthesia requires drugs that act predictably and allow for titration of effect. These drugs must also provide durations of action sufficient for field procedures while also facilitating rapid and smooth recovery.

Recovery from general anesthesia is a significant consideration in choosing an anesthetic or anesthesia protocol. In a major study on perianesthetic mortality in the horse, fractures and the development of myopathies during recovery were the second and third most common causes of perianesthetic death of noncolic horses [1]. In some cases, current techniques and procedures can obviate the need for general anesthesia in the field by using medications that allow for standing chemical restraint, possibly in combination with local anesthesia.

Clinical pharmacology of equine anesthetic drugs

Sedatives
Alpha-2 adrenergic agonists

Alpha-2 adrenergic agonists (A-2 agonists) are the backbone of premedication protocols in equine anesthesia.

A-2 agonists act by binding to alpha adrenergic receptors in the central nervous system (CNS) and the periphery, producing sedation, muscle relaxation, analgesia, and other adrenergic effects (Table 3.1) [2, 3]. A-2 agonists are commonly used alone and in combination with other agents to produce sedation and analgesia in horses to facilitate standing procedures. Table 3.2 presents some of the common protocols used for standing sedation and analgesia in horses. There are four A-2 agonists that are commonly used in equine anesthesia: xylazine, detomidine, dexmedetomidine, and romifidine. The activity of these drugs depends on their relative specificity for the A-2 and A-1 receptors. Specificity is important because it imparts the unique effects and side effects of the individual A-2 agonists and determines the most appropriate reversal agent. For example, activation of the A-1 receptor can cause excitement and increased locomotor activity, whereas activation of the A-2 receptor produces sedation and muscle relaxation. Of the agents listed earlier, xylazine has the least specificity for A-2 receptor with an A-2:A-1 binding ratio of 160:1, followed by detomidine at 260:1 and romifidine at 340:1 [4]. Dexmedetomidine has the highest specificity for A-2 receptors at 1620:1; however, it is used more commonly as an adjunct to equine general anesthesia than as a sedative agent and, as such, will be discussed later in this chapter [5].

The hemodynamic effects of A-2 agonists have been well studied in horses [11–18]. When administered intravenously, A-2 agonists cause dose-dependent vasoconstriction, which, in turn, leads to a reflex bradycardia. This bradycardia can cause AV nodal blockade, with development of first- and second-degree blockade, which is far more common in the horse than third-degree blockade [11, 12, 19, 20]. The bradycardia, combined

Equine Pharmacology, First Edition. Edited by Cynthia Cole, Bradford Bentz and Lara Maxwell.
© 2015 John Wiley & Sons, Inc. Published 2015 by John Wiley & Sons, Inc.

Table 3.1 Expected effects of administration of A-2 adrenergic agonists to the horse.

System	Effects/side effects
CNS	–Decreased dopamine and norepinephrine release leading to sympatholysis
Nerves and nerve terminals	–Decreased norepinephrine release leading to sympatholysis –Inhibition of PNS
Cardiovascular	–Vasoconstriction –Bradycardia: reflex and from sympatholysis –Decreased cardiac output
Gastrointestinal	–Decreased motility of the cecum and colon –Intestinal muscle relaxation
Others	–Hyperglycemia (inhibition of insulin release) –Polyuria (inhibition of ADH in DCT/CD)

Table 3.2 Sedation/analgesia for standing procedures in the horse.

Drug(s)	Loading dose(s)	Infusion rate(s)	Effects	Reference
Detomidine	10 µg/kg		Sedation (~45 min)	[6]
Detomidine + buprenorphine	10 µg/kg + 5 µg/kg		Prolonged sedation (~60 min) and increased ataxia over detomidine alone	[6]
Detomidine	10 µg/kg	0.12 µg/kg/min	Good sedation, minimal ataxia, rapid recovery	[7]
Romifidine	80 µg/kg	30 µg/kg/h	Ataxia + sedation	[8]
Romifidine + butorphanol	80 µg/kg + 18 µg/kg	29 µg/kg/h + 25 µg/kg/h	Prolonged sedation and increased ataxia over romifidine alone	[8]
Xylazine	1 mg/kg	0.69 mg/kg/h	Ataxia + sedation	[9]
Xylazine + butorphanol	1 mg/kg + 18 µg/kg	0.65 mg/kg/h + 25 µg/kg/h	Increased ataxia and response to stimuli over xylazine alone	[9]
Medetomidine + morphine	5 µg/kg + 50 µg/kg	5 µg/kg/h + 30 µg/kg/h	Good sedation for standing laparoscopy	[10]

with sympatholysis in the CNS, leads to a decrease in cardiac output. Vasoconstriction causes an initial increase in blood pressure, with romifidine and detomidine causing a longer period of increased arterial blood pressure than xylazine [17, 18]. With all agents, however, blood pressure eventually falls and hypotension may occur secondary to sympatholysis and decreased cardiac output.

Respiratory changes secondary to A-2 agonists are not nearly as profound as the cardiovascular effects. All of the A-2 agonists decrease respiratory rate, tidal volume, and minute ventilation, resulting in mild hypercapnia and a slight decrease in PaO$_2$ in the awake horse [11, 12, 21, 22]. A-2 agonists are also associated with decreases in pulmonary resistance and increases in compliance [23].

In the gastrointestinal system, A-2 agonists decrease myoelectrical activity and organized propulsive motility while increasing gastrointestinal transit time [24–33]. These gastrointestinal effects are reported to outlast sedation and analgesia. Detomidine and romifidine are reported to produce longer durations of intestinal stasis than xylazine [24, 25, 27, 29, 31]. Despite their effects on intestinal motility, A-2 agonists are the cornerstone of analgesic therapy for colic. Their sympatholysis provides substantial smooth muscle relaxation, and the analgesic effects of xylazine have been shown to be superior to both opioids and nonsteroidal anti-inflammatory drugs in controlling visceral pain in the horse [24, 34, 35]. Ataxia produced by A-2 agonists occurs in a dose-dependent manner but is reported to be minimized by the selective use of romifidine [19].

Xylazine

The duration of sedation and analgesia achieved with xylazine is dose dependent. In one study when xylazine was administered intravenously at a dose of 0.4 mg/kg, maximal analgesia and sedation was observed within 10 min, and most appreciable effects had disappeared by 30 min postinjection [12]. In additional studies when a dose of 1.1 mg/kg was administered IV, sedation and maximal analgesia was achieved within 5 min and lasted for approximately 30 min [4, 19, 36, 37]. The magnitude of sedation is dose dependent but with a ceiling effect, which is the phenomenon in which a drug reaches a maximum effect, and further increases in the dose are not associated with increases in effectiveness.

As with all drugs, there are limitations and adverse events associated with xylazine administration. For example, in excited, agitated, or painful horses, clinically appropriate doses of xylazine may result in inadequate sedation, and any additional doses may actually result in potentiation of the excitement. Accidental intracarotid administration of xylazine often results in seizure activity and a prolonged duration of sedation after cessation of the seizures. In addition, sudden death due to ventricular fibrillation has been reported after administration of xylazine to horses [38]. In the original Confidential Enquiry of Perioperative Equine Fatalities (CEPEF), administration of xylazine as a monotherapeutic premedication was a factor associated with increased mortality. This troubling finding, however, was not reported in the second study that used greater patient numbers [1, 39].

Detomidine

Detomidine has a slower onset of action than xylazine, but the duration of action is longer. In studies evaluating detomidine administered IV at a dose of 20 µg/kg, maximal sedation and analgesia were achieved in approximately 15 min and were maintained for approximately 1 h [19, 40]. These studies also demonstrated that the sedation and analgesia associated with the

administration of detomidine were similar to that provided by a 1.1 mg/kg dose of xylazine. Although detomidine shares the same cardiovascular effects as other A-2 agonists, one study evaluating organ perfusion in ponies found that during detomidine-mediated sedation, perfusion to reproductive organs was maintained at normal levels, making it a reasonable choice for use in pregnant mares [41]. Although no comparable studies have been performed using xylazine or romifidine, it is reasonable to expect similar results.

In addition to the parenteral formulation, detomidine is also available as a gel for sublingual administration to the horse (Dormosedan Gel®, Zoetis Animal Health, Florham Park, NJ). In one study, a dose of 40 µg/kg of detomidine gel produced sedation within 40 min of administration and that sedation lasted approximately 2 h [42]. Another study evaluated sedation and analgesia in 10 horses receiving 40 µg/kg of the detomidine gel sublingually and reported that sedation lasted for up to 1 h and analgesia lasted for up to 100 min [43]. Ataxia was noted to occur with sedation in both studies.

Romifidine

Romifidine has a rapid onset of action of approximately 2 min after IV dosing and a duration of effect lasting between 40 and 80 min [4, 19]. While romifidine provides similar levels of sedation and analgesia as equipotent doses of xylazine and detomidine, it is less likely to cause ataxia [19]. In two studies evaluating the level of sedation and responsiveness to noxious stimuli, the combination of romifidine and butorphanol was more reliable than romifidine alone [14, 44]. The administration of romifidine as a premedication either alone or in combination with other premedicants was a factor associated with increased mortality in the second CEPEF study [1].

A-2 antagonists

Although not routinely used, the effects of A-2 agonists can be antagonized with A-2 antagonists. Yohimbine, a selective A-2 receptor antagonist, has been studied for reversal of xylazine and detomidine in the horse [45–47]. IV administration of yohimbine resulted in effective reversal of the sedative and cardiovascular effects of both drugs [45, 47]. Atipamezole, a highly selective A-2 receptor antagonist, has also been evaluated for reversal of both xylazine and detomidine in the horse [48–50]. An early study demonstrated some reversal of sedation, but no improvement in cardiovascular function, when atipamezole was administered IV following xylazine sedation in ponies [48]. In contrast, in two recent studies, atipamezole administration failed to fully reverse the sedative effects of detomidine but did help to reverse the effects of a detomidine overdose in a horse [49, 50].

Acepromazine

Acepromazine is a phenothiazine derivative that provides sedation and muscle relaxation in the horse. The use of acepromazine alone or in combination with an A-2 agonist was found to reduce the risk of perioperative mortality in the first CEPEF study [39]. The sedative effects are largely attributed to the blockade of dopaminergic receptors in the CNS. Acepromazine also blocks serotonergic receptors in the CNS, which may affect behavior [51]. Acepromazine, through dopamine antagonism in conjunction with its effects on norepinephrine in the CNS, may be helpful in limiting the excitatory effects produced by opioids in the horse [52]. Acepromazine also blocks histamine receptors, glandular muscarinic receptors, and A-1 adrenergic receptors. A-1 adrenergic blockade causes vasodilation, which can cause hypotension following acepromazine administration.

Acepromazine is a water-soluble drug and can be administered by oral, intramuscular (IM), and IV routes. It has a slow onset of action, with peak sedation occurring 10–30 min after IV administration. The duration of action is dose dependent but may last up to 2 h [53–55]. When compared to xylazine, acepromazine produces less intense sedation and horses can easily become aroused by loud noises or painful stimuli [21]. Unlike A-2 agonists, acepromazine does not produce analgesia.

The A-1 adrenoceptor blockade, which produces vascular smooth muscle relaxation and vasodilation, is dose dependent. Low doses (0.009 mg/kg) of acepromazine administered IV resulted in transient decreases in mean arterial pressure of approximately 20 mmHg, while higher doses (0.1 mg/kg) reduced systolic blood pressure by approximately 40 mmHg [16, 56]. Low doses of acepromazine are not associated with clinically relevant hypotension in normal horses, but hypotension may occur when acepromazine is administered with other hypotensive agents, such as inhalant anesthetics.

Beneficial effects of acepromazine administration include an antiarrhythmic effect on the myocardium. It has been suggested to help prevent arrhythmias due to catecholamine sensitization in anesthetized dogs [57]. The respiratory effects of acepromazine are minimal and are generally clinically insignificant. Adverse effects of acepromazine administration are related to its A-1 adrenoceptor and muscarinic receptor blockades. A reduction in gastrointestinal motility may lead to increases in intestinal transit time. A reduction in packed cell volume is reported to occur due to sequestration of the red blood cells in the spleen. Acepromazine often causes penile protrusion and has the potential to cause priapism and penile paralysis in geldings and particularly in stallions. This effect is reported to occur without respect to age or dose. The exact mechanism of penile protrusion remains unclear but may be attributed to the A-1 adrenoceptor and dopamine blockade [58, 59]. Due to concerns that priapism may occur, acepromazine administration should be avoided in intact males.

Analgesics
Opioids

Opioids, which are used in the horse to provide analgesia, act by binding to one or more of the opioid receptors present in the CNS and some peripheral tissue locations. The opioid receptors are traditionally referred to by their Greek nomenclature as μ, κ, and δ, with the μ receptor considered the most important for analgesia in mammals [60]. Opioid drugs are classified based on their activity at the receptor as full or partial agonists, mixed agonist–antagonists, and opioid antagonists. Full agonists bind to and can cause maximal activation of the μ receptor; however, they may also activate other opioid receptors. Partial agonists also bind to the μ receptor but only result in partial activation and therefore can never achieve the efficacy of full agonists. Mixed agonist–antagonists, such as butorphanol, bind to and block the μ receptor while binding to and activating the κ receptor. Finally, opioid antagonists bind to and block the μ receptor.

In general, opioid administration to the horse provides analgesia; however, in a model of both superficial and visceral pain, xylazine produced a greater increase in the pain threshold than either morphine or butorphanol, and in a colic model, xylazine produced more profound visceral analgesia than butorphanol [34, 35]. Although opioids provide CNS-mediated sedation in a number of species, horses tend to exhibit CNS stimulation and an increase in spontaneous locomotor activity, especially when they are administered alone [61–64]. Opioids have the potential to cause respiratory depression; however, this does not appear to be clinically relevant in horses [65–67]. Nevertheless, in very sick horses or in horses that have been profoundly sedated with other agents, respiratory depression may occur. Opioids also have the potential to cause cardiac depression, particularly bradycardia, but at clinically relevant doses, they do not produce significant changes in heart rate, blood pressure, or other cardiac and hemodynamic parameters in horses [66–69].

Perhaps the most important side effect of opioid administration in the horse is their inhibition of gastrointestinal motility. Although different agents and different doses will lead to varying degrees of dysfunction, all of the opioids cause a reduction in propulsive motility of the equine gastrointestinal tract [67, 70–74]. Combined with a potential for producing increased smooth muscle sphincter tone, opioids have the potential to lead to ileus and abdominal discomfort in the horse [70, 75].

Butorphanol

Butorphanol is a mixed agonist–antagonist opioid that is commonly used in the horse. It exhibits a rapid onset of activity following IV administration, and the duration of analgesia is dose dependent, lasting between 15 and 90 min [76]. In one study evaluating the effect of butorphanol administered at a dose of 0.22 mg/kg IM in a model of visceral pain in ponies, the pain threshold was elevated for 4 h postdosing [35]. In another study, however, a dose of 0.2 mg/kg only provided visceral analgesia for 60 min [34]. The disparity between these study results may be a reflection of the methodology used in testing analgesic efficacy.

In general, butorphanol produces less profound changes in gastrointestinal function and transit time than other opioids [77, 78]. As with other opioids, however, butorphanol can cause CNS excitement, which is commonly manifested as exaggerated responses to external stimuli, as well as increased spontaneous locomotor activity. Muscle twitching is also commonly observed even when A-2 agonists or acepromazine is concurrently administered with the butorphanol.

Buprenorphine

Buprenorphine is a partial μ opioid agonist that is gaining popularity for analgesic use in the horse. Unlike most opioids, buprenorphine has a slow onset of action, even after IV dosing. Although the onset time has not been well defined in the horse, in most species,

45 min or more is required to reach maximal effect. Although the onset of activity is slow, the duration of effect is prolonged for buprenorphine in comparison to other opioids. In the only equine study to evaluate buprenorphine as a sole analgesic agent, a dose of 0.01 mg/kg IV provided analgesia for up to 11 h [79]. In another study, buprenorphine, administered at various doses, combined with acepromazine produced analgesia for approximately 7.5–9.5 h [80]. Like other opioids, buprenorphine causes excitement, increases spontaneous locomotor activity, and decreases gastrointestinal function [79, 81, 82].

Morphine

IV administration of the pure μ opioid agonist morphine to horses has a rapid onset of action but a short duration of effect. In one study, a dose of 0.66 mg/kg IV produced 30 min of analgesia for superficial pain and 1 h of mild analgesia for visceral pain [35]. In a recent study in which morphine was administered both IV and IM at doses of 0.05 and 0.1 mg/kg, it failed to produce significant analgesia based on the response to noxious stimuli [67]. As with other opioids, morphine causes CNS excitement, increased locomotor activity, and decreased gastrointestinal function. Finally, caution should be exercised when administering morphine IV as it has the potential to cause histamine release, which can result in urticaria and potentially severe vasodilation.

Opioid antagonists

Naloxone is an opioid antagonist with a rapid onset of action following IV administration. While it is effective in reversing all of the opioids, its duration of action is only about 30 min [52]. As a result, if the agonist has a longer duration of effect than naloxone, "renarcotization" can occur and the administration of additional doses of the antagonist may be necessary. Because buprenorphine has such a high affinity for the μ receptor, larger doses of naloxone may be necessary to outcompete the buprenorphine for the binding site on the μ receptor. Naloxone is also reported to reverse endogenous endorphins and enkephalins, which can result in pain and distress in normal, nonpainful horses [83].

N-methylnaltrexone is a peripherally acting opioid antagonist that is used in human medicine to treat opioid-induced constipation. Because it does not cross the blood–brain barrier, it preserves the analgesic effects of the opioids while reversing the unwanted peripheral effects, including reduced gastrointestinal motility. In one study in which *N*-methylnaltrexone was administered at a dose of 0.75 mg/kg IV concurrently with 0.5 mg/kg of morphine IV, horses exhibited increased frequency of defecation, decreased signs of colic, increased fecal weight, and more normal intestinal transit times in comparison to horses that receive only morphine [84]. While not currently a mainstay in equine anesthesia, additional studies on *N*-methylnaltrexone are warranted.

Muscle relaxants

Benzodiazepines

Benzodiazepines produce muscle relaxation by enhancing the binding of gamma-aminobutyric acid (GABA) to its receptors in the CNS. In some species, the benzodiazepines also produce sedation when administered as sole agents, but in the adult horse, their administration is more likely to produce CNS excitement and ataxia. In the foal, however, benzodiazepines provide excellent sedation. (For more information, see Chapter 7.) When they are administered to adult horses concurrently with other sedatives or anesthetic agents, however, benzodiazepines do enhance the degree of sedation. The benzodiazepines commonly used in equine anesthesia include diazepam and midazolam. At clinically relevant doses, neither drug produces significant cardiac or respiratory changes [85, 86].

Diazepam

Diazepam is the most commonly used benzodiazepine in equine anesthesia. It is most frequently used in combination with ketamine to provide muscle relaxation during induction of general anesthesia. When administered IV, diazepam has a rapid onset of action and a dose-dependent duration of effect. In one study, after a dose of 0.2 mg/kg of diazepam was administered IV, ataxia occurred and persisted for 2–3 h after dosing [55]. Diazepam should only be administered IV because it is poorly water soluble. IM administration of diazepam causes inflammation and unpredictable, generally incomplete, absorption.

Midazolam

Midazolam can be used in the place of diazepam for muscle relaxation while inducing or maintaining general anesthesia in the horse. IV administration may cause agitation and ataxia as observed with diazepam. Although the efficacy of midazolam has not been determined in the horse, a pharmacokinetic study reported a median terminal half-life of 408 min after a 0.1 mg/kg dose was administered IV. Ataxia and agitation, however, occurred postdosing and persisted for approximately 60 min [87]. Midazolam, in contrast to diazepam, is water soluble, making it an attractive option for IM administration.

Guaifenesin

Guaifenesin is a centrally acting muscle relaxant that is commonly used in equine anesthesia for muscle relaxation during induction and maintenance of anesthesia. It is administered as an IV infusion to effect, prior to the administration of an IV anesthetic. It is typically diluted in 5% dextrose solution to a final concentration of 50 mg/ml. At clinically relevant doses, guaifenesin does not produce significant cardiac or respiratory effects [88, 89]. Anesthetic protocols using guaifenesin are described in conjunction with ketamine, thiopental, propofol, and alfaxalone anesthetic inductions [90–98]. Guaifenesin is also commonly used to help maintain a surgical plane of anesthesia in many protocols that use only injectable anesthetic agents.

Premedication protocols

Premedications are agents administered prior to induction of general anesthesia with the goal of improving the quality of induction of anesthesia and its maintenance. They may include any one or a combination of agents previously discussed, and they are typically administered IV to horses. If a horse is needle shy or difficult to handle, some premedication combinations may be administered IM; however, this will result in a slower onset of sedation and potentially a less intense sedation than the IV route. For longer procedures, additional doses of the premedications may be administered at 1/4–1/2 of the original dose. Table 3.3 lists anesthetic premedication protocols that are commonly used in horses and their indication and side effects.

General anesthesia induction agents

Induction is the initial introduction of anesthesia to the animal. When induction of anesthesia is applied

Table 3.3 Commonly used equine anesthetic premedications.

Drug(s)	Indications	Side effects or contraindications
Xylazine (1 mg/kg) + butorphanol (0.02 mg/kg)	Appropriate for most premedication scenarios Combination provides synergistic sedation and analgesia	Mild to moderate ataxia Bradycardia with decreased cardiac output First- or second-degree AV block
Detomidine (20–40 µg/kg) + butorphanol (0.02 mg/kg)	Appropriate for procedures of longer duration Provides sedation and analgesia	More likely to cause ataxia than xylazine Cardiovascular effects as aforementioned
Romifidine (80–100 µg/kg) + butorphanol (0.02 mg/kg)	Appropriate for procedures of longer duration Provides sedation and analgesia	Less likely than xylazine or detomidine to cause ataxia Cardiovascular effects as aforementioned
Acepromazine (0.02–0.05 mg/kg) + A-2 agonist 15–20 min later	Appropriate for procedures > 45 min and high-spirited horses This combination will provide profound sedation	Will likely result in moderate ataxia Potential for severe hypotension due to additive effect of drugs

Butorphanol can be replaced with morphine (0.02–0.05 mg/kg), buprenorphine (0.006 mg/kg), or methadone (0.1 mg/kg) in any of the aforementioned combinations.

Table 3.4 Equine induction protocols.

Drug(s)	Indications	Side effects or contraindications
Diazepam/midazolam (0.04–0.1 mg/kg) + ketamine (2.2–3 mg/kg)	Acceptable for nearly any equine induction scenario Smooth induction with recumbency 30–60 s after drug administration Suitable alone for short surgical procedures	Diazepam may cause excitement. Administer with ketamine to alleviate excitement that may be experienced with diazepam Avoid in horses with increased intracranial pressure
Guaifenesin (50–100 mg/kg—to effect) + ketamine (0.5–1 mg/kg)	Guaifenesin is administered until horse is visibly relaxed and then bolus of ketamine is given Recumbency within 60 s of ketamine administration Suitable for short surgical procedures	Ataxia is likely with guaifenesin Potential for hypoventilation due to neuromuscular weakness of diaphragm from guaifenesin Prolonged recovery when compared to diazepam/ketamine
Guaifenesin (50–100 mg/kg—to effect) + thiopental (1–2 mg/kg)	Administration as aforementioned except that thiopental bolus is administered rather than ketamine Recumbency within 30 s of thiopental administration Suitable for short surgical procedures	Ataxia as aforementioned Hypoventilation as aforementioned Potential for cardiovascular depression secondary to thiopental Prolonged recovery as aforementioned
Thiopental (6–10 mg/kg)	Recumbency within 30–45 s Suitable for short surgical procedures	Induction is abrupt and uncoordinated when compared to ketamine Will result in cardiorespiratory depression Recovery may be prolonged and uncoordinated

effectively, it provides rapid and safe muscle relaxation, analgesia, and unconsciousness that facilitate recumbency and safe positioning for surgery with time to connect to a continuous intravenous (IV) infusion and/or to a breathing circuit connected to an appropriate inhalant anesthetic vaporizer. Table 3.4 summarizes a number of induction protocols commonly used for the horse.

Dissociative anesthetics: Ketamine and tiletamine

Ketamine is arguably the most commonly used equine anesthetic induction agent. Along with tiletamine, they represent the two dissociative anesthetics used in equine anesthesia. While their specific mechanism of action is only partly understood, they are known to antagonize the *N*-methyl-*D*-aspartate (NMDA) receptors in the CNS. The NMDA receptor is important in sensitization of central pain pathways, and this antagonism provides explanation of the antihyperalgesic properties attributed to these agents.

Ketamine and tiletamine induce anesthesia by blocking sensory input to the CNS, and because of this, reflexes, such as swallowing or palpebral, may persist. Anesthesia provided by these agents is characterized by very poor muscle relaxation, and therefore, they are generally always administered in conjunction with muscle relaxing agents. Tiletamine is only available in combination with the benzodiazepine agent zolazepam (Telazol®, Zoetis Animal Health, Florham Park, NJ), whereas ketamine is commonly administered with either guaifenesin or diazepam.

These dissociative anesthetics are unique among the induction agents used in horses in that they stimulate the sympathetic nervous system and increase circulating catecholamines [99]. Catecholamines increase heart rate, blood pressure, and cardiac output in the anesthetized horse, although the effect may be compromised in sick or debilitated horses [99]. In these cases, dissociative anesthetics may act as direct myocardial depressants [100]. While the dissociative agents have minimal effects on ventilation and oxygenation, they can cause a transient apneustic respiratory pattern. Apneustic breathing is characterized by a deep, gasping inspiration with a pause at full inspiration followed by a brief, insufficient release. The effect of ketamine or tiletamine on intracranial and intraocular pressure is controversial, and further research is necessary to determine the safety of their administration to horses at risk for development of elevated intracranial or intraocular pressures.

Ketamine and Telazol are most effective when administered to horses that are already sedated [101]. Numerous studies report the use of ketamine and Telazol in combination with a variety of agents for induction and maintenance of anesthesia in the horse. The typical induction dose of ketamine ranges from 1.5 to 3 mg/kg, while the recommended induction dose of Telazol (100 mg/ml) is 1.65–2.2 mg/kg IV [102]. Both ketamine and Telazol are typically administered IV at a precalculated dose, and there is usually a 30–60 s delay from the time the injection is complete to anesthetic induction. One study compared the duration of anesthesia following induction with ketamine versus Telazol with xylazine as a premedication. This study reported that the mean duration of anesthesia after ketamine administration was 18 min compared to 33 min after Telazol administration [103].

Thiopental

Thiopental was a mainstay of equine anesthesia for many years; however, its use has largely been replaced by that of dissociative anesthetics. It is an ultrashort-acting barbiturate that induces general anesthesia by enhancing the conduction of chloride ions at GABA channels in the CNS. Thiopental causes CNS depression and decreases cerebral metabolic oxygen demands, the latter factor making its use appealing in horses with intracranial lesions. Anesthetic doses result in cardiovascular and respiratory depression with transient ventricular bigeminy and apnea reported to occur [104]. In addition, leukopenia and hyperglycemia have been described in horses following administration of doses of thiopental between 9 and 17 mg/kg [105].

Thiopental administered at a dose of 6–10 mg/kg IV can be used as a sole induction agent following sedation with an appropriate premedication [105, 106]. Excitement and muscle tremors may occur if horses are not appropriately sedated prior to administration. Recumbency is typically achieved within 30–45 s after administration. Unlike ketamine-based protocols, horses tend to drop to the ground in a rapid, uncoordinated manner. Therefore, care should be taken to support the horse's head during the induction period. Recovery to standing occurs within 20–30 min of induction, and horses may experience uncoordinated recovery attempts, including rolling and significant ataxia. Typically, recovery from dissociative anesthesia is smoother than recovery from thiopental anesthesia. Thiopental can also be administered in conjunction with guaifenesin infused at a dose of 5 mg/kg [94, 107].

Propofol

Propofol is a short-acting general anesthetic that enhances GABA receptor activity. Despite its popularity in human and small animal anesthesia, propofol has yet to gain mainstream use in equine anesthesia.

In early studies when propofol was administered at doses varying from 2 to 8 mg/kg IV, the quality of the inductions was reported as variable, but the recoveries were reported as generally good. These inductions were associated with significant increases in arterial carbon dioxide and decreases in arterial oxygen tension [108, 109]. A more recent study evaluated administration of propofol at doses of 1, 2, and 4 mg/kg IV in comparison to a standard ketamine induction and concluded that the 2 mg/kg propofol dose most closely approximated the anesthesia quality of the ketamine protocol [110]. Recovery times following administration of a single induction dose of propofol range from 30 to 40 min. The variable quality of the induction combined with the potential for hypoventilation and hypoxemia has prevented the routine use of propofol in equine anesthesia. A recent study reported that the quality of the induction was improved when guaifenesin was administered prior to the propofol [97]. This combination prevented paddling and other manifestations of excitement previously reported with propofol. Propofol has also been used in combination with other medications for total or partial IV anesthesia.

Alfaxalone

Alfaxalone is a neurosteroid general anesthetic that functions as an agonist at the GABA receptor. It is not routinely used in the horse owing to a number of factors, including cost. One study compared 1 mg/kg IV of alfaxalone with 2.2 mg/kg IV of ketamine for induction in ponies undergoing surgical castration [111]. The mean induction time was 18 s with alfaxalone, and the recovery score was slightly lower in comparison to that with ketamine. Another study compared ketamine and alfaxalone using the same induction doses but with different premedications [98]. In that study, muscle tremors were reported at induction with alfaxalone administration. Although the times for recovery to standing were similar, horses receiving alfaxalone exhibited prolonged ataxia.

General anesthesia maintenance agents
Total intravenous anesthesia (TIVA)

Total intravenous anesthesia (TIVA) describes the technique of maintaining general anesthesia using only injectable drugs. TIVA techniques are commonly used in equine practice. IV anesthetics may be administered as intermittent boluses using the same medications as used for premedication and/or induction or as continuous rate infusions. Table 3.5 lists the drugs, dosages, indications, and side effects of commonly employed protocols for equine TIVA based on expected durations of anesthesia.

Table 3.5 Maintenance anesthesia using TIVA.

Procedure duration	Drugs	Indications	Side effects or contraindications
<15 min	Most induction combinations will provide reliable anesthesia for surgical procedures lasting less than 15 min		
15–30 min	Ketamine (1 mg/kg)	Extends duration of anesthesia with no additional side effects	Muscle relaxation may not be adequate
	Xylazine (0.25–0.5 mg/kg) + ketamine (0.25–1 mg/kg)	Extends duration of anesthesia and provides additional muscle relaxation	May prolong recovery compared to ketamine alone; *Do not top up with romifidine or detomidine*
30–90 min	Guaifenesin + ketamine + xylazine (GKX) *Triple drip*	Dosed to effect Good muscle relaxation Minimal cardiovascular depression Smooth recovery	Respiratory depression worsens with longer infusions—consider supplemental oxygen Longer durations lead to prolonged recoveries
	Guaifenesin + ketamine + detomidine (GKD) Guaifenesin + ketamine + romifidine (GKR)	As aforementioned As aforementioned	Recovery is prolonged when compared to GKX Recovery is prolonged when compared to GKX
>90 min	Not recommended. Longer procedures should be performed in an operating theater with appropriate ventilatory support		

Ketamine/Xylazine

Boluses of ketamine administered at doses of 0.25–1.0 mg/kg combined with xylazine administered at doses of 0.25–0.5 mg/kg can be used to prolong anesthesia following an induction with either ketamine/diazepam or ketamine/guaifenesin. With this approach, cardiopulmonary parameters are unaffected and recovery is typically smooth. One study reported the use of multiple boluses of ketamine and xylazine, both administered at doses of 0.25 mg/kg, following a ketamine/diazepam induction [112]. This protocol maintained surgical anesthesia for approximately 40 min and resulted in recovery by approximately 20 min after the final injection. The investigators of that study suggested, however, that muscle relaxation and analgesia with this protocol may be inferior to that produced by the more traditional combination of xylazine, ketamine, and guaifenesin, which is often referred to as "triple-drip" anesthesia.

Mama *et al.* reported the use of a maintenance infusion of ketamine and xylazine to facilitate up to 60 min of surgical anesthesia [113]. They evaluated several combinations of the two drugs, xylazine administered at 35 or 70 µg/kg/min and ketamine administered at 90, 120, or 150 µg/kg/min, in association with various concentrations of inspired oxygen. They concluded that the protocols were associated with acceptable cardiopulmonary performance in the study animals and good quality recoveries that ranged between 45 and 70 min to standing.

Guaifenesin/ketamine/xylazine

A mixture of guaifenesin/ketamine/xylazine (GKX) given as a continuous infusion is one of the most common protocols used for maintaining general anesthesia in the horse. The combined formulation, often referred to as "triple drip," is achieved by combining 1 g of ketamine with 500 mg of xylazine and 1 l of a 5% guaifenesin solution. Variations of the concentration of each drug are reportedly used in practice. The infusion is administered either at a rate of 1–2 ml/kg/h or, more frequently, "to effect," in order to achieve a sufficient plane of anesthesia and muscle relaxation. Despite an appropriate anesthetic plane, palpebral reflexes often remain intact.

Triple drip has been evaluated in a number of studies with varying induction protocols. One study used the triple-drip combination described previously for both induction and maintenance [91]. With this approach, minimal cardiopulmonary changes were observed, with

the most significant changes reported to occur during administration of the initial induction bolus. In another investigation, all three drugs were doubled in concentration in the final formulation and administered at a rate of 1 ml/kg/h [114]. Minimal change in cardiopulmonary performance was observed, and the mean time to standing time was 38 min following discontinuation of the infusion.

Guaifenesin/ketamine/detomidine

Taylor *et al.* described the use of an infusion of ketamine and guaifenesin combined with detomidine, rather than xylazine, for castration of colts [93]. The formulation was achieved by adding 4 g of ketamine and 40 mg of detomidine to 1 l of 10% guaifenesin. This solution was administered to effect at an initial rate of 0.6–0.8 ml/kg/h. The cardiorespiratory parameters were reported to be more stable using this protocol compared to horses maintained on the inhalant anesthetic agent halothane. The reported time to recovery was approximately 45 min following discontinuation of the infusion.

Guaifenesin/ketamine/romifidine

McMurphy *et al.* investigated the use of an infusion of ketamine and guaifenesin combined with romifidine, rather than xylazine [115]. Rather than administering the infusion to effect, this study used a specific dosing regimen. Ketamine and romifidine were administered at rates of 6.6 mg/kg/h and 82.5 µg/kg/h, respectively, and guaifenesin was administered initially at a rate of 100 mg/kg/h, followed by a reduction in the rate to 50 mg/kg/h after 30 min of infusion. In comparison to horses maintained on halothane, the guaifenesin/ketamine/romifidine (GKR) combination resulted in superior cardiopulmonary stability over the course of 75 min of anesthesia.

Inhalant anesthetics

Inhalant anesthetics are at the center of many equine hospital general anesthesia protocols. They are unique in that, despite long and widespread use in both human and veterinary medicine, their exact mechanism of action remains unknown. We do know that they work at the level of the CNS to produce general anesthesia and that they also have peripheral effects that contribute to both wanted and unwanted effects.

Inhalant anesthetics require specialized equipment, including vaporizers and anesthetic machines, for their delivery, which makes them impractical for use outside of the operating theater. They are delivered to the patient in a vaporized state within a carrier gas, usually oxygen and occasionally other gases. Inhalants diffuse from the lungs into the bloodstream where they are carried to the CNS and throughout the body. The uptake and the related speed of induction of the inhalant from the alveoli to the blood are dependent on its solubility, the horse's cardiac output, and the alveolar to venous partial pressure gradient of the inhalant. The gradient between the partial pressure of the inhalant in the alveoli and in the blood will determine uptake, with larger gradients favoring more uptake of inhalant by the blood. Although it seems counterintuitive, inhalant anesthetics that are less soluble, such as sevoflurane and desflurane, will be taken up faster than those that are more soluble, such as isoflurane and halothane. This is because the concentration of less soluble anesthetics will actually increase in the alveoli causing a larger partial pressure gradient and favoring diffusion between the alveoli and the blood. Finally, a horse with a poor cardiac output will have a faster anesthetic uptake than a horse with an elevated cardiac output because the blood will spend more time in contact with the alveoli in the horse with poor cardiac output, so the inhalant anesthetic will have more time to equilibrate between the alveoli and the blood. The inhalant anesthetics in use currently have very similar solubilities between the blood and the brain, and as a result, the uptake at the level of the lungs is the primary determinant of how quickly an anesthetic will work.

Although all inhalants are administered to effect, there are some guidelines and rationales to dictate dosing. The minimum alveolar concentration (MAC) of an inhaled anesthetic is essentially an inverse measure of its potency; the higher the MAC value, the larger the amount of anesthetic that must be delivered to the horse to achieve anesthesia. The MAC is defined as the minimum alveolar concentration of an inhaled anesthetic necessary to prevent 50% of animals from responding to a supramaximal noxious stimulus. This value is determined experimentally and the values of common inhalant anesthetics used in the horses are listed in Table 3.6. It is important for the practitioner to realize, however, that MAC values are determined in horses that have received no other medications, which differs significantly from most clinical scenarios. Despite this limitation, a delivered concentration of inhalant anesthetic 1.5 times the MAC is usually

Table 3.6 MAC values of inhalant anesthetics in the horse.

Inhalant anesthetic	MAC (%)	References
Halothane	0.88	[116]
	0.95	[117]
	1.02	[118]
	1.05	[119]
Isoflurane	1.31	[116]
	1.43	[120]
	1.44	[121]
	1.64	[122]
Sevoflurane	2.31	[123]
	2.84	[124]
Desflurane	7.02	[125]
	8.06	[126]

sufficient to provide surgical anesthesia without other medication. In practice, MAC values are usually used to guide the practitioner to vaporizer settings. Initial vaporizer settings at the MAC of the inhalant, instead of 1.5 × MAC, usually provide adequate surgical anesthesia in the clinical setting due to the additive effects provided by premedication and induction agents. Other physiologic effects of anesthesia, such as CNS depression, hypotension, hypoxemia, hypercapnia, and hypothermia, may also potentiate the development of a surgical plane of anesthesia at inhaled concentrations at or below MAC.

The effects of the inhalant anesthetics are not limited to the CNS. For example, all of the inhalant anesthetics are negative inotropes, and therefore, they cause dose-dependent reductions in cardiac output [127–132]. This reduction in cardiac output may also cause a decrease in arterial blood pressure in horses receiving inhaled anesthetics. Inhalants also decrease both the depth and frequency of respiration, which may cause hypoventilation [133, 116, 134, 135]. As CNS depressants, inhaled anesthetics also depress the medullary respiratory centers, reducing the horse's reflexive response to increased blood carbon dioxide tensions. Depression of the respiratory center compounds the direct respiratory depression caused by inhalants, further potentiating hypercapnia. All of the modern inhalants also have the potential to cause malignant hyperthermia in horses [136–138]. Lastly, while the majority of any inhaled anesthetic is exhaled unchanged, all modern inhalants also undergo some degree of metabolism. While the specifics of the rates of metabolism of inhaled anesthetics are unknown in horses, in human patients, about 0.2% of isoflurane, 2–5% of sevoflurane, and 20–46% of halothane undergo biotransformation in the liver [139–144].

Sevoflurane and isoflurane are currently the most commonly used inhalant anesthetics in equine practice. While sevoflurane is considerably more expensive than isoflurane, it is less soluble, which offers the theoretical advantages of more rapid induction and recovery. Despite these theoretical advantages, one study evaluating horses anesthetized for magnetic resonance imaging concluded that there was no significant difference in recovery time between the two gases [145].

Perioperative infusions

Perioperative infusions are used in conjunction with inhalant anesthesia to provide analgesia and to reduce the dose of inhalants necessary to maintain a surgical plane of anesthesia. These ancillary medications often prove to be very useful in the face of the cardiorespiratory suppression caused by inhalant anesthetics. Several drugs or drug combinations have been studied in the horse.

Dexmedetomidine

Infusions of dexmedetomidine have been evaluated for use in horses receiving inhalant anesthesia. An infusion rate of 1.75 µg/kg/h reduced the MAC of sevoflurane in ponies by approximately 53% [146]. In horses anesthetized with isoflurane, this infusion rate improved the quality of recovery as compared to horses that received a saline infusion [147].

Lidocaine

Infusions of lidocaine have been studied in the horse for MAC reduction, analgesia, and their effects on intestinal motility. Infusions of lidocaine reduced the MAC of halothane in horses in a dose-dependent fashion [148]. An infusion of 50 µg/kg/min reduced the MAC of sevoflurane by approximately 26.7%. This infusion rate, however, was also reported to increase ataxia during recovery from both sevoflurane and isoflurane anesthesia [149, 150].

Opioids

Although no study has evaluated the effect of morphine infusions on the MAC of any inhalant anesthetics in the horse, a study evaluating two different bolus doses of morphine failed to find any significant reduction in

the MAC of isoflurane [120]. Another study evaluated three different infusion rates of fentanyl in isoflurane-anesthetized horses and found only an 18% reduction in MAC at the highest infusion rate evaluated, which produced a mean plasma concentration of 16 ng/ml. No significant reduction in MAC was observed at lower infusion rates [151]. Another study that evaluated the effect of even higher plasma fentanyl concentrations failed to show any reduction in the MAC of isoflurane [152]. A more recent study evaluated the effect of fentanyl administered at a loading dose of 5 µg/kg followed by a continuous infusion at a rate of 0.1 µg/kg/min in sevoflurane-anesthetized horses and found that the concentration of the inhalant necessary to maintain surgical anesthesia decreased by 13% compared to horses that did not receive fentanyl [153]. In addition, Clark *et al.* showed that in halothane-anesthetized horses, morphine administered as a perioperative infusion at a rate of 0.1 mg/kg/h was associated with a significantly faster recovery to standing times compared to horses that did not receive the morphine infusion [154].

Ketamine

While ketamine is used frequently as an adjunct to equine inhalant anesthesia, there is only one experimental study in which its use was evaluated for MAC reduction as a supplement to an inhalant anesthetic [155]. Although the authors did not publish the doses that they administered, they did report that plasma concentrations of ketamine greater than 1 ng/ml resulted in a mean reduction in the MAC of halothane of 37%. Infusion rates of 1–3.6 mg/kg/h have been reported in studies where ketamine infusions are used in addition to other drugs [156–159].

Combinations

A multitude of drug combinations have been used to provide partial IV anesthesia supplementation to inhalant anesthetics in the horse. In one study, an infusion of ketamine administered initially at a rate of 60 µg/kg/min and then reduced to 39 µg/kg/min, combined with an infusion of lidocaine, administered initially at a rate of 40 µg/kg/min and then reduced to 26 µg/kg/min evaluated in isoflurane-anesthetized horses. This protocol reduced the mean concentration of isoflurane required to maintain a surgical plane of anesthesia from 1.57 to 0.97%, and it decreased the mean dose of dobutamine required for cardiovascular support [158]. Valverde *et al.* reported that the addition of a medetomidine infusion at a rate of

5 µg/kg/h to isoflurane- and lidocaine-induced anesthesia improved recovery quality when compared to recoveries following a combination of isoflurane and lidocaine alone [160]. In another study, the MAC of isoflurane was reduced by 49% by adding an infusion of lidocaine, administered at a rate of 3 mg/kg/h, and ketamine, administered at a rate of 3 mg/kg/h [157]. When an infusion of morphine, administered at a rate of 0.1 mg/kg/h, was added to the lidocaine and ketamine infusions, the isoflurane MAC decreased by 53%. A recent study has also reported that infusions of combinations of guaifenesin and ketamine or romifidine and ketamine produced stable anesthetic events, smooth recoveries, and reductions in isoflurane requirements [161].

Foal anesthesia

Foals differ from adult horses not only in size but physiologically as well, and therefore, their anesthetic needs are more complicated than simple dose reductions. The following sections offer several accepted anesthetic protocols for foals.

Premedications and sedatives

Unlike in the adult horse, benzodiazepine drugs are CNS depressants and provide sedation in foals less than 2 months of age [162, 163]. After about 2 months of age, however, foals will likely experience CNS excitement with the administration of a benzodiazepine, and therefore, the A-2 agonists are the preferred sedatives in this age group [55, 162–165]. Xylazine administration has been linked to hypothermia in the foal, and steps should be taken to monitor and provide temperature support if necessary [166]. If pain is expected, the sedation can be supplemented with an opioid that may also potentiate sedation [165]. Acepromazine can be used to provide mild sedation in foals; however, it should be used with caution in this age group because it can produce prolonged sedation and is not reversible. It may not be appropriate at any dose in neonatal foals because of their immature hepatic metabolism [162].

Induction and maintenance of anesthesia in foals

The ideal induction protocol for neonatal foals has not been determined. It has been suggested that inhalant anesthetics delivered in oxygen via either a facemask or a nasotracheal tube are the most appropriate induction agents in neonatal foals that have immature liver function. Inhalants are only minimally metabolized and they allow

for rapid changes in the depth of anesthesia. However, evaluations of the safety of inhalant inductions in foals have produced conflicting results. In the first CEPEF study, the authors noted that in neonatal foals, induction of anesthesia with halothane carried a 4.5 times greater risk of perianesthetic mortality than induction with ketamine [39]. In contrast, another clinical study evaluating both halothane and isoflurane inductions concluded that both agents could be used safely for induction and maintenance in the foal [167].

As in adult horses, ketamine can be used to induce general anesthesia in foals [162, 165]. The distribution and elimination of ketamine in foals have not been studied, but in the adult horse, ketamine is rapidly redistributed and largely metabolized by the liver [155, 168, 169]. Therefore, it is possible that ketamine metabolism might be prolonged in neonatal foals with immature liver function. Propofol has gained popularity as an injectable induction agent in foals, but respiratory depression has been reported to occur with its use [162, 165, 170, 171]. Although not studied extensively in horses, one potential benefit to the use of propofol in foals is that, in other species, it appears to be metabolized by an extrahepatic pathway.

Maintenance of general anesthesia in the foal for procedures lasting longer than about 15–20 min is usually best accomplished using an inhalant anesthetic. There are no known differences in the MAC values between adult horses and foals. Practitioners need to be aware that administration of an inhalant anesthetic to a foal less than 150 kg requires the use of a small animal anesthesia machine, while larger foals can be safely anesthetized on a large animal anesthesia machine.

References

1 Johnston, G.M., Eastment, J.K., Wood, J.L.N. & Taylor, P.M. (2002) The confidential enquiry into perioperative equine fatalities (CEPEF): Mortality results of Phases 1 and 2. *Veterinary Anaesthesia and Analgesia*, **29**, 159–170.

2 Virtanen, R., Ruskoaho, H. & Nyman, L. (1985) Pharmacological evidence for the involvement of alpha-2 adrenoceptors in the sedative effect of detomidine, a novel sedative-analgesic. *Journal of Veterinary Pharmacology and Therapeutics*, **8**, 30–37.

3 Doze, V.A., Chen, B.X. & Maze, M. (1989) Dexmedetomidine produces a hypnotic-anesthetic action in rats via activation of central alpha-2 adrenoceptors. *Anesthesiology*, **71**, 75–79.

4 Moens, Y., Lanz, F., Doherr, M.G. & Schatzmann, U. (2003) A comparison of the antinociceptive effects of xylazine,

detomidine and romifidine on experimental pain in horses. *Veterinary Anaesthesia and Analgesia*, **30**, 183–190.

5 Virtanen, R. (1989) Pharmacological profiles of medetomidine and its antagonist, atipamezole. *Acta Veterinaria Scandinavica Supplementum*, **85**, 29–37.

6 Taylor, P., Coumbe, K., Henson, F., Scott, D. & Taylor, A. (2013) Evaluation of sedation for standing clinical procedures in horses using detomidine combined with buprenorphine. *Veterinary Anaesthesia and Analgesia*, **41** (1), 14–24.

7 Scicluna C. (1999) Clinical evaluation of detomidine infusion for laparoscopy in standing horses. Proceedings of the Association of Veterinary Anaesthetists, Newcastle, March 29.

8 Ringer, S.K., Portier, K.G., Fourel, I. & Bettschart-Wolfensberger, R. (2012) Development of a romifidine constant rate infusion with or without butorphanol for standing sedation of horses. *Veterinary Anaesthesia and Analgesia*, **39**, 12–20.

9 Ringer, S.K., Portier, K.G., Fourel, I. & Bettschart-Wolfensberger, R. (2012) Development of a xylazine constant rate infusion with or without butorphanol for standing sedation of horses. *Veterinary Anaesthesia and Analgesia*, **39**, 1–11.

10 Solano, A.M., Valverde, A., Desrochers, A., Nykamp, S. & Boure, L.P. (2009) Behavioural and cardiorespiratory effects of a constant rate infusion of medetomidine and morphine for sedation during standing laparoscopy in horses. *Equine Veterinary Journal*, **41**, 153–159.

11 Wagner, A.E., Muir, W.W. & Hinchcliff, K.W. (1991) Cardiovascular effects of xylazine and detomidine in horses. *American Journal of Veterinary Research*, **52**, 651–657.

12 Bueno, A.C., Cornick-Seahorn, J., Seahorn, T.L., Hosgood, G. & Moore, R.M. (1999) Cardiopulmonary and sedative effects of intravenous administration of low doses of medetomidine and xylazine to adult horses. *American Journal of Veterinary Research*, **60**, 1371–1376.

13 Sarazan, R.D., Starke, W.A., Krause, G.F. & Garner, H.E. (1989) Cardiovascular effects of detomidine, a new alpha 2-adrenoceptor agonist, in the conscious pony. *Journal of Veterinary Pharmacology and Therapeutics*, **12**, 378–388.

14 Clarke, K.W., England, G.C. & Goossens, L. (1991) Sedative and cardiovascular effects of romifidine, alone and in combination with butorphanol, in the horse. *Journal of Veterinary Anaesthesia*, **18**, 25–29.

15 Freeman, S.L., Bowen, I.M., Bettschart-Wolfensberger, R., Alibhai, H.I.K. & England, C.G.W. (2002) Cardiovascular effects of romifidine in the standing horse. *Research in Veterinary Science*, **72**, 123–129.

16 Muir, W.W., Skarda, R.T. & Sheehan, W. (1979) Hemodynamic and respiratory effects of a xylazine-acetylpromazine drug combination in horses. *American Journal of Veterinary Research*, **40**, 1518–1522.

17 Yamashita, K., Tsubakishita, S., Futaok, S. *et al.* (2000) Cardiovascular effects of medetomidine, detomidine and xylazine in horses. *Journal of Veterinary Medical Science*, **62**, 1025–1032.

18 Figueiredo, J.P., Muir, W.W., Smith, J. & Wolfrom, G.W. (2005) Sedative and analgesic effects of romifidine in horses. *International Journal of Applied Research in Veterinary Medicine*, **3**, 249–258.

19 England, G.C., Clarke, K.W. & Goossens, L. (1992) A comparison of the sedative effects of three alpha 2-adrenoceptor agonists (romifidine, detomidine and xylazine) in the horse. *Journal of Veterinary Pharmacology and Therapeutics*, **15**, 194–201.

20 Gasthuys, F., Parmentier, D., Goossens, L. & Demoor, A. (1990) A preliminary study on the effects of atropine sulphate on bradycardia and heart blocks during romifidine sedation in the horse. *Veterinary Research Communications*, **14**, 489–502.

21 Kerr, D.D., Jones, E.W., Holbert, D. & Huggins, K. (1972) Comparison of the effects of xylazine and acetylpromazine maleate in the horse. *American Journal of Veterinary Research*, **33**, 777–784.

22 Reitemeyer, H., Klein, H.J. & Deegen, E. (1986) The effect of sedatives on lung function in horses. *Acta Veterinaria Scandinavica Supplementum*, **82**, 111–120.

23 Broadstone, R.V., Gray, P.R., Robinson, N.E. & Derksen, F.J. (1992) Effects of xylazine on airway function in ponies with recurrent airway obstruction. *American Journal of Veterinary Research*, **53**, 1813–1817.

24 Roger, T. & Ruckebusch, Y. (1987) Colonic alpha 2-adrenoceptor-mediated responses in the pony. *Journal of Veterinary Pharmacology and Therapeutics*, **10**, 310–318.

25 Stick, J.A., Chou, C.C., Derksen, F.J. & Arden, W.A. (1987) Effects of xylazine on equine intestinal vascular resistance, motility, compliance, and oxygen consumption. *American Journal of Veterinary Research*, **48**, 198–203.

26 Rutkowski, J.A., Ross, M.W. & Cullen, K. (1989) Effects of xylazine and/or butorphanol or neostigmine on myoelectric activity of the cecum and right ventral colon in female ponies. *American Journal of Veterinary Research*, **50**, 1096–1101.

27 Watson, T.D. & Sullivan, M. (1991) Effects of detomidine on equine oesophageal function as studied by contrast radiography. *Veterinary Record*, **129**, 67–69.

28 Singh, S., Young, S.S., McDonell, W.N. & O'Grady, M. (1997) Modification of cardiopulmonary and intestinal motility effects of xylazine with glycopyrrolate in horses. *Canadian Journal of Veterinary Research*, **61**, 99–107.

29 Grubb, T.L., Muir, W.W., 3rd, Bertone, A.L., Beluche, L.A. & Garcia-Calderon, M. (1997) Use of yohimbine to reverse prolonged effects of xylazine hydrochloride in a horse being treated with chloramphenicol. *Journal of the American Veterinary Medical Association*, **210**, 1771–1773.

30 Lester, G.D., Merritt, A.M., Neuwirth, L. *et al.* (1998) Effect of alpha 2-adrenergic, cholinergic, and nonsteroidal anti-inflammatory drugs on myoelectric activity of ileum, cecum, and right ventral colon and on cecal emptying of radiolabeled markers in clinically normal ponies. *American Journal of Veterinary Research*, **59**, 320–327.

31 Merritt, A.M., Furrow, J.A. & Hartless, C.S. (1998) Effect of xylazine, detomidine, and a combination of xylazine and

butorphanol on equine duodenal motility. *American Journal of Veterinary Research*, **59**, 619–623.

32 Sutton, D.G., Preston, T., Christley, R.M. *et al.* (2002) The effects of xylazine, detomidine, acepromazine and butorphanol on equine solid phase gastric emptying rate. *Equine Veterinary Journal*, **34**, 486–492.

33 Zullian, C., Menozzi, A., Pozzoli, C., Poli, E. & Bertini, S. (2011) Effects of α2-adrenergic drugs on small intestinal motility in the horse: An in vitro study. *Veterinary Journal*, **187**, 342–346.

34 Muir, W.W. & Robertson, J.T. (1985) Visceral analgesia: Effects of xylazine, butorphanol, meperidine, and pentazocine in horses. *American Journal of Veterinary Research*, **46**, 2081–2084.

35 Kalpravidh, M., Lumb, W.V., Wright, M. & Heath, R.B. (1984) Effects of butorphanol, flunixin, levorphanol, morphine, and xylazine in ponies. *American Journal of Veterinary Research*, **45**, 217–223.

36 Kerr, D.D., Jones, E.W., Huggins, K. & Edwards, W.C. (1972) Sedative and other effects of xylazine given intravenously to horses. *American Journal of Veterinary Research*, **33**, 525–532.

37 Hoffman, P.E. (1974) Clinical evaluation of xylazine as a chemical restraining agent, sedative, and analgesic in horses. *Journal of the American Veterinary Medical Association*, **164**, 42–45.

38 Fuentes, V.O. (1978) Sudden death in a stallion after xylazine medication. *Veterinary Record*, **102**, 106.

39 Johnston, G.M., Taylor, P.M., Holmes, M.A. & Wood, J.L.N. (1995) Confidential enquiry of perioperative equine fatalities (CEPEF-1): Preliminary results. *Equine Veterinary Journal*, **27**, 193–200.

40 Jochle, W. & Hamm, D. (1986) Sedation and analgesia with Domosedan (detomidine hydrochloride) in horses: Dose response studies on efficacy and its duration. *Acta Veterinaria Scandinavica Supplementum*, **82**, 69–84.

41 Araujo, R.R. & Ginther, O.J. (2009) Vascular perfusion of reproductive organs in pony mares and heifers during sedation with detomidine or xylazine. *American Journal of Veterinary Research*, **70**, 141–148.

42 Dimaio Knych, H.K. & Stanley, S.D. (2011) Pharmacokinetics and pharmacodynamics of detomidine following sublingual administration to horses. *American Journal of Veterinary Research*, **72**, 1378–1385.

43 L'Ami, J.J., Vermunt, L.E., van Loon, J.P. & Sloet van Oldruitenborgh-Oosterbaan, M.M. (2012) Sublingual administration of detomidine in horses: Sedative effect, analgesia and detection time. *Veterinary Journal*, **196** (2), 253–259.

44 Browning, A.P. & Collins, J.A. (1994) Sedation of horses with romifidine and butorphanol. *Veterinary Record*, **134**, 90–91.

45 DiMaio Knych, H.K., Covarrubias, V. & Steffey, E.P. (2012) Effect of yohimbine on detomidine induced changes in behavior, cardiac and blood parameters in the horse. *Veterinary Anaesthesia and Analgesia*, **39**, 574–583.

46 Knych, H.K., Steffey, E.P. & Stanley, S.D. (2012) The effects of yohimbine on the pharmacokinetic parameters of detomidine in the horse. *Veterinary Anaesthesia and Analgesia*, **39**, 221–229.

47 Kollias-Baker, C.A., Court, M.H. & Williams, L.L. (1993) Influence of yohimbine and tolazoline on the cardiovascular, respiratory, and sedative effects of xylazine in the horse. *Journal of Veterinary Pharmacology and Therapeutics*, **16**, 350–358.

48 Luna, S.P., Beale, N.J. & Taylor, P.M. (1992) Effects of atipamezole on xylazine sedation in ponies. *Veterinary Record*, **130**, 268–271.

49 Hubbell, J.A. & Muir, W.W. (2006) Antagonism of detomidine sedation in the horse using intravenous tolazoline or atipamezole. *Equine Veterinary Journal*, **38**, 238–241.

50 Di Concetto, S., Michael Archer, R., Sigurdsson, S.F. & Clarke, K. (2007) Atipamezole in the management of detomidine overdose in a pony. *Veterinary Anaesthesia and Analgesia*, **34**, 67–69.

51 Baldessarini, R.J. & Tarazi, F.I. (2006) Pharmacology of psychosis and mania. In: L.S. Goodman & S. Gilman (eds), *The Pharmacological Basis of Therapeutics*, 11 edn, pp. 461–481. McGraw-Hill, New York.

52 Combie, J., Shults, T., Nugent, E.C., Dougherty, J. & Tobin, T. (1981) Pharmacology of narcotic analgesics in the horse: Selective blockade of narcotic-induced locomotor activity. *American Journal of Veterinary Research*, **42**, 716–721.

53 Ballard, S., Shults, T., Kownacki, A.A., Blake, J.W. & Tobin, T. (1982) The pharmacokinetics, pharmacological responses and behavioral effects of acepromazine in the horse. *Journal of Veterinary Pharmacology and Therapeutics*, **5**, 21–31.

54 Marroum, P.J., Webb, A.I., Aeschbacher, G. & Curry, S.H. (1994) Pharmacokinetics and pharmacodynamics of acepromazine in horses. *American Journal of Veterinary Research*, **55**, 1428–1433.

55 Muir, W.W. (2009) Anxiolytics, nonopioid sedative-analgesics, and opioid analgesics. In: W.W. Muir & J.A. Hubbell (eds), *Equine Anesthesia: Monitoring and Emergency Therapy*, 2 edn, pp. 185–209. Saunders Elsevier, St. Louis.

56 Parry, P.W., Anderson, G.A. & Gay, C.G. (1982) Hypotension in the horse induced by acepromazine maleate. *Australian Veterinary Journal*, **59**, 148–152.

57 Muir, W.W., Werner, L.L. & Hamlin, R.L. (1975) Effects of xylazine and acetylpromazine upon induced ventricular fibrillation in dogs anesthetized with thiamylal and halothane. *American Journal of Veterinary Research*, **36**, 1299–1303.

58 Gerring, E.L. (1981) Priapism and ACP in the horse. *Veterinary Record*, **109**, 64.

59 Nie, G.J. & Pope, K.C. (1997) Persistent penile prolapse associated with acute blood loss and acepromazine maleate administration in a horse. *Journal of the American Veterinary Medical Association*, **211**, 587–589.

60 Kieffer, B.L. (1999) Opioids: First lessons from knockout mice. *Trends in Pharmacological Sciences*, **20**, 19–26.

61 Combie, J., Dougherty, J., Nugent, E.C. & Tobin, T. (1979) The pharmacology of narcotic analgesics in the horse. IV. Dose and time response relationships for behavioral responses to morphine, meperidine, pentazocine, anileridine, methadone, and hydromorphone. *Journal of Equine Medical and Surgical*, **3**, 377–385.

62 Tobin, T. & Woods, W.E. (1979) Pharmacology review: Actions of central stimulant drugs in the horse. *Equine Veterinary Journal*, **3**, 60–66.

63 Tobin, T., Combie, J., Shults, T. & Doughtery, J. (1979) The pharmacology of narcotic analgesics in the horse. III. Characteristics of the locomotor effects of fentanyl and apomorphine. *Journal of Equine Medical and Surgery*, **3**, 284–288.

64 Kamerling, S.G., DeQuick, D.J., Weckman, T.J. & Tobin, T. (1985) Dose-related effects of fentanyl on autonomic and behavioral responses in performance horses. *General Pharmacology*, **16**, 253–258.

65 Clark, L., Clutton, R.E., Blissitt, K.J. & Chase-Topping, M.E. (2005) Effects of peri-operative morphine administration during halothane anaesthesia in horses. *Veterinary Anaesthesia and Analgesia*, **32**, 10–15.

66 Nolan, A.M., Chanbers, J.P. & Hale, G.J. (1991) The cardiorespiratory effects of morphine and butorphanol in horses anaesthetized under clinical conditions. *Journal of Veterinary Anaesthesia*, **18**, 19–24.

67 Figueiredo, J.P., Muir, W.W. & Sams, R. (2012) Cardiorespiratory, gastrointestinal, and analgesic effects of morphine sulfate in conscious healthy horses. *American Journal of Veterinary Research*, **73**, 799–808.

68 Muir, W.W., Skarda, R.T. & Sheehan, W.C. (1978) Cardiopulmonary effects of narcotic agonists and a partial agonist in horses. *American Journal of Veterinary Research*, **39**, 1632–1635.

69 Robertson, J.T., Muir, W.W. & Sams, R. (1981) Cardiopulmonary effects of butorphanol tartrate in horses. *American Journal of Veterinary Research*, **42**, 41–44.

70 Boscan, P., Van Hoogmoed, L.M., Farver, T.B. & Snyder, J.R. (2006) Evaluation of the effects of the opioid agonist morphine on gastrointestinal tract function in horses. *American Journal of Veterinary Research*, **67**, 992–997.

71 Adams, S.B., Lamar, C.H. & Masty, J. (1984) Motility of the distal portion of the jejunum and pelvic flexure in ponies: Effects of six drugs. *American Journal of Veterinary Research*, **45**, 795–799.

72 Kohn, C.W. & Muir, W.W., 3rd. (1988) Selected aspects of the clinical pharmacology of visceral analgesics and gut motility modifying drugs in the horse. *Journal of Veterinary Internal Medicine*, **2**, 85–91.

73 Menozzi, A., Pozzoli, C., Zullian, C., Poli, E., Serventi, P. & Bertini, S. (2012) Inhibition of motility in isolated horse small intestine is mediated by kappa but not mu opioid receptors. *Equine Veterinary Journal*, **44**, 368–370.

74 Sellon, D.C., Monroe, V.L., Roberts, M.C. & Papich, M.G. (2001) Pharmacokinetics and adverse effects of butorphanol administered by single intravenous injection or continuous intravenous infusion in horses. *American Journal of Veterinary Research*, **62**, 183–189.

75 Taguchi, A., Sharma, N., Saleem, R.M. *et al.* (2001) Selective postoperative inhibition of gastrointestinal opioid receptors. *New England Journal of Medicine*, **345**, 935–940.

76 Kalpravidh, M., Lumb, W.V., Wright, M. & Heath, R.B. (1984) Analgesic effects of butorphanol in horses: Dose-response studies. *American Journal of Veterinary Research*, **45**, 211–216.

77 Sellon, D.C., Roberts, M.C., Blikslager, A.T., Ulibarri, C. & Papich, M.G. (2004) Effects of continuous rate intravenous infusion of butorphanol on physiologic and outcome variables in horses after celiotomy. *Journal of Veterinary Internal Medicine*, **18**, 555–563.

78 Sojka, J.E., Adams, S.B., Lamar, C.H. & Eller, L.L. (1988) Effect of butorphanol, pentazocine, meperidine, or metoclopramide on intestinal motility in female ponies. *American Journal of Veterinary Research*, **49**, 527–529.

79 Carregaro, A.B., Luna, S.P., Mataqueiro, M.I. & de Queiroz-Neto, A. (2007) Effects of buprenorphine on nociception and spontaneous locomotor activity in horses. *American Journal of Veterinary Research*, **68**, 246–250.

80 Love, E.J., Taylor, P.M., Murrell, J. & Whay, H.R. (2012) Effects of acepromazine, butorphanol and buprenorphine on thermal and mechanical nociceptive thresholds in horses. *Equine Veterinary Journal*, **44**, 221–225.

81 Davis, J.L., Messenger, K.M., LaFevers, D.H., Barlow, B.M. & Posner, L.P. (2012) Pharmacokinetics of intravenous and intramuscular buprenorphine in the horse. *Journal of Veterinary Pharmacology and Therapeutics*, **35**, 52–58.

82 Messenger, K.M., Davis, J.L., LaFevers, D.H., Barlow, B.M. & Posner, L.P. (2011) Intravenous and sublingual buprenorphine in horses: Pharmacokinetics and influence of sampling site. *Veterinary Anaesthesia and Analgesia*, **38**, 374–384.

83 Kamerline, S.B., Harma, J.G. & Bagwell, C.A. (1990) Naloxone-induced abdominal distress in the horse. *Equine Veterinary Journal*, **22**, 241–243.

84 Boscan, P., Van Hoogmoed, L.M., Pypendop, B.H., Farver, T.B. & Snyder, J.R. (2006) Pharmacokinetics of the opioid antagonist N-methylnaltrexone and evaluation of its effects on gastrointestinal tract function in horses treated or not treated with morphine. *American Journal of Veterinary Research*, **67**, 998–1004.

85 Muir, W.W., 3rd & Mason, D.E. (1993) Effects of diazepam, acepromazine, detomidine, and xylazine on thiamylal anesthesia in horses. *Journal of the American Veterinary Medical Association*, **203**, 1031–1038.

86 Muir, W.W., Sams, R.A., Huffman, R.H. & Noonan, J.S. (1982) Pharmacodynamic and pharmacokinetic properties of diazepam in horses. *American Journal of Veterinary Research*, **43**, 1756–1762.

87 Hubbell, J.A., Kelly, E.M., Aarnes, T.K. *et al.* (2013) Pharmacokinetics of midazolam after intravenous administration to horses. *Equine Veterinary Journal*, **45** (6), 721–5.

88 Tavernor, W.D. (1970) The influence of guaiacol glycerol ether on cardiovascular and respiratory function in the horse. *Research in Veterinary Science*, **11**, 91–93.

89 Hubbell, J.A., Muir, W.W. & Sams, R.A. (1980) Guaifenesin: Cardiopulmonary effects and plasma concentrations in horses. *American Journal of Veterinary Research*, **41**, 1751–1755.

90 Muir, W.W., Skarda, R.T. & Sheehan, W. (1978) Evaluation of xylazine, guaifenesin, and ketamine hydrochloride for restraint in horses. *American Journal of Veterinary Research*, **39**, 1274–1278.

91 Greene, S.A., Thurmon, J.C., Tranquilli, W.J. & Benson, G.J. (1986) Cardiopulmonary effects of continuous intravenous

infusion of guaifenesin, ketamine, and xylazine in ponies. *American Journal of Veterinary Research*, **47**, 2364–2367.

92 Muir, W.W., Skarda, R.T., Sheehan, W. & Gates, B.R. (1979) Evaluation of thiamylal, guaifenesin, and ketamine hydrochloride combinations administered prior to halothane anesthesia in horses. *Journal of Equine Medical and Surgery*, **3**, 178–184.

93 Taylor, P.M., Kirby, J.J., Shrimpton, D.J. & Johnson, C.B. (1998) Cardiovascular effects of surgical castration during anaesthesia maintained with halothane or infusion of detomidine, ketamine and guaifenesin in ponies. *Equine Veterinary Journal*, **30**, 304–309.

94 Bennett, R.C., Taylor, P.M., Brearley, J.C., Johnson, C.B. & Luna, S.P. (1998) Comparison of detomidine/ketamine and guaiphenesin/thiopentone for induction of anaesthesia in horses maintained with halothane. *Veterinary Record*, **142**, 541–545.

95 Gangl, M., Grulke, S., Detilleux, J., Caudron, I. & Serteyn, D. (2001) Comparison of thiopentone/guaifenesin, ketamine/guaifenesin and ketamine/midazolam for the induction of horses to be anaesthetised with isoflurane. *Veterinary Record*, **149**, 147–151.

96 Oku, K., Kakizaki, M., Ono, K. & Ohta, M. (2011) Clinical evaluation of total intravenous anesthesia using a combination of propofol and medetomidine following anesthesia induction with medetomidine, guaifenesin and propofol for castration in Thoroughbred horses. *Journal of Veterinary Medical Science*, **73**, 1639–1643.

97 Brosnan, R.J., Steffey, E.P., Escobar, A., Palazoglu, M. & Fiehn, O. (2011) Anesthetic induction with guaifenesin and propofol in adult horses. *American Journal of Veterinary Research*, **72**, 1569–1575.

98 Keates, H.L., van Eps, A.W. & Pearson, M.R. (2012) Alfaxalone compared with ketamine for induction of anaesthesia in horses following xylazine and guaifenesin. *Veterinary Anaesthesia and Analgesia*, **39**, 591–598.

99 Muir, W.W., 3rd, Gadawski, J.E. & Grosenbaugh, D.A. (1999) Cardiorespiratory effects of a tiletamine/zolazepam-ketamine-detomidine combination in horses. *American Journal of Veterinary Research*, **60**, 770–774.

100 Muir, W.W., Skarda, R.T. & Milne, D.W. (1977) Evaluation of xylazine and ketamine hydrochloride for anesthesia in horses. *American Journal of Veterinary Research*, **38**, 195–201.

101 Trim, C.M., Adams, J.G. & Hovda, L.R. (1987) Failure of ketamine to induce anesthesia in two horses. *Journal of the American Veterinary Medical Association*, **190**, 201–202.

102 Hubbell, J.A., Bednarski, R.M. & Muir, W.W. (1989) Xylazine and tiletamine-zolazepam anesthesia in horses. *American Journal of Veterinary Research*, **50**, 737–742.

103 Cuvelliez, S., Rosseel, G., Blais, D., Salmon, Y., Troncy, E. & Larivière, N. (1995) Intravenous anesthesia in the horse: Comparison of xylazine-ketamine and xylazine-tiletamine-zolazepam combinations. *Canadian Veterinary Journal*, **36**, 613–618.

104 Butera, S.T., Garner, H.E., Moore, J.N. & Amend, J.F. (1980) Xylazine/sodium thiopental combination for short-term anesthesia in the horse. *Veterinary Medicine, Small Animal Clinician*, **75**, 765–770.

105 Tyagi, R.P., Arnold, J.P., Usenik, E.A. & Fletchers, T.F. (1964) Effects of thiopental sodium (pentothal sodium) anesthesia on the horse. *Cornell Veterinarian*, **54**, 584–602.

106 Jones, E.W., Johnson, L. & Heinze, C.D. (1960) Thiopental sodium anesthesia in the horse: A rapid induction technique. *Journal of the American Veterinary Medical Association*, **137**, 119–122.

107 Hubbell, J.A., Hinchcliff, K.W., Schmall, L.M., Muir, W.W., Robertson, J.T. & Sams, R.A. (2000) Anesthetic, cardiorespiratory, and metabolic effects of four intravenous anesthetic regimens induced in horses immediately after maximal exercise. *American Journal of Veterinary Research*, **61**, 1545–1552.

108 Mama, K.R., Steffey, E.P. & Pascoe, P.J. (1995) Evaluation of propofol as a general anesthetic for horses. *Veterinary Surgery*, **24**, 188–194.

109 Mama, K.R., Steffey, E.P. & Pascoe, P.J. (1996) Evaluation of propofol for general anesthesia in premedicated horses. *American Journal of Veterinary Research*, **57**, 512–516.

110 Frias, A.F., Marsico, F., Gomez de Segura, I.A. *et al* (2003) Evaluation of different doses of propofol in xylazine pre-medicated horses. *Veterinary Anaesthesia and Analgesia*, **30**, 193–201.

111 Kloppel, H. & Leece, E.A. (2011) Comparison of ketamine and alfaxalone for induction and maintenance of anaesthesia in ponies undergoing castration. *Veterinary Anaesthesia and Analgesia*, **38**, 37–43.

112 Muir, W.W., 3rd, Lerche, P., Robertson, J.T. *et al.* (2000) Comparison of four drug combinations for total intravenous anesthesia of horses undergoing surgical removal of an abdominal testis. *Journal of the American Veterinary Medical Association*, **217**, 869–873.

113 Mama, K.R., Wagner, A.E., Steffey, E.P. *et al.* (2005) Evaluation of xylazine and ketamine for total intravenous anesthesia in horses. *American Journal of Veterinary Research*, **66**, 1002–1007.

114 Young, L.E., Bartram, D.H., Diamond, M.J., Gregg, A.S. & Jones, R.S. (1993) Clinical evaluation of an infusion of xylazine, guaifenesin and ketamine for maintenance of anaesthesia in horses. *Equine Veterinary Journal*, **25**, 115–119.

115 McMurphy, R.M., Young, L.E., Marlin, D.J. & Walsh, K. (2002) Comparison of the cardiopulmonary effects of anesthesia maintained by continuous infusion of romifidine, guaifenesin, and ketamine with anesthesia maintained by inhalation of halothane in horses. *American Journal of Veterinary Research*, **63**, 1655–1661.

116 Steffey, E.P., Howland, D., Jr, Giri, S. & Eger, E.I., 2nd (1977) Enflurane, halothane, and isoflurane potency in horses. *American Journal of Veterinary Research*, **38**, 1037–1039.

117 Steffey, E.P., Willits, N. & Woliner, M. (1992) Hemodynamic and respiratory responses to variable arterial partial pressure

of oxygen in halothane-anesthetized horses during spontaneous and controlled ventilation. *American Journal of Veterinary Research*, **53**, 1850–1858.

118 Pascoe, P.J., Steffey, E.P., Black, W.D., Claxton, J.M., Jacobs, J.R. & Woliner, M.J. (1993) Evaluation of the effect of alfentanil on the minimum alveolar concentration of halothane in horses. *American Journal of Veterinary Research*, **54**, 1327–1332.

119 Bennett, R.C., Steffey, E.P., Kollias-Baker, C. & Sams, R. (2004) Influence of morphine sulfate on the halothane sparing effect of xylazine hydrochloride in horses. *American Journal of Veterinary Research*, **65**, 519–526.

120 Steffey, E.P., Eisele, J.H. & Baggot, J.D. (2003) Interactions of morphine and isoflurane in horses. *American Journal of Veterinary Research*, **64**, 166–175.

121 Steffey, E.P. & Pascoe, J.R. (2002) Detomidine reduces isoflurane anesthetic requirement (MAC) in horses. *Veterinary Anaesthesia and Analgesia*, **29**, 223–227.

122 Steffey, E.P., Pascoe, P.J., Woliner, M.J. & Berryman, E.R. (2000) Effects of xylazine hydrochloride during isoflurane-induced anesthesia in horses. *American Journal of Veterinary Research*, **61**, 1225–1231.

123 Aida, H., Mizuno, Y., Hobo, S., Yoshida, K. & Fujinaga, T. (1994) Determination of the minimum alveolar concentration (MAC) and physical response to sevoflurane inhalation in horses. *Journal of Veterinary Medical Science*, **56**, 1161–1165.

124 Steffey, E.P., Mama, K.R., Galey, F.D. *et al.* (2005) Effects of sevoflurane dose and mode of ventilation on cardiopulmonary function and blood biochemical variables in horses. *American Journal of Veterinary Research*, **66**, 606–614.

125 Tendillo, F.J., Mascias, A., Santos, M. *et al.* (1997) Anesthetic potency of desflurane in the horse: Determination of the minimum alveolar concentration. *Veterinary Surgery*, **26**, 354–357.

126 Steffey, E.P., Woliner, M.J., Puschner, B. & Galey, F.D. (2005) Effects of desflurane and mode of ventilation on cardiovascular and respiratory functions and clinicopathologic variables in horses. *American Journal of Veterinary Research*, **66**, 669–677.

127 Eger, E.I., 2nd (1985) *Isoflurane (Forane): A compendium and reference*. Madison, WI, Anaquest.

128 Eger, E.I., 2nd (1993) *Desflurane (Suprane): A Compendium and Reference*. Healthpress, Rutherford.

129 Warltier, D.C. & Pagel, P.S. (1992) Cardiovascular and respiratory actions of desflurane: Is desflurane different from isoflurane? *Anesthesia & Analgesia*, **75**, S17–S29 discussion S29-31.

130 Pagel, P.S., Kampine, J.P., Schmeling, W.T. & Warltier, D.C. (1993) Evaluation of myocardial contractility in the chronically instrumented dog with intact autonomic nervous system function: Effects of desflurane and isoflurane. *Acta Anaesthesiologica Scandinavica*, **37**, 203–210.

131 Pagel, P.S., Kampine, J.P., Schmeling, W.T. & Warltier, D.C. (1991) Influence of volatile anesthetics on myocardial contractility in vivo: Desflurane versus isoflurane. *Anesthesiology*, **74**, 900–907.

132 Boban, M., Stowe, D.F., Buljubasic, N., Kampine, J.P. & Bosnjak, Z.J. (1992) Direct comparative effects of isoflurane and desflurane in isolated guinea pig hearts. *Anesthesiology*, **76**, 775–780.

133 Steffey, E.P. & Howland, D., Jr (1980) Comparison of circulatory and respiratory effects of isoflurane and halothane anesthesia in horses. *American Journal of Veterinary Research*, **41**, 821–825.

134 Steffey, E.P., Kelly, A.B. & Woliner, M.J. (1987) Time-related responses of spontaneously breathing, laterally recumbent horses to prolonged anesthesia with halothane. *American Journal of Veterinary Research*, **48**, 952–957.

135 Steffey, E.P., Hodgson, D.S., Dunlop, C.I. *et al.* (1987) Cardiopulmonary function during 5 hours of constant-dose isoflurane in laterally recumbent, spontaneously breathing horses. *Journal of Veterinary Pharmacology and Therapeutics*, **10**, 290–297.

136 Aleman, M., Brosnan, R.J., Williams, D.C. *et al.* (2005) Malignant hyperthermia in a horse anesthetized with halothane. *Journal of Veterinary Internal Medicine*, **19**, 363–366.

137 Aleman, M., Riehl, J., Aldridge, B.M., Lecouteur, R.A., Stott, J.L. & Pessah, I.N. (2004) Association of a mutation in the ryanodine receptor 1 gene with equine malignant hyperthermia. *Muscle & Nerve*, **30**, 356–365.

138 Hildebrand, S.V. & Howitt, G.A. (1983) Succinylcholine infusion associated with hyperthermia in ponies anesthetized with halothane. *American Journal of Veterinary Research*, **44**, 2280–2284.

139 Holaday, D.A., Fiserova-Bergerova, V., Latto, I.P. & Zumbiel, M.A. (1975) Resistance of isoflurane to biotransformation in man. *Anesthesiology*, **43**, 325–332.

140 Holaday, D.A. & Smith, F.R. (1981) Clinical characteristics and biotransformation of sevoflurane in healthy human volunteers. *Anesthesiology*, **54**, 100–106.

141 Shiraishi, Y. & Ikeda, K. (1990) Uptake and biotransformation of sevoflurane in humans: A comparative study of sevoflurane with halothane, enflurane, and isoflurane. *Journal of Clinical Anesthesia*, **2**, 381–386.

142 Carpenter, R.L., Eger, E.I., 2nd, Johnson, B.H., Unadkat, J.D. & Sheiner, L.B. (1986) The extent of metabolism of inhaled anesthetics in humans. *Anesthesiology*, **65**, 201–205.

143 Rehder, K., Forbes, J., Alter, H., Hessler, O. & Stier, A. (1967) Halothane biotransformation in man: A quantitative study. *Anesthesiology*, **28**, 711–715.

144 Cascorbi, H.F., Blake, D.A. & Helrich, M. (1970) Differences in the biotransformation of halothane in man. *Anesthesiology*, **32**, 119–123.

145 Leece, E.A., Corletto, F. & Brearley, J.C. (2008) A comparison of recovery times and characteristics with sevoflurane and isoflurane anaesthesia in horses undergoing magnetic resonance imaging. *Veterinary Anaesthesia and Analgesia*, **35**, 383–391.

146 Gozalo-Marcilla, M., Hopster, K., Gasthuys, F., Hatz, L., Krajewski, A.E. & Schauvliege, S. (2013) Effects of a constant-rate infusion of dexmedetomidine on the

minimal alveolar concentration of sevoflurane in ponies. *Equine Veterinary Journal*, **45**, 204–208.

147 Marcilla, M.G., Schauvliege, S., Segaert, S., Duchateau, L. & Gasthuys, F. (2012) Influence of a constant rate infusion of dexmedetomidine on cardiopulmonary function and recovery quality in isoflurane anaesthetized horses. *Veterinary Anaesthesia and Analgesia*, **39**, 49–58.

148 Doherty, T.J. & Frazier, D.L. (1998) Effect of intravenous lidocaine on halothane minimum alveolar concentration in ponies. *Equine Veterinary Journal*, **30**, 300–303.

149 Rezende, M.L., Wagner, A.E., Mama, K.R., Ferreira, T.H. & Steffey, E.P. (2011) Effects of intravenous administration of lidocaine on the minimum alveolar concentration of sevoflurane in horses. *American Journal of Veterinary Research*, **72**, 446–451.

150 Valverde, A., Gunkelt, C., Doherty, T.J., Giguère, S. & Pollak, A.S. (2005) Effect of a constant rate infusion of lidocaine on the quality of recovery from sevoflurane or isoflurane general anaesthesia in horses. *Equine Veterinary Journal*, **37**, 559–564.

151 Thomasy, S.M., Steffey, E.P., Mama, K.R., Solano, A. & Stanley, S.D. (2006) The effects of i.v. fentanyl administration on the minimum alveolar concentration of isoflurane in horses. *British Journal of Anaesthesia*, **97**, 232–237.

152 Knych, H.K., Steffey, E.P., Mama, K.R. & Stanley, S.D. (2009) Effects of high plasma fentanyl concentrations on minimum alveolar concentration of isoflurane in horses. *American Journal of Veterinary Research*, **70**, 1193–1200.

153 Ohta, M., Wakuno, A., Okada, J. *et al.* (2010) Effects of intravenous fentanyl administration on end-tidal sevoflurane concentrations in thoroughbred racehorses undergoing orthopedic surgery. *Journal of Veterinary Medical Science*, **72**, 1107–1111.

154 Clark, L., Clutton, R.E., Blissitt, K.J. & Chase-Topping, M.E. (2008) The effects of morphine on the recovery of horses from halothane anaesthesia. *Veterinary Anaesthesia and Analgesia*, **35**, 22–29.

155 Muir, W.W., 3rd & Sams, R. (1992) Effects of ketamine infusion on halothane minimal alveolar concentration in horses. *American Journal of Veterinary Research*, **53**, 1802–1806.

156 Kempchen, S., Kuhn, M., Spadavecchia, C. & Levionnois, O.L. (2012) Medetomidine continuous rate intravenous infusion in horses in which surgical anaesthesia is maintained with isoflurane and intravenous infusions of lidocaine and ketamine. *Veterinary Anaesthesia and Analgesia*, **39**, 245–255.

157 Villalba, M., Santiago, I. & Gomez de Segura, I.A. (2011) Effects of constant rate infusion of lidocaine and ketamine, with or without morphine, on isoflurane MAC in horses. *Equine Veterinary Journal*, **43**, 721–726.

158 Enderle, A.K., Levionnois, O.L., Kuhn, M. & Schatzmann, U. (2008) Clinical evaluation of ketamine and lidocaine intravenous infusions to reduce isoflurane requirements in horses under general anaesthesia. *Veterinary Anaesthesia and Analgesia*, **35**, 297–305.

159 Kushiro, T., Yamashita, K., Umar, M.A. *et al.* (2005) Anesthetic and cardiovascular effects of balanced anesthesia using constant rate infusion of midazolam-ketamine-medetomidine with inhalation of oxygen-sevoflurane (MKM-OS anesthesia) in horses. *Journal of Veterinary Medical Science*, **67**, 379–384.

160 Valverde, A., Rickey, E., Sinclair, M. *et al.* (2010) Comparison of cardiovascular function and quality of recovery in isoflurane-anaesthetised horses administered a constant rate infusion of lidocaine or lidocaine and medetomidine during elective surgery. *Equine Veterinary Journal*, **42**, 192–199.

161 Nannarone, S. & Spadavecchia, C. (2012) Evaluation of the clinical efficacy of two partial intravenous anesthetic protocols, compared with isoflurane alone, to maintain general anesthesia in horses. *American Journal of Veterinary Research*, **73**, 959–967.

162 Robertson, S.A. (2005) Sedation and general anesthesia of the foal. *Equine Veterinary Education*, **7**, 94–101.

163 Dunlop, C.I. (1994) Anesthesia and sedation of foals. *Veterinary Clinics of North America: Equine Practice*, **10**, 67–85.

164 Tranquilli, W.J. & Thurmon, J.C. (1990) Management of anesthesia in the foal. *Veterinary Clinics of North America: Equine Practice*, **6**, 651–663.

165 Mama KR. (2006) *Anesthetic Management of Foals*. North American Veterinary Conference—Large Animal Proceedings, Orlando, FL, January 7–11, 2006, p. 150.

166 Robertson, S.A., Carter, S.W., Donovan, M. & Steele, C. (1990) Effects of intravenous xylazine hydrochloride on blood glucose, plasma insulin and rectal temperature in neonatal foals. *Equine Veterinary Journal*, **22**, 43–47.

167 Steffey, E.P., Willits, N., Wong, P. *et al.* (1991) Clinical investigations of halothane and isoflurane for induction and maintenance of foal anesthesia. *Journal of Veterinary Pharmacology and Therapeutics*, **14**, 300–309.

168 Kaka, J.S., Klavano, P.A. & Hayton, W.L. (1979) Pharmacokinetics of ketamine in the horse. *American Journal of Veterinary Research*, **40**, 978–981.

169 Waterman, A.E., Robertson, S.A. & Lane, J.G. (1987) Pharmacokinetics of intravenously administered ketamine in the horse. *Research in Veterinary Science*, **42**, 162–166.

170 Chaffin, M.K., Walker, M.A., McArthur, N.H., Perris, E.E. & Matthews, N.S. (1997) Magnetic resonance imaging of the brain of normal neonatal foals. *Veterinary Radiology & Ultrasound*, **38**, 102–111.

171 Matthews, N.S., Chaffin, M.K., Erickson, S.W. & Overhulse, W.A. (1995) Propofol anesthesia for non-surgical procedures of neonatal foals. *Equine Practice*, **17**, 15.

CHAPTER 4

Clinical application of equine analgesics

Sheilah A. Robertson and L. Chris Sanchez

Department of Large Animal Clinical Sciences, University of Florida College of Veterinary Medicine, Gainesville, FL, USA

The prevention and alleviation of pain in horses increases patient and personnel safety, results in less disruption of normal physiologic functions, enhances return to normal function, and is an important welfare issue. Colic and lameness are the most common painful conditions affecting horses worldwide. As these conditions represent manifestations of visceral and somatic pain, respectively, their management can be used as a template for other similar presentations. Therapeutic options in this chapter will be discussed by drug class. Nonsteroidal anti-inflammatory drugs (NSAIDs) are commonly used analgesics and are reviewed in Chapters 5 and 13.

Use of systemic analgesics

Opioids

The use of opioids for the treatment of pain in horses has been more controversial than in other species for several reasons. In horses, there seems to be a narrow margin between achieving analgesia and producing arousal or excitement. In addition, other possible undesirable side effects include increased locomotor activity and gastrointestinal stasis. Equine clinicians should note, however, that the effects of opioids on healthy, pain-free research horses are often remarkably different from those observed in clinical cases where horses are in pain and are often receiving sedative agents concurrently with the opioids. In addition, several nociceptive testing modalities, such as thermal threshold or thermal latency testing and mechanical and electrical threshold testing, do not always produce the consistent results in horses that are reported in other species after administration of opioids, making preclinical assessment of potentially useful drugs difficult [1].

However, armed with an understanding that horses may respond differently to opioids and with newer methods for assessing clinical analgesia, including composite pain scoring tools based on behavior, there has been a renewed interest in the use of opioids in equine patients.

Opioid receptor binding in the horse

Opioid receptor binding studies have been conducted on horse brain [2, 3]. These studies show that there are differences between horses and other species with regard to distribution and density of opioid receptors, but the clinical significance of these data is still unclear.

Systemic administration of opioids

Butorphanol, one of the most widely used opioid in horses, exhibits partial agonist and antagonist activity at the μ-opioid receptor, as well as competitive antagonist and partial agonist activity at the κ-opioid receptor. Approved in the USA for intravenous (IV) administration in horses at a dose of 0.1 mg/kg bwt q3–4 h, it is often given intramuscularly or as a continuous rate infusion (CRI), because IV dosing has been associated with excitement, ataxia, increased locomotion, and decreased gut sounds. If used IM, it may need to be given more frequently or at higher doses because systemic availability after this route is only about 37%, but dose and dosing interval should be based on the response to treatment in each individual patient. In normal horses, a CRI of butorphanol administered at a loading dose of 17.8 μg/kg bwt followed by an infusion rate of 23.7 μg/kg/h for 24 h minimized the behavioral side effects associated with a single bolus injection (e.g., staggering and ataxia) administered at a dose of 0.1–0.13 mg/kg bwt and achieved plasma concentrations

Equine Pharmacology, First Edition. Edited by Cynthia Cole, Bradford Bentz and Lara Maxwell.

thought to be therapeutic [4]. However, the number of fecal piles produced in horses treated with either a single bolus or a continuous infusion of butorphanol over a 24 h period was significantly less than in control horses. The authors recommended that caution was still warranted, however, and suggested that treatment should be restricted to 12–24 h. If a longer duration of therapy is needed, doses should be titrated to the lowest effective dose, and in some cases, treatment with mineral oil may be indicated. In another study, Sanchez *et al.* found no significant decrease in duodenal motility in research horses administered a loading dose of butorphanol of 18 µg/kg bwt, followed by an infusion at rate of 13 µg/kg/h for 2 h [5]. In a clinical study, the effects of butorphanol administered at 13 µg/kg/h for 24 h were compared to a saline control CRI after celiotomy [6]. Horses that received butorphanol lost significantly less weight, had improved recovery characteristics, and on average were discharged 3 days earlier than control horses. The latter finding represented an overall significant financial saving for the client.

Morphine administration to horses is controversial, and there are both those who oppose its use and those that wonder why it is not used routinely in equine pain management. Because morphine, when administered at doses of 0.25 or 2.0 mg/kg bwt IV, was not anesthetic sparing in research horses and because the high dose resulted in undesirable recoveries, Steffey and others did not advise its use as an anesthetic adjuvant, and for several years, its use went out of favor [7]. More recently, however, lower doses of 0.5 and 0.1 mg/kg bwt, IV or IM, were administered to conscious healthy horses with no clinically relevant changes in behavior or intestinal motility [1]. Nevertheless, in that same study, morphine did not result in an antinociceptive effect to thermal or electrical stimuli.

In the clinical arena, very different experiences from those in a research setting have been reported. For example, Love and colleagues reported that the addition of IV morphine to a standard anesthetic protocol in horses undergoing upper airway surgery, at doses lower than those used in the study by Steffey (e.g., 0.1–0.2 mg/kg bwt), significantly improved the quality of anesthetic recovery [8]. Two other studies also reported favorable results when morphine was used perioperatively in horses [9, 10]. In one study, horses received a single intraoperative dose of morphine at 0.10–0.17 mg/kg bwt IV, and in the other, the loading dose of 0.15 mg/kg

bwt was followed by an infusion of 0.1 mg/kg/h. In these studies, horses that received morphine required fewer attempts to stand successfully and overall had shorter recovery times compared to untreated controls. No adverse effects were noted, and thus, the results of these studies support the use of morphine in clinical cases. The difference between research and clinical studies should be noted. Clinical cases usually receive sedative agents in addition to morphine and undergo painful procedures. As such, their physiological state is different from normal, nonpainful research horses, and thus, their responses to the morphine appear to be different as well.

Efficacy aside, the gastrointestinal effects of morphine in the horse must also be considered. Boscan and colleagues studied the effects of morphine administered to normal horses at a dose of 0.5 mg/kg bwt IV every 12 h for 6 days [11]. Gastrointestinal function was altered for 6 h following each treatment; defecation frequency decreased, as did fecal moisture content and gastrointestinal sounds. The conclusion of the study was that morphine can contribute to ileus and constipation. The same authors studied the combination of *N*-methylnaltrexone, an opioid antagonist that does not cross the blood–brain barrier, and morphine administered at the same dose as in the previously described study and found that the antagonist largely, but not completely, reversed the adverse effects of morphine on the gastrointestinal tract [12]. When a single lower dose of morphine (i.e., <0.5 mg/kg bwt) was administered to horses, the observed change in intestinal motility was minimal and clinically irrelevant [1].

What we really need to know in the clinical arena, however, is whether or not the administration of morphine at commonly used clinical doses is a risk factor for developing colic. Two retrospective studies have evaluated risk factors for the development of colic in horses following general anesthesia with or without surgery [13, 14]. When the records of 496 horses that underwent orthopedic surgery were analyzed, 14 developed colic, and the authors found that the administration of morphine to horses was associated with a fourfold increased risk of colic compared to the use of no opioids or butorphanol [13]. Andersen and others looked at 553 anesthetic records of horses that either underwent MRI, but no surgery, or that underwent nonabdominal surgery to revisit the role of morphine as a risk factor for colic [14]. In that study, 20 (e.g., 3.6%) of horses developed colic within 7 days of anesthesia, and significantly more of those horses were in the group that underwent surgery. Perianesthetic use of morphine, however, was not associated with an increased risk of the development of colic. Other factors identified in the study that increased the risk of colic included the use of isoflurane as the anesthetic agent and the administration of the antimicrobials benzylpenicillin and/or ceftiofur. The risks of morphine in horses remain unclear, but they appear to be dose related. In the clinical arena, however, morphine does appear to have benefits for the treatment of pain in horses.

Fentanyl used in horses increased with the development of the transdermal patch formulation because the patches were simple to use, provided a slow-release formulation, and were "hands-off." The pharmacokinetics of fentanyl both after IV, bolus and infusion, and transdermal administrations have been well described in the horse [15–17]. However, after a more critical look at this opioid in horses, the efficacy of fentanyl in general and the patches in particular are now being questioned. For example, absorption of fentanyl from the patches appears to be unreliable. The results of one study demonstrated that uptake of fentanyl from a transdermal patch is highly variable in horses when applied to the middorsal thorax [18]. Consistent with this finding, the results of an *in vitro* study by Mills and Cross showed that uptake of fentanyl varied according to the area of skin where the patch was applied. Absorption from the leg region was lowest, and this lack of bioavailability could affect systemic levels of drug [19].

The efficacy of fentanyl has also been evaluated in several studies. For example, in one study that used a minimal alveolar concentration (MAC) model for assessing analgesia, only high plasma concentrations of fentanyl had any significant analgesic effect. The results of this study also demonstrated that the pharmacokinetics of fentanyl were altered by general anesthesia [16, 20]. In a different study, conducted in conscious research horses, fentanyl failed to produce significant visceral or somatic antinociception at serum concentrations above the nociceptive threshold in other species [17]. In addition, when high plasma concentrations were attained (i.e., >5 ng/ml), some, but not all, of the horses became agitated. Finally, in a small clinical study of horses with pain that was refractory to NSAID therapy alone, the addition of a fentanyl transdermal therapeutic system appeared to be effective based on subjective evaluation of pain behaviors [21]. In summary, the usefulness of fentanyl as an analgesic in horses remains to be determined, and more study is needed on its effects in painful horses.

Methadone is a μ-opioid agonist that also has antagonistic activity at *N*-methyl-*D*-aspartate (NMDA) receptors, which are involved in the development of central sensitization. This latter unique activity may provide additional benefits when used to treat pain in horses [22]. Currently, there are only a few reports of the use of methadone in horses, and these are restricted to the research arena. When given IV or intraorally (i.e., squirted directly into the mouth) at a dose of 0.15 mg/kg bwt, the resulting plasma concentrations were in the range that would be considered analgesic in humans, and no changes in behavior were observed [23, 24]. Intraoral administration would be useful in a clinical setting, and methadone appears to have a favorable bioavailability when given by this route. Intragastric administration was less effective, perhaps because more of the drug was subjected to hepatic metabolism, often referred to as a first-pass effect, resulting in a significantly decreased bioavailability compared to intraoral administration [24]. Methadone is available both in a racemic mixture formulation and in one that only contains the active isomer levomethadone. Levomethadone was shown in one study to increase and prolong the antinociceptive effects of detomidine [25]. Reports of methadone use in clinical equine settings are currently anecdotal, but this opioid shows great promise.

Tramadol is an analog of codeine that is used in humans, dogs, and cats both acutely, for perioperative analgesia, for example, and chronically to alleviate maladaptive or chronic pain. Some of its analgesic effects are related to its opioid properties, but it has less abuse potential and fewer cardiorespiratory side effects than drugs classified as true opioids. Tramadol could be an important addition to the list of drugs used for alleviating pain in equine patients, if efficacy could be shown. The pharmacokinetic profiles of tramadol and its active M1 metabolite have been described after IV, intramuscular, and oral, immediate-release and sustained-release formulations [26]. Compared to other species, tramadol in horses had a short half-life and a very low oral bioavailability of approximately 3% [26]. In addition, formation of the active M1 metabolite was extremely limited. These findings led the authors to conclude that tramadol may be of limited usefulness in horses. Dhanjal and colleagues, using hoof withdrawal and skin twitch latencies to a thermal stimulus as a measure of antinociception, determined the pharmacodynamics of tramadol following administration of doses ranging from 0.1 to 1.6 mg/kg bwt IV [27]. Although minimal side effects were reported, there was no prolongation of the response to the thermal stimulus, indicating a lack of analgesic effects. However, in a clinical setting, although tramadol alone failed to provide pain relief to horses with naturally occurring laminitis, significant improvement was noted in combination with subanesthetic doses of ketamine [28]. Thus, tramadol may be more valuable as part of a multimodal approach to pain in horses than as a sole analgesic agent.

Alpha-2 adrenergic agonists

The alpha-2 adrenergic agonists are among the most frequently used drugs in equine medicine for both sedation and short-term analgesia. These drugs are not ideal for prolonged analgesic therapy, however, as they cause an immediate and profound decrease in gastrointestinal motility, negative cardiovascular effects, and have a relatively short duration of action. Importantly, equine clinicians should note that with the majority of drugs in this class, the sedative effects may occur at lower dosages and may persist longer than the analgesic effects [29].

Analgesic effects of the alpha-2 agonists, along with sedation and anxiolysis, are primarily mediated through centrally located alpha-2 adrenergic receptors. Many of the perceived untoward effects of these drugs are mediated through modulation of the sympathetic nervous system. Activation of presynaptic alpha-2 adrenergic receptors causes bradycardia, decreased systemic vascular resistance, and decreased cardiac contractility, while activation of postsynaptic receptors increases the systemic vascular resistance [30]. These effects manifest clinically as decreased heart rate, increased then decreased blood pressure and systemic vascular resistance, and an initial decrease in cardiac output [31–34].

Alpha-2 adrenergic agonists provide dose-dependent visceral and somatic antinociception of varying durations, as well as an opioid-sparing effect. Thus, the combination of an alpha-2 adrenergic agonist and an opioid is used in a variety of commonly used multimodal analgesic protocols.

Xylazine provides excellent dose-dependent visceral analgesia for short durations, typically 15–20 but occasionally up to 90 min, as determined in some experimental pain models [35–37]. Somatic antinociception is also provided, but the duration is very short [38]. Adverse effects associated with its administration include decreased gastrointestinal motility [39–42].

Detomidine has been shown to provide visceral antinociception in models of cecal, duodenal, and colorectal distention [43, 44]. Importantly, plasma concentrations required to demonstrate significant visceral antinociception were substantially higher than those required to produce sedation and decreased gastrointestinal motility [44].

Medetomidine infusions have been used successfully in horses as part of a balanced anesthetic protocol [45]. Medetomidine was administered at a dose of 5 µg/kg bwt IV, followed 10 min later by morphine at a dose of 50 µg/kg bwt IV and then 10 min later by a CRI of medetomidine and morphine at 5 and 30 µg/kg bwt/h, respectively, provided suitable conditions for standing laparoscopy in horses [32].

The relative potency of the alpha-2 adrenergic agonists is correlated primarily, but not completely, with their alpha-2/alpha-1 receptor selectivity. For example, medetomidine and dexmedetomidine with alpha-2/alpha-1 ratios of 1620 are the most potent, followed by detomidine, clonidine, and xylazine, with ratios of 260, 220, and 160, respectively [46–49]. Clinically, with all factors considered, a dose of 1 mg/kg bwt of xylazine administered IV corresponds to 5–10 µg/kg bwt of medetomidine, 3.5 µg/kg bwt dexmedetomidine, 25 µg/kg bwt clonidine, 80–120 µg/kg bwt romifidine, or 20–40 µg/kg bwt detomidine.

Sodium channel blockers

Lidocaine is an aminoamide local anesthetic that prevents propagation of action potentials by binding to voltage-gated sodium channels. Lidocaine, administered as an CRI, is commonly used in horses for its analgesic, prokinetic, and anti-inflammatory properties [50–55]. Variable doses of IV lidocaine have been reported; loading doses vary from 1.3 to 5.0 mg/kg bwt, and infusion rates vary from 25 to 100 µg/kg/min. Clinical signs of toxicity in conscious horses include skeletal muscle tremors, altered visual function, anxiety, ataxia, collapse, and electrocardiographic changes. Most commonly, signs of toxicity are observed when serum concentrations are between 1.65 and 4.53 µg/ml (mean 3.24 ± SD 0.74 µg/ml) [56]. It is important to note that the neurologic manifestations of toxicosis may be masked by general anesthesia.

Using electroencephalographic changes as an objective measure of nociception in anesthetized ponies, an IV loading dose of lidocaine of 5 mg/kg bwt followed by a CRI at 100 µg/kg/min obtunded the response to castration, lending support to the effectiveness of lidocaine as a visceral analgesic [57]. Lidocaine administrations following exploratory laparotomies were associated with reduced small intestinal size and peritoneal fluid accumulation, as well as improved survival [54, 58]. In one hospital setting, the intraoperative use of lidocaine was associated with a reduction in the incidence of postoperative ileus of approximately 50% [59]. In a different multicenter study of horses with enteritis or postoperative ileus, lidocaine infusions decreased the volume and duration of reflux compared to saline-treated controls [53]. Lidocaine was also shown to improve mucosal healing following experimentally induced small intestinal ischemia [60]. Although the mechanism for this effect is unknown, the authors of the study hypothesized that it may be related to the decreased production of inflammatory cytokines.

Because treatment of horses with gastrointestinal disease may need to be prolonged, it is important to understand how the duration of infusion affects the disposition of lidocaine and how the pharmacokinetics of lidocaine might be altered by disease or general anesthesia, so that appropriate changes in the infusion rate can be made if necessary to avoid toxicosis. Based on the results of one study, the target steady-state serum concentration of lidocaine for the treatment of ileus should be between 1.0 and 2.0 µg/ml [61]. In healthy horses, a CRI at 50 µg/kg/min, with no loading dose, produced steady-state serum concentrations slightly below this suggested target with a mean of 0.98 µg/ml after approximately 3 h of infusion, and no bioaccumulation was evident over a 96 h infusion period [62]. In a clinical setting, however, accumulation was demonstrated at that same infusion rate, so clinicians need to adjust the rate as necessary to prevent toxicity [63]. In addition, ceftiofur sodium and flunixin meglumine can decrease the protein binding of lidocaine, which can increase the unbound or active fraction of the drug in the blood. Therefore, lower infusion rates of lidocaine should be used in horses receiving those or other highly protein-bound drugs [63]. Plasma concentrations may also be affected by liver disease or changes in liver blood

flow, which occur under general anesthesia. For example, a loading dose of 1.3 mg/kg bwt followed by an infusion of 50 µg/kg/min resulted in higher serum concentrations in anesthetized compared to awake horses, and the serum concentrations produced in the anesthetized horses were within the range reported to be toxic in conscious horses [56, 64].

Lidocaine: Other applications

Many horses that present with abdominal pain will undergo a rectal palpation, which can be uncomfortable and in some cases painful. Fifteen ml of a 2% solution of lidocaine, administered intrarectally, increased rectal wall compliance, facilitated rectal palpation, and likely decreased the risk of rectal tears [65]. The pain associated with other diagnostic procedures, such as thoracocentesis and abdominocentesis, can also be decreased by local infiltration with lidocaine or another local anesthetic. In mares undergoing laparoscopic ovariectomy, the addition of 10 ml of 2% lidocaine injected into the mesovarium to a protocol of IV xylazine and butorphanol and epidural detomidine resulted in fewer pain responses compared to intraovarian injection of saline [66].

N-methyl-D-aspartate antagonists

Ketamine was traditionally considered solely a dissociative anesthetic, but its role as a potential analgesic has evolved over the years in both human and veterinary medicine. Ketamine is a noncompetitive NMDA receptor antagonist and therefore can modulate central sensitization and exert an antihyperalgesic effect [67, 68]. Ketamine may also have activity at opioid, monoaminergic, and muscarinic receptors and at voltage-sensitive Ca^{++} channels, and although these actions are not fully understood, they may also contribute to its analgesic effects, which occur at subanesthetic doses. In addition, there is interest in ketamine for its immunomodulating effects in animals with endotoxemia [69].

The pharmacokinetics and clinical effects of CRIs of subanesthetic doses of ketamine, ranging from 0.4 to 1.6 mg/kg/h, have been determined in healthy horses [70–72]. In one study, doses less than 0.8 mg/kg/h did not cause any adverse behavioral effects, such as sedation, excitation, or increased locomotor activity, or changes in heart rate, respiratory rate, or blood pressure [72]. In a different study, when horses received ketamine at a rate of 1.2 mg/kg/h for up to 96 h, Elfenbein and others reported no changes in heart rate, respiratory rate, rectal temperature, or behavior scores, but did note a significant delay in gastrointestinal transit time [70].

Although antinociception was not demonstrated in healthy horses receiving infusions of ketamine, in clinical settings, there seem to be some beneficial effects [28, 73]. For example, when ketamine, administered at a dose of 0.2 mg/kg bwt IV was added to a protocol of xylazine and butorphanol, it did not increase the level of sedation, but it did make insertion of a dental float easier than xylazine alone or xylazine plus butorphanol. In addition, horses treated with ketamine/xylazine/ butorphanol permitted arthrocentesis with minimal response and tolerated more pressure applied to their withers using an algometer [73]. However, the horses treated with ketamine were more responsive to a sharp needle prick, and the authors concluded that more studies were needed to determine which clinical procedures would be facilitated by the addition of ketamine to a standard sedation protocol.

Ketamine has shown some promise for the treatment of chronic laminitis, a common ailment in horses that is usually associated with severe, often unremitting pain and impaired mobility. The etiology of the disease is still poorly understood, making treatment and provision of effective pain relief challenging for the clinician. In addition, many laminitic horses are refractory to traditional anti-inflammatory therapy. As a neuropathic component of the pain associated with this disease has been demonstrated, ketamine is a suitable candidate drug for therapy [74]. In a randomized crossover study using horses with naturally occurring laminitis, the effect of oral tramadol alone, administered at 5 mg/kg bwt q12 h, was compared to the same dose of tramadol given concurrently with ketamine at a dose of 0.6 mg/ kg/h IV for 6 h for the first 3 days of a 7-day treatment [28]. Tramadol alone provided little pain relief, but the combination of tramadol and ketamine resulted in decreased blood pressure, decreased forelimb "off-loading" frequency, and increased forelimb load as measured by a force plate. In addition, these benefits persisted for 3 days after the end of the 7-day treatment period. Based on auscultation assessments, no changes in gastrointestinal motility scores were noted with either treatment. Although the clinical significance of the finding is unknown, plasma concentrations of tumor necrosis factor-α and thromboxane B_2 also decreased when ketamine was added to the protocol. This study showed that ketamine could provide some pain relief in laminitic horses and that a 3-day treatment produced effects that could be measured for up to 7 days. Based on these results, more studies on the use of ketamine in painful equine conditions are encouraged.

Antispasmodic medications

N-butylscopolammonium bromide (NBB) has both anticholinergic and antispasmodic properties and is labeled for the treatment of spasmodic colic. In an experimental model of cecal balloon distention, NBB administered at a dose of 0.3 mg/kg bwt IV had an analgesic effect in six of the eight ponies studied [75]. In another similar trial, NBB administered at a dose of 20 mg/100 kg bwt had a brief analgesic effect, as well as a transient negative effect on cecal contractions [76]. In horses, administration of NBB produced visceral antinociception, as indicated by a significantly increased colorectal distention threshold and a small but nonsignificant increase in duodenal distention threshold [5]. The administration of NBB also decreased rectal tone for facilitation of a rectal examination [77]. In all reports, duration of effect was short at 15–20 min.

Use of intra-articular analgesics

Recent reports in the human literature have raised concerns over the use of local anesthetic drugs in joints due to the potential for chondrotoxicity. *In vitro* studies report deleterious effects on chondrocytes exposed to lidocaine and bupivacaine but less so with mepivacaine and ropivacaine. This topic remains controversial, and single injections of local anesthetics *in vivo* continue to be used [78]. In humans, intra-articular opioids are used to provide analgesia following arthroscopic surgery and joint replacement and in patients with osteoarthritis. The rationale behind this practice is that opioid receptors are present in many peripheral tissues and are upregulated under inflammatory states. μ-Opioid receptors have been identified in equine synovial tissue, and the authors of that study advocate the practice of intra-articular administration of opioids to relieve pain related to arthroscopic surgery [79]. In horses and ponies, intra-articular injections of morphine and saline induced the release of large molecular size proteoglycan subunits into the synovial fluid [80]. Morphine injected at a dose of 0.05 mg/kg bwt was detectable in synovial fluid for 24 h after treatment, whereas serum concentrations were very low and only detectable for 6 h after administration [81]. In this same study, white blood cell counts and protein concentrations were increased, and hyaluronate concentrations were decreased in synovial fluid samples at 24 h following the injection of morphine or saline with no differences between treatments [81].

Using an experimentally induced equine synovitis model, Santos and colleagues compared the analgesic effects of the local anesthetic ropivacaine and morphine alone and in combination when administered intra-articularly [82]. Ropivacaine alone resulted in some pain relief, but the duration was short at less than 3.5 h. In contrast, morphine alone or combined with the local anesthetic produced a good analgesic effect for up to 24 h. The explanation for this may be that local anesthetics are less effective in the acidic environment associated with synovitis, whereas opioid receptors may be upregulated in the same environment, making them good targets for opioid agonists, such as morphine.

Epidural administration of analgesic drugs

Caudal epidural injections at the sacrococcygeal or C1–C2 space of various drugs can be performed in horses to facilitate surgery on the hind end (e.g., rectal, anal, perineal, urethral, bladder, vulvar, and vaginal procedures) or to treat painful hindlimb conditions. Single or repeated injections may be made, and epidural catheters can be placed for long-term treatment. Instructions for placement of epidural catheters have been well described in an article by Ball and others [83].

Local anesthetic agents, such as lidocaine, mepivacaine, and ropivacaine, produce loss of both sensory and motor function. Recumbency must be avoided because horses tend to panic when they lose motor control of their hindlimbs. Therefore, the volume administered, which dictates cranial spread, must be carefully calculated. Lidocaine (2%) is the most common local anesthetic administered epidurally, and recommended doses are 0.2–0.25 mg/kg bwt, which equates to 1–1.25 ml/100 kg bwt. Onset of anesthesia usually occurs within 5 min and lasts 45–60 min. When other

analgesic agents, including opioids, tramadol, alpha-2 adrenergic agonists, and ketamine, are used, motor function is maintained, but mild ataxia may be observed. Although the sensory blockade achieved with these drugs alone is insufficient for surgery, it provides pain relief. These drugs can be used epidurally in combination with injection of a local anesthetic into the flank and/ or into intra-abdominal structures, such as the mesovarium or cryptorchid testes, for flank laparoscopic techniques.

The epidural administration of butorphanol, morphine [84, 85], and methadone has all been reported in horses [84–86]. Morphine is the most popular opioid given by this route at a typical dose of 0.1–0.2 mg/kg bwt. It has a slow onset of action, requiring 1–5 h, but a long duration, lasting from 16 to 28 h. In an acute synovitis model, epidural morphine decreased lameness, improved weight bearing at rest, and improved range of motion during locomotion [84]. When tramadol was administered epidurally at a dose of 1 mg/kg bwt, diluted to a final volume of 20–30 ml for horses weighing 450–500 kg, it had an onset time of approximately 30 min and a duration of effect of 5 h [85].

The alpha-2 adrenergic agonists have also been administered epidurally to provide analgesia. Xylazine is administered at 0.17–0.22 mg/kg bwt and detomidine at 0.01–0.06 mg/kg bwt [87–90]. Both produce sensory blockade, but the duration of effect is longer with xylazine, and it produces fewer systemic effects including sedation [87]. Epidural ketamine provided analgesia to the tail, perineum, and upper hindlimbs with a duration of effect that was dose dependent; doses of 0.5 and 1.0 mg/kg bwt lasted 30 min, while a dose of 2.0 mg/kg bwt lasted 75 min [91]. Dose-dependent sedation was also observed with epidural ketamine administration, but cardiopulmonary effects were minimal.

Combinations of drugs can also be administered epidurally, and this approach may be the most clinically relevant. Effective combinations include an alpha-2 adrenergic agonist, such as detomidine administered at a dose of 0.02–0.03 mg/kg bwt and morphine administered at a dose of 0.2 mg/kg bwt [92, 93]. These combinations provide the benefit of more rapid onset and prolonged activity. This is a good combination to produce long-lasting hindlimb analgesia, for example, in cases of septic arthritis. This technique also decreased postoperative pain in horses after bilateral stifle surgery [93]. An alpha-2 agonist combined with a local anesthetic can also be used for standing surgery and has a longer duration of action than the use of a local anesthesia alone [94].

Long-term administration of analgesic agents using epidural catheters can be a lifesaving technique for horses with severe hindlimb orthopedic pain. Long-term catheterization is associated with changes in cerebrospinal fluid, red blood cell values, protein content, and evidence of mild inflammation; however, these do not cause adverse clinical signs [95]. In a clinical setting, complications related to long-term placement of epidural catheters were short lived and minor [96].

Complications related to epidural administration of drugs

Sedation is often seen soon after epidural injection of alpha-2 adrenergic agonists, but it is short lived compared to the analgesia obtained. Ataxia and recumbency can be prevented by avoiding oversedation, injecting slowly, limiting the volume of local anesthetic injected, and using caution in weak or debilitated horses. As in other species, including humans, pruritus has been reported after epidural administration of morphine [97].

Analgesic use in foals

It is important to anticipate and prevent noxious stimuli in this population of patients, because pain in the neonatal and pediatric period can alter pain processing, leading to altered pain thresholds and responses, as well as aversive behaviors later in life. Many foals develop painful medical (meconium retention, gastroenteritis, infectious synovitis, flexural deformity, gastric ulceration) and surgical conditions ("colic," angular limb deformities, fractures, uroperitoneum). In addition, many foals are nursed in critical care units, where, although they may have a nonpainful disease, they may be subjected to potentially painful diagnostic or nursing procedures, including abdominocentesis, venipuncture, arteriopuncture, and placement of IV catheters, nasogastric tubes, and urinary catheters. Although there is information on the pharmacokinetics of a few analgesic drugs in foals, there is little information on their pharmacodynamic effects. This lack of information combined with a lack of validated pain scoring systems has made the treatment of pain in foals largely empirical. However, some recommendations can be made, and new information continues to be published.

Opioids

Pharmacokinetic data are available in foals for the agonist–antagonist opioid butorphanol, which has been widely used in equine practice. In healthy 3–12-day-old foals, 0.05 mg/kg bwt given IV or IM had minimal effects on heart rate and respiratory rate but did cause an increase in rectal temperature. Although there was a significant decrease in the gastrointestinal motility score, it was not associated with any obvious ill effects [98]. Unlike adult horses treated with butorphanol, foals became calm and sedate and showed no increase in locomotor activity. Foals also showed a marked increase in nursing behavior, which may prove to be a beneficial drug effect. Clearance of butorphanol in foals is faster, and systemic uptake is greater compared to adults, suggesting that higher doses may be required in this age group. Plasma concentrations associated with analgesia in adults were not achieved in foals when a dose of 0.05 mg/kg bwt was administered IV [98]. The thermal antinociceptive effects of butorphanol administered IV at 0.05 mg/kg bwt and 0.1 mg/kg bwt were evaluated in healthy neonatal pony foals, aged 1–2 weeks, and older pony foals, aged 4–8 weeks [99]. An increase in thermal threshold was found in both age groups following administration of butorphanol at 0.1 mg/kg, but not following administration of the lower dose. No adverse behaviors were reported at the effective dose.

Systemic morphine and fentanyl at doses similar to those used in adults have been administered to foals, but little is known about the pharmacokinetics or pharmacodynamics of these drugs in this age group. Pharmacokinetic data of transdermal fentanyl are available, however, and in 4–8-day-old foals, fentanyl was detected in plasma as early as 20 min after application of a 100 µg/h patch, but peak plasma fentanyl concentrations and the time to reach that peak varied widely from 0.1 to 28.7 ng/ml and 14.3 ± 7.6 h, respectively [100]. Rectal temperature rose above 38.5°C in all foals, but the authors stated that the patch was well tolerated and there were no changes in fecal output, urine production, or activity associated with patch application. Further studies are needed to fully evaluate the role of systemic opioids for pain management in equine neonates, but at present, butorphanol has the most evidence to support its use.

Local anesthetic agents

Local anesthetics are versatile, likely underutilized, agents that have multiple applications in the treatment of pain in foals. Neuraxial (e.g., epidural or spinal) or peripheral nerve blocks with local anesthetics are simple to perform and provide complete analgesia with few side effects, and in many cases, they can be repeated as needed. It is not unusual for foals to respond to a painful stimulus more abruptly and profoundly than adults. Even under general anesthesia, they may respond to the initial incision, although the anesthetic depth appears adequate [101]. Simply infiltrating the incision site with local anesthetic is an effective technique to block the initial response to surgery and will continue to provide analgesia in the early postoperative period.

Lidocaine skin patches containing 5% lidocaine with a total dose of 700 mg per patch and measuring 10×14 cm have been developed for treatment of postherpetic neuralgia in humans but are also used to relieve musculoskeletal pain. Lidocaine penetrates intact skin providing dermal analgesia, but there is minimal systemic absorption. In adult horses, lidocaine was undetectable in serum samples collected for 12 h after application of two patches to the medial side of each carpus. Local anesthetic patches have potential to alleviate wound and musculoskeletal pain [102].

Topical application of local anesthetic creams facilitates catheter placement and venipuncture. Two are readily available: lidocaine in a liposome-encapsulated formulation and a eutectic mixture of lidocaine and prilocaine. In cats, the success rate of jugular catheterization increased from 38 to 60%, when the eutectic mixture was used, and similar protocols could be used in foals [103]. The benefit of topical creams over subcutaneous infiltration is that there is no disruption of the local tissues and the vein is not obscured by a "bleb." The time to onset of action with these products can range from 10 to 30 min; therefore, they may not be applicable in an emergent situation.

Lidocaine jelly that has a rapid onset of action when used on mucous membranes could be used for placement of nasogastric tubes, nasal oxygen cannulas, and urinary catheters.

Alpha-2 adrenergic agonists

This group of drugs produces sedation, muscle relaxation, and analgesia. Xylazine (0.5–1.0 mg/kg IV or IM) and romifidine (40–80 µg/kg IV or IM) are excellent choices in foals, as they produce fewer cardiopulmonary changes than detomidine [104]. They can be used as premedicant agents and for short invasive procedures, such as passage of a nasogastric tube. Both xylazine and romifidine can be used in combination with butorphanol

to provide additional analgesia, and subjectively, these combinations result in a more cooperative foal. It is important to note, however, that the duration of analgesia achieved with alpha-2 adrenergic agonists is shorter than sedation and, as in adults, the plasma concentrations that equate with sedation are much lower than those needed to produce analgesia [44, 105].

References

1 Figueiredo, J.P., Muir, W.W. & Sams, R. (2012) Cardiorespiratory, gastrointestinal, and analgesic effects of morphine sulfate in conscious healthy horses. *American Journal of Veterinary Research*, **73**, 799–808.

2 Hellyer, P.W., Bai, L., Supon, J. *et al.* (2003) Comparison of opioid and alpha-2 adrenergic receptor binding in horse and dog brain using radioligand autoradiography. *Veterinary Anaesthesia and Analgesia*, **30**, 172–182.

3 Thomasy, S.M., Moeller, B.C. & Stanley, S.D. (2007) Comparison of opioid receptor binding in horse, guinea pig, and rat cerebral cortex and cerebellum. *Veterinary Anaesthesia and Analgesia*, **34**, 351–358.

4 Sellon, D.C., Monroe, V.L., Roberts, M.C. & Papich, M.G. (2001) Pharmacokinetics and adverse effects of butorphanol administered by single intravenous injection or continuous intravenous infusion in horses. *American Journal of Veterinary Research*, **62**, 183–189.

5 Sanchez, L.C., Elfenbein, J.R. & Robertson, S.A. (2008) Effect of acepromazine, butorphanol, or N-butylscopolammonium bromide on visceral and somatic nociception and duodenal motility in conscious horses. *American Journal of Veterinary Research*, **69**, 579–585.

6 Sellon, D.C., Roberts, M.C., Blikslager, A.T., Ulibarri, C. & Papich, M.G. (2004) Effects of continuous rate intravenous infusion of butorphanol on physiologic and outcome variables in horses after celiotomy. *Journal of Veterinary Internal Medicine*, **18**, 555–563.

7 Steffey, E.P., Eisele, J.H. & Baggot, J.D. (2003) Interactions of morphine and isoflurane in horses. *American Journal of Veterinary Research*, **64**, 166–175.

8 Love, E.J., Lane, J.G. & Murison, P.J. (2006) Morphine administration in horses anaesthetized for upper respiratory tract surgery. *Veterinary Anaesthesia and Analgesia*, **33**, 179–188.

9 Mircica, E., Clutton, R.E., Kyles, K.W. & Blissitt, K.J. (2003) Problems associated with perioperative morphine in horses: A retrospective case analysis. *Veterinary Anaesthesia and Analgesia*, **30**, 147–155.

10 Clark, L., Clutton, R.E., Blissitt, K.J. & Chase-Topping, M.E. (2008) The effects of morphine on the recovery of horses from halothane anaesthesia. *Veterinary Anaesthesia and Analgesia*, **35**, 22–29.

11 Boscan, P., Van Hoogmoed, L.M., Farver, T.B. & Snyder, J.R. (2006) Evaluation of the effects of the opioid agonist

morphine on gastrointestinal tract function in horses. *American Journal of Veterinary Research*, **67**, 992–997.

12 Boscan, P., Van Hoogmoed, L.M., Pypendop, B.H., Farver, T.B. & Snyder, J.R. (2006) Pharmacokinetics of the opioid antagonist N-methylnaltrexone and evaluation of its effects on gastrointestinal tract function in horses treated or not treated with morphine. *American Journal of Veterinary Research*, **67**, 998–1004.

13 Senior, J.M., Pinchbeck, G.L., Dugdale, A.H. & Clegg, P.D. (2004) Retrospective study of the risk factors and prevalence of colic in horses after orthopaedic surgery. *Veterinary Record*, **155**, 321–325.

14 Andersen, M.S., Clark, L., Dyson, S.J. & Newton, J.R. (2006) Risk factors for colic in horses after general anaesthesia for MRI or nonabdominal surgery: Absence of evidence of effect from perianaesthetic morphine. *Equine Veterinary Journal*, **38**, 368–374.

15 Maxwell, L.K., Thomasy, S.M., Slovis, N. & Kollias-Baker, C. (2003) Pharmacokinetics of fentanyl following intravenous and transdermal administration in horses. *Equine Veterinary Journal*, **35**, 484–490.

16 Thomasy, S.M., Mama, K.R., Whitley, K., Steffey, E.P. & Stanley, S.D. (2007) Influence of general anaesthesia on the pharmacokinetics of intravenous fentanyl and its primary metabolite in horses. *Equine Veterinary Journal*, **39**, 54–58.

17 Sanchez, L.C., Robertson, S.A., Maxwell, L.K., Zientek, K. & Cole, C. (2007) Effect of fentanyl on visceral and somatic nociception in conscious horses. *Journal of Veterinary Internal Medicine*, **21**, 1067–1075.

18 Orsini, J.A., Moate, P.J., Kuersten, K., Soma, L.R. & Boston, R.C. (2006) Pharmacokinetics of fentanyl delivered transdermally in healthy adult horses—variability among horses and its clinical implications. *Journal of Veterinary Pharmacology and Therapeutics*, **29**, 539–546.

19 Mills, P.C. & Cross, S.E. (2007) Regional differences in transdermal penetration of fentanyl through equine skin. *Research in Veterinary Science*, **82**, 252–256.

20 Thomasy, S.M., Steffey, E.P., Mama, K.R., Solano, A. & Stanley, S.D. (2006) The effects of i.v. fentanyl administration on the minimum alveolar concentration of isoflurane in horses. *British Journal of Anaesthesia*, **97**, 232–237.

21 Thomasy, S.M., Slovis, N., Maxwell, L.K. & Kollias-Baker, C. (2004) Transdermal fentanyl combined with nonsteroidal anti-inflammatory drugs for analgesia in horses. *Journal of Veterinary Internal Medicine*, **18**, 550–554.

22 Gorman, A.L., Elliott, K.J. & Inturrisi, C.E. (1997) The d- and l-isomers of methadone bind to the non-competitive site on the N-methyl-D-aspartate (NMDA) receptor in rat forebrain and spinal cord. *Neuroscience Letters*, **223**, 5–8.

23 Linardi, R.L., Stokes, A.M., Barker, S.A., Short, C., Hosgood, G. & Natalini, C.C. (2009) Pharmacokinetics of the injectable formulation of methadone hydrochloride administered orally in horses. *Journal of Veterinary Pharmacology and Therapeutics*, **32**, 492–497.

24 Linardi, R.L., Stokes, A.M., Keowen, M.L., Barker, S.A., Hosgood, G.L. & Short, C.R. (2012) Bioavailability and pharmacokinetics of oral and injectable formulations of methadone after intravenous, oral, and intragastric administration in horses. *American Journal of Veterinary Research*, **73**, 290–295.

25 Schatzman, U., Armbruster, S., Stucki, F., Busato, A. & Kohler, I. (2001) Analgesic effect of butorphanol and levo-methadone in detomidine sedated horses. *Journal of Veterinary Medicine A*, **48**, 337–342.

26 Shilo, Y., Britzi, M., Eytan, B., Lifschitz, T., Soback, S. & Steinman, A. (2008) Pharmacokinetics of tramadol in horses after intravenous, intramuscular and oral administration. *Journal of Veterinary Pharmacology and Therapeutics*, **31**, 60–65.

27 Dhanjal, J.K., Wilson, D.V., Robinson, E., Tobin, T.T. & Dirikolu, L. (2009) Intravenous tramadol: Effects, nociceptive properties, and pharmacokinetics in horses. *Veterinary Anaesthesia and Analgesia*, **36**, 581–590.

28 Guedes, A.G., Matthews, N.S. & Hood, D.M. (2012) Effect of ketamine hydrochloride on the analgesic effects of tramadol hydrochloride in horses with signs of chronic laminitis-associated pain. *American Journal of Veterinary Research*, **73**, 610–619.

29 England, G.C.W. & Clarke, K.W. (1996) Alpha(2) adrenoceptor agonists in the horse: A review. *British Veterinary Journal*, **152**, 641–657.

30 Valverde, A. (2010) Alpha-2 agonists as pain therapy in horses. *Veterinary Clinics of North America Equine Practice*, **26**, 515–532.

31 Freeman, S.L., Bowen, I.M., Bettschart-Wolfensberger, R. & England, G.C. (2000) Cardiopulmonary effects of romifidine and detomidine used as premedicants for ketamine/halothane anaesthesia in ponies. *Veterinary Record*, **147**, 535–539.

32 Solano, A.M., Valverde, A., Desrochers, A., Nykamp, S. & Boure, L.P. (2009) Behavioural and cardiorespiratory effects of a constant rate infusion of medetomidine and morphine for sedation during standing laparoscopy in horses. *Equine Veterinary Journal*, **41**, 153–159.

33 Yamashita, K., Tsubakishita, S., Futaoka, S. *et al.* (2000) Cardiovascular effects of medetomidine, detomidine and xylazine in horses. *Journal of Veterinary Medical Science*, **62**, 1025–1032.

34 Bettschart-Wolfensberger, R., Freeman, S.L., Bowen, I.M. *et al.* (2005) Cardiopulmonary effects and pharmacokinetics of i.v. dexmedetomidine in ponies. *Equine Veterinary Journal*, **37**, 60–64.

35 Brunson, D.B. & Majors, L.J. (1987) Comparative analgesia of xylazine, xylazine/morphine, xylazine/butorphanol, and xylazine/nalbuphine in the horse, using dental dolorimetry. *American Journal of Veterinary Research*, **48**, 1087–1091.

36 Muir, W.W. & Robertson, J.T. (1985) Visceral analgesia: Effects of xylazine, butorphanol, meperidine, and pentazocine in horses. *American Journal of Veterinary Research*, **46**, 2081–2084.

37 Kalpravidh, M., Lumb, W.V., Wright, M. & Heath, R.B. (1984) Effects of butorphanol, flunixin, levorphanol, morphine, and xylazine in ponies. *American Journal of Veterinary Research*, **45**, 217–223.

38 Moens, Y., Lanz, F., Doherr, M.G. & Schatzmann, U. (2003) A comparison of the antinociceptive effects of xylazine, detomidine and romifidine on experimental pain in horses. *Veterinary Anaesthesia and Analgesia*, **30**, 183–190.

39 Clark, E.S., Thompson, S.A., Becht, J.L. & Moore, J.N. (1988) Effects of xylazine on cecal mechanical activity and cecal blood flow in healthy horses. *American Journal of Veterinary Research*, **49**, 720–723.

40 Lester, G.D., Merritt, A.M., Neuwirth, L., Vetro-Widenhouse, T., Steible, C. & Rice, B. (1998) Effect of alpha 2-adrenergic, cholinergic, and nonsteroidal anti-inflammatory drugs on myoelectric activity of ileum, cecum, and right ventral colon and on cecal emptying of radiolabeled markers in clinically normal ponies. *American Journal of Veterinary Research*, **59**, 320–327.

41 Merritt, A.M., Burrow, J.A. & Hartless, C.S. (1998) Effect of xylazine, detomidine, and a combination of xylazine and butorphanol on equine duodenal motility. *American Journal of Veterinary Research*, **59**, 619–623.

42 Sutton, D.G., Preston, T., Christley, R.M., Cohen, N.D., Love, S. & Roussel, A.J. (2002) The effects of xylazine, detomidine, acepromazine and butorphanol on equine solid phase gastric emptying rate. *Equine Veterinary Journal*, **34**, 486–492.

43 Lowe, J.E. & Hilfiger, J. (1986) Analgesic and sedative effects of detomidine compared to xylazine in a colic model using i.v. and i.m. routes of administration. *Acta Veterinaria Scandinavica Supplementum*, **82**, 85–95.

44 Elfenbein, J.R., Sanchez, L.C., Robertson, S.A., Cole, C.A. & Sams, R. (2009) Effect of detomidine on visceral and somatic nociception and duodenal motility in conscious adult horses. *Veterinary Anaesthesia and Analgesia*, **36**, 162–172.

45 Ringer, S.K., Kalchofner, K., Boller, J., Fürst, A. & Bettschart-Wolfensberger, R. (2007) A clinical comparison of two anaesthetic protocols using lidocaine or medetomidine in horses. *Veterinary Anaesthesia and Analgesia*, **34**, 257–268.

46 Faber, E.S.L., Chambers, J.P. & Evans, R.H. (1998) Depression of NMDA receptor-mediated synaptic transmission by four alpha(2) adrenoceptor agonists on the in vitro rat spinal cord preparation. *British Journal of Pharmacology*, **124**, 507–512.

47 Ossipov, M.H., Suarez, L.J. & Spaulding, T.C. (1988) A comparison of the antinociceptive and behavioral-effects of intrathecally administered opiates, alpha-2-adrenergic agonists, and local-anesthetics in mice and rats. *Anesthesia & Analgesia*, **67**, 616–624.

48 Virtanen, R. (1986) Pharmacology of detomidine and other alpha-2-adrenoceptor agonists in the brain. *Acta Veterinaria Scandinavica*, 35–46.

49 Virtanen, R. & Macdonald, E. (1985) Comparison of the effects of detomidine and xylazine on some alpha-2-adrenoceptor-mediated responses in the central and peripheral nervous systems. *European Journal of Pharmacology*, **115**, 277–284.

50 Robertson, S.A., Sanchez, L.C., Merritt, A.M. & Doherty, T.J. (2005) Effect of systemic lidocaine on visceral and somatic nociception in conscious horses. *Equine Veterinary Journal*, **37**, 122–127.

51 Van Hoogmoed, L.M., Nieto, J.E., Snyder, J.R. & Harmon, F.A. (2004) Survey of prokinetic use in horses with gastrointestinal injury. *Veterinary Surgery*, **33**, 279–285.

52 Milligan, M., Beard, W., Kukanich, B., Sobering, T. & Waxman, S. (2007) The effect of lidocaine on postoperative jejunal motility in normal horses. *Veterinary Surgery*, **36**, 214–220.

53 Malone, E., Ensink, J., Turner, T. *et al.* (2006) Intravenous continuous infusion of lidocaine for treatment of equine ileus. *Veterinary Surgery*, **35**, 60–66.

54 Brianceau, P., Chevalier, H., Karas, A. *et al.* (2002) Intravenous lidocaine and small-intestinal size, abdominal fluid, and outcome after colic surgery in horses. *Journal of Veterinary Internal Medicine*, **16**, 736–741.

55 Cook, V.L. & Blikslager, A.T. (2008) Use of systemically administered lidocaine in horses with gastrointestinal tract disease. *Journal of the American Veterinary Medical Association*, **232**, 1144–1148.

56 Meyer, G.A., Lin, H.C., Hanson, R.R. & Hayes, T.L. (2001) Effects of intravenous lidocaine overdose on cardiac electrical activity and blood pressure in the horse. *Equine Veterinary Journal*, **33**, 434–437.

57 Murrell, J.C., White, K.L., Johnson, C.B., Taylor, P.M., Doherty, T.J. & Waterman-Pearson, A.E. (2005) Investigation of the EEG effects of intravenous lidocaine during halothane anaesthesia in ponies. *Veterinary Anaesthesia and Analgesia*, **32**, 212–221.

58 Torfs, S., Delesalle, C., Dewulf, J., Devisscher, L. & Deprez, P. (2009) Risk factors for equine postoperative ileus and effectiveness of prophylactic lidocaine. *Journal of Veterinary Internal Medicine*, **23**, 606–611.

59 Cohen, N.D., Lester, G.D., Sanchez, L.C., Merritt, A.M. & Roussel, A.J., Jr (2004) Evaluation of risk factors associated with development of postoperative ileus in horses. *Journal of the American Veterinary Medical Association*, **225**, 1070–1078.

60 Cook, V.L., Jones, S.J., McDowell, M., Campbell, N.B., Davis, J.L. & Blikslager, A.T. (2008) Attenuation of ischaemic injury in the equine jejunum by administration of systemic lidocaine. *Equine Veterinary Journal*, **40**, 353–357.

61 Malone, E.D., Turner, T.A. & Wilson, J.H. (1998) Intravenous lidocaine for the treatment of equine ileus. *Proceedings of the Equine Colic Research Symposium*, **6**, 42.

62 Dickey, E.J., McKenzie, H.C., III, Brown, J.A. & de Solis, C.N. (2008) Serum concentrations of lidocaine and its metabolites

after prolonged infusion in healthy horses. *Equine Veterinary Journal*, **40**, 348–352.

63 Milligan, M., Kukanich, B., Beard, W. & Waxman, S. (2006) The disposition of lidocaine during a 12-hour intravenous infusion to postoperative horses. *Journal of Veterinary Pharmacology and Therapeutics*, **29**, 495–499.

64 Feary, D.J., Mama, K.R., Wagner, A.E. & Thomasy, S. (2005) Influence of general anesthesia on pharmacokinetics of intravenous lidocaine infusion in horses. *American Journal of Veterinary Research*, **66**, 574–580.

65 Sanchez, L.C. & Merritt, A.M. (2005) Colorectal distention in the horse: Visceral sensitivity, rectal compliance and effect of i.v. xylazine or intrarectal lidocaine. *Equine Veterinary Journal*, **37**, 70–74.

66 Farstvedt, E.G. & Hendrickson, D.A. (2005) Intraoperative pain responses following intraovarian versus mesovarian injection of lidocaine in mares undergoing laparoscopic ovariectomy. *Journal of the American Veterinary Medical Association*, **227**, 593–596.

67 Muir, W.W. (2012) NMDA receptor antagonists and pain: Ketamine. *Veterinary Clinics of North America Equine Practice*, **26**, 565–578.

68 Pozzi, A., Muir, W.W. & Traverso, F. (2006) Prevention of central sensitization and pain by N-methyl-D-aspartate receptor antagonists. *Journal of the American Veterinary Medical Association*, **228**, 53–60.

69 Alcott, C.J., Sponseller, B.A., Wong, D.M. *et al.* (2011) Clinical and immunomodulating effects of ketamine in horses with experimental endotoxemia. *Journal of Veterinary Internal Medicine*, **25**, 934–943.

70 Elfenbein, J.R., Robertson, S.A., Corser, A.A., Urion, R.J. & Sanchez, L.C. (2011) Systemic effects of a prolonged continuous infusion of ketamine in healthy horses. *Journal of Veterinary Internal Medicine*, **25**, 1134–1137.

71 Lankveld, D.P., Driessen, B., Soma, L.R. *et al.* (2006) Pharmacodynamic effects and pharmacokinetic profile of a long-term continuous rate infusion of racemic ketamine in healthy conscious horses. *Journal of Veterinary Pharmacology and Therapeutics*, **29**, 477–488.

72 Fielding, C.L., Brumbaugh, G.W., Matthews, N.S., Peck, K.E. & Roussel, A.J. (2006) Pharmacokinetics and clinical effects of a subanesthetic continuous rate infusion of ketamine in awake horses. *American Journal of Veterinary Research*, **67**, 1484–1490.

73 Wagner, A.E., Mama, K.R., Contino, E.K., Ferris, D.J. & Kawcak, C.E. (2011) Evaluation of sedation and analgesia in standing horses after administration of xylazine, butorphanol, and subanesthetic doses of ketamine. *Journal of the American Veterinary Medical Association*, **238**, 1629–1633.

74 Jones, E., Vinuela-Fernandez, I., Eager, R.A. *et al.* (2007) Neuropathic changes in equine laminitis pain. *Pain*, **132**, 321–331.

75 Boatwright, C.E., Fubini, S.L., Grohn, Y.T. & Goossens, L. (1996) A comparison of N-butylscopolammonium bromide and butorphanol tartrate for analgesia using a balloon model of abdominal pain in ponies. *Canadian Journal of Veterinary Research*, **60**, 65–68.

76 Roelvink, M.E., Goossens, L., Kalsbeek, H.C. & Wensing, T. (1991) Analgesic and spasmolytic effects of dipyrone, hyoscine-N-butylbromide and a combination of the two in ponies. *Veterinary Record*, **129**, 378–380.

77 Luo, T., Bertone, J.J., Greene, H.M. & Wickler, S.J. (2006) A comparison of N-butylscopolammonium and lidocaine for control of rectal pressure in horses. *Veterinary Therapeutics*, **7**, 243–248.

78 Baker, J.F. & Mulhall, K.J. (2012) Local anaesthetics and chondrotoxicity: What is the evidence? *Knee Surgery, Sports Traumatology, Arthroscopy* , **20**, 2294–2301.

79 Sheehy, J.G., Hellyer, P.W., Sammonds, G.E. *et al.* (2001) Evaluation of opioid receptors in synovial membranes of horses. *American Journal of Veterinary Research*, **62**, 1408–1412.

80 Tulamo, R.M., Raekallio, M., Taylor, P., Johnson, C.B. & Salonen, M. (1996) Intra-articular morphine and saline injections induce release of large molecular weight proteoglycans into equine synovial fluid. *Zentralblatt für Veterinärmedizin A*, **43**, 147–153.

81 Raekallio, M., Taylor, P., Johnson, C.B., Tulamo, R.M. & Ruprah, M. (1996) The disposition and local effects of intra-articular morphine in normal ponies. *Journal of Veterinary Anaesthesia*, **23**, 23–26.

82 Santos, L.C., de Moraes, A.N. & Saito, M.E. (2009) Effects of intraarticular ropivacaine and morphine on lipopolysaccharide-induced synovitis in horses. *Veterinary Anaesthesia and Analgesia*, **36**, 280–286.

83 Ball, M.A., Cable, C.S. & Kirker, E.J. (1998) How to place an epidural catheter and indications for its use. Proceedings of the 44th Annual Convention of the American Association of Equine Practitioners, Baltimore, MD, pp. 182–185.

84 van Loon, J.P., Menke, E.S., L'Ami, J.J., Jonckheer-Sheehy, V.S., Back, W. & René van Weeren, P. (2012) Analgesic and anti-hyperalgesic effects of epidural morphine in an equine LPS-induced acute synovitis model. *Veterinary Journal*, **193**, 464–470.

85 Natalini, C.C. & Robinson, E.P. (2000) Evaluation of the analgesic effects of epidurally administered morphine, alfentanil, butorphanol, tramadol, and U50488H in horses. *American Journal of Veterinary Research*, **61**, 1579–1586.

86 Olbrich, V.H. & Mosing, M. (2003) A comparison of the analgesic effects of caudal epidural methadone and lidocaine in the horse. *Veterinary Anaesthesia and Analgesia*, **30**, 156–164.

87 Skarda, R.T. & Muir, W.W., 3rd. (1996) Comparison of antinociceptive, cardiovascular, and respiratory effects, head ptosis, and position of pelvic limbs in mares after caudal epidural administration of xylazine and detomidine hydrochloride solution. *American Journal of Veterinary Research*, **57**, 1338–1345.

88 Skarda, R.T. & Muir, W.W., 3rd. (1996) Analgesic, hemody-namic, and respiratory effects of caudal epidurally adminis-tered xylazine hydrochloride solution in mares. *American Journal of Veterinary Research*, **57**, 193–200.

89 LeBlanc, P.H. & Caron, J.P. (1990) Clinical use of epidural xylazine in the horse. *Equine Veterinary Journal*, **22**, 180–181.

90 LeBlanc, P.H., Caron, J.P., Patterson, J.S., Brown, M. & Matta, M.A. (1988) Epidural injection of xylazine for peri-neal analgesia in horses. *Journal of the American Veterinary Medical Association*, **193**, 1405–1408.

91 Gomez de Segura, I.A., De Rossi, R., Santos, M., López San-Roman, J., Tendillo, F.J. & San-Roman, F. (1998) Epidural injection of ketamine for perineal analgesia in the horse. *Veterinary Surgery*, **27**, 384–391.

92 Sysel, A.M., Pleasant, R.S., Jacobson, J.D. *et al.* (1996) Efficacy of an epidural combination of morphine and deto-midine in alleviating experimentally induced hindlimb lameness in horses. *Veterinary Surgery*, **25**, 511–518.

93 Goodrich, L.R., Nixon, A.J., Fubini, S.L. *et al.* (2002) Epidural morphine and detomidine decreases postoperative hindlimb lameness in horses after bilateral stifle arthroscopy. *Veterinary Surgery*, **31**, 232–239.

94 Grubb, T.L., Riebold, T.W. & Huber, M.J. (1992) Comparison of lidocaine, xylazine, and xylazine/lidocaine for caudal epi-dural analgesia in horses. *Journal of the American Veterinary Medical Association*, **201**, 1187–1190.

95 Sysel, A.M., Pleasant, R.S., Jacobson, J.D. *et al.* (1997) Systemic and local effects associated with long-term epidural catheterization and morphine-detomidine administration in horses. *Veterinary Surgery*, **26**, 141–149.

96 Martin, C.A., Kerr, C.L., Pearce, S.G., Lansdowne, J.L. & Bouré, L.P. (2003) Outcome of epidural catheterization for delivery of analgesics in horses: 43 cases (1998–2001). *Journal of the American Veterinary Medical Association*, **222**, 1394–1398.

97 Burford, J.H. & Corley, K.T. (2006) Morphine-associated pruritus after single extradural administration in a horse. *Veterinary Anaesthesia and Analgesia*, **33**, 193–198.

98 Arguedas, M.G., Hines, M.T., Papich, M.G., Farnsworth, K.D. & Sellon, D.C. (2008) Pharmacokinetics of butorpha-nol and evaluation of physiologic and behavioral effects after intravenous and intramuscular administration to neo-natal foals. *Journal of Veterinary Internal Medicine*, **22**, 1417–1426.

99 McGowan, K.T., Elfenbein, J.R., Robertson, S.A. & Sanchez, L.C. (2013) Effect of butorphanol on thermal nociceptive threshold in healthy pony foals. *Equine Veterinary Journal*, **45**, 503–506.

100 Eberspacher, E., Stanley, S.D., Rezende, M. & Steffey, E.P. (2008) Pharmacokinetics and tolerance of transdermal fentanyl administration in foals. *Veterinary Anaesthesia and Analgesia*, **35**, 249–255.

101 Dunlop, C.I. (1994) Anesthesia and sedation of foals. *Veterinary Clinics of North America Equine Practice*, **10**, 67–85.

102 Bidwell, L.A., Wilson, D.V. & Caron, J.P. (2007) Lack of systemic absorption of lidocaine from 5% patches placed on horses. *Veterinary Anaesthesia and Analgesia*, **34**, 443–446.

103 Wagner, K.A., Gibbon, K.J., Strom, T.L., Kurian, J.R. & Trepanier, L.A. (2006) Adverse effects of EMLA (lidocaine/prilocaine) cream and efficacy for the placement of jugular catheters in hospitalized cats. *Journal of Feline Medicine and Surgery*, **8**, 141–144.

104 Robertson, S.A. (2006) Anesthesia and analgesia for foals. In: J.A. Auer & J.A. Stick (eds), *Equine Surgery*, 3rd edn, pp. 227–238. Saunders, St Louis.

105 Naylor, J.M., Garven, E. & Fraser, L. (1997) A comparison of romifidine and xylazine in foals: The effects on sedation and analgesia. *Equine Veterinary Education*, **9**, 329–334.

CHAPTER 5

Pharmacology of nonsteroidal anti-inflammatory drugs

Cynthia Cole

Mars Veterinary, Portland, OR, USA

The objective of this chapter is to provide a thorough, but concise, review of the pharmacology of nonsteroidal anti-inflammatory drugs (NSAIDs). NSAIDs are some of the most commonly used medications in equine practice but are associated with a significant risk of adverse events. The pharmacology of specific nonsteroidal agents is covered in Chapter 13.

The inflammatory cascade

The term inflammation comes from the Latin word "inflammo," meaning to ignite or set alight. The inciting cause of all inflammation is some form of cellular injury, such as microbial invasion or nonorganic thermal, chemical, or physical damage. At the onset of injury, the cells already present in the tissues, such as resident macrophages, dendritic cells, and mastocytes, release inflammatory mediators including bradykinins (BK), prostaglandins (PGs), and leukotrienes (LT). These mediators produce a myriad of responses that culminate in the cardinal signs of inflammation. Redness (*rubor*) and heat (*calor*) are produced by vasodilation, which results in increased blood flow, and swelling (*tumor*) is produced by increased permeability of the blood vessels, which results in exudation of plasma proteins and fluid. Some mediators increase sensitivity to pain (*dolor*), and pain and swelling at the site of injury lead to loss of use (*functio laesa*), the final cardinal sign of inflammation. If the inciting stimulus is removed by the response, the inflammation will resolve and tissue healing will be initiated. If the stimulus is not eliminated, however, the inflammation may transition into a chronic response, which is often associated with excessive fibroblast activity and scar formation.

Although the inflammatory cascade is complex, members of the family of compounds referred to as eicosanoids, which include the PG, LT, and thromboxanes (TX), have been shown to play key roles in the process [1]. Any injury that perturbs the cell membrane releases phospholipids that are rapidly converted to arachidonic acid (AA) by phospholipase A2 and other acyl hydrolases. Once released, AA forms the substrate for a number of enzyme systems. Products that contain ring structures (PG and TX) are the result of metabolism by the PG G/H synthases that are more commonly referred to as cyclooxygenase (COX) enzymes. LT are straight-chain fatty acids formed by the 5-lipoxygenase enzymatic pathway [1]. Currently, two isoforms of the COX enzyme, known as COX1 and COX2, have been well described [2]. COX1 is constitutively expressed in most normal tissues, where COX2 expression is generally low. COX2 expression is highly inducible, however, and production increases dramatically in the presence of inflammation. For example, in quiescent unstimulated rat macrophages, COX1, but not COX2, can be readily detected [3]. When macrophages are exposed to bacterial lipopolysaccharides, however, COX2 expression significantly increases, while COX1 levels remain unchanged or increase to a lesser degree [3, 4]. Unfortunately, the activities of COX1 and COX2 in the body cannot be neatly divided into respective homeostatic and inflammatory roles. It appears that the constitutively produced COX1 enzyme plays a key

Equine Pharmacology, First Edition. Edited by Cynthia Cole, Bradford Bentz and Lara Maxwell.
© 2015 John Wiley & Sons, Inc. Published 2015 by John Wiley & Sons, Inc.

role in the initial acute inflammatory response, and in humans and laboratory animals, it has been shown that constitutively produced COX2 enzymes produce PGs critical in cardiovascular and renal homeostasis [5]. The homeostatic and inflammatory roles of the COX1 and COX2 isoforms have not been well defined in any veterinary species, particularly the horse.

The four PGs that provide the majority of biological activity are PGE_2, PGI_2, PGD_2, and $PGF_2\alpha$. Their common precursor is PGH_2, which is produced by both COX1 and COX2 [5]. PGs are ubiquitously produced, but each cell type usually only generates one or two of the PG subtypes. As previously discussed, they are constitutively produced at low levels in many tissues and serve as autocrine and paracrine mediators to maintain local homeostatic processes. With activation of the inflammatory cascade, their synthesis increases dramatically [5]. PGs produce their effects by binding to G protein-coupled receptors that are in turn coupled to numerous intracellular signaling pathways including, but not limited to, adenyl cyclase, phosphatidylinositol metabolism, and alterations in intracellular free calcium.

Each PG has unique roles in homeostatic and inflammatory processes. PGE_2 is one of the most abundant PGs produced in the body, and it plays critical roles in many physiological processes within the immune, gastrointestinal (GI), and reproductive systems. It also plays a particularly critical role in the inflammatory process, as it causes arterial dilation, increased microvascular permeability, and sensitization of peripheral and central sensory neurons. The COX2 isoform in endothelial and vascular smooth muscle cells are the major source of PGI_2, which is a primary regulator of cardiovascular homeostasis [5]. PGI_2 is a potent vasodilator and inhibitor of platelet aggregation, leukocyte adhesion, and proliferation of vascular smooth muscle cells [6]. In addition to homeostatic roles in the cardiovascular system, however, PGI_2 is also an important mediator in the setting of acute inflammation, causing edema and pain. PGD_2 plays homeostatic roles in sleep and other CNS activities but is also produced in large amounts by activated mast cells, and as such, it plays critical roles in IgE-mediated type I acute allergic responses and asthma. Finally, $PGF_2\alpha$ is derived primarily from COX1 activity and is an important mediator in the female reproductive cycle. In addition, it plays roles in renal function and acute and chronic inflammation [5].

Both COX isoforms also mediate the formation of TXA_2, which is an unstable AA metabolite with a half-life of approximately 30 s. The COX1 enzyme in platelets is the major source of TXA_2 in the body under normal conditions, but during inflammation, it is also produced by COX2 in inflammatory cells. TXA_2 is a primary mediator of platelet adhesion and aggregation, smooth muscle cell contraction and proliferation, and activation of endothelial inflammatory responses. Because so many of its effects are antagonist to those mediated by PGI_2, TXA_2 is often thought of as an opposing mediator.

NSAIDs are competitive site inhibitors of both COX isoforms. Although the numerous classes of NSAIDs are structurally distinct, they all share the capacity to inhibit eicosanoid production. Their clinical efficacy demonstrates the importance of eicosanoids in the inflammatory pathway. Because the COX2 isoform plays such a critical role in the inflammatory process and was thought to play only minor roles in homeostatic processes, agents that selectively inhibit that isoform were proposed as safer alternatives to nonselective NSAIDs. In humans, COX2 selective NSAIDs were found to cause significantly fewer GI side effects but were unfortunately associated with an increase in the incidence of thromboembolic events, such as heart attack and stroke [7]. It has been proposed that the mechanism of these adverse events is directly related to decreased production of COX2-mediated PGI_2 in cardiovascular tissues [8]. Because of these adverse events, only one COX2 selective agent labeled for use in humans remains in the US market at this point in time. Fortunately, ischemic cardiovascular events have not been observed in veterinary species, and COX2 selective agents have been reported to have a much wider safety margin in these species than nonselective NSAIDs. Nevertheless, equine practitioners need to be aware that the physiological roles of the COX1 and COX2 isoforms have not been well characterized in the horse. In addition, it should be remembered that agents that are considered COX2 selective inhibitors will also inhibit COX1 at higher concentrations. Therefore, the true safety of COX2 selective agents in horses has yet to be determined, and more study is needed. In addition, cost, particularly in equine medicine, often limits the adoption of new drugs, and the COX2 selective agents are no exception. For this reason alone, nonselective NSAIDs will continue to be used extensively in equine medicine for some time to come, and equine practitioners need to understand their pharmacology so as to maximize their efficacy and minimize the risks associated with their use.

Indications and use of NSAIDs in horses

NSAIDs are most commonly administered to horses for relief of musculoskeletal pain and inflammation, and phenylbutazone is the agent most frequently prescribed for this purpose. Flunixin meglumine is the NSAID of choice for acute GI distress or colic, fever, and soft tissue inflammation, but it can also be used for musculoskeletal issues. In addition, flunixin meglumine is often administered to counteract the systemic effects of endotoxemia; however, there is some experimental evidence that other NSAIDs, such as ketoprofen, aspirin, and phenylbutazone, may also possess anti-endotoxic properties [9, 10].

There are a number of misperceptions regarding the use of NSAIDs in horses. First, in terms of efficacy, despite anecdotal reports to the contrary, there is very little evidence that any one of the NSAIDs commonly used in horses is any more or less effective than another [11–14]. The results of studies comparing one NSAID to another are highly variable. The agent that appears most efficacious in any particular study depends largely on the model used and the dose and frequency of the NSAID administered. Another misperception held by some practitioners is that potency of an NSAID correlates with efficacy. Potency refers to the drug's strength, and it is the relationship between the amount of drug administered and the therapeutic effect it produces. Efficacy, in contrast, is the ability of a drug to produce the desired therapeutic effect. If two NSAIDs are equally efficacious, differences in potency are rarely clinically important, because it is generally not difficult to administer a larger total dose to a horse. There is also some question as to whether administering more than one NSAID concomitantly produces effects that are additive or synergistic in terms of efficacy. The scientific literature provides evidence both to support and refute this common clinical practice often referred to as "stacking." For example, the results of one study that evaluated the drugs in naturally occurring lamenesses found a synergistic effect of the concomitant administration of phenylbutazone

and flunixin meglumine compared to the effects of phenylbutazone alone [15]. However, in another study that used an inducible model of foot pain, no synergistic effect was observed when concomitant flunixin meglumine and phenylbutazone administration was compared to administration of each NSAID alone [16]. The conflicting results may be due to differences in the pain models used in each study and/or the dosing regimens. In the former Keegan *et al.* study, for example, efficacy was determined after 5 days of NSAID administration, whereas in the latter Foreman *et al.* study, efficacy was first determined 20 min after the horses were administered a single dose of the NSAID and additional evaluations were conducted for up to 12 h after dosing. Based on the results of these studies, it remains to be determined whether stacking is actually more efficacious than administration of a single NSAID. There is, however, evidence that the duration of action of an NSAID can be prolonged by concurrent administration of another NSAID. For example, in one study, concurrent administration of flunixin meglumine and phenylbutazone did not alter the pharmacokinetics of either agent in plasma, but the combination of the two inhibited serum TXB_2 production for a significantly longer period (24 h) than either flunixin meglumine (12 h) or phenylbutazone (8 h) alone [17]. There is also evidence that concurrent administration of NSAIDs is associated with an increased risk of gastric ulcer development [18]. Whether the increased risk of ulcer formation is any greater than that associated with administration of higher doses of a single NSAID alone has not been determined.

Pharmacokinetics of NSAIDs in horses

Although NSAIDs are a large and structurally diverse group of compounds, they share a number of common features in horses. For example, most NSAIDs are administered either intravenously or orally (PO). Occasionally, they are administered intramuscularly, but necrotizing myositis has been associated with this route of administration [19]. In addition, some formulations, particularly the injectable formulation of phenylbutazone, can be extremely irritating when administered IM and should only be administered IV.

Although most, but not all, NSAIDs are well absorbed following oral administration, there is some variability in the bioavailability among different horses [20]. In addition, the presence of ingesta in the proximal GI tract of the horse has been shown to decrease the rate and the extent of absorption of NSAIDs, such as flunixin meglumine, meclofenamic acid, and phenylbutazone, following oral administration.

As one might expect from such a structurally diverse group, the pharmacokinetic parameters of NSAIDs in the horse are highly variable. For example, the plasma elimination half-lives of meclofenamic acid and ketoprofen are relatively short at 1–2 h in the horse, while the half-lives of firocoxib and carprofen are long at over 18 and 40 h, respectively [21–24]. Although phenylbutazone has a variable plasma elimination half-life, most commonly, it is determined to be in the range of 6–8 h [25]. Somewhat paradoxically, however, the duration of effect of many, but not all, NSAIDs in horses is fairly long, even those with short plasma elimination half-lives. For example, ketoprofen has been shown to be an effective NSAID in horses when administered only once per day, despite its short half-life [13]. This may be due in part to the tendencies of most NSAIDs to bind with very high avidity to the COX enzyme, to concentrate in areas of inflammation, and to exhibit prolonged clearance from inflammatory loci [13, 22]. For example, 1 h after administration of ketoprofen IV, the synovial fluid concentration of the NSAID was 6.5 times higher in horses with carrageenan-induced synovitis than in normal control horses [22]. In a similar manner, the half-life of flunixin in carrageenan-induced inflammatory exudates collected from subcutaneously implanted tissue cages was approximately 16 h, whereas the plasma half-life of the NSAID in the same horses was only 4 h [13]. It is also important to note that in the presence of inflammation, the plasma pharmacokinetics of NSAIDs may be altered. For example, in one study, the clearance and volume of distribution (V_d) of phenylbutazone were increased in horses with experimentally induced inflammatory loci compared to normal horses [26]. The rate of elimination of ketoprofen in horses with experimentally induced inflammation was also more rapid than in normal horses [22]. Whether the more rapid clearance of the NSAID is important clinically, however, is unknown, because as previously discussed in horses,

the plasma elimination half-life does not directly correlate with the duration of effect of most NSAIDs.

Adverse effects of the use of NSAIDs in horses

Gastrointestinal effects

In the horse, the most frequently reported side effect of NSAID therapy is GI ulceration, which results primarily from the inhibition of cytoprotective PG production. For example, ponies administered phenylbutazone alone developed multifocal GI ulceration, while those administered PGE_2 concurrently with phenylbutazone did not develop significant GI lesions [27]. The roles of the COX1 and COX2 isoforms in GI cytoprotection are complex. Although COX1 is the predominant isoform expressed in the GI tract of every species studied, including the horse, it appears that inhibition of COX1 and COX2 is required to produce GI ulceration. For example, in mice, small intestinal ulceration was observed when the COX2 selective agent celecoxib and the COX1 selective inhibitor SC-560 were administered concurrently, but not when either compound was administered alone [28]. Nevertheless, in all of the species examined, including the horse, NSAIDs that selectively inhibit COX2 produce less GI ulceration than nonselective COX inhibitors [29].

In the GI tract, PGs protect the integrity of the gastric mucosa by a number of different mechanisms. For example, they inhibit gastric acid secretion stimulated by feeding, gastrin, and histamine, and they increase blood flow to the gastric mucosa. PGs also induce mucus and electrolyte secretion into the GI lumen. In addition to inhibiting the production of cytoprotective PG, NSAIDs are weak acids that can directly injure the gastric mucosa.

The erosive effects of NSAIDs in the GI tract are dose related, with higher doses increasing the likelihood that ulceration will develop. For example, when horses were administered three times the recommended dosage of flunixin meglumine (1.1 mg/kg bwt), ketoprofen (2.2 mg/kg bwt), and phenylbutazone (4.4 mg/kg bwt) for 12 days, all the horses developed significant GI ulceration, with the glandular portion of the stomach being the most severely affected [30]. Ponies appear to be more susceptible to the erosive effects of NSAIDs, with signs of toxicity occurring at dosages usually well tolerated by horses [31]. In the horse, the right dorsal colon also appears to be particularly susceptible to the ulcerogenic effects of NSAIDs [32]. Prolonged treatment with even moderate doses of phenylbutazone and the use of any NSAIDs in the presence of concurrent hypovolemia appear to predispose the horse to development of ulceration of the right dorsal colon. It has not been determined why the right dorsal colon is more susceptible to the effects of NSAIDs, although it has been hypothesized that blood flow to this area is more dependent on PG-mediated vasodilation than other regions of the colon [32]. In one study examining the effects of phenylbutazone on the right dorsal colon, horses treated with the high doses of phenylbutazone (8.8 mg/kg bwt, PO, q24 h for 21 days) developed hypoalbuminemia, hypoproteinemia, and neutropenia, although histological evidence of colitis was not apparent on postmortem examination [32]. Monitoring serum albumin concentrations may be a particularly sensitive method of detecting early signs of colonic mucosal dysfunction associated with phenylbutazone toxicity, but whether this monitoring is applicable to other NSAIDs remains to be determined.

The results from human and canine studies provide good evidence that COX2 selective NSAIDs cause less GI side effects than nonselective NSAIDs. Firocoxib (Equioxx®, Merial Limited, Duluth, GA) is the only COX2 selective inhibitor approved for use in the horse in the USA, and there is evidence that it causes less GI side effects than other commonly used nonselective agents, such as phenylbutazone [11]. Firocoxib is not entirely devoid of adverse effects, however, particularly at higher doses. In addition, the results of studies in humans and laboratory animals suggest that the COX2 isoform plays a significant role in the healing of GI ulcers [33]. Whether this is true in the horse has not been determined, but if GI ulceration is suspected, it may be prudent to allow a washout period of several days when transitioning a horse off of a nonselective COX inhibitor, such as phenylbutazone, to firocoxib.

Renal effects

In normal horses, therapeutic doses of NSAIDs have little effect on renal function or blood flow. The administration of high doses of NSAIDs to normal animals, however, can cause acute renal failure [34]. Even therapeutic doses of NSAIDs can result in the development of acute renal failure in patients who are volume depleted, are hypotensive, or have preexisting renal disease [35]. As

in the GI tract, the negative effects of NSAIDs on the kidneys are thought to result from inhibition of the production of protective PGs. Across numerous species, COX1 is the most abundant isoform expressed in the kidney, and it is regionally localized in the renal vasculature, collecting ducts, and papillary interstitial cells, although the horse has not been well studied [29]. Although under normal conditions, COX2 expression is minimal, it still appears to play an important role in normal renal function. For example, COX2-deficient mice exhibit severely impaired renal development and function [36]. Determining the physiological roles of each COX isoform, however, is complicated, because expression can be affected by inflammation, as well as other factors, such as high-salt diets, hypovolemia, and hypotension [37]. PGI_2 and PGE_2, produced during periods of hypovolemia and hypotension, cause afferent arteriolar dilation, which acts to maintain renal blood flow and glomerular filtration rate. The PGs also counteract the effects of systemic vasoconstrictor agents, such as angiotensin II and antidiuretic hormone. There is also evidence that PGs help to maintain blood flow and glomerular filtration in the surviving nephrons in human patients suffering from chronic renal failure. The COX isoforms responsible for these protective processes in the kidney are not well defined, particularly in the horse, but based on the results of studies carried out in humans and laboratory animals, COX2 does appear to play a role [38].

In the horse, renal papillary necrosis can be a sequela to NSAID therapy [39–42]. It is, however, less common than GI ulceration and most commonly occurs when NSAIDs are administered to animals that are dehydrated or have decreased renal perfusion. There is some disagreement as to the clinical importance of renal papillary necrosis. For example, one report indicates that renal papillary necrosis is most often an incidental finding and not associated with clinical renal disease [39, 40]. In another study, however, in which large doses of phenylbutazone were given to normal horses, renal papillary necrosis was associated with renal failure, indicated by progressive increases in serum creatinine, blood urea nitrogen, and phosphorus and decreases in serum calcium concentrations [41]. It has been hypothesized that blood flow to the renal pelvis is marginal in the horse and in the presence of even mild dehydration or hypotension, maintaining adequate blood flow may require PG-mediated vasodilation [41]. Under these conditions, the renal pelvis of the horse may be exquisitely sensitive to ischemic necrosis induced by the anti-PG effects of NSAIDs. Nevertheless, the physiological roles of the COX1 and COX2 isoforms in the horse renal pelvis have not been well defined.

In summary, PGs play important roles in maintaining renal blood flow and thus renal function. The inhibition of these responses by NSAIDs can have significant effects on renal function and viability during periods of hypoperfusion or concurrent renal damage. The risk of developing analgesic nephropathy is highest in geriatric cases and in those with preexisting renal, cardiac, or liver disease, dehydration, and shock or those undergoing concurrent therapy with nephrotoxic drugs. Because the renal effects of COX2 selective agents have not been determined, at this point in time, it is not known whether they are safer than nonselective NSAIDs in terms of this organ system. Therefore, they should be used with caution in the at-risk horse until more information is available.

Plasma protein binding

Most NSAIDs are highly bound to plasma proteins, with the bound fraction approaching 99% for some agents. Care should be taken when administering NSAIDs concurrently with other compounds that are also highly protein bound, such as other NSAIDs, sulfonamides, and gentamicin, because these compounds will compete for binding sites on the plasma proteins. The ultimate effect of this displacement is difficult to predict. As it is the unbound fraction (or free drug) in the plasma that is responsible for the drug's activity, this displacement could result in an increase in the drug's observed clinical effect. However, an increase in the unbound fraction can also be associated with a parallel increase in the rate of elimination. For example, when phenylbutazone and gentamicin were concurrently administered to horses, the plasma half-life and the V_d for gentamicin decreased by 23 and 26%, respectively, while the kinetic parameters of phenylbutazone were unaffected [43]. Phenylbutazone has also been shown to enhance the anticoagulation properties of warfarin. Studies in humans, however, suggest that this effect is primarily mediated through differential inhibition of the metabolism of the more active S isomer of warfarin rather than interference with albumin binding [44]. The study, however, has not been duplicated in the horse, so whether the same differential effect on metabolism

occurs in this species is unknown. Therefore, although the clinical relevance of protein binding displacement in the interaction between warfarin and NSAIDs may have been overstated, it has not been eliminated, and a significant effect may be more likely in the presence of high concentrations of NSAIDs in patients with slow elimination of warfarin (e.g., those with severe heart failure or impaired liver function) [45]. Because it is hard to predict the outcome when NSAIDs are administered concurrently with other highly protein-bound drugs, relevant pharmacokinetic or pharmacodynamic parameters should be monitored. For example, when an aminoglycoside and an NSAID are administered concurrently, serum concentrations of the aminoglycoside should be monitored to ensure that they are within the desired therapeutic range. Doses should be adjusted based on changes in the monitored parameters and not on hypothetically predicted sequelae.

Hepatic effects

Nearly all NSAIDs have the potential to induce hepatic injury, although this effect has not been documented in the horse. In other species, hepatic injury associated with most NSAIDs is an idiosyncratic reaction with a low incidence of occurrence. The hepatotoxicity of carprofen in dogs, for example, was not observed until the NSAID was in widespread use in the USA [46]. The hepatotoxicity of a few compounds, such as aspirin and acetaminophen (paracetamol), however, is a dose-dependent side effect that is well described in some species [47].

Although the horse appears to be refractory to the hepatic effects of most NSAIDs, their hepatotoxic potential should be considered, especially when they are concomitantly administered with other potentially hepatotoxic agents, such as fluoroquinolones, potentiated sulfonamides, or anabolic steroids. In addition, many herbal preparations are potential hepatotoxins, and clients may administer these compounds concomitantly with prescribed NSAIDs without consulting their veterinarian. Echinacea and kava kava products, for example, are reported to be potential hepatotoxins, and both are used in herbal remedies that claim to produce calming or sedating effects in horses [48].

Coagulation effects

Because of their inhibition of COX1 activity, NSAIDs can inhibit platelet aggregation. The extent and the duration of this inhibition, and thus its clinical relevancy, vary with the NSAID. For example, aspirin irreversibly inactivates platelet COX1, making it a very effective antithrombotic agent in most species [49]. In contrast, neither flunixin meglumine nor phenylbutazone had any significant effect on bleeding times in horses. The effect of other commonly used NSAIDs on coagulation in horses is less clear. For example, in dogs, ketoprofen has been shown to prolong the bleeding time significantly in some studies, but not in others. The effects of ketoprofen on coagulation have not been determined in horses [50, 51]. In contrast, multiple studies in dogs have failed to detect any clinically significant effects of carprofen on coagulation profiles [50, 52]. Nevertheless, because the effects of these NSAIDs on bleeding parameters in horses have not been determined, the use of any NSAID in the presence of a bleeding tendency should be carefully considered.

Novel targets of classic NSAIDs

As previously discussed, PG and TX are crucial mediators in the development of inflammation, pain, and fever. Consequently, blocking the synthesis of PG and TX has been accepted as the major mechanism by which NSAIDs produce their effects. There is a growing body of evidence, however, that some NSAIDs produce anti-inflammatory and analgesic effects independent of COX inhibition. For example, in humans, low doses of aspirin trigger synthesis of lipoxins, which are generated from AA but which have a number of immunomodulatory and anti-inflammatory actions. Lipoxins are high-affinity ligands for the lipoxin A_4 receptor (ALX), and activation of this receptor inhibits chemotaxis, transmigration, superoxide generation, and nuclear factor kappa-light-chain-enhancer of activated B cell (NF-κB) synthesis [53]. NF-κB is a protein complex that controls transcription of DNA. NF-κB, which is found in almost all cells, plays a critical role in cellular responses to stimuli, such as stress, cytokines, free radicals, and bacterial or viral antigens. Dysregulation of NF-κB has been linked to cancer, inflammatory and autoimmune diseases, septic shock, and viral infections. Other NSAIDs have been shown to inhibit the actions of other key inflammatory mediators. For example, nimesulide and ibuprofen inhibit TNFα, and other NSAIDs affect the responses of T cells to IL-2 [54, 55]. The effects of other inflammatory mediators, such protein kinase C,

substance P, and BK, have also been shown to be modulated by various NSAIDs [56, 57].

New NSAIDs

The recognition that at least some of the anti-inflammatory effects of NSAIDs are produced through modulation of intracellular signaling pathways has led to the search for specific and potent inhibitors of those pathways. Unlike classical NSAIDs, these new therapeutic agents are not small molecules, but are peptides and antibodies. For example, the recombinant molecule etanercept is a fusion protein produced by recombinant DNA technology that acts as a TNF inhibitor. It is a large molecule, with a molecular weight of 150 kDa, which binds to TNFα, decreasing its activity. In humans and other animals, etanercept has been effective in the treatment of disorders involving excess inflammation, including autoimmune diseases such as ankylosing spondylitis, juvenile rheumatoid arthritis, psoriasis, psoriatic arthritis, rheumatoid arthritis, and, potentially, in a variety of other diseases mediated by excess TNFα [58]. In a similar manner, infliximab is a chimeric human–murine anti-TNFα monoclonal antibody, and adalimumab is a fully human anti-TNF monoclonal antibody. These agents have shown great promise in treating severe autoimmune diseases in humans, although they also produce significant immunosuppression. Whether or not similar therapeutic approaches could be developed in a cost-effective manner for use in the horse remains to be determined.

References

1 Flower RJ, Moncada S, Vane JR. Analgesic, antipyretic, and anti-inflammatory agents. In: Gilman AG, Goodman L, Rall TW, Murad F, eds. *Goodman and Gilman's the Pharmacological Basis of Therapeutics*, 7th ed. New York: Macmillan, 1985;674–715.

2 Vane, J.R. & Botting, R.M. (1995) New insights into the mode of action of anti-inflammatory drugs. *Inflammation Research*, **44**, 1–10.

3 Lee, S.H., Soyoola, E., Chanmugam, P. *et al.* (1992) Selective expression of mitogen-inducible cyclooxygenase in macrophages stimulated with lipopolysaccharide. *Journal of Biological Chemistry*, **267**, 25934–25938.

4 McAdam, B.F., Mardini, I.A., Habib, A. *et al.* (2000) Effect of regulated expression of human cyclooxygenase isoforms on eicosanoid and isoeicosanoid production in inflammation. *Journal of Clinical Investigation*, **105**, 1473–1482.

5 Ricciotti, E. & FitzGerald, G.A. (2011) Prostaglandins and inflammation. *Arteriosclerosis, Thrombosis, and Vascular Biology*, **31**, 986–1000.

6 McAdam, B.F., Catella-Lawson, F., Mardini, I.A., Kapoor, S., Lawson, J.A. & FitzGerald, G.A. (1999) Systemic biosynthesis of prostacyclin by cyclooxygenase (COX)-2: The human pharmacology of a selective inhibitor of COX-2. *Proceedings of the National Academy of Sciences of the USA*, **96**, 272–277.

7 Mukherjee, D., Nissen, S.E. & Topol, E.J. (2001) Risk of cardiovascular events associated with selective COX-2 inhibitors. *JAMA*, **286**, 954–959.

8 McGettigan, P., Han, P. & Henry, D. (2006) Cyclooxygenase-2 inhibitors and coronary occlusion—exploring dose-response relationships. *British Journal of Clinical Pharmacology*, **62**, 358–365.

9 Jackman, B.R., Moore, J.N., Barton, M.H. & Morris, D.D. (1994) Comparison of the effects of ketoprofen and flunixin meglumine on the in vitro response of equine peripheral blood monocytes to bacterial endotoxin. *Canadian Journal of Veterinary Research*, **58**, 138–143.

10 King, J.N. & Gerring, E.L. (1989) Antagonism of endotoxin-induced disruption of equine bowel motility by flunixin and phenylbutazone. *Equine Veterinary Journal Supplement*, 38–42.

11 Doucet, M.Y., Bertone, A.L., Hendrickson, D. *et al.* (2008) Comparison of efficacy and safety of paste formulations of firocoxib and phenylbutazone in horses with naturally occurring osteoarthritis. *Journal of the American Veterinary Medical Association*, **232**, 91–97.

12 Foreman, J.H., Grubb, T.L., Inoue, O.J., Banner, S.E. & Ball, K.T. (2010) Efficacy of single-dose intravenous phenylbutazone and flunixin meglumine before, during and after exercise in an experimental reversible model of foot lameness in horses. *Equine Veterinary Journal Supplement*, 601–605.

13 Landoni, M.F. & Lees, P. (1995) Comparison of the anti-inflammatory actions of flunixin and ketoprofen in horses applying PK/PD modelling. *Equine Veterinary Journal*, **27**, 247–256.

14 Owens, J.G., Kamerling, S.G., Stanton, S.R., Keowen, M.L. & Prescott-Mathews, J.S. (1996) Effects of pretreatment with ketoprofen and phenylbutazone on experimentally induced synovitis in horses. *American Journal of Veterinary Research*, **57**, 866–874.

15 Keegan, K.G., Messer, N.T., Reed, S.K., Wilson, D.A. & Kramer, J. (2008) Effectiveness of administration of phenylbutazone alone or concurrent administration of phenylbutazone and flunixin meglumine to alleviate lameness in horses. *American Journal of Veterinary Research*, **69**, 167–173.

16 Foreman, J.H. & Ruemmler, R. (2011) Phenylbutazone and flunixin meglumine used singly or in combination in experimental lameness in horses. *Equine Veterinary Journal Supplement*, 12–17.

17 Semrad, S.D., Sams, R.A., Harris, O.N. & Ashcraft, S.M. (1993) Effects of concurrent administration of phenylbutazone and flunixin meglumine on pharmacokinetic variables and in vitro generation of thromboxane B2 in mares. *American Journal of Veterinary Research*, **54**, 1901–1905.

18 Reed, S.K., Messer, N.T., Tessman, R.K. & Keegan, K.G. (2006) Effects of phenylbutazone alone or in combination with flunixin meglumine on blood protein concentrations in horses. *American Journal of Veterinary Research*, **67**, 398–402.

19 Kahn, L.H. & Styrt, B.A. (1997) Necrotizing soft tissue infections reported with nonsteroidal antiinflammatory drugs. *Annals of Pharmacotherapy*, **31**, 1034–1039.

20 Sullivan, M. & Snow, D.H. (1982) Factors affecting absorption of non-steroidal anti-inflammatory agents in the horse. *Veterinary Record*, **110**, 554–558.

21 Letendre, L.T., Tessman, R.K., McClure, S.R., Kvaternick, V.J., Fischer, J.B. & Hanson, P.D. (2008) Pharmacokinetics of firocoxib after administration of multiple consecutive daily doses to horses. *American Journal of Veterinary Research*, **69**, 1399–1405.

22 Owens, J.G., Kamerling, S.G. & Barker, S.A. (1995) Pharmacokinetics of ketoprofen in healthy horses and horses with acute synovitis. *Journal of Veterinary Pharmacology and Therapeutics*, **18**, 187–195.

23 Snow, D.H., Baxter, P. & Whiting, B. (1981) The pharmacokinetics of meclofenamic acid in the horse. *Journal of Veterinary Pharmacology and Therapeutics*, **4**, 147–156.

24 Lees, P., McKellar, Q., May, S.A. & Ludwig, B. (1994) Pharmacodynamics and pharmacokinetics of carprofen in the horse. *Equine Veterinary Journal*, **26**, 203–208.

25 Lees, P. & Higgins, A.J. (1985) Clinical pharmacology and therapeutic uses of non-steroidal anti-inflammatory drugs in the horse. *Equine Veterinary Journal*, **17**, 83–96.

26 Mills, P.C., Ng, J.C. & Auer, D.E. (1996) The effect of inflammation on the disposition of phenylbutazone in thoroughbred horses. *Journal of Veterinary Pharmacology and Therapeutics*, **19**, 475–481.

27 Collins, L.G. & Tyler, D.E. (1985) Experimentally induced phenylbutazone toxicosis in ponies: Description of the syndrome and its prevention with synthetic prostaglandin E2. *American Journal of Veterinary Research*, **46**, 1605–1615.

28 Sigthorsson, G., Simpson, R.J., Walley, M. *et al.* (2002) COX-1 and 2, intestinal integrity, and pathogenesis of nonsteroidal anti-inflammatory drug enteropathy in mice. *Gastroenterology*, **122**, 1913–1923.

29 Radi, Z.A. (2009) Pathophysiology of cyclooxygenase inhibition in animal models. *Toxicologic Pathology*, **37**, 34–46.

30 MacAllister, C.G., Morgan, S.J., Borne, A.T. & Pollet, R.A. (1993) Comparison of adverse effects of phenylbutazone, flunixin meglumine, and ketoprofen in horses. *Journal of the American Veterinary Medical Association*, **202**, 71–77.

31 Tobin, T., Chay, S., Kamerling, S. *et al.* (1986) Phenylbutazone in the horse: A review. *Journal of Veterinary Pharmacology and Therapeutics*, **9**, 1–25.

32 McConnico, R.S., Morgan, T.W., Williams, C.C., Hubert, J.D. & Moore, R.M. (2008) Pathophysiologic effects of phenylbutazone on the right dorsal colon in horses. *American Journal of Veterinary Research*, **69**, 1496–1505.

33 Peskar, B.M. (2005) Role of cyclooxygenase isoforms in gastric mucosal defense and ulcer healing. *Inflammopharmacology*, **13**, 15–26.

34 Henry, D. & McGettigan, P. (2003) Epidemiology overview of gastrointestinal and renal toxicity of NSAIDs. *International Journal of Clinical Practice Supplement*, 43–49.

35 Stillman, M.T. & Schlesinger, P.A. (1990) Nonsteroidal anti-inflammatory drug nephrotoxicity. Should we be concerned? *Archives of Internal Medicine*, **150**, 268–270.

36 Dinchuk, J.E., Car, B.D., Focht, R.J. *et al.* (1995) Renal abnormalities and an altered inflammatory response in mice lacking cyclooxygenase II. *Nature*, **378**, 406–409.

37 Yang, T., Singh, I., Pham, H. *et al.* (1998) Regulation of cyclooxygenase expression in the kidney by dietary salt intake. *American Journal of Physiology*, **274**, F481–F489.

38 Lopez, R., Roig, F., Llinas, M.T. & Salazar, F.J. (2003) Role of cyclooxygenase-2 in the control of renal haemodynamics and excretory function. *Acta Physiologica Scandinavica*, **177**, 429–435.

39 Gunson, D.E. (1983) Renal papillary necrosis in horses. *Journal of the American Veterinary Medical Association*, **182**, 263–266.

40 Gunson, D.E. & Soma, L.R. (1983) Renal papillary necrosis in horses after phenylbutazone and water deprivation. *Veterinary Pathology*, **20**, 603–610.

41 MacKay, R.J., French, T.W., Nguyen, H.T. & Mayhew, I.G. (1983) Effects of large doses of phenylbutazone administration to horses. *American Journal of Veterinary Research*, **44**, 774–780.

42 Ramirez, S., Seahorn, T.L. & Williams, J. (1998) Renal medullary rim sign in 2 adult quarter horses. *Canadian Veterinary Journal*, **39**, 647–649.

43 Whittem, T., Firth, E.C., Hodge, H. & Turner, K. (1996) Pharmacokinetic interactions between repeated dose phenylbutazone and gentamicin in the horse. *Journal of Veterinary Pharmacology and Therapeutics*, **19**, 454–459.

44 Lewis, J., Tragewr, W.F., Chan, K.K. *et al.* (1974) Warfarin: Stereochemical aspects of its metabolism and the interaction with phenylbutazone. *Journal of Clinical Investigation*, **53**, 1607–1617.

45 Chan, T.Y. (1995) Adverse interactions between warfarin and nonsteroidal antiinflammatory drugs: Mechanisms, clinical significance, and avoidance. *Annals of Pharmacotherapy*, **12**, 1274–1283.

46 MacPhail, C.M., Lappin, M.R., Meyer, D.J., Smith, S.G., Webster, C.R. & Armstrong, P.J. (1998) Hepatocellular toxicosis associated with administration of carprofen in 21 dogs. *Journal of the American Veterinary Medical Association*, **212**, 1895–1901.

47 Fry, S.W. & Seeff, L.B. (1995) Hepatotoxicity of analgesics and anti-inflammatory agents. *Gastroenterology Clinics of North America*, **24**, 875–905.

48 Abebe, W. (2002) Herbal medication: Potential for adverse interactions with analgesic drugs. *Journal of Clinical Pharmacy and Therapeutics*, **27**, 391–401.

49 Kopp, K.J., Moore, J.N., Byars, T.D. & Brooks, P. (1985) Template bleeding time and thromboxane generation in the horse: Effects of three non-steroidal anti-inflammatory drugs. *Equine Veterinary Journal*, **17**, 322–324.

50 Grisneaux, E., Pibarot, P., Dupuis, J. & Blais, D. (1999) Comparison of ketoprofen and carprofen administered prior to orthopedic surgery for control of postoperative pain in dogs. *Journal of the American Veterinary Medical Association*, **215**, 1105–1110.

51 Mathews, K.A., Pettifer, G., Foster, R. & McDonell, W. (2001) Safety and efficacy of preoperative administration of meloxicam, compared with that of ketoprofen and butorphanol in dogs undergoing abdominal surgery. *American Journal of Veterinary Research*, **62**, 882–888.

52 Hickford, F.H., Barr, S.C. & Erb, H.N. (2001) Effect of carprofen on hemostatic variables in dogs. *American Journal of Veterinary Research*, **62**, 1642–1646.

53 Chiang, N., Arita, M. & Serhan, C.N. (2005) Anti-inflammatory circuitry: Lipoxin, aspirin-triggered lipoxins and their receptor ALX. *Prostaglandins Leukot Essent Fatty Acids*, **73**, 163–177.

54 Hall, V.C. & Wolf, R.E. (1997) Effects of tenidap and nonsteroidal antiinflammatory drugs on the response of cultured human T cells to interleukin 2 in rheumatoid arthritis. *Journal of Rheumatology*, **24**, 1467–1470.

55 Jiang, C., Ting, A.T. & Seed, B. (1998) PPAR-gamma agonists inhibit production of monocyte inflammatory cytokines. *Nature*, **391**, 82–86.

56 Matsumoto, M., Inoue, M. & Ueda, H. (2006) NSAID zaltoprofen possesses novel anti-nociceptive mechanism through blockage of B2-type bradykinin receptor in nerve endings. *Neuroscience Letters*, **397**, 249–253.

57 Vellani, V., Franchi, S., Prandini, M. *et al.* (2013) Effects of NSAIDs and paracetamol (acetaminophen) on protein kinase C epsilon translocation and on substance P synthesis and release in cultured sensory neurons. *Journal of Pain Research*, **6**, 111–120.

58 Rainsford, K.D. (2007) Anti-inflammatory drugs in the 21st century. *Subcellular Biochemistry*, **42**, 3–27.

CHAPTER 6

Parasiticides for use in horses

Tad Coles[1] and Randy Lynn[2]

[1] Kansas City, MO, USA
[2] Greensboro, NC, USA

Introduction

As our understanding of the ecological relationship of host and parasite has evolved, so have preventative and treatment recommendations. In the days before ivermectin, horses were evaluated for parasite burdens and the veterinarian administered deworming agents only when indicated. Early deworming agents had to be administered by nasogastric tube either because the product was irritating to oral mucous membranes, such as with carbon disulfide, or because the volume that had to be administered was very large, as with a piperazine, carbon disulfide, and phenothiazine mixture used in the 1950s and 1960s [1]. One advantage of this approach was that the veterinarian played an integral role in development of anthelmintic control strategies on the farm. With time and the introduction of newer anthelmintics, that changed. In the mid-1960s, it became standard practice to treat all the horses in the herd every other month. Known as interval dosing, this protocol was based on the life cycle and egg reappearance period (ERP) of the highly pathogenic large strongyle, *Strongylus vulgaris*, after thiabendazole treatment.

The advent of the macrocyclic lactones (or macrolides) made highly effective broad-spectrum anthelmintics widely available to veterinarians and horse owners, which led to regular herd treatment without regard to the parasite burdens of specific animals or pastures. As a result of that approach, the veterinarian was no longer integral in development of anthelmintic treatment plans and all classes of equine anthelmintics became associated with resistant parasitic strains. Also, as a result of that approach, disease due to *S. vulgaris* infections

became uncommon. Currently, cyathostomes (small strongyles) have become the primary parasitic problem in mature horses [2] and ascarids have emerged as a problem in young horses.

Looking across the road to the small ruminant situation, parasite resistance issues have become so severe that sheep and goats are dying because none of the currently marketed anthelmintics are efficacious. Therefore, it is in the best interest of both horse owners and equine practitioners to manage horses and anthelmintic use so as to delay, as long as possible, the apparently inevitable emergence of parasite drug resistance. Veterinary parasitologists have advocated for decades that parasite burdens should be determined in individual horses and only those with high worm burdens should be treated. While some equine practitioners agree with this approach, they have found it difficult to convince horse owners, because anthelmintic products are so inexpensive that it is often cheaper to treat the whole herd than to conduct fecal egg counts (FEC) on every horse.

This short-term thinking will certainly lead to long-term problems when macrolide anthelmintic resistance eventually becomes pervasive. The time for veterinary practitioners to educate horse owners that minimal-use anthelmintic programs are in the best interest of the horse and the horse owner is long overdue. Moving toward the goal of widespread acceptance of sustainable, evidence-based parasite control programs can be accomplished through continuing education of veterinary practitioners and distribution of high-quality information to horse owners [3, 4]. The objective of this chapter is to provide the veterinary

Equine Pharmacology, First Edition. Edited by Cynthia Cole, Bradford Bentz and Lara Maxwell.
© 2015 John Wiley & Sons, Inc. Published 2015 by John Wiley & Sons, Inc.

practitioner with the tools and information needed to achieve that goal. The literature on equine anthelmintics is voluminous, and therefore, references are cited only as needed to guide the practicing veterinarian toward more specific information on topics or products, favoring citation of open-access material whenever possible. An excellent starting point that every equine practitioner should be familiar with is the American Association of Equine Practitioners (AAEP) Parasite Control Guidelines [5]. The AAEP formed a task force that developed this excellent source of baseline information. While the guidelines may not necessarily represent a consensus among practitioners or equine parasitologists, they are freely available online and provide a starting point for discussion.

Resistance issues

There have been only 11 new endoparasiticides developed for horses since 1917 [6]. For various reasons, including toxicity and resistance, many have become obsolete including febantel, levamisole, trichlorfon, dichlorvos, phenothiazine, and carbon disulfide [6]. Prior to the availability of broad-spectrum anthelmintics, rotation of drug classes was used to achieve control of various equine gastrointestinal parasites. There was a valid purpose for setting up rotation programs at that time, which was to provide good efficacy against large and small strongyles, ascarids, and pinworms, but with the introduction of broad-spectrum anthelmintics, rotation was no longer necessary at least for that purpose. Rotation was still recommended though, as it was thought at the time that it would prevent the development of resistance. While this approach may have been based on a logical hypothesis, it was without scientific proof [3, 7].

Wide availability of macrocyclic lactones led to routine anthelmintic treatment of every horse in the herd every 4–8 weeks, regardless of need, which became standard practice and resulted in the emergence and escalation of anthelmintic resistance [4]. Resistance to all classes of equine anthelmintics is emerging and has been well documented in the southeastern USA [5]. For example, there is evidence that small strongyles are resistant to pyrantel [8], ivermectin [9], fenbendazole [10], and oxibendazole [11] and that ascarids are becoming resistant to pyrantel pamoate [9], ivermectin,

and moxidectin [12]. The occurrence of resistance varies tremendously, however, and there may be large differences between local farms. Therefore, testing is needed to determine resistance on any given farm [5].

Once resistance develops to an anthelmintic, reversion to susceptibility will not occur as long as use of that anthelmintic continues [6]. Studies that suggest otherwise are not universally accepted by the scientific community [13–15]. For example, repeated 8-week interval treatments with oxibendazole can induce small strongyle resistance to that drug [7]. Once oxibendazole resistance occurs, continuing to use the drug, even as part of a rotation program that alternates treatments with a nonbenzimidazole, does not decrease or slow the development of parasite resistance to oxibendazole [16]. It is not rational to continue to use a drug when there is evidence of helminth resistance to that drug on that particular farm [3].

Ongoing testing for resistance is important. It is logical that, with the passage of time, reversion to susceptibility may occur if pests are no longer exposed to chemicals to which they are resistant. While to the authors' knowledge such reversion to susceptibility has not been proven with anthelmintics, insect resistance to DDT and organophosphates showed rapid reversion upon cessation of use of those chemicals, presumably due to decreased evolutionary selection pressure on insects [17]. Depending on the level of introduction of new individuals, susceptibility of the population of helminths on a particular farm may be affected more by introduction of different strains of helminths that may or may not tolerate a particular anthelmintic, rather than by "resistance" *per se*. Resistance can be defined as the selection of a specific heritable trait (or traits) in a population of helminths, due to that population's contact with a chemical, that results in a significant increase in the percentage of the population that will survive a standard dose of that chemical (or a closely related chemical in the case of cross-resistance). The scientific literature, however, is rife with evidence of decreased susceptibility or increased tolerance being labeled as "resistance." The important point is that the only way to know if the helminth population in question is susceptible to an anthelmintic is to gather evidence and treat appropriately.

An important principle for evidence-based management of parasite populations is maintenance of healthy herd refugia. The refugium (singular of refugia) is the portion of a helminth population that is not exposed to anthelmintics. It includes all stages of the life cycle and provides a reservoir of anthelmintic-susceptible genes because there is no selection pressure on these unexposed individuals. Experts claim increasing helminth refugium populations will delay the emergence of anthelmintic resistance [3, 18].

Treating only the horses with dangerously high parasite burdens rather than treating the entire herd will spare refugia and allow healthy populations of nonresistant parasites to flourish. Parasite burdens are not uniformly distributed among herd members. It is common to find that a relatively small percentage of the herd bears the majority of the internal parasites. About 20–30% of horses carry about 80% of the worms [19]. Parasite load is heaviest in foals and young adult horses. An individual horse's shedding level, high or low, tends to be consistent from 1 year to the next [20].

The McMaster procedure or the more sensitive modified Wisconsin technique can be used to perform a quantitative FEC, the result of which will determine which horses to treat. Horses with an FEC of less than 500 eggs per gram (EPG) should not be treated because (i) the risk of clinical signs due to parasitic disease is low and (ii) the parasites that low-shedding horses harbor will maintain refugia on the farm, which is healthier for the entire herd [5].

While FEC is a useful tool to manage parasite burdens in adult horses, it is important to note that it primarily monitors strongyle eggs and it may not correlate with total worm burden (encysted and nonencysted parasites) or with other pathogenic species (tapeworms and adult ascarids). It is also important to note that all foals and weanlings should be considered high shedders and treated accordingly.

Another evidence-based principle for managing parasites is to determine the efficacy of currently used anthelmintics on each and every farm. Since tremendous differences in efficacy of a specific anthelmintic may occur from farm to farm, even in the same region, it is important to perform a fecal egg count reduction test (FECRT) at least every 1–2 years to determine anthelmintic efficacy for each and every herd [19]. To accomplish this, the EPG should be determined in each horse before treatment and again 10–14 days after treatment; if anthelmintic treatment does not reduce the FEC by ≥85% for pyrantel pamoate, ≥90% for benzimidazoles, or ≥95% for macrolides, then parasites on

that farm are considered resistant to that anthelmintic [3, 5]. Since a reduction in the time it takes for eggs to reappear after anthelmintic treatment precedes development of resistance [21], monitoring the ERP will be helpful in detecting emerging resistance to ivermectin and moxidectin.

If the anthelmintic is effective on that farm, then it is important to continue its use for as long as possible. There is nothing to be gained by rotating to a less effective anthelmintic. Conversely, rotating from a macrolide to a drug that is efficacious for tapeworms could be important, because macrolides will not kill cestodes.

Tapeworms may be causing more pathology in horses than was previously appreciated, because they can be difficult to diagnose [22, 23]. The fact that tapeworms are ubiquitous and challenging to diagnose contributes to ongoing discussions among parasitologists regarding their pathogenicity [24, 25]. Horses harboring large numbers of tapeworms may be difficult to identify because the parasites shed eggs sporadically and clinical signs associated with tapeworm infections, such as colic, are erratically manifested, confounding efforts to accurately estimate parasite load and the effect that load has on clinical disease. While serological and molecular methods of cestode detection have been evaluated [26], FEC from samples collected just prior to treatment, 24–48 h after treatment, and 16–21 days after treatment provide cost-effective and valuable information about the prevalence of tapeworms and the efficacy of cestodicidal treatments [24]. Many tapeworm-infected horses are negative on fecal exam prior to treatment but positive 24–48 h after treatment, revealing a higher prevalence than was previously suspected [24, 27]. The use of centrifugal fecal floatation increases the likelihood of finding tapeworm eggs compared to gravitational fecal flotation.

While small strongyles represent the major health issue in adult horses, young horses less than 3 years of age have a different problem because ascarids (*Parascaris equorum*) are ubiquitous in breeding horses. Also, resistance to ivermectin and moxidectin is common and pyrantel resistance is developing. Young horses should be considered high shedders and treated for ascarids with fenbendazole or oxibendazole. These horses should be treated for ascarids initially as foals at 2–3 months of age, again at weaning, and at 9 months of age. They should also be treated for small strongyles at 1 year of age. A FECRT should be performed at least annually on breeding farms to confirm efficacy [5].

There are several other key components to an effective parasite management program. First, proper dosing is important to maximize efficacy. Veterinarians and horse owners are notoriously inaccurate in estimating body weight, which can lead to underdosing, decreased efficacy, and increased resistance. Therefore, use of a weight tape or scale to determine body weight is highly recommended. In addition, fresh manure should not be spread on pastures, because this practice seeds the pastures with parasites. Instead, equine manure should be composted prior to spreading. Removing feces from pastures twice a week will also help decrease the spread of parasites. Other recommended management practices include:
- Avoiding high stocking densities
- Refraining from feeding hay or concentrates directly on the ground
- Rotating nonequid species through the pasture to graze, which will allow the host-specific horse parasites to die off
- Refraining from dragging currently occupied pastures, which disrupts natural fecal avoidance tendencies
- Quarantining all arriving horses until their shedding status can be determined and treated as needed

These simple management techniques can help prolong the efficacy of currently available anthelmintics.

Although unpopular with some owners, culling the high shedders will make parasite control easier, as will selection of low shedders for breeding stock, both of which should eventually result in a more genetically vigorous and parasite-resistant herd.

Specific anthelmintics

An exhaustive review of the pharmacology, mechanism of action, pharmacokinetics, and efficacy of all anthelmintics is outside the scope of this book. Those anthelmintics that are approved by the FDA for use in the USA and are still commercially available at this time are grouped together by class according to their generic names. In this text, the nonproprietary names are used to identify the products and one or more of the trade names may be mentioned, usually parenthetically. No discrimination is intended and no endorsement is implied when trade names appear. Practitioners should always refer to the manufacturer's recommendations concerning dosing, spectrum of activity, efficacy, safety, and contraindications, because availability and labeling claims vary between countries and change over time (Table 6.1).

Table 6.1 Summary of common equine anthelmintics, doses, and indications.

Drug	Class	Dose	Frequency*	Indications
Moxidectin	M	0.4 mg/kg	10–12-week ERP	Adult and encysted small strongyles, adult and larval large strongyles, and bots; may be used for ascarids if favorable FECRT confirmed
Ivermectin	M	0.2 mg/kg	6–8-week ERP	Adult small strongyles, adult and larval large strongyles, and bots; may be used for ascarids if favorable FECRT confirmed
Fenbendazole	B	10 mg/kg (once or daily for 5 days)	4–5 weeks	Ascarid control in foals; approved for all stages of encysted small strongyles; may be used for small strongyles if favorable FECRT confirmed
Oxibendazole	B	10 mg/kg		Ascarid control in foals; may be used for small strongyles if favorable FECRT confirmed
Pyrantel pamoate	T	6.6 mg/kg[†,‡] 13.2 mg/kg[§]	4–6 weeks[†,‡]	Ascarid control in foals; may be used for small strongyles if favorable FECRT confirmed; tapeworm control (praziquantel alternative)
Praziquantel	I	1–1.5 mg/kg		Tapeworm control

M, macrocyclic lactone; B, benzimidazole; T, tetrahydropyrimidine; I, isoquinolone.
*Avoid administering dewormer more frequently than its ERP and use actual ERP to help determine treatment frequency.
[†]Ascarid.
[‡]Small strongyle.
[§]Tapeworm.
Adapted from Refs [19, 98].

The goal is to provide the information necessary for the reader to develop effective antiparasite programs for clients. For those who wish to delve deeper, a few key citations are included in the text. For more exhaustive information about specific anthelmintics, such as mechanism of action, the reader is advised to seek other references [28–31]. It is hoped that new therapeutic agents will result from research into anthelmintic mechanisms of action. Several reviews discuss exciting new areas of research that may be of interest to equine practitioners [32–36].

Macrocyclic lactone anthelmintics

Macrocyclic lactones (or macrolides) have revolutionized the control of parasites in both man and animal. Ivermectin is the best-known agent in this class, which includes avermectins (ivermectin) and milbemycins (moxidectin). Macrocyclic lactones bind to glutamate receptors, triggering a chloride influx that hyperpolarizes the parasite neuron and prevents initiation or propagation of normal action potentials. The net effect is paralysis and death of target nematodes and arthropods. Macrocyclic lactones are effective against a wide range of nematodes as well as bots but are ineffective against cestodes and trematodes.

Ivermectin

Ivermectin was the first commercially available macrolide, released for animal use by Merck & Co., Inc., in 1981, just 6 years after the discovery of avermectins [37, 38]. The avermectins were isolated from the fermentation broth of *Streptomyces avermitilis*. The discovery of anthelmintic activity was made after administering actinomycetic broth to mice infected with the nematode *Nematospiroides dubius*. Although ivermectin was originally believed to act by disturbing GABA-mediated neurotransmission, it is now known that it binds with high affinity to glutamate-gated chloride channels, triggering chloride influx, hyperpolarization, paralysis, and death [28, 34, 37, 39–41].

The commercial success of ivermectin inspired other companies to develop analogs, including moxidectin, milbemycin oxime, doramectin, selamectin, abamectin, and eprinomectin [38]. The current literature contains reports of use against hundreds of species of parasites in a very long list of hosts including many exotic and wild animal species.

Ivermectin has a broad spectrum of activity against nematodes and arthropod parasites of horses and is administered orally at 0.2 mg/kg of body weight. It is available in a variety of products formulated as a 1.87% paste for oral administration or 10 mg/ml liquid for administration by nasogastric tube or oral drench. It is also available as a 1.87% paste in combination with praziquantel, a formulation that is discussed later in the section on broad-spectrum combination products. Ivermectin was previously available for horses as an injectable for intramuscular administration but was withdrawn from the market due to adverse reactions, such as pain and clostridial infection at the injection site [42].

Ivermectin is used for the treatment and control of large strongyles (*Strongylus equinus*: adults; *S. vulgaris*: adults and early forms in blood vessels; *Strongylus edentatus*: adults and tissue stages; *Craterostomum acuticaudatum*: adults; *Triodontophorus* spp. including *Triodontophorus brevicauda*: adults; and *T. serratus*: adults), small strongyle adults including those resistant to some benzimidazoles (*Coronocyclus* spp., *Cyathostomum* spp., *Cylicocyclus* spp., *Cylicodontophorus* spp., *Cylicostephanus* spp., and *Petrovinema poculatum*), small strongyle fourth-stage larvae, pinworms (*Oxyuris equi*: adults and fourth-stage larvae), ascarids (*P. equorum*: adult and larval stages), hairworms (*Trichostrongylus axei*: adults), large-mouth stomach worms (*Habronema muscae*: adults), bots (oral and gastric stages of *Gasterophilus* spp. including *Gasterophilus intestinalis* and *G. nasalis*), lungworms (*Dictyocaulus arnfieldi*: adults and fourth-stage larvae), intestinal threadworms (*Strongyloides westeri*: adults), summer sores caused by cutaneous third-stage larvae of *Draschia* and *Habronema* spp., and dermatitis caused by microfilariae of neck threadworm *Onchocerca* spp [43]. Since macrocyclic lactone resistance to many of these parasites has been documented in the USA, especially in *P. equorum*, young horses should be treated primarily with benzimidazole anthelmintics [5].

When used to treat horses with onchocerciasis, a single ivermectin dose often results in clinical remission within 2–3 weeks, but sometimes 2–3 monthly treatments are needed [44]. On occasion, treated horses exhibit edematous reactions caused by a massive release of parasitic antigens. About a quarter of horses treated for onchocerciasis have an adverse reaction, which may occur more frequently in horses with a large burden of neck threadworm microfilariae, presumably as a result of death of a large number of microfilariae and massive release of parasitic antigens. The signs of ventral midline edema or pruritus occur 1–10 days posttreatment and may necessitate therapy with prednisolone or phenylbutazone. When left untreated, edema usually resolves in a week to 10 days and pruritus in about 3 weeks [45]. Administering a glucocorticoid just prior to ivermectin treatment and repeating it 1–2 days after treatment prevents this adverse reaction [45].

According to package inserts, ivermectin may be used in horses of all ages, including mares at any stage of pregnancy and breeding stallions, although foals should not be treated until they are 6–8 weeks of age [43, 46]. Treating foals that are younger is ill-advised because toxicity can occur, presumably due to the immaturity of the blood–brain barrier [47]. Disruption of the blood–brain barrier is suspected, but not proven, as the cause of ivermectin toxicity in adult horses given the labeled dose of ivermectin after having access to silver nightshade (*Solanum elaeagnifolium*) [48, 49].

Pregnant mares treated orally with 0.6 mg of ivermectin per kilogram body weight throughout the organogenesis period gave birth to normal, healthy foals. Treatment with 0.6 mg of ivermectin per kilogram body weight did not affect the sexual behavior of stallions or the quality of their semen. Thus, oral administration of three times the recommended dose of ivermectin was well tolerated by horses. Horses orally dosed at 1.8 mg/kg (9× the recommended dose) did not have signs of toxicity, but when dosed at 2 mg/kg (10× the recommended dose), visual impairment, depression, and ataxia were noted [45].

Ivermectin paste and liquid labels indicate the products are for oral use in horses only and caution that the product may cause severe adverse reactions when administered to other species, which may include death in dogs [43, 46]. It is not unusual for macrocyclic lactone (ivermectin and moxidectin) toxicity to be reported in dogs that were in close proximity to horses during deworming, because horses may spit the paste out during administration [50]. Coprophagic dogs with an ivermectin-sensitive genetic makeup (e.g., carrying the multidrug resistance gene) are also at risk for ivermectin toxicity if they eat the feces of a recently treated horse. Ivermectin reaches maximum fecal concentration 2–3 days after oral treatment [51]. By 4 days posttreatment, 90% of the drug has been excreted in the feces. Owners of ivermectin-sensitive coprophagic dogs should be advised to treat feces from horses administered ivermectin as toxic waste, disposing it in a manner that will prevent their dog from eating it [50].

Moxidectin

Moxidectin is available in a 20 mg/ml formulation designed to deliver 0.4 mg/kg to horses and ponies for the treatment and control of large strongyles (*S. vulgaris*, adult and L4/L5 arterial stages; *S. edentatus*, adult and tissue stages; *T. brevicauda*, adults; *T. serratus*, adults), small strongyle, adults (*Cyathostomum* spp., *Cylicostephanus* spp., *Cylicocyclus* spp., *Coronocyclus* spp., *Gyalocephalus capitatus*, *Petrovinema poculatus*, and undifferentiated luminal larvae), ascarids (*P. equorum*, adults and L4 larval stages), pinworms (*O. equi*, adults and L4 larval stages), hairworms (*T. axei*, adults), stomach worms (*H. muscae*), and botfly larva (*G. intestinalis* and *G. nasalis*) [52–54]. The moxidectin product is particularly effective against encysted small strongyles and is labeled to suppress strongyle egg production through 84 days. Since it is fat soluble and very effective against a broad range of parasites, it should not be the first choice product for heavily parasitized thin horses [55]. While moxidectin is labeled as safe for use in mares during breeding, gestation, and lactation, and for foals older than 6 months, it should be dosed carefully, especially in foals. Overdoses of moxidectin and treatment of very young (<4 months of age), emaciated, or debilitated animals may result in neurological signs, such as ataxia, incoordination, lethargy, depression, tremors, seizures, and rarely, death. These clinical signs generally resolved with supportive care [56, 57]. As previously noted, since macrocyclic lactone resistance to many of these parasites has been documented in the USA, especially in *P. equorum*, young horses should be treated primarily with benzimidazole anthelmintics [5].

Benzimidazole anthelmintics

The benzimidazoles represent a large family of broad-spectrum agents that have been widely used for many years in a vast array of animal species. Excellent review articles are available that discuss the history, mode of action, and spectrum of activity of this useful class of anthelmintics [58–61].

Thiabendazole, the first benzimidazole discovered, represented a major step forward when it became available more than 50 years ago [62]. At the time of its introduction, thiabendazole was a true broad-spectrum product that was very safe to the host animal. Since that time, safer and broader-spectrum benzimidazoles have been introduced and parasite resistance to the benzimidazoles has been discovered in several species.

Considerable effort has been devoted to determining the mechanism by which the benzimidazoles act on parasites. Conventional wisdom holds that benzimidazoles bind to tubulin molecules, which inhibits the formation of microtubules and disrupts cell division [63–65]. It has a much higher affinity for nematode tubulin versus mammalian tubulin, thus providing selective activity against parasites. Evidence also indicates that the benzimidazoles can inhibit fumarate reductase, which blocks mitochondrial function, depriving the parasite of energy and thus resulting in death.

The benzimidazoles are poorly soluble in water and, therefore, are generally administered by mouth. They tend to be more effective in horses and ruminants because of slow transit of gastrointestinal contents through the cecum and rumen. The dose is usually more effective when divided, thus prolonging the contact time with the parasite.

Fenbendazole

Fenbendazole is a commercially successful benzimidazole that is widely used in domestic animals. The oral LD_{50} for rats and mice is >10 000 mg/kg. Fenbendazole does not have embryotoxic or teratogenic effects in rats, sheep, and cattle. In the rabbit, fenbendazole was fetotoxic, but not teratogenic. It is generally considered safe to use in pregnancy in all species, making it the extralabel drug of choice for treating pregnant animals.

Fenbendazole suspension, granules, pellets, or paste (Panacur) is administered orally to horses at 5 mg/kg for the control of large strongyles (*S. edentatus*, *S. equinus*, *S. vulgaris*, and *Triodontophorus* spp.), small strongyles (*Cyathostomum* spp., *Cylicocyclus* spp., *Cylicostephanus* spp., and *Cylicodontophorus* spp.), and pinworms (*O. equi*). For the removal of ascarids (*P. equorum*), a dose of 10 mg/kg is recommended. For the control of fourth-stage larvae of *S. vulgaris*, the dosage is 10 mg/kg daily for 5 days [66, 67]. This is the only approved treatment that kills all stages of encysted small strongyles and controls larval stages of *P. equorum* [68]. Pregnant mares, stallions, and foals may be treated safely with fenbendazole at the recommended dosages. When treating foals with a large burden of ascarids, practitioners should consider an initial treatment at a dose of 5 mg/kg followed by 10 mg/kg to

try to avoid colic or impactions that occur secondary to rapid killing of a large number of ascarids [62]. Fenbendazole has been evaluated for safety in pregnant mares during all stages of gestation and in stallions at doses up to 25 mg/kg. No adverse reproductive effects were found.

While benzimidazole resistance has been documented in the southeastern USA, improved efficacy against strongyles results when using 10 mg/kg for 5 consecutive days. There are farms in other regions of the USA where a single dose of 5 mg/kg is still effective. The results of an FECRT will reveal the effectiveness on a given farm. Fenbendazole has emerged as a cornerstone for control of ascarids in young horses, especially in areas where resistance has emerged to other classes of anthelmintic [69].

Oxibendazole

Oxibendazole paste or suspension is administered orally to horses at 10 mg/kg for the removal and control of large strongyles (*S. edentatus*, *S. equinus*, *S. vulgaris*), small strongyles (species of the genera *Cylicostephanus*, *Cylicocyclus*, *Cyathostomum*, *Triodontophorus*, *Cylicodontophorus*, and *Gyalocephalus*), large roundworms (*P. equorum*), and pinworms (*O. equi* including various larval stages) [70–72]. The dose must be increased to 15 mg/kg for treatment of threadworms [73]. Historically, it has been one of the last of the benzimidazoles to remain effective against helminths and has been used successfully against parasites resistant to fenbendazole. A study of 44 farms in the southern USA revealed cyathostomins were resistant to fenbendazole on 98% of farms and resistant to oxibendazole at 74% on farms [11]. Oxibendazole may have good activity in farms outside of the southeastern USA; FECRT test results should be used to guide its use. Recently, a study of horses in Kentucky demonstrated that oxibendazole had good efficacy against ascarids, but not strongyles when used at a dose of 10 mg/kg [9]. It is useful for treating and controlling ascarid infections in young horses, but it should not be used in severely debilitated horses or in horses suffering from colic, toxemia, or infectious disease.

Tetrahydropyrimidine anthelmintics

The tetrahydropyrimidines include the numerous salts of pyrantel, morantel, and oxantel, the latter of which is only available outside the USA. They all act as nicotinic agonists, which disrupt the neuromuscular system, causing contraction and subsequent tonic paralysis by their action at synaptic and extrasynaptic nicotinic acetylcholine receptors on nematode muscle cells [28, 34, 65, 74, 75]. *In vitro* experiments indicate that pyrantel is 100 times more potent than acetylcholine. It seems that the nicotinic acetylcholine receptors of invertebrate parasites are essential for neural function but different in physiology and distribution from mammals [32].

Introduced in 1966, pyrantel is the most widely used of all the tetrahydropyrimidine anthelmintics and is the only one marketed for use in horses in the USA [65]. Pyrantel is currently available under a wide variety of trade names as a paste, oral suspension, medicated pellet, and medicated feed for use in horses [76]. Pyrantel salts are stable in solid form but degrade when suspended in water, resulting in a reduction in potency.

Pyrantel tartrate

The tartrate salt of pyrantel is a white powder, soluble in water, and absorbed more readily than the pamoate salt [65]. Pyrantel tartrate is rapidly metabolized. Pyrantel tartrate (Strongid C) is fed at a dose of 2.6 mg/kg daily for the prevention of *S. vulgaris* larval infection and control of adult large strongyles (*S. vulgaris*, *S. edentatus*) and adult and 4th-stage larval small strongyles (*Cyathostomum* spp., *Cylicocyclus* spp., *Cylicostephanus* spp., *Cylicodontophorus* spp., *Poteriostomum* spp., *Triodontophorus* spp.), pinworms (*O. equi*), and ascarids (*P. equorum*) [77–79]. Pyrantel tartrate is safe for use in horses and ponies of all ages, including foals and pregnant mares. Foals may be treated as soon as they take grain. Stallion fertility is not affected by the use of pyrantel tartrate.

One downside of treating with pyrantel daily is development of parasite resistance to the drug. Another downside is that foals raised on daily pyrantel do not develop acquired resistance to subsequent strongyle infections [80]. So while this medicated feed is safe and easy to administer, indiscriminate use throughout a herd, without focusing use toward particular horses in need, will decrease the immune response to strongyles, be detrimental to the maintenance of healthy refugia, and eventually lead to increased parasite resistance. One practitioner using an FEC-based parasite control program found that stables relying upon daily pyrantel administration had a higher number of high-shedding horses and that those horses required ivermectin or moxidectin administration to reduce the FEC [81].

Pyrantel pamoate

Pyrantel pamoate is poorly absorbed from the gastrointestinal tract and is primarily eliminated through the feces with less than 15% excretion through the urinary tract [82]. The pamoate salt of pyrantel is a yellow powder that is insoluble in water. It is available as a ready-to-use suspension or paste in horses. The fact that pyrantel pamoate is poorly absorbed from the intestine adds to its safety in very young or weak animals but should be used with caution in foals with heavy burdens of *P. equorum*, because intestinal impaction may occur.

Several manufacturers have pyrantel pamoate products approved by the FDA for use in horses. It is available as a paste in concentrations of 171, 180, or 226 mg(base)/ml. It is also available as a flavored suspension with 50 mg(base)/ml (e.g., Strongid T), which is FDA approved for administration at 6.6 mg(base)/kg to remove and control adult populations of large strongyles (*S. vulgaris*, *S. edentatus*, *S. equinus*), small strongyles, pinworms (*O. equi*), and large roundworms (*P. equorum*) in horses and ponies. Ordinarily, other drugs are used to eliminate tapeworms, but a single oral pyrantel pamoate dose of 13.2 mg/kg has been shown to be 83–98% effective against tapeworms [27, 83]. In 2005, the same dose was FDA approved for removal and control of tapeworms (*Anoplocephala perfoliata*) in horses and ponies for a Phoenix Scientific, Inc., pyrantel pamoate paste product, but as that product is not currently on the market, 13.2 mg/kg for tapeworms is considered an extralabel dose for currently marketed products [84]. Small strongyles resistant to pyrantel pamoate are commonly reported in the southeastern USA [4, 5, 8].

Praziquantel

Praziquantel was the first cestodicidal isoquinolone that was FDA approved in the USA. It disrupts parasitic neuromuscular junction and tegument and causes increased cell membrane permeability to calcium with resulting loss of intracellular calcium. This effect causes an instantaneous contraction and paralysis of the parasite [85, 86]. The second effect is a devastating vacuolization and destruction of the protective tegument [29, 63]. The combined effects of paralysis and tegmental destruction provide excellent activity against cestodes.

Praziquantel has marked anthelmintic activity against a wide range of adult and larval cestodes and trematodes of the genus *Schistosoma*. Oral administration results in nearly complete absorption and rapid distribution throughout the body and across the blood–brain barrier. Praziquantel has high oral bioavailability, high protein binding, and a marked first-pass effect [87]. Although 80% of the drug is excreted in the urine, the main site of inactivation is the liver, with only trace amounts of the unchanged drug excreted intact [88]. Both the parent compound and metabolite are roughly similar in pharmacological activity. Praziquantel is a very safe anthelmintic. Rats tolerated daily administration of up to 1000 mg/kg for 4 weeks, and dogs tolerated up to 180 mg/kg/day for 13 weeks. It can be used safely in breeding and pregnant animals without restriction. Praziquantel did not induce embryotoxicity, teratogenesis, mutagenesis, or carcinogenesis, nor did it affect the reproductive performance of test animals [65].

Although not FDA approved as a sole ingredient in any equine products, praziquantel may be used for *A. perfoliata* tapeworm infections. Praziquantel has been administered to horses as a single extralabel dose of 1.23 mg/kg using the dog and cat injectable product (56.8 mg/ml Droncit) delivered via nasogastric intubation, not by injection [83]. Praziquantel is FDA approved in combination with the macrocyclic lactones moxidectin and ivermectin for use in horses. See the following section on combination products for more information.

Broad-spectrum combination anthelmintic products

Ivermectin and praziquantel

Two oral paste products (Equimax® paste, Bimeda, Dublin, Ireland, and Zimecterin® Gold paste, Merial Ltd, Duluth, GA) containing ivermectin and praziquantel are FDA approved for use in horses. The addition of praziquantel extends the parasitic spectrum of ivermectin to include the tapeworm (*A. perfoliata*). The formulation of the active ingredients and dosing is different for these products. Equimax paste (ivermectin 1.87%/praziquantel 14.03%) is given orally at a dose of 0.2 mg/kg for ivermectin and 1.5 mg/kg body weight for praziquantel. Zimecterin Gold (ivermectin 1.55%/praziquantel 7.75%) is given orally at a dose of 0.2 mg/kg body weight for ivermectin and 1 mg/kg body weight for praziquantel.

Both combination products are FDA approved for the treatment and control of *A. perfoliata*, large strongyles, small strongyles, pinworms, ascarids, hairworms,

large-mouth stomach worms, bots, lungworms, and threadworms. They are also used to treat summer sores caused by *Draschia* and *Habronema* spp. larvae and dermatitis caused by neck threadworm (*Onchocerca* spp.) microfilariae (onchocerciasis).

When used to treat onchocerciasis, a single dose often results in clinical remission of signs within 2–3 weeks, but sometimes, 2–3 monthly ivermectin treatments are needed [44]. As previously discussed, about a quarter of the horses treated for onchocerciasis will have an adverse reaction, which may occur more frequently in horses with a large burden of neck threadworm microfilariae, presumably as a result of death of a large number of microfilariae and massive release of parasitic antigens. The signs, ventral midline edema or pruritus, occur 1–10 days posttreatment and may necessitate therapy with prednisolone or phenylbutazone. If untreated, the edema usually resolves in a week to 10 days and the pruritus subsides in approximately 3 weeks [45]. Administering a glucocorticoid just prior to ivermectin treatment and repeating 1–2 days after treatment reportedly prevents this adverse reaction [45].

Oral administration of 10× the recommended dose of Zimecterin Gold was well tolerated by 5-month-old foals. The package insert states that Zimecterin Gold has not been tested in pregnant mares, in breeding stallions, or in foals less than 5 months of age but also reports it was found safe when given at 3× the recommended dose in 2-month-old foals. On the other hand, the Equimax paste package insert safety section indicates it can be used in horses as young as 4 weeks of age, breeding stallions, and breeding, pregnant, or lactating mares. Neither product should be used in horses intended for food.

Moxidectin and praziquantel

An oral paste containing moxidectin and praziquantel is FDA approved for use in horses and ponies. The product has 20 mg/ml of moxidectin and 125 mg/ml of praziquantel formulated to provide 0.4 mg/kg of moxidectin and 2.5 mg/kg of praziquantel when given as directed. The addition of praziquantel extends the parasitic spectrum of moxidectin to include the tapeworm plus the parasites that moxidectin treats and controls: large strongyles, small strongyles, ascarids, pinworms, hairworms, stomach worms, and botfly larva. The moxidectin combination product is particularly effective against encysted small strongyles and is labeled to suppress strongyle egg production through 84 days. Since moxidectin is fat sol-uble and very effective against a broad range of parasites, this product should not be the first choice for heavily par-asitized thin horses [55]. This combination product has not been tested in mares during breeding, gestation, and lactation or in breeding stallions, although moxidectin as a sole agent is labeled as safe for use in mares during breeding, gestation, and lactation and for foals older than 6 months. Nevertheless, it should be dosed carefully, espe-cially in foals. Overdoses of moxidectin and treatment of very young (<4 months of age), emaciated, or debilitated animals may result in neurological reactions such as ataxia, incoordination, lethargy, depression, tremors, sei-zures, and rarely death. These clinical signs generally resolved with supportive care [56, 57].

General Recommendations

The bottom line is that meaningful advice can be given to horse owners about parasite control only after it is apparent which individual horses are high shedders, which parasites are prominent, and which anthelmin-tics are still effective for those parasites. The answers to those questions are unknown without FEC and FECRT data. Knowledge of the specific ERP will allow more fine-tuning, since decreasing ERP will occur before par-asites become completely resistant to a particular anthelmintic. There are many excellent articles that the interested practitioner can refer to for more information on this topic [3, 5, 12, 18, 69, 89–96]. A recently pub-lished text has a wealth of information about parasite control in horses including interesting case reports [97].

When formulating a FEC-based program, it is also important to consider the interval between ingestion of the infective stage of the parasite and appearance of eggs in the stool (the prepatent period) (Table 6.2).

Rational use of equine anthelmintics should be based upon proper therapy of horses in need and should be balanced to avoid and delay the development of anthel-mintic resistance. Implementation of FEC-based parasite control programs presents challenges. For example, sending fecal samples to a commercial laboratory for testing, rather than performing the service in-house, will obviously result in a fee that is much greater than what it costs to treat the horse with over-the-counter (OTC) dewormers. One practitioner addressed this by setting the charge for the fecal at just under what it would cost

Table 6.2 Common equine parasite prepatent periods.

Ascarids	10–15 weeks
Small strongyles	6 weeks to several years
Large strongyles	6–11 months
Tapeworms	6–16 weeks
Pinworms	<5 months
Threadworms	10–14 days

Adapted from Ref. [98].

for a benzimidazole anthelmintic dose [81]. This hospi-tal's commitment to the program included training technicians in the McMaster technique and allocating time for processing in the evening and even overnight if the daytime staff was busy. This practice also shared the software they used to identify high-shedding individuals with other practices in their region in an effort to improve the FEC processing capacity of area practices [81]. While there is a shift occurring with more and more practices coming on board the last few years, encouraging surrounding practices to adopt FEC-based programs is important because when a recently educated client calls another practice that is unknowledgeable or unsupportive of the FEC-based approach, many clients will drop it right there and head to the feed store for a tube of OTC dewormer (R. Kaplan, pers. comm.). Client education is essential because the status quo of clients administering whatever anthelmintic is on sale every 6 weeks without paying attention to other important management strategies is the history given on presenta-tion of some of the most severely diseased horses harboring tremendous parasite burdens (R. Kaplan, pers. comm.). The owners of such horses have been lulled into a sense of security by routinely giving an ineffective anthelmintic. If this occurs during a wet season and is combined with mismanagement such as nutritional compromise and overgrazing on a poor-quality pasture with high fecal concentration, all the ingredients are there to create a perfect storm of dangerous parasitic disease due to negligence (R. Kaplan, pers. comm.).

Treatment should be based upon determination of quantitative egg counts in each individual horse. Adult horses that exceed the therapeutic threshold (>500 EPG) should be treated and the egg count reduction should be determined 10–14 days after treatment. All foals and yearlings should be considered high shedders and treated accordingly.

Anthelmintics that do not reduce the quantitative strongyle FEC by at least 85% for pyrantel and 90% for benzimidazoles should be considered ineffective [5]. Macrolides that do not reduce strongyle FEC by at least 95–98% may be ineffective [5].

Anthelmintic resistance patterns vary widely by geographic area and from farm to farm. Monitoring FECRT results after treatment can provide the equine practitioner with the information necessary to administer anthelmintics properly. Proper pasture management and herd husbandry should be used in addition to rational anthelmintic therapy. It is only with a combined approach that we can prolong the useful life of these important therapeutic molecules.

References

1 Briggs, K., Reinemyer, C., French, D. & Kaplan, R. (2004) *Bad bug basics: Parasite primer—Parts 1–12*, p. 57. http://www.thehorse.com/Parasites/Parasites_ALL.pdf [accessed on August 21, 2012].

2 Love, S., Murphy, D. & Mellor, D. (1999) Pathogenicity of cyathostome infection. *Veterinary Parasitology*, **85**, 113–121. discussion 121–112, 215–125.

3 Kaplan, R.M. & Nielsen, M.K. (2010) An evidence-based approach to equine parasite control: It ain't the 60s anymore. *Equine Veterinary Education*, **22**, 306–316.

4 Kaplan, R.M. (2002) Anthelmintic resistance in nematodes of horses. *Veterinary Research*, **33**, 491–507.

5 Nielsen, M.K., Mittel, L., Grice, A. *et al.* (2013) *AAEP parasite control guidelines*. http://www.researchgate.net/publication/235976120_AAEP_Parasite_Control_Guidelines [accessed on July 16, 2013].

6 Love, S. & Christley, R.M. (2004) Parasiticides. In: J.J. Bertone & L.J.I. Horspool (eds), *Equine Clinical Pharmacology*, pp. 63–74. Saunders, Edinburgh.

7 Drudge, J.H., Lyons, E.T., Tolliver, S.C. & Swerczek, T.W. (1985) Use of oxibendazole for control of cambendazole-resistant small strongyles in a band of ponies: A six -year study. *American Journal of Veterinary Research*, **46**, 2507–2511.

8 Brazik, E.L., Luquire, J.T. & Little, D. (2006) Pyrantel pamoate resistance in horses receiving daily administration of pyrantel tartrate. *Journal of the American Veterinary Medical Association*, **228**, 101–103.

9 Lyons, E.T., Tolliver, S.C., Ionita, M. & Collins, S.S. (2008) Evaluation of parasiticidal activity of fenbendazole, ivermectin, oxibendazole, and pyrantel pamoate in horse foals with emphasis on ascarids (Parascaris equorum) in field studies on five farms in Central Kentucky in 2007. *Parasitology Research*, **103**, 287–291.

10 Authier, S. (2000) Strongyle resistance to fenbendazole in horses. *Canadian Veterinary Journal*, **41**, 268.

11 Kaplan, R.M., Klei, T.R., Lyons, E.T. *et al.* (2004) Prevalence of anthelmintic resistant cyathostomes on horse farms. *Journal of the American Veterinary Medical Association*, **225**, 903–910.

12 Reinemeyer, C.R. (2009) Diagnosis and control of anthelmintic-resistant Parascaris equorum. *Parasites and Vectors*, **2** (Suppl 2), S8.

13 Blanek, M., Brady, H.A. & Nichols, W.T. (2008) Equine anthelmintic resistance and rotational deworming regimens. Paper presented at: *International Symposium on Equine Parasitology*. Copenhagen, Denmark, August 2008.

14 Brady, H.A., Nichols, W.T., Blanek, M. & Hutchison, D.P. (2008) Parasite resistance and the effects of rotational deworming regimens in horses. Paper presented at: *American Association of Equine Practitioners*. San Diego, CA.

15 Blanek, M., Brady, H.A., Nichols, W.T. *et al.* (2006) Investigation of anthelmintic resistance and deworming regimens in horses. *Professional Animal Scientist*, **22**, 346–352.

16 Uhlinger, C. & Kristula, M. (1992) Effects of alternation of drug classes on the development of oxibendazole resistance in a herd of horses. *Journal of the American Veterinary Medical Association*, **201**, 51–55.

17 Yu, S.J. (ed) (2008) Insecticide resistance. In: *The Toxicology and Biochemistry of Insecticides*, pp. 201–230. CRC Press/Taylor & Francis, Boca Raton.

18 Nielsen, M.K., Kaplan, R.M., Thamsborg, S.M., Monrad, J. & Olsen, S.N. (2007) Climatic influences on development and survival of free-living stages of equine strongyles: Implications for worm control strategies and managing anthelmintic resistance. *Veterinary Journal*, **174**, 23–32.

19 Taylor, D.R. (2010) Equine parasite control in the new century (V420). *Western Veterinary Conference*, February 14–18, 2010, Mandalay Bay Resort & Casino, Las Vegas, NV.

20 Nielsen, M.K., Haaning, N. & Olsen, S.N. (2006) Strongyle egg shedding consistency in horses on farms using selective therapy in Denmark. *Veterinary Parasitology*, **135**, 333–335.

21 Sangster, N.C. (1999) Pharmacology of anthelmintic resistance in cyathostomes: Will it occur with the avermectin/milbemycins? *Veterinary Parasitology*, **85**, 189–201 discussion 201–184, 215–125.

22 Proudman, C.J., French, N.P. & Trees, A.J. (1998) Tapeworm infection is a significant risk factor for spasmodic colic and ileal impaction colic in the horse. *Equine Veterinary Journal*, **30**, 194–199.

23 Jordan, M.E., DiPietro, J.A. & Courtney, C.H. (1999) Equine tapeworms implicated in colic. *DVM Newsmagazine*, **30**, 1E–4E.

24 Elsener, J. & Villeneuve, A. (2011) Does examination of fecal samples 24 hours after cestocide treatment increase the sensitivity of Anoplocephala spp. detection in naturally infected horses? *Canadian Veterinary Journal*, **52**, 158–161.

25 Matthews, J.B., Hodgkinson, J.E., Dowdall, S.M. & Proudman, C.J. (2004) Recent developments in research into the Cyathostominae and Anoplocephala perfoliata. *Veterinary Research*, **35**, 371–381.

26 Traversa, D., Fichi, G., Campigli, M. *et al.* (2008) A comparison of coprological, serological and molecular methods for the diagnosis of horse infection with Anoplocephala perfoliata (Cestoda, Cyclophyllidea). *Veterinary Parasitology*, **152**, 271–277.

27 Slocombe, J.O. (1979) Prevalence and treatment of tapeworms in horses. *Canadian Veterinary Journal*, **20**, 136–140.

28 Martin, R.J. (1997) Modes of action of anthelmintic drugs. *Veterinary Journal*, **154**, 11–34.

29 Arundel, J.H., Vanden Bossche, H., Thienpoint, D. *et al.* (1985) *Chemotherapy of Gastrointestinal Helminths*. Springer-Verlag, New York.

30 Campbell, W.C. & Rew, R.S. (1985) *Chemotherapy of Parasitic Diseases*. Plenum Press, New York.

31 Riviere, J.E. & Papich, M.G. (2009) *Veterinary Pharmacology and Therapeutics*, 9th edn, p. 1524. Wiley-Blackwell, Ames.

32 Londershausen, M. (1996) Approaches to new parasiticides. *Pesticide Science*, **48**, 269–292.

33 Martin, R. (1997) Target sites of anthelmintics. *Parasitology Research*, **114**, 111–124.

34 Martin, R.J. (1993) Neuromuscular transmission in nematode parasites and antinematodal drug action. *Pharmacology and Therapeutics*, **58**, 13–50.

35 Martin, R.J., Robertson, A.P., Buxton, S.K., Beech, R.N., Charvet, C.L. & Neveu, C. (2012) Levamisole receptors: A second awakening. *Trends in Parasitology*, **28**, 289–296.

36 Behnke, J.M., Buttle, D.J., Stepek, G., Lowe, A. & Duce, I.R. (2008) Developing novel anthelmintics from plant cysteine proteinases. *Parasites and Vectors*, **1**, 29.

37 Shoop, W.L., Mrozik, H. & Fisher, M.H. (1995) Structure and activity of avermectins and milbemycins in animal health. *Veterinary Parasitology*, **59**, 139–156.

38 Holden-Dye, L. & Walker, R.J. (2007) Anthelmintic drugs. In: WormBook (ed), *WormBook: The Online Review of C. elegans Biology*, Pasadena. http://www.wormbook.org/chapters/www_anthelminticdrugs/anthelminticdrugs.pdf [accessed on January 7, 2013].

39 Arena, J.P., Liu, K.K., Paress, P.S. & Cully, D.F. (1991) Avermectin-sensitive chloride channels induced by Caenorhabditis elegans RNA in Xenopus oocytes. *Molecular Pharmacology*, **40**, 368–374.

40 Vercruysse, J. & Rew, R. (2002) *Macrocyclic Lactones in Antiparasitic Therapy*. New York, CAB International.

41 Wolstenholme, A.J. & Rogers, A.T. (2005) Glutamate-gated chloride channels and the mode of action of the avermectin/milbemycin anthelmintics. *Parasitology*, **131** (Suppl), S85–S95.

42 Barragry, T.B. (1987) A review of the pharmacology and clinical uses of ivermectin. *Canadian Veterinary Journal*, **28**, 512–517.

43 Merial Limited. (2008) *EQVALAN Paste 1.87%—package insert*. http://dailymed.nlm.nih.gov/dailymed/lookup.cfm?setid=4605c7bc-224f-4a8a-90bf-d57950b6e424 [accessed on May 15, 2014].

44 Rees, C.A. (2010) Disorders of the skin. In: S.M. Reed, W.M. Bayly & D.C. Sellon (eds), *Equine Internal Medicine*, 3rd edn, pp. 682–729. Saunders, St. Louis.

45 Plumb, D.C. (2008) *Plumb's Veterinary Drug Handbook*, 6th edn. Blackwell Publishing, Ames.

46 RXV Products. *Ivermax Equine Oral Liquid—package insert*. http://http://dailymed.nlm.nih.gov/dailymed/lookup.cfm?setid=d533ff10-3ca1-455f-a28b-b6b2fdbf8849 [accessed on May 15, 2014].

47 Godber, L.M., Derksen, F.J., Williams, J.F. & Mahmoud, B. (1995) Ivermectin toxicosis in a neonatal foal. *Australian Veterinary Journal*, **72**, 191–192.

48 Swor, T.M., Whittenburg, J.L. & Chaffin, M.K. (2009) Ivermectin toxicosis in three adult horses. *Journal of the American Veterinary Medical Association*, **235**, 558–562.

49 Garland, T., Bailey, E.M., Reagor, J.C. & Binford, E. (1998) Probable interaction between Solanum eleagnifolium and ivermectin in horses. In: T. Garland & A.C. Barr (eds), *Toxic Plants and Other Natural Toxicants*, pp. 423–427. CABI Publishing, New York.

50 Coles, T.B. & Lynn, R.C. (2012) Drugs for the treatment of helminth infections: Anthelmintics. In: D.M. Boothe (ed), *Small Animal Clinical Pharmacology and Therapeutics*, 2nd edn, pp. 451–468. Elsevier, St. Louis.

51 Perez, R., Cabezas, I., Sutra, J.F., Galtier, P. & Alvinerie, M. (2001) Faecal excretion profile of moxidectin and ivermectin after oral administration in horses. *Veterinary Journal*, **161**, 85–92.

52 Bello, T.R. & Laningham, E.T. (1994) A controlled trial evaluation of three oral dosages of moxidectin against equine parasites. *Journal of Equine Veterinary Science*, **14**, 483–488.

53 Slocombe, O. & Lake, M.C. (July, 1997) Dose confirmation trial of moxidectin equine oral gel against Gasterophilus spp. in equines. Paper presented at: *American Association of Veterinary Parasitologists*. Reno, Nevada.

54 Fort Dodge Animal Health (2006) *Quest 2% Equine Oral Gel—package insert*. http://http://vetlabel.com/lib/vet/meds/quest/page/2/ [accessed on May 15, 2014].

55 Bertone, J.J. & Horspool, L.J.I. (2004) *Equine Clinical Pharmacology*. Saunders, New York.

56 Khan, S.A., Kuster, D.A. & Hansen, S.R. (2002) A review of moxidectin overdose cases in equines from 1998 through 2000. *Veterinary and Human Toxicology*, **44**, 232–235.

57 Johnson, P.J., Mrad, D.R., Schwartz, A.J. & Kellam, L. (1999) Presumed moxidectin toxicosis in three foals. *Journal of the American Veterinary Medical Association*, **214**, 678–680.

58 Loukas, A. & Hotez, P. (2006) Chemotherapy of helminth infections. In: L. Brunton (ed), *Goodman & Gilman's the Pharmacological Basis of Therapeutics*, 11th edn, pp. 1073–1093. McGraw-Hill, New York.

59 McKellar, Q.A. & Scott, E.W. (1990) The benzimidazole anthelmintics: A review. *Journal of Veterinary Pharmacology and Therapeutics*, **13**, 223–247.

60 Campbell, W.C. (1990) Benzimidazoles: Veterinary uses. *Parasitology Today*, **6**, 130–133.

61 Lacey, E. (1990) Mode of action of benzimidazoles. *Parasitology Today*, **6**, 112–115.

62 Duckett, W.M. (2009) Equine parasite control strategies: Anthelmintics—past, present, resistant (V435). *Western Veterinary Conference*, February 15–19, 2009, Mandalay Bay Resort & Casino, Las Vegas, NV.

63 Frayha, G.J., Smyth, J.D., Gobert, J.G. & Savel, J. (1997) The mechanisms of action of antiprotozoal and anthelmintic drugs in man. *General Pharmacology*, **28**, 273–299.

64 Reinemeyer, C.E. & Courtney, C.H. (2001) Antinematodal drugs. In: H.R. Adams (ed), *Veterinary Pharmacology and Therapeutics*, 8th edn, pp. 947–979. Iowa State University Press, Ames.

65 Lanusse, C.E., Alvarez, L.I., Sallovitz, J.M., Mottier, L. & Sanchez Bruni, S. (2009) Antinematodal drugs. In: J.E. Riviere & M.G. Papich (eds), *Veterinary Pharmacology and Therapeutics*, 9th edn, pp. 1053–1094. Iowa State University Press, Ames.

66 Leneau, H., Haig, M. & Ho, I. (1985) Safety of larvicidal doses of fenbendazole in horses. *Modern Veterinary Practice*, **66**, B17–B19.

67 Plumb, D.C. (2011) *Plumb's Veterinary Drug Handbook*, 7th edn. Blackwell Publishing, Ames.

68 Vandermyde, C.R., DiPietro, J.A., Todd, K.S., Jr & Lock, T.F. (1987) Evaluation of fenbendazole for larvacidal effect in experimentally induced Parascaris equorum infections in pony foals. *Journal of the American Veterinary Medical Association*, **190**, 1548–1549.

69 Tarigo-Martinie, J.L., Wyatt, A.R. & Kaplan, R.M. (2001) Prevalence and clinical implications of anthelmintic resistance in cyathostomes of horses 1. *Journal of the American Veterinary Medical Association*, **218**, 1957.

70 Drudge, J.H., Lyons, E.T., Tolliver, S.C. & Kubis, J.E. (1981) Further clinical trials on strongyle control with some contemporary anthelmintics. *Equine Practice*, **3**, 27–36.

71 Drudge, J.H., Lyons, E.T., Tolliver, S.C. & Kubis, J.E. (1981) Clinical trials of oxibendazole for control of equine internal parasites. *Modern Veterinary Practice*, **62**, 679–682.

72 Drudge, J.H., Lyons, E.T. & Tolliver, S.C. (1985) Clinical trials comparing oxfendazole with oxibendazole and pyrantel for strongyle control in thoroughbreds featuring benzimidazole-resistant small strongyles. *Equine Practice*, **7**, 23–31.

73 DiPetro, J.A. & Todd, K.S. (1987) Anthelmintics used in treatment of parasitic infections of horses. *Veterinary Clinics of North America Equine Practice*, **3**, 1–14.

74 Eyre, P. (1970) Some pharmacodynamic effects of the nematocides: Methyridine, tetramisole and pyrantel. *Journal of Pharmacy and Pharmacology*, **22**, 26–36.

75 Aubry, M.L., Cowell, P., Davey, M.J. & Shevde, S. (1970) Aspects of the pharmacology of a new anthelmintic: Pyrantel. *British Journal of Pharmacology*, **38**, 332–344.

76 North American Compendiums (2012) *Compendium of Veterinary Products (CVP)*. North American Compendiums, Port Huron.

77 Cornwell, R.L. & Jones, R.M. (1968) Critical tests in the horse with the anthelmintic pyrantel tartrate. *Veterinary Record*, **82**, 483–484.

78 Lyons, E.T., Drudge, J.H. & Tolliver, S.C. (1975) Field tests of three salts of pyrantel against internal parasites of the horse. *American Journal of Veterinary Research*, **36**, 161–166.

79 Drudge, J.H., Lyons, E.T., Tolliver, S.C. & Kubis, J.E. (1982) Pyrantel in horses, clinical trials with emphasis on a paste formulation and activity on benzimidazole-resistant small strongyles. *Veterinary Medicine, Small Animal Clinician*, **77**, 957–967.

80 Monahan, C.M., Chapman, M.R., Taylor, H.W., French, D.D. & Klei, T.R. (1997) Foals raised on pasture with or without daily pyrantel tartrate feed additive: Comparison of parasite burdens and host responses following experimental challenge with large and small strongyle larvae. *Veterinary Parasitology*, **73**, 277–289.

81 True, C.K., DeWitt, S.F., Dennison, L.F., Bashton, E.F., Fulton, C.M. & Berry, D.B., II (2010) How to implement an internet parasite-control program based on fecal egg counts. *American Association of Equine Practitioners Convention Proceedings*, **56**, 258–260.

82 United States Pharmacopeia (2005) *USP monograph—tetrahydropyrimidines (veterinary—oral-local)*. The United States Pharmacopeial Convention, Inc. https://www.yumpu.com/en/document/view/19384272/tetrahydropyrimidines [accessed on May 15, 2014].

83 Craig, T., Scrutchfield, W., Thompson, J. & Bass, E.E. (2003) Comparison of anthelmintic activity of pyrantel, praziquantel, and nitazoxanide against Anoplocephala perfoliata in horses. *Journal of Equine Veterinary Science*, **23**, 68–70.

84 Food and Drug Administration. (2005) *Freedom of Information Summary*, Supplemental NADA 200-342, Pyrantel Pamoate Paste (Pyrantel Pamoate). http://www.fda.gov/downloads/AnimalVeterinary/Products/ApprovedAnimalDrugProducts/FOIADrugSummaries/ucm061808.pdf [accessed on May 15, 2014].

85 Andrews, P., Thomas, H., Pohlke, R. & Seubert, J. (1983) Praziquantel. *Medicinal Research Reviews*, **3**, 147–200.

86 Redman, C.A., Robertson, A., Fallon, P.G. *et al.* (1996) Praziquantel: An urgent and exciting challenge. *Parasitology Today*, **12**, 14–20.

87 Lanusse, C.E., Virkel, G.L. & Alvarez, L.I. (2009) Anticestodal and antitrematodal drugs. In: J.E. Riviere & M.G. Papich (eds), *Veterinary Pharmacology and Therapeutics*, 9th edn, pp. 1095–1115. Iowa State University Press, Ames.

88 Roberson, E.L. & Courtney, C.H. (1995) Anticestodal and antitrematodal drugs. In: H.R. Adams (ed), *Veterinary Pharmacology and Therapeutics*, 7th edn, pp. 933–954. Iowa State University Press, Ames.

89 Vidyashankar, A.N., Hanlon, B.M. & Kaplan, R.M. (2012) Statistical and biological considerations in evaluating drug

efficacy in equine strongyle parasites using fecal egg count data. *Veterinary Parasitology*, **185**, 45–56.

90 Kaplan, R.M. & Vidyashankar, A.N. (2012) An inconvenient truth: Global warming and anthelmintic resistance. *Veterinary Parasitology*, **186**, 70–78.

91 Kaplan, R.M. (2004) Drug resistance in nematodes of veterinary importance: A status report. *Trends in Parasitology*, **20**, 477–481.

92 Reinemeyer, C.R. (2012) Anthelmintic resistance in non-strongylid parasites of horses. *Veterinary Parasitology*, **185**, 9–15.

93 Reinemeyer, C.R. (2004) Rational approaches to equine parasite control. Paper presented at: *Equine Nutrition Conference for Feed Manufacturers*, October 18–19, 2004, Lexington, KY.

94 Nielsen, M.K. (2009) Restrictions of anthelmintic usage: Perspectives and potential consequences. *Parasites and Vectors*, **2** (Suppl 2), S7.

95 Nielsen, M.K., Fritzen, B., Duncan, J.L. *et al.* (2010) Practical aspects of equine parasite control: A review based upon a workshop discussion consensus. *Equine Veterinary Journal*, **42**, 460–468.

96 Nielsen, M.K. (2012) Sustainable equine parasite control: Perspectives and research needs. *Veterinary Parasitology*, **185**, 32–44.

97 Reinemeyer, C.R. & Nielsen, M.K. (2013) *Handbook of Equine Parasite Control*. Wiley-Blackwell, Ames.

98 Reeder, D.B. (2011) Equine parasitology: Parasites, protocols and resistance. *Atlantic Coast Veterinary Conference*, October 10–13, 2011, Atlantic City, NJ.

CHAPTER 7

Foals are not just mini horses

K. Gary Magdesian

School of Veterinary Medicine, University of California, Davis, CA, USA

Unique aspects of foal pharmacology

Neonatal foal physiology is unique, and there exist important physiological differences between foals and mature horses that have clinical implications in terms of drug absorption, distribution, metabolism, and/or elimination. Many of the recommendations regarding the use of specific drugs in foals have been extrapolated from other species or adult horses, which may or may not be applicable. Data specific to foal pharmacology are scarce. Using an evidence-based approach, however, some generalized observations and recommendations can be made regarding pharmacodynamics and pharmacokinetics in foals:

1 Dynamic dosage regimens: Foals can typically gain 1.15 ± 0.17 kg/day (1.5–3.3 lb/day), and therefore, as they age, they require frequent dosage adjustments, particularly for drugs with narrow therapeutic indexes, such as the aminoglycosides, amikacin, and gentamicin [1, 2].

2 Increased oral bioavailability of drugs: While many drugs are poorly absorbed following oral administration in adult horses, they may have a relatively high bioavailability in foals. For example, ampicillin, amoxicillin, and many first-generation cephalosporins are well absorbed in foals, whereas their bioavailability in adult horses is insufficient to achieve therapeutic plasma concentrations [3–5].

3 Variability in the volume of distribution: Compared to the adult horse, the neonatal foal's body content is relatively high in water and low in fat. As a result, the volume of distribution for some drugs varies significantly with the age of the horse [6]. In general, compared with adult horses, polar drugs have larger volumes of distribution in foals, whereas nonpolar drugs have smaller volumes of distribution. For example, in foals, gentamicin has an increased volume of distribution compared to mature horses. Therefore, when the same dose per unit of body weight is administered, it will result in lower plasma concentrations in foals than adult horses [7]. The clinical significance of this difference is that higher doses of water-soluble drugs are often required to reach the same plasma and tissue concentrations as adults. For example, gentamicin and amikacin doses recommended for neonatal foals are higher than those for adult horses.

4 Lower serum total protein concentrations: Compared to adult horses, foals have a lower total serum protein concentration [8]. The clinical significance of this difference is that for drugs that are highly protein bound, the total serum drug concentrations may be the same in neonatal foals and mature adults, but the concentration of free or unbound drug in the serum will be higher in the foal. Because it is the free or unbound fraction that is active, and potentially toxic, this is particularly important for drugs with narrow therapeutic indexes, such as nonsteroidal anti-inflammatory drugs (NSAID). With an increased unbound fraction, elimination and metabolism may increase, because it is the unbound fraction that is metabolized and/or excreted. This may reduce some of the impact of higher concentrations of the unbound fraction. However, in the neonatal foal with relatively reduced metabolism/elimination as compared to adult horses, the potential pharmacologic and therapeutic effects could be increased to a clinically relevant degree. Therefore, drugs with a relatively low therapeutic index, such as NSAID, may need to be administered as lower doses in significantly hypoproteinemic foals.

Equine Pharmacology, First Edition. Edited by Cynthia Cole, Bradford Bentz and Lara Maxwell.

5 Decreased metabolic and excretory capacity: Although foals are physiologically precocious at birth, additional maturation of hepatic and renal function occurs, primarily in the first 1–2 weeks postpartum. In particular, compared to adults, neonates have poorly developed hepatic microsomal enzyme pathways, including reduced oxidative and glucuronide activities that are important in the metabolism of many drugs. For drugs that are eliminated from the body primarily by hepatic metabolism, the decreased metabolic capacity of neonatal foals will result in longer elimination half-lives and decreased rates of clearance, compared to adult horses. Examples of drugs eliminated by hepatic metabolism include chloramphenicol, methylxanthines, trimethoprim, sulfonamides, erythromycin, rifampin, metronidazole, and barbiturates. The maturation of hepatic metabolism in neonatal foals is well illustrated by the decreasing elimination half-life of chloramphenicol observed in foals as they age. For example, the mean elimination half-life for chloramphenicol was 5.29 h in 1-day-old foals, 1.35 h in 3-day-old foals, 0.61 h in 7-day-old foals, and 0.51 h in 14-day-old foals [9]. Another example of a drug with delayed elimination due to the limited capacity of biliary excretion in foals, compared to adult horses, is ceftriaxone, a third-generation cephalosporin, which undergoes partial biliary excretion [10, 11]. The elimination half-life of ceftriaxone in adult horses is 1.62 ± 0.42 h, while in the foal it is 3.25 ± 3.22 h [10, 11].

Glomerular filtration rates (GFR) and effective renal plasma flows in foals appear to be similar to those in adult horses, even at 1–2 days of age [12, 13]. This highlights the relatively rapid maturation of renal function in foals as compared to neonates of other species. For example, adult values of glomerular filtration and renal tubular function progressively increase in puppies, but may not reach adult values until 2.5 months of age [14, 15]. Therefore, renal immaturity may not be as significant to equine neonatal pharmacology as is hepatic. Active, carrier-mediated tubular secretion, however, may be incompletely developed in newborn foals, and it is unknown how long it takes to reach adult capacity. What role this plays in altered elimination of drugs in foals is unknown.

6 Urine pH: Foals generally have an acidic urine pH, in contrast to the alkaline pH of adult horses [16]. This favors tubular reabsorption of drugs that are weak acids, particularly those with a relatively high lipid solubility. In contrast, weak bases such as trimethoprim become ion trapped in acid urine and are more readily eliminated.

Clinical pharmacology for neonatal diseases

Sepsis

Sepsis in foals is one of the most common reasons for referral to neonatal intensive care units (ICU) and is often a medical emergency. Foals with sepsis experience a systemic inflammatory response syndrome (SIRS) with increased circulating levels of cytokines. Cytokinemia is associated with tachycardia, tachypnea, fever or hypothermia, and immune dysregulation. Cardiovascular derangements, including hypotension resulting in tissue hypoperfusion, are also common. Clinical signs of sepsis include depressed mentation, weakness, lack of or reduced nursing, injected sclera, mucosal hemorrhages such as petechial hemorrhages of the mucous membranes, and signs of hypoperfusion. Localized sepsis includes umbilical infections, osteomyelitis, septic physitis or arthritis, pneumonia, uveitis, and meningitis. The treatment triad for sepsis is antimicrobial, hemodynamic, and supportive therapy.

Antimicrobial therapy for sepsis should be administered intravenously (IV) because the bioavailability of drugs administered intramuscularly, orally (PO), and subcutaneously may be decreased during sepsis due to hypoperfusion. In addition, bactericidal, rather than bacteriostatic, antibiotics should be used because septic foals are immunocompromised and often neutropenic [17]. Broad-spectrum agents should be administered initially, until results of blood culture and susceptibility testing are available. Blood cultures should not be solely relied upon to make a diagnosis of sepsis, however, because they are not particularly sensitive diagnostic tests, with false-negative results occurring fairly frequently [18]. Antimicrobials should be administered as early as possible to foals exhibiting signs of sepsis, even before confirmation is obtained. Any delay in institution of antibiotic therapy can have severe consequences, such as the development of septic physitis and osteomyelitis. In human patients with septic shock, institution of effective antibiotic therapy within the first hour of hypotension resulted in a significant reduction in mortality [19]. Antimicrobials should not be withheld for the sake of obtaining blood cultures prior to initiating therapy, even when referral to a hospital for neonatal intensive care is planned.

The equine literature has consistently documented that Gram-negative microbes, particularly enteric bacteria such as *E. coli*, *Enterobacter*, and *Klebsiella*, are the most common isolates among foals with sepsis [18, 20–23]. Gram-negative nonenteric bacteria, including *Actinobacillus* and *Pasteurella*, are also common, as are mixed infections, with Gram-negative and Gram-positive bacteria, such as streptococci, enterococci, or staphylococci. Therefore, initial selection of broad-spectrum antimicrobial therapy is essential.

There are several drugs or drug combinations commonly used to provide broad-spectrum antimicrobial coverage in foals. Responsible antimicrobial use dictates reservation of higher generation and newer antimicrobials for infections with bacterial isolates that are multidrug resistant. There are a number of efficacious and cost-effective, first-line antimicrobials available for use in foals with sepsis.

Antibiotic therapy
First-line antimicrobial treatment of sepsis

One of the most commonly used antibiotic combinations that has excellent activity against isolates commonly obtained from septic foals, as described earlier, is that of an aminoglycoside and a beta-lactam, specifically amikacin and ampicillin (Table 7.1) [12, 18, 21, 24]. Other aminoglycosides, such as gentamicin or netilmicin, can be used in place of amikacin; however, the Gram-negative spectrums of activity of these drugs are not as broad as amikacin, and they may not be as efficacious. Amikacin also has excellent activity against staphylococci, including many methicillin-resistant *Staphylococcus aureus* (MRSA) isolates. In addition, amikacin was less likely than beta-lactam antibiotics, such ceftiofur, ampicillin, or imipenem, to induce endotoxin and tumor necrosis factor (TNF)α synthesis during bactericidal activity against *E. coli* in mononuclear cell cultures [25]. However, aminoglycosides should not be used in foals with renal compromise.

Beta-lactam antimicrobials other than ampicillin, including penicillin, first-generation cephalosporins, and ceftiofur, can also be used in combination with amikacin. However, many of these agents are less efficacious than ampicillin against *Enterococcus* isolates.

When aminoglycosides including amikacin are used, particularly in sick or premature foals, monitoring for adverse effects should be diligent. Aminoglycosides are potentially nephrotoxic, particularly when coupled with hypoperfusion or reduced oxygen delivery from any cause. In addition, the pharmacokinetics of aminoglycosides can be altered by the presence of hypoxia, prematurity, and sepsis [26]. Concurrent prematurity and hypoxia led to an increase in half-life and a smaller elimination rate constant in one study [26]. However, a more recent study had different results, where sepsis, prematurity, and hypoxemia did not alter amikacin concentrations [27]. These conflicting results likely reflect differences in disease severity, foal populations, and GFR. This variability makes it difficult for the clinician to empirically predict pharmacokinetics in sick foals and emphasizes the importance of therapeutic drug monitoring (TDM) in critically ill foals. Concurrent azotemia and hypoxia in critically ill foals were associated with decreased clearance and increased peak and trough serum concentrations of amikacin [28]. Interestingly, amikacin-induced nephrotoxicity was not indicated by conventional laboratory testing, nor was it suspected at postmortem examination [28]. Despite these findings, the author recommends that aminoglycosides not be used in azotemic foals as there are other options available, such as third-generation cephalosporins. It should therefore be anticipated that the clearance of amikacin will be reduced, with a resulting increase in the elimination half-life, in some critically ill foals [29]. Plasma creatinine concentrations should be monitored at least every 3–5 days in foals undergoing treatment with aminoglycosides, and more often, even daily, in those with hypotension or reduced peripheral oxygen delivery, such as those with sepsis, hypoxic–ischemic injury, or prematurity. A trend of increasing serum creatinine concentrations, even if they are within the normal range, should warrant reassessment of the dosing protocol; one should not wait until creatinine is above the reference range. Urine output and urinalysis can also aid in monitoring foals on aminoglycoside therapy. Hematuria; glucosuria; proteinuria, with the exception of the first 24 h of life; or the presence of casts can indicate nephrotoxicosis.

TDM is a practical means of ensuring adequate dosing to maximize efficacy and appropriate dosing intervals to minimize the potential for toxicity when administering aminoglycosides. TDM for aminoglycosides consists of

Table 7.1 Dosing guidelines for medications commonly used in foals.

Drug	Dosage	Comment
Antimicrobial agents		
Aminoglycosides		
Amikacin	25 mg/kg, IV, q24 h	TDM recommended (monitor creatinine + UA)
Gentamicin	8–12 mg/kg, IV, q24 h	TDM recommended (monitor creatinine + UA)
Beta-lactams		
Ampicillin	22–30 mg/kg, IV or PO, q6–8 h	(Oral pivampicillin 19.9 mg/kg)
Amoxicillin	13–30 mg/kg, PO, q8 h	
Penicillin, potassium, or sodium	22 000–44 000 IU/kg, IV, q6 h	
Ticarcillin–clavulanic acid	50 mg/kg, IV, q6 h	(Dose based on ticarcillin)
Imipenem	15 mg/kg, IV, q6–8 h	Slow and dilute infusion
First-generation cephalosporins		
Cefazolin	15–22 mg/kg, IV, q6–8 h	
Cephalothin	10–20 mg/kg, IV, q6 h	
Cefadroxil	20–40 mg/kg, PO, q8–12 h	
Cephalexin	25–30 mg/kg, PO, q6–8 h	
Second-generation cephalosporins		
Cefuroxime	16–33 mg/kg, IV, q8 h	
Cefoxitin	20 mg/kg, IV, q6 h	
Third-generation cephalosporins:		
Ceftazidime	20–50 mg/kg, IV, q6 h, slow infusion	
Cefoperazone	30 mg/kg, IV, q8 h, slow infusion	
Cefotaxime	40–50 mg/kg, IV, q6 h, slow infusion	
Ceftizoxime	20–50 mg/kg, IV, q6 h, slow infusion	
Cefpodoxime proxetil	10 mg/kg, PO, q6–8–12 h	
Ceftriaxone	25–50 mg/kg, IV, q12 h	
Ceftiofur	2.2–10 mg/kg, IV, SC, IM, q12 h	
Fourth-generation cephalosporins		
Cefepime	11 mg/kg, IV, q8 h	
Cefquinome	1 mg/kg, IM or IV, q12 h	
Macrolides		
Azithromycin	10 mg/kg, PO, q24 and q48 h after 5 days	Keep foal out of sunlight/heat
Clarithromycin	7.5 mg/kg, PO, q12 h	Keep foal out of sunlight/heat
Erythromycin	15–25 mg/kg, PO, q8 h	Keep foal out of sunlight/heat
Other antimicrobials		
Chloramphenicol*	40–50 mg/kg, PO, q12 h day 1–2 and q8 h day 3–5 or older	Handlers should wear gloves (Should be used with caution in first few days of life)
Doxycycline	10 mg/kg, PO, q12 h	May cause tendon laxity
Rifampin	5 mg/kg, PO, q12 h	
Metronidazole for enteric clostridiosis	10–15 mg/kg, PO, IV, q8 h	
Trimethoprim–sulfonamide	25–30 mg/kg, PO, q12 h	
Antifungal agents		
Fluconazole	8.8–14 mg/kg loading dose once, then 5 mg/kg, PO, q24 h	
Itraconazole	5 mg/kg, PO, q24 h	
Voriconazole	4 mg/kg, PO, q24 h	
Antivirals		
Valacyclovir	20–30 mg/kg, PO, q12 h	Herpes infections

Table 7.1 (*Continued*)

Drug	Dosage	Comment
Other drugs		
Bethanechol	0.22–0.45 mg/kg, PO, q6–8 h	
	0.025–0.04 mg/kg, SC, q6–8 h	
Caffeine	10 mg/kg loading, then 2.5–3 mg/kg, PO, q24 h	
Cimetidine	6.6 mg/kg, IV, q6–8 h	Watch for seizures
	15–25 mg/kg, PO, q8 h	Watch for seizures
Clenbuterol	0.8–3.2 µg/kg, PO, q12 h	
Diazepam	0.04–0.4 mg/kg, IV	Good sedative; seizure control
Di-tri-octahedral smectite	0.5–1 ml/kg, PO, q12 h	Interferes with colostral IgG absorption
Doxapram	0.01–0.05 mg/kg/min CRI; start with low dose	Monitor for excitation and seizures
Epinephrine	0.01–0.02 mg/kg, IV, slow or dilute of 1 : 1000 form	For CPR q3–5 min
Esomeprazole	0.5 mg/kg, IV, slow, q24 h	
Famotidine	0.23–0.5 mg/kg, IV, q8–12 h	
	2.8–4 mg/kg, PO, q8–12 h	
Flunixin meglumine	0.25–1 mg/kg, IV, PO, q12–24 h	Monitor creatinine and urinalysis
		Use concurrent ulcer prevention
Firocoxib	0.1 mg/kg, PO, q24 h	Monitor creatinine and urinalysis
	0.09 mg/kg, IV, q24 h	Not compatible with heparin flush or any other drug
Insulin, regular form	0.005–0.01 IU/kg/h to start, up to 0.1 IU/kg/h	Monitor glucose closely
Ketoprofen	1.1–2.2 mg/kg, IV, q24 h	Monitor creatinine and urinalysis
Lactase	120 U/kg, PO, q3–8 h	
Lidocaine	0.05 mg/kg/min	Watch for seizures, excitation, CNS signs
Metoclopramide	0.02–0.04 mg/kg/h, IV, CRI	Monitor for extrapyramidal signs
	0.6 mg/kg, PO, q4–6 h	
Midazolam	0.04–0.2 mg/kg, IV	Use lowest dose possible, for seizures, sedation
	0.02–0.1 mg/kg/h, IV, CRI	For longer-term seizure control
Neostigmine	0.005–0.01 mg/kg, SC	
Omeprazole	4 mg/kg, PO, q24 h	
Oxytetracycline	For tendon contracture: 30–60 mg/kg, IV 1–3 treatments only, every other day, administer with fluids	Give in fluids, check renal function pre and post Renal failure is a risk
Pantoprazole	1.5 mg/kg, IV, slow and dilute q24 h	
Paromomycin	100 mg/kg, PO, q24 h	Antiprotozoal (*Cryptosporidium* spp.), efficacy unproven
Phenobarbital	2–10 mg/kg, IV, slow, q8–24 h	Give slow infusion, watch for respiratory depression
	3–10 mg/kg, PO, q12 h	and hypotension
Pentoxifylline	7.5–8 mg/kg, PO, q12 h	
Potassium bromide	60 mg/kg, PO, q24 h	For long-term seizure control
Ranitidine	1.5 mg/kg, IV, q8–12 h	
	6.6 mg/kg, PO, q8 h	
Sucralfate	20 mg/kg, PO, q6 h	Stagger 2 h with other medications
Inhaled treatments		
Albuterol inhaler	1–2 µg/kg via inhaler or nebulizer q8–12 h	
Albuterol nebulizer (0.5%)	1 µg/kg (0.2–0.5 ml total for 50 kg foal)	Dilute in sterile saline
Clenbuterol inhaler	0.5 µg/kg nebulized	
Ipratropium bromide inhaler	0.5–3 µg/kg nebulized/inhaled q8–12 h	Nebulized or inhaled
Salmeterol inhaler	0.5 µg/kg via inhaler q6–12 h	

(*Continued*)

Table 7.1 (*Continued*)

Drug	Dosage	Comment
Nebulized antimicrobials		
Gentamicin (nebulized)	2.2 mg/kg as a 50 mg/ml solution, q24 h	
Ceftiofur (nebulized)	1 mg/kg as a 25 mg/ml solution in sterile water, q12 h	
Inotropes/pressors for blood pressure support		
Dobutamine	2–10 µg/kg/min, IV	Titrate to effect
Norepinephrine	0.01–1 µg/kg/min, IV	Must be diluted in 5% dextrose
Vasopressin	0.25–1.0 mU/kg/min	

CRI, continuous rate infusion; TDM, therapeutic drug monitoring; UA, urinalysis.
*Risk of aplastic anemia to human handlers.

collecting two serum samples. The first is collected soon after administration of the once-daily dose and is considered the peak serum concentration. The second sample is collected 20–24 h after administration (i.e., just before the next dose is administered) and is considered the trough serum concentration. Obtaining the peak concentration at 1 h postadministration will ensure adequate time for tissue distribution. The goal is to achieve a peak concentration that is 8- to 10-fold over the minimum inhibitory concentrations (MICs) of the cultured pathogen. For example, if 2 µg/ml of amikacin is the MIC for the cultured pathogen, the desired peak serum concentration would be 16–20 µg/ml. If culture and susceptibility results are not available, the targeted goal should be a serum amikacin concentration ≥40 µg/ml, because most of the common and susceptible bacterial agents associated with sepsis in horses have MICs ≤4 µg/ml. Although the Clinical Laboratory Standards Institute (CLSI) considers bacteria with MIC ≤ 16 µg/ml to be susceptible to amikacin, the results of several studies have found that most Gram-negative microbes isolated from horses and foals had MIC_{90} ≤4 µg/ml [27, 30–32]. Based on these study results, a peak serum amikacin concentration of 40 µg/ml would be a reasonable goal in the absence of a culture and sensitivity test indicating that a higher concentration is needed. To decrease the risk of nephrotoxicity, the trough serum amikacin concentration should ideally be less than 1 µg/ml. By collecting the trough sample 20 h after dosing and targeting the 1 µg/ml concentration for that time period, an additional 4 h is provided for the tubular epithelium to eliminate accumulated aminoglycoside prior to administration of the next dose.

If half-life calculations are desired, additional samples will need to be collected between the peak and trough samples, as serum concentrations 20–24 h postadministration are often below the limit of quantification of the analytical method. To estimate the elimination half-life collection of a sample, 8 h postadministration has been suggested. At that time period, target serum amikacin concentrations should be between 15 and 20 µg/ml. If gentamicin is used instead of amikacin, the targeted peak, 8 h, and trough target concentrations are ≥20, 3–5, and ≤1 µg/ml, respectively.

The beta-lactam of choice, in the author's experience, to combine with an aminoglycoside in order to produce the broadest spectrum of antimicrobial activity is ampicillin. It is one of the few antimicrobials with efficacy against some of the resistant isolates of *Enterococcus faecalis* and *Enterococcus faecium*, although some isolates of *Pseudomonas aeruginosa* and enterococci, other than *E. faecalis* and *E. faecium*, are resistant. Penicillin or first- or second-generation cephalosporins can all be used in combination with an aminoglycosides. Although the third-generation cephalosporin ceftiofur can also be paired with amikacin, it is not as efficacious as ampicillin against many enterococci.

Third- and fourth-generation cephalosporins

As indicated earlier, first- and second-generation cephalosporins can be used to treat sepsis in foals, but they must be combined with aminoglycosides because of their limited activity against Gram-negative organisms (Table 7.1). Third- and fourth-generation cephalosporins, however, are alternatives to aminoglycoside–beta-lactam combinations for treatment of sepsis in foals. They are indicated in foals with acute kidney injury where use of aminoglycosides is contraindicated and in foals with bacterial isolates that are resistant to amikacin. Two of these agents, ceftiofur and cefquinome, are labeled for use in horses in the USA and European Union, respectively.

The third-generation cephalosporin ceftiofur is bactericidal with a relatively broad spectrum of activity that includes many Gram-positive and Gram-negative aerobic and anaerobic organisms and is an excellent alternative to aminoglycoside–beta-lactam combinations in foals with renal azotemia (Table 7.1). Resistance to ceftiofur, however, is more common than resistance to aminoglycoside–beta-lactam combinations. For example, literature reports indicate that as many as 30% of the isolates obtained from septic foals may be resistant to ceftiofur [12, 18, 21, 24, 33]. Therefore, the decision to use it should be made based on culture and susceptibility testing results or if they are not available historical local antimicrobial susceptibility data, particularly any data obtained on bacterial isolates from septic foals. In addition, because the labeled dose of ceftiofur, 2.2 mg/kg bwt, q24 h targets *Streptococcus* spp., which are generally considered particularly sensitive to ceftiofur, and because it has a wide margin of safety, ceftiofur can be administered to septic foals at higher than labeled doses [34]. In fact, doses as high as 10 mg/kg bwt q6–12 h have been administered in order to achieve serum concentrations likely to be efficacious against the Gram-negative microbes often associated with sepsis in foals [35, 36]. A recent study showed that ceftiofur administered at a dose of 5 mg/kg bwt q12 h was efficacious against 90% of the *E. coli, Pasteurella, Klebsiella*, and *Streptococcus* organisms isolated from blood cultures from foals and a few from other equine clinical samples (i.e., MIC≤2 µg/ml) [37]. Nevertheless, even at that dose, which is over 2× the labeled dose, 27% of *Salmonella* isolates and most *Enterococcus* isolates were resistant to ceftiofur. Another study found that 23% of all bacterial isolates obtained from septic neonatal foals were resistant to ceftiofur [33]. In addition, ceftiofur is not optimal for treatment of infections caused by *Proteus* or *Staphylococcus* spp., because its intermediate metabolite, desfuroylceftiofur (DCA), is less active than the parent drug against these species and therefore predicting efficacy is difficult.

A recent study evaluated the pharmacokinetics of ceftiofur administered to foals as a continuous rate infusion (CRI) [38]. The potential advantage of CRI administration is maintenance of plasma concentrations of the antimicrobial above the MIC of the offending microbe 100% of the time, which would be optimal for time-dependent antimicrobials such as the beta-lactams. Based on the pharmacokinetic values from this study, the authors predicted that a bolus loading dose of 1.26 mg/kg followed immediately by a CRI of 2.86 µg/kg/min would maintain plasma concentrations of DCA≥2 µg/ml [38]. This is equal to a daily dose of 5.4 mg/kg/day. For bacteria with higher MIC values (up to 4 µg/ml for DCA), higher doses may be required. When switching from a CRI to intermittent bolus administration as the foal improves, the bolus dose should be started 12 h after the end of the CRI.

Other third- and fourth-generation cephalosporins can be used in foals infected with multidrug-resistant bacteria that are not susceptible to ceftiofur (Table 7.1). Concern for the development of antimicrobial resistance, as well as their cost, dictates that these antimicrobials should be used judiciously, only when antimicrobial susceptibility data indicate that other options are limited. In general, the third-generation cephalosporins are very broad spectrum, with some individual variations among the specific drugs. For example, cefotaxime is among those with the highest anaerobe coverage. Ceftazidime and cefoperazone have the most potent activity against *Pseudomonas* spp. isolates, but ceftazidime has poor anaerobic coverage. Recently, a third-generation cephalosporin, cefpodoxime, that is formulated for oral administration has been studied in foals [39]. It may be particularly useful in the field when MIC data justify its use.

A recent study compared CRI and intermittent bolus administration of cefotaxime in 1-day-old pony foals [40]. In the intermittent bolus dosing group, the dose administered was 40 mg/kg bwt, IV, q6 h. In the CRI dosing group, an initial loading dose of 40 mg/kg bwt, IV, was administered followed by a CRI at 160 mg/kg/day (6.7 mg/kg/h). With CRI dosing, mean plasma concentrations were constantly maintained above the MIC of most susceptible pathogens (16 µg/ml), whereas intermittent dosing allowed for concentrations to decrease to as low as 0.78 µg/ml 6 h after dosing. While many Gram-negative and Gram-positive bacteria are susceptible to cefotaxime, many *Pseudomonas* and MRSA and some *E. coli* isolates are not susceptible, even with CRI dosing. The CRI dosing protocol is particularly indicated for foals with sepsis and septic arthritis, as synovial fluid concentrations were significantly higher with CRI dosing as compared to those achieved by intermittent dosing. Cefotaxime is compatible with 0.9% saline as a diluent, and the diluted formulation is stable for at least 24 h at room temperature as long as it is protected from light.

A limited number of fourth-generation cephalosporins, including cefquinome and cefepime, have been studied in horses (Table 7.1) [41, 42]. Cefquinome is actually labeled for use in foal septicemia in the European Union. It has a very broad spectrum of activity, including good activity against *Actinobacillus equuli*, streptococci, enteric bacteria, *Clostridium perfringens*, and staphylococci [42, 43]. Cefepime requires further study in foals but may be potentially useful for treatment of sepsis. The MICs of cefepime for equine isolates of enteric microbes have not been reported; however, *E. coli*, *Klebsiella pneumonia*, and *C. perfringens* isolated from humans are often considered susceptible to cefepime (i.e., MIC ≤ 8 µg/ml). *E. faecalis* and MRSA are considered resistant.

On occasion, bacterial meningitis is the unfortunate sequel of sepsis in the foal. There are a limited number of antimicrobial agents that can be used to treat bacterial meningitis, because few agents are able to penetrate the blood–brain barrier (BBB) sufficiently to produce therapeutic concentrations within the cerebrospinal fluid (CSF). For example, ceftiofur does not penetrate the BBB to a clinically significant degree [37]. A number of other third-generation cephalosporins have greater BBB penetration than ceftiofur, and among these, ceftriaxone achieves the highest concentration within the CSF. Because ceftizoxime, cefotaxime, and ceftazidime penetrate the BBB to a greater extent than both ceftiofur and amikacin they are superior choices for the treatment of meningitis in foals.

It should be pointed out that doses of cephalosporins may need to be lowered in foals with renal insufficiency, as has been recommended for humans, because of reduced renal clearance.

Carbapenems: Imipenem and meropenem
Carbapenems are a group of modified beta-lactams that have the broadest spectrum of activity of any of the commercially available antimicrobials. The class includes imipenem, meropenem, and doripenem. Imipenem, which is the only carbapenem that has been evaluated in the horse, has activity against many bacteria that are resistant to older, first-line antimicrobials including

enterococci, *Pseudomonas* spp., and anaerobic isolates (Table 7.1) [44]. MRSA organisms are typically resistant to imipenem as are some *Enterobacter* and *Pseudomonas* isolates and *E. faecium*. Its activity is synergistic with aminoglycosides against *Pseudomonas*.

Imipenem, which can only be administered IV, is formulated with cilastatin, a compound that inhibits the imipenem-degrading renal enzyme dehydropeptidase. Cilastatin prolongs the elimination half-life of imipenem, but does not have any antibiotic activity itself. In adult horses, imipenem–cilastatin was well tolerated with no significant adverse events reported, but it had a short elimination half-life requiring administrations every 6–8 h to maintain serum concentrations likely to be effective against common equine pathogens [44]. Because of concerns over the increasing development of antimicrobial resistance, imipenem should be used judiciously, only when culture and susceptibility testing dictates its use or when cultures are not available in neonatal foals with infections that are not responding to first-line antimicrobials. Foals undergoing treatment with imipenem should be monitored for adverse effects, including rarely seizures, antimicrobial-induced diarrhea, and thrombophlebitis if not diluted properly. Dilution should occur as per label instructions but briefly should include resuspension of vials with 10 ml diluent, with subsequent transfer of the vial contents into 100 ml of infusion solution prior to intravenous infusion. Compatible solutions include 0.9% sodium chloride and 5 or 10% dextrose.

Enrofloxacin
Fluoroquinolones, such as enrofloxacin, have excellent spectrums of activity against Gram-negative bacteria and some *Staphylococcus* isolates. However, enrofloxacin should not be used in foals or pregnant mares, because it is associated with cartilage toxicity and subsequent arthropathy [45, 46].

Duration of antibiotic therapy
The duration of antimicrobial treatment will vary with each case, but in general, a 14-day course is recommended for foals with septicemia. As previously discussed, initial therapy should be a bactericidal antimicrobial administered IV because septic foals may have difficulty absorbing drugs administered via other routes and are likely to have dysfunctional immune function, including neutropenia and failure of passive

transfer of colostral antibodies [47]. Once the foal is hemodynamically stable and a positive clinical response to the antimicrobial therapy is apparent, the mode of administration of the antimicrobial can be changed to an oral drug based ideally on current or if necessary historical MIC data.

Foals with localized sepsis, such as those with bone, physeal, or umbilical infections, often require more prolonged durations of treatment; often, a minimum of a 30-day course or longer in these cases is required.

Supportive care

Supportive care is critically important for septic foals. Such care includes fluid therapy and nutritional support, and excellent reviews on these topics are available [48–53]. Additional supportive care of neonatal foals with sepsis includes ocular and umbilical care, physical therapy for limbs, and recumbency management. Finally, antiendotoxin therapy is controversial, but many agents including flunixin meglumine, pentoxifylline, polymyxin B, and plasma containing antiendotoxin antibody have been used in attempts to modify pathological responses to endotoxemia.

Several studies have evaluated the use of plasma in clinically ill foals, and the results of these studies generally support its use. For example, in one clinical study, septic foals that received hyperimmune plasma rich in antiendotoxin antibodies had increased survival rates compared to foals that received conventional hyperimmune equine plasma [54]. In addition, the results of another study showed that plasma administration enhanced *in vitro* neutrophil function in septic, but not healthy, normal foals [17]. Despite the findings of these studies, it should be noted that plasma is not unequivocally accepted as a treatment of endotoxemia in foals, and there is some evidence that it could have detrimental effects. For example, in an experimental model of endotoxemia, 3–5-month-old foals receiving *Salmonella* antiserum had an increase in plasma interleukin-6 (IL-6) and TNF concentrations compared to untreated control foals [55]. IL-6 and TNF are inflammatory cytokines associated with negative hemodynamic effects. In this same study, foals pretreated with polymyxin B prior to administration of endotoxin had significantly (P<0.05) lower maximum plasma TNF and IL-6 activities and significantly lower rectal temperatures and respiratory rates compared to foals administered endotoxin alone [55].

Flunixin meglumine is commonly used in adult horses with endotoxemia or Gram-negative sepsis as a means to decrease prostaglandin and thromboxane production [56]. Its use in neonatal foals with endotoxemia has not been critically evaluated, however, and there is wide variability in its use among equine practitioners and neonatologists. This is due in large part to a concern over the increased susceptibility of neonates to the adverse effects of NSAID, which include gastrointestinal ulceration and renal injury. Even in healthy neonatal foals, the elimination and clearance rates of flunixin meglumine are longer, compared to older foals and adult horses [56]. In addition, foals with sepsis and other critical illnesses suffer from hemodynamic derangements, malperfusion, and multiple organ dysfunctions that further increase their risk of developing NSAID-associated adverse events. For example, in one study when flunixin meglumine was administered daily at the labeled dose of 1.1 mg/kg bwt for 30 days, all 10 treated foals developed gastric erosions and 1 developed gastric ulcers, whereas none of the untreated control foals developed erosions or ulcers [57]. In addition, the three foals that were administered flunixin meglumine PO also developed oral ulcerations. Therefore, if NSAID are administered to neonatal foals, the concurrent administration of gastroprotectants, such as omeprazole, is strongly recommended.

To detect renal and gastrointestinal injury as early as possible, serum creatinine and total protein, or albumin, concentrations should be determined if possible every few days in the neonatal foal on NSAID therapy. Foals with mal- or hypoperfusion, such as foals with septic or endotoxic shock, should be monitored more often, even daily, if flunixin meglumine is used. In general, the author avoids the use of NSAID in such cases. In addition, urinalyses can be conducted to detect microscopic hematuria as a marker of renal papillary necrosis from NSAID toxicity. In adult horses, a low dose of flunixin meglumine at 0.25 mg/kg bwt, IV, mitigated eicosanoid production in an experimental model of endotoxemia [58]. Although this treatment regimen has not specifically evaluated in foals, this dose administered daily to twice daily may be associated with fewer adverse effects.

Firocoxib is a selective COX2 inhibitor available for use in horses, unlike the more commonly used NSAID, such as phenylbutazone and flunixin meglumine, which are nonselective agents that inhibit both COX1 and

COX2 enzymes [59]. Firocoxib is available in both an oral paste and an IV formulation that are administered at slightly different dose rates (Table 7.1). Although the safety profile for firocoxib in adult horses appears superior to any of the nonselective NSAID, its safety and efficacy have not been determined in neonatal foals nor in the presence of endotoxemia.

Blood pressure support: Inotropes and pressors

Foals with severe sepsis, SIRS, and septic shock often experience hypotension and derangements in tissue perfusion. Affected foals are often hypovolemic and may have myocardial dysfunction, increased vascular permeability, and loss of vasomotor tone as a result of circulating cytokines and inflammatory mediators. Therefore, in addition to antimicrobial therapy, improvement of tissue perfusion is one of the cornerstones of sepsis therapy. Blood pressure correlates directly with systemic vascular resistance and cardiac output and is the driving force for adequate tissue perfusion. Therefore, in order to improve tissue perfusion, blood pressure must be maintained or restored to normal. Targeting a specific arterial mean blood pressure number should not be the goal, because "normal" blood pressure varies widely among neonatal foals. In general, a mean arterial pressure of 60 mmHg is associated with end-organ perfusion. However, some premature and small foals appear to perfuse adequately at lower pressures. Therefore, the blood pressure number should be interpreted in light of the foal's clinical picture, including perfusion parameters (e.g., mentation, pulse quality, capillary refill time, extremity temperature, mucous membrane color), laboratory indicators of perfusion status (e.g., lactate, oxygen extraction ratio, central venous oxygen saturation), and urine output.

The first step to improve tissue perfusion is IV fluid therapy in order to maximize stroke volume and cardiac output [49, 51, 53]. Once fluid volume has been maximized (as evidenced by increases in central venous pressure [maximum 12 cm H_2O; 8.9 mmHg]) and if signs of hypoperfusion, such as cold extremities, poor mucous membrane color, poor pulse quality, and prolonged capillary refill time, have not yet abated, stroke volume should be further enhanced with the use of positive inotropic agents. In foals, the most commonly used inotrope is dobutamine, a primarily beta-1 agonist that increases the force of contraction and thus cardiac

output, administered at a dose of 3–10 µg/kg/min, IV (Table 7.1). Dobutamine infusions have a low rate of adverse effects, with monitoring directed primarily at ensuring tachyarrhythmias do not develop. Dobutamine can be diluted in isotonic saline, lactated Ringer's solution, or 5% dextrose in water.

If hypotension and signs of hypoperfusion are refractory to the combination of IV fluids and dobutamine, then pressor therapy, which will increase system vascular resistance, should be added to the regimen. Because of the potential for excessive vasoconstriction with a consequent decrease in stroke volume, pressors should not be used without concurrent inotropes. In neonatal foals, the two most commonly used pressor agents are the catecholamines norepinephrine and vasopressin. Because of the potential for reduction in splanchnic circulation with vasopressin, it is recommended that pressor therapy be initiated with norepinephrine at a dose of 0.01–0.1 titrated up to 1.0 µg/kg/min to effect. For example, in a study of healthy 1–5-day-old foals that were maintained at a hypotensive state induced by isoflurane anesthesia, vascular resistance was increased by both norepinephrine and vasopressin administration [60]. However, the gastric to arterial CO_2 gap, a marker of splanchnic hypoperfusion, was significantly increased during administration of vasopressin at a high infusion rate of 1.0 mU/kg/min. In this same study, both dobutamine and norepinephrine improved cardiac performance and enhanced oxygen delivery to the tissues, whereas vasopressin did not [60].

Norepinephrine is primarily an alpha-1 adrenergic receptor agonist, but it also has weak beta-1 receptor activity. It primarily raises blood pressure through increasing vascular tone and systemic vascular resistance. It should be diluted in 5% dextrose as it is incompatible with electrolyte-containing crystalloids. Norepinephrine should be initiated at a low dose rate and carefully titrated while monitoring arterial blood pressure, urine output, and other cardiovascular indicators, such as plasma lactate concentration and clinical perfusion parameters [61]. Any deterioration of these parameters (e.g., decrease in urine output or increase in plasma lactate concentration), despite an increase in arterial blood pressure, should warrant reconsideration of pressor administration, because an excessive increase in systemic vascular resistance will lead to increased cardiac afterload and subsequent decreased stroke volume. Vasopressin at a dose of 0.25–1.0 mU/kg/min can be initiated in foals in which fluids, dobutamine, and norepinephrine fail to improve perfusion. Vasopressin can be added to the regimen of fluids, dobutamine, and norepinephrine.

Foals with septic or SIRS shock that is refractory to fluid therapy are candidates for referral to a center that treat critically ill foals. The use of inotropes and pressors is generally beyond the scope of field treatment.

Gastrointestinal pharmacology: Enteritis, ulcer prophylaxis, and ileus

Neonatal foals are susceptible to a number of gastrointestinal disorders, including enterocolitis and colic. In a study of 410 sick neonatal foals, enterocolitis ranked only behind sepsis and perinatal asphyxia as the third most common clinical diagnosis [62].

Enteritis/enterocolitis
Enterocolitis is treated with the triad of hemodynamic support, specific antiagent therapy, and supportive care. Hemodynamic support consists primarily of IV crystalloid and colloid fluid administration, as well as inotrope and pressor therapy in fluid-refractory shock states (see Section "Blood Pressure Support: Inotropes and Pressors") [49, 51, 53].

All neonatal foals with enterocolitis should be treated with parenteral, broad-spectrum antimicrobials because of the high risk of bacteremia. Approximately 50% of foals with diarrhea are blood culture positive [51, 63].

Specific antiagent therapy refers to medications targeting one or more of the many potentially causative agents of diarrhea. Clostridial enterocolitis, including *C. difficile* and *C. perfringens*, can be treated with metronidazole at a dose of 10–15 mg/kg bwt, PO or IV, q8 h (Table 7.1). Foals with ileus and resultant reflux should be treated with metronidazole IV. Di-tri-octahedral smectite (Bio-Sponge, Platinum Performance, Inc., Buellton, CA), which has been shown to bind clostridial toxins and endotoxins *in vitro*, may also be helpful in these foals. Fortunately, it does not appear to impact the efficacy of metronidazole, at least *in vitro*; however, it does bind immunoglobulins [64, 65]. Therefore, it should not be administered within the first 8 h of initial nursing in newborn foals. It also binds basic drugs, and

therefore, administration should be staggered with other medications. The recommended dose of di-tri-octahedral smectite for a 45–50 kg foal is 30–60 ml, PO, q12 h. Although nitazoxanide (NZT), which is labeled for use in human patients with *Cryptosporidium* and *Giardia* infections, has shown some promising effects in preliminary studies where it was administered to humans with *C. difficile* infections, it has yet to be evaluated in foals for this purpose [66].

Salmonellosis cases in foals should be treated with systemic antimicrobials because of the high risk of bacterial translocation and sepsis. However, it should be kept in mind that antimicrobial treatment does not alter the course of enteric salmonellosis and there are no specific treatments for this form of enteritis.

Viral diarrheas in foals are treated primarily with supportive care. The results of recent studies in human patients indicate, however, that NTZ may have efficacy against rotavirus. For example, in a randomized double-blinded trial in children with rotavirus infections, NZT reduced the time to resolution of illness and produced no significant adverse events [67]. It should be noted, however, that NTZ has been associated with severe diarrhea in adult horses and, therefore, it should be used with caution even in foals.

Enteritis caused by *Cryptosporidium* spp. is also primarily treated with supportive care. Foals with severe forms of *Cryptosporidium*-induced diarrhea that do not respond to supportive care should be treated with drugs that have shown efficacy in humans with cryptosporidiosis. These include NTZ, azithromycin, and paromomycin (Table 7.1). Foals suffering from enteritis caused by *Giardia* spp. should be treated with fenbendazole or metronidazole (Table 7.1).

Supportive treatment of the foal with enterocolitis consists of ulcer prophylaxis, nutritional support, and use of anti-inflammatory or antiendotoxic measures. Foals with enteritis often benefit from transient withholding of nursing and provision of parenteral nutrition to allow time for the gut to rest and heal. Administration of lactase enzyme may also be helpful in foals suffering from enteritis. Agents, such as *C. difficile* and rotavirus, can cause small intestinal microvillus destruction that can lead to secondary lactase deficiency [68]. Supplementation with lactase at a dose of 120 U/kg, PO, q3–8 h is helpful in minimizing the osmotic contribution to diarrhea from undigested lactose. The adsorbent material di-tri-octahedral smectite can also be administered to foals with diarrhea and is especially useful for clostridial diarrheas (Table 7.1). Please see Chapter 11 for more detail.

Ulcer prophylaxis and treatment of existing ulcers in foals

Ulcer prophylaxis in neonatal foals currently is controversial in equine neonatology, because of concerns of an increased susceptibility to bacterial enteric infections associated with the loss of gastric acidity [69]. In a recent multicenter retrospective study, the use of histamine type 2 receptor antagonists and omeprazole increased the risk of diarrhea in neonatal foals treated in ICU [69]. The risk of gastric ulceration in foals with gastrointestinal diseases, however, is also documented, and therefore, it is highly recommended that gastric ulcer prophylaxis be instituted in every neonatal foal with GI signs, including diarrhea and colic [70, 71].

For the prevention of gastric ulceration, proton-pump inhibitors, including omeprazole (4 mg/kg, PO, q24 h), pantoprazole (1.5 mg/kg, IV, slow and dilute, q24 h), and esomeprazole (recently studied in adult horses at 0.5 mg/kg, IV, q24 h), are the preferred medications (Table 7.1) [72]. Although esomeprazole has not been evaluated in foals, omeprazole and pantoprazole have been well characterized in this age group [73, 74]. When administered PO to neonatal foals, omeprazole resulted in a significant increase in gastric pH within 2 h [74]. Critically ill foals exhibited a blunted response to the histamine H2 receptor antagonist ranitidine, and therefore, this class of antacids may not be as effective in foals as the proton-pump inhibitors [75].

Sucralfate may be an effective adjunctive medication for ulcer prophylaxis/treatment in foals. It inhibits pepsin, buffers hydrogen ion, and stimulates production of prostaglandin E, sodium bicarbonate, and mucus. A dose of 20 mg/kg bwt, PO, q6–8 h is typically used in foals, and its administration should be staggered with other medications due to its nonspecific adsorbent qualities. Sucralfate may be particularly useful for prophylaxis when NSAID are administered [76].

Ileus

Neonatal foals develop ileus for many reasons, often secondary to gastrointestinal injury associated with peripartum asphyxia, sepsis, prematurity, endotoxemia, and shock of any origin. Hypoperfusion, hypoxemia, hypothermia, hypoglycemia, acidosis, or electrolyte

disturbances can also contribute to ileus. Finally, botulism also causes ileus.

Treatment of ileus consists primarily of addressing the underlying cause, as well as providing supportive care, including IV fluids, blood pressure support, and oxygen insufflation. Withholding of enteral nutrition while providing alternate (parenteral) nutrition may also prove helpful. Sucralfate, which has been shown to aid in reducing the risk of bacterial translocation in laboratory animals with ileus due to gut injury, can be administered, provided that significant amounts of reflux are not present [77].

The use of prokinetics for ileus in neonatal foals is controversial, because no studies have been conducted on the effects of these agents in this age group. In human infants, erythromycin, a motilin receptor agonist, is commonly used as a prokinetic. In randomized clinical trials, erythromycin, when administered at low doses prophylactically to preterm infants, did not demonstrate a clear benefit for preventing ileus [78]. In contrast, a high-dose administration protocol of erythromycin, considered "rescue therapy," has shown consistent results in treating gastrointestinal dysmotility in human infants, but again, this has not been evaluated in foals [78].

A number of prokinetic agents have been used in neonatal foals, including metoclopramide, lidocaine, neostigmine, and bethanechol (Table 7.1). Nevertheless, it is generally advisable not administer prokinetic agents to foals unless the ileus persists for prolonged periods. Rather the preference is to wait on initiating enteral feeding until the gut has healed enough to adequately digest milk. After metabolic and fluid derangements have been corrected and the gut has been allowed to rest for one or more days, if progressive gastrointestinal motility does return, then prokinetic therapy should be considered.

Respiratory pharmacology

Foal pneumonia

Bacterial pneumonia is the most common respiratory disease in foals. Antimicrobial selection for treatment of foal pneumonia should be based on culture and sensitivity results of tracheal aspirates, when possible, as well as the age of the foal, because causative agents, to some degree, vary with age. For example, neonatal foal pneumonia is often caused by the same microbes associated with septicemia, including enteric bacteria (e.g., *E. coli, Klebsiella, Enterobacter, Enterococcus*), nonenteric Gram-negative (e.g., *Actinobacillus, Pasteurella*), and Gram-positive bacteria (e.g., *Streptococcus*) [21, 79]. This is because pneumonia is often of hematogenous origin in these foals, developing secondary to septicemia. Aspiration pneumonia, however, also occurs, particularly in foals with pharyngeal paresis or dysphagia. In these cases, oropharyngeal agents, including *Actinobacillus, Streptococcus*, and enteric and anaerobic bacteria, should be considered as possible causative agents.

In neonatal foals, transtracheal aspiration is not performed as commonly as in older foals and adult horses. Therefore, antimicrobial selection in neonatal foals should be empiric until culture and susceptibility results of blood cultures are available (see Section "Sepsis").

In the older foal, 1–6 months of age, inhalation pneumonia is more common than pneumonia secondary to septicemia or aspiration. The most common bacteria affecting this age group include *Streptococcus equi* subsp. *zooepidemicus, Actinobacillus* spp., *Pasteurella* spp., *Rhodococcus equi* (on endemic premises), enterics, *Bordetella bronchiseptica*, and *Staphylococcus* spp., and the less common *S. equi* subsp. *equi* and anaerobes. *Pneumocystis carinii*, a protozoal agent, and *Mycoplasma* spp. are uncommon to rare causes of pneumonia in foals [79–81]. Particularly in this age group of foals, antimicrobial selection should be based on culture of transtracheal aspirate fluid and antimicrobial susceptibility testing of cultured isolates whenever possible. Because of the delay associated with culture and susceptibility testing, however, antimicrobial selection is initially empiric and based on knowledge of the common historical isolates found on a particular farm or in a specific geography.

One of the most difficult and important decisions in treating foals is determining whether the pneumonia is likely due to *R. equi* or some other bacteria, because the treatment for these will likely be very different. *R. equi* should be suspected on endemic premises, whenever foals exhibit signs of pneumonia and have ultrasonographic or radiographic evidence of pulmonary abscesses, and specific antirhodococcal treatment should be initiated [81]. A factor that increases the level of suspicion of a subclinical *R. equi* infection on an endemic farm is a WBC count > 15 000/µl [82]. Another study showed that a fibrinogen >700 mg/dl and a WBC > 20 000/µl in foals with clinical pneumonia were

highly predictive of *R. equi* infections, as opposed to an infection caused by other bacteria. In that same study, a fibrinogen concentration >900 and WBC >28 000 each had a specificity of 100% for predicting an *R. equi* infection [81]. Interestingly, foals with *R. equi* pneumonia are less likely to have nasal discharge than foals infected with other bacteria, such as *Streptococcus* [79].

Currently, the most common antimicrobial therapy used for treatment of *R. equi* pneumonia is a combination of a macrolide and rifampin. Historically, erythromycin was the most common macrolide used, but because of its side effects and a perceived loss of efficacy, it has largely been replaced with azithromycin or clarithromycin [83]. The perceived lack of efficacy, however, has not been confirmed in any randomized well-controlled clinical trials. In a retrospective study, however, foals treated with clarithromycin–rifampin had higher short- and long-term treatment success rates compared to those treated with erythromycin–rifampin [83]. Reported side effects of macrolides, though less common for azithromycin and clarithromycin, include diarrhea, hyperthermia with respiratory distress syndrome, and lethargy [84]. In a retrospective study by Giguere *et al.*, there was a tendency toward a higher incidence of diarrhea in foals treated with clarithromycin–rifampin (5/18) compared to those treated with azithromycin–rifampin (1/20). Gamithromycin was recently studied in foals and may represent an alternative and long-acting macrolide for use in foals in the future [85]. Currently, tulathromycin and tilmicosin have no role in the treatment of *R. equi* infection due to poor *in vitro* activity [86, 87].

Recently, a small percentage of *R. equi* isolates have been reported to be resistant to macrolides and/or rifampin [88]. In that retrospective study, foals infected with these isolates suffered a higher mortality than foals infected with susceptible isolates. The optimal treatment of foals infected with macrolide- or rifampin-resistant *R. equi* is currently unknown. Suggested treatments include doxycycline/rifampin, trimethoprim–sulfonamide/rifampin, and chloramphenicol, although the efficacy of the latter is variable, with some reports indicating as many as 30% of isolates are resistant. Vancomycin has reportedly been used in some cases of resistant *R. equi* infections; however, because of legitimate concerns over the development of vancomycin-resistant isolates, its use in horses should be limited. Foals treated with vancomycin should be housed in strict isolation.

Foals suspected of having infections with non-*R. equi* bacteria should initially be treated with bactericidal, broad-spectrum antimicrobials until transtracheal wash culture and susceptibility results are available. Similar to the treatment of sepsis, often a combination of a beta-lactam drug (e.g., penicillin or cephalosporin) and an aminoglycoside (e.g., gentamicin) or a third- or fourth-generation cephalosporin (e.g., ceftiofur, cefquinome, respectively) is the most appropriate initial antimicrobials for foals with established broncho- or pleuropneumonia. Early or mild cases often respond to trimethoprim–sulfonamide combinations. It should also be noted that some *Actinobacillus* and *Pasteurella* isolates are relatively more susceptible to ceftiofur than to aminoglycosides. Most *Bordetella* isolates are susceptible to aminoglycosides (92–100% to gentamicin, 90–92% to amikacin) and slightly fewer to trimethoprim–sulfonamides (75–77%) and tetracycline (75–100%) [89]. Foals with *P. carinii* should be treated with trimethoprim–sulfonamides. Recently, successful treatment of *Pneumocystis* pneumonia with dapsone was described in one foal [80]. Finally, macrolides, azithromycin, and doxycycline can be used to treat *Mycoplasma* pneumonia.

Antimicrobials may also be administered through the inhalational or aerosol route in conjunction with systemic antibiotics. Antimicrobials that are conducive to use via an aerosol route through nebulization include ceftiofur and aminoglycosides. Gentamicin should be administered at a dose of 2.2 mg/kg bwt q24 h, using a 50 mg/ml solution (diluted in sterile water or 0.9% saline), whereas ceftiofur should be administered at a dose of 1 mg/kg bwt q12 h using a 25 mg/ml solution of the ceftiofur diluted in sterile water (1:1 in sterile water to make a final concentration of 25 mg/ml) [90, 91]. It should be noted that aerosol administration of a gentamicin solution at 50 mg/ml in sterile water caused mild pulmonary inflammation within 24 h of administration to horses [92]. Ideally, nebulized medications should be isotonic and have a neutral pH, in order to avoid induction of bronchoconstriction and coughing. A report has recommended that antimicrobial aerosolization solutions should be formulated in a saline solution of 0.23–0.45% concentration, to get as close to isotonic as possible [93]. This has not been studied in foals and horses, and ceftiofur is not compatible with saline solutions.

Bronchodilators may decrease the work of breathing, particularly in foals with auscultable wheezes indicating some degree of bronchoconstriction. Available bronchodilators include beta-2 agonists (e.g., albuterol, clenbuterol, salmeterol), which are formulated for oral or inhalational administration to foals (Table 7.1). In addition to bronchodilation, beta-2 agonists have the added benefit of enhancing mucociliary clearance. Compared to oral administration, inhalation of beta-2 agonists causes fewer adverse effects, such as tachycardia, tremors, and sweating. The anticholinergic agent ipratropium bromide also has bronchodilatory effects and can be administered via an inhaler or nebulizer (Table 7.1). The narrow therapeutic index of methylxanthines (aminophylline and theophylline) limits their usefulness in foals, and they should not be considered first-line bronchodilatory agents. Expectorant formulations containing guaifenesin and iodides are commercially available for horses and may be used in foals as well.

Treatment of hypoventilation in neonatal foals

Hypoventilation is a common cause of hypoxemia and hypercapnia in neonatal foals that are presented for intensive care, including those with sepsis, hypoxic–ischemic encephalopathy, and prematurity/dysmaturity. These syndromes are believed to cause hypoventilation through depression of the central respiratory centers. While other causes of hypoventilation, such as neuromuscular disease or severe respiratory disease, are best treated with positive-pressure ventilation, hypoventilation associated with depressed neurologic function initially should be treated with chemical stimulation. Treatment options are doxapram administered at a dose of 0.01–0.05 mg/kg/min, IV, or caffeine administered at a loading dose of 10 mg/kg bwt, PO, followed by 2.5–3 mg/kg bwt, PO, q24 h (Table 7.1). In a retrospective study, doxapram was more effective than caffeine for rapid correction of hypercapnia in foals with a clinical diagnosis of hypoxic–ischemic encephalopathy [94]. In a similar manner, in an experimental study, doxapram in a dose-dependent manner was more effective than caffeine at restoring ventilation in 1–3-day-old healthy foals with isoflurane-induced hypercapnia [95]. It should be noted, however, that both of these agents cause CNS stimulation and can exacerbate seizures in foals with a propensity toward them.

Seizure control

One of the most common causes of seizures in foals is neonatal maladjustment syndrome. Diazepam (0.04–0.2 mg/kg, IV, up to 0.4 mg/kg if needed, IV) or midazolam (0.04–0.1 mg/kg, IV, up to 0.2 mg/kg, IV) should be administered initially to terminate the seizures (Table 7.1). These benzodiazepines act rapidly but have short durations of effect. Midazolam is more water soluble and, therefore, does not bioaccumulate to the same extent as diazepam. Midazolam can be administered IM but has poor oral bioavailability due to a large hepatic first-pass effect. In contrast, diazepam is so poorly absorbed following intramuscular administration that it should not be administered via this route; however, unlike midazolam, it can be administered PO, although not for termination of status epilepticus. Both agents can also be administered as a CRI, and because it bioaccumulates less than diazepam, midazolam is more conducive to this route of administration at a rate of 0.02–0.1 mg/kg/h. Administration of these agents should be titrated slowly, starting with the lowest effective dose, because they can cause hypoventilation or even apnea when injected too rapidly. Benzodiazepines are among the safest sedatives for use in neonatal foals from a hemodynamic standpoint, although respiratory depression can still occur.

Foals that have multiple seizures despite benzodiazepine administration are candidates for barbiturate therapy. Phenobarbital is the most common drug used to treat refractory seizures in foals. Typically, it is administered at a dose of 2–4 mg/kg bwt, slow IV over 15–20 min, q12 h, but doses as high as 10 mg/kg bwt may be needed and the dosing frequency can range from q8 to q24 h (Table 7.1). High doses and/or rapid administration of phenobarbital are associated with respiratory depression, hypothermia, and hypoperfusion. The onset of action of phenobarbital is slow, with peak activity occurring as long as 45 min after administration, making it unsuitable for treatment of status epilepticus or for ongoing, active seizures.

Foals with recurrent seizures, such as those with epilepsy (e.g., juvenile epilepsy of Arabian foals), can be treated with oral phenobarbital at a dose of 3–10 mg/kg bwt, PO, q12 h or potassium bromide at a dose of 60 mg/kg bwt, PO, q24 h, up to 90 mg/kg bwt, if necessary, for long-term seizure control. TDM can be used when treating foals with these agents. In other species, target plasma bromide concentrations are 70–240 mg/dl (700–2400 µg/ml); however, the efficacy of these concentrations has not been confirmed in horses. In a similar manner, the most efficacious plasma target concentrations for phenobarbital in foals have not been determined, but in other species, a range of 14–40 µg/ml is recommended (range to include both peak and troughs). What is most important when treating foals with recurrent seizures is to use the lowest effective dose that controls the seizures, without causing excessive sedation. In the author's experience, seizures are often controlled in horses with peak phenobarbital concentrations less than 15 µg/ml.

Bromide therapy has fewer side effects than phenobarbital, and therefore, it is preferred for long-term treatment. Potassium bromide, however, has a long half-life of 75 ± 14 h (3.1 ± 0.6 day), although this is quite a bit shorter than the half-life of potassium bromide in other species (11.2 days in cat, 37 days in dog) [96]. This half-life was similar to that obtained for sodium bromide in horses, which was 126 h or 5.2 days, and therefore, it can be difficult to obtain therapeutic plasma concentrations in a short period of time without administration of large loading doses [97]. To circumvent this problem when long-term therapy is required, it should be initiated with both phenobarbital and potassium bromide. Once steady-state therapeutic concentrations of potassium bromide are reached, after approximately 16–25 days of therapy, the dose of phenobarbital can slowly be tapered and eliminated all together if possible.

References

1 Heidler, B., Aurich, J.E., Pohl, W. & Aurich, C. (2004) Body weight of mares and foals, estrous cycles and plasma glucose concentration in lactating and non-lactating Lipizzaner mares. *Theriogenology*, **61**, 883–893.

2 Magdesian, K.G., Wilson, W.D. & Mihalyi, J. (2004) Pharmacokinetics of a high dose of amikacin administered at extended intervals to neonatal foals. *American Journal of Veterinary Research*, **65**, 473–479.

3 Baggot, J.D., Love, D.N., Stewart, J. & Raus, J. (1988) Bioavailability and disposition kinetics of amoxicillin in neonatal foals. *Equine Veterinary Journal*, **20**, 125–127.

4 Duffee, N.E., Stang, B.E. & Schaeffer, D.J. (1997) The pharmacokinetics of cefadroxil over a range of oral doses and animal ages in the foal. *Journal of Veterinary Pharmacology and Therapeutics*, **20**, 427–433.

5 Love, D.N., Rose, R.J., Martin, I.C. & Bailey, M. (1981) Serum levels of amoxycillin following its oral administration to thoroughbred foals. *Equine Veterinary Journal*, **13**, 53–55.

6 Fielding, C.L., Magdesian, K.G. & Edman, J.E. (2011) Determination of body water compartments in neonatal foals by use of indicator dilution techniques and multifrequency bioelectrical impedance analysis. *American Journal of Veterinary Research*, **72**, 1390–1396.

7 Cummings, L.E., Guthrie, A.J., Harkins, J.D. & Short, C.R. (1990) Pharmacokinetics of gentamicin in newborn to 30-day-old foals. *American Journal of Veterinary Research*, **51**, 1988–1992.

8 Runk, D.T., Madigan, J.E., Rahal, C.J., Allison, D.N. & Fredrickson, K. (2000) Measurement of plasma colloid osmotic pressure in normal thoroughbred neonatal foals. *Journal of Veterinary Internal Medicine*, **14**, 475–478.

9 Adamson, P.J., Wilson, W.D., Baggot, J.D., Hietala, S.K. & Mihalyi, J.E. (1991) Influence of age on the disposition kinetics of chloramphenicol in equine neonates. *American Journal of Veterinary Research*, **52**, 426–431.

10 Ringger, N.C., Brown, M.P., Kohlepp, S.J., Gronwall, R.R. & Merritt, K. (1998) Pharmacokinetics of ceftriaxone in neonatal foals. *Equine Veterinary Journal*, **30**, 163–165.

11 Ringger, N.C., Pearson, E.G., Gronwall, R. & Kohlepp, S.J. (1996) Pharmacokinetics of ceftriaxone in healthy horses. *Equine Veterinary Journal*, **28**, 476–479.

12 Brewer, B.D., Clement, S.F., Lotz, W.S. & Gronwall, R. (1990) A comparison of inulin, para- aminohippuric acid, and endogenous creatinine clearances as measures of renal function in neonatal foals. *Journal of Veterinary Internal Medicine*, **4**, 301–305.

13 Holdstock, N.B., Ousey, J.C. & Rossdale, P.D. (1998) Glomerular filtration rate, effective renal plasma flow, blood pressure and pulse rate in the equine neonate during the first 10 days post partum. *Equine Veterinary Journal*, **30**, 335–343.

14 Cowan, R.H., Jukkola, A.F. & Arant, B.S., Jr (1980) Pathophysiologic evidence of gentamicin nephrotoxicity in neonatal puppies. *Pediatric Research*, **14**, 1204–1211.

15 Horster, M. & Valtin, H. (1971) Postnatal development of renal function: Micropuncture and clearance studies in the dog. *Journal of Clinical Investigation*, **50**, 779–795.

16 Edwards, D.J., Brownlow, M.A. & Hutchins, D.R. (1990) Indices of renal function: Values in eight normal foals from birth to 56 days. *Australian Veterinary Journal*, **67**, 251–254.

17 McTaggart, C., Penhale, J. & Raidala, S.L. (2005) Effect of plasma transfusion on neutrophil function in healthy and septic foals. *Australian Veterinary Journal*, **83**, 499–505.

18 Wilson, W.D. & Madigan, J.E. (1989) Comparison of bacteriologic culture of blood and necropsy specimens for determining the cause of foal septicemia: 47 cases (1978–1987). *Journal of the American Veterinary Medical Association*, **195**, 1759–1763.

19 Kumar, A., Haery, C., Paladugu, B. *et al.* (2006) The duration of hypotension before the initiation of antibiotic treatment is a critical determinant of survival in a murine model of Escherichia coli septic shock: Association with serum lactate and inflammatory cytokine levels. *Journal of Infectious Diseases*, **193**, 251–258.

20 Koterba, A.M., Brewer, B.D. & Tarplee, F.A. (1984) Clinical and clinicopathological characteristics of the septicaemic neonatal foal: Review of 38 cases. *Equine Veterinary Journal*, **16**, 376–382.

21 Marsh, P.S. & Palmer, J.E. (2001) Bacterial isolates from blood and their susceptibility patterns in critically ill foals: 543 cases (1991–1998). *Journal of the American Veterinary Medical Association*, **218**, 1608–1610.

22 Raisis, A.L., Hodgson, J.L. & Hodgson, D.R. (1996) Equine neonatal septicaemia: 24 cases. *Australian Veterinary Journal*, **73**, 137–140.

23 Stewart, A.J., Hinchcliff, K.W., Saville, W.J. *et al.* (2002) Actinobacillus sp. bacteremia in foals: Clinical signs and prognosis. *Journal of Veterinary Internal Medicine*, **16**, 464–471.

24 Henson, S. & Barton, M. (2001) Bacterial isolates and antibiotic susceptibility patterns from septicemic neonatal foals: One 15 year retrospective study (1986–2000). Dorothy Havemeyer Foundation Third Neonatal Septicemia Workshop, October 2001, Talliores, France, pp. 50–52.

25 Bentley, A.P., Barton, M.H., Lee, M.D., Norton, N.A. & Moore, J.N. (2002) Antimicrobial-induced endotoxin and cytokine activity in an in vitro model of septicemia in foals. *American Journal of Veterinary Research*, **63**, 660–668.

26 Green, S.L. & Conlon, P.D. (1993) Clinical pharmacokinetics of amikacin in hypoxic premature foals. *Equine Veterinary Journal*, **25**, 276–280.

27 Bucki, E.P., Giguere, S., Macpherson, M. & Davis, R. (2004) Pharmacokinetics of once-daily amikacin in healthy foals and therapeutic drug monitoring in hospitalized equine neonates. *Journal of Veterinary Internal Medicine*, **18**, 728–733.

28 Green, S.L., Conlon, P.D., Mama, K. & Baird, J.D. (1992) Effects of hypoxia and azotaemia on the pharmacokinetics of amikacin in neonatal foals. *Equine Veterinary Journal*, **24**, 475–479.

29 Adland-Davenport, P., Brown, M.P., Robinson, J.D. & Derendorf, H.C. (1990) Pharmacokinetics of amikacin in critically ill neonatal foals treated for presumed or confirmed sepsis. *Equine Veterinary Journal*, **22**, 18–22.

30 Adamson, P.J., Wilson, W.D., Hirsh, D.C., Baggot, J.D. & Martin, L.D. (1985) Susceptibility of equine bacterial isolates to antimicrobial agents. *American Journal of Veterinary Research*, **46**, 447–450.

31 Jacks, S.S., Giguere, S. & Nguyen, A. (2003) In vitro susceptibilities of Rhodococcus equi and other common equine pathogens to azithromycin, clarithromycin, and 20 other antimicrobials. *Antimicrobial Agents and Chemotherapy*, **47**, 1742–1745.

32 Orsini, J.A., Soma, L.R., Rourke, J.E. & Park, M. (1985) Pharmacokinetics of amikacin in the horse following intravenous and intramuscular administration. *Journal of Veterinary Pharmacology and Therapeutics*, **8**, 194–201.

33 Sanchez, L.C., Giguere, S. & Lester, G.D. (2008) Factors associated with survival of neonatal foals with bacteremia and racing performance of surviving thoroughbreds: 423 cases (1982–2007). *Journal of the American Veterinary Medical Association*, **233**, 1446–1452.

34 Wilson, W. & Mihalyi, J. (1998) Comparative pharmacokinetics of ceftiofur in neonatal foals and adult horses. Dorothy R Havemeyer Foundation Neonatal Septicemia Workshop, October 2001, Talliores, France, pp. 34–35.

35 Wilkins, P.A. (2004) Disorders of foal. In: S. Reed, W.M. Bayly & D. Sellon (eds), *Equine Internal Medicine*, pp. 1381–1440. Saunders, St. Louis.

36 Wilson, W. (2001) Rational selection of antimicrobials for use in horses. *Proceedings of the American Association of Equine Practitioners*, **47**, 75–93.

37 Meyer, S., Giguere, S., Rodriguez, R., Zielinski, R.J., Grover, G.S. & Brown, S.A. (2009) Pharmacokinetics of intravenous ceftiofur sodium and concentration in body fluids of foals. *Journal of Veterinary Pharmacology and Therapeutics*, **32**, 309–316.

38 Wearn, J.M., Davis, J.L., Hodgson, D.R., Raffetto, J.A. & Crisman, M.V. (2012) Pharmacokinetics of a continuous rate infusion of ceftiofur sodium in normal foals. *Journal of Veterinary Pharmacology and Therapeutics*, **36**, 99–101.

39 Carrillo, N.A., Giguere, S., Gronwall, R.R., Brown, M.P., Merritt, K.A. & O'Kelley, J.J. (2005) Disposition of orally administered cefpodoxime proxetil in foals and adult horses and minimum inhibitory concentration of the drug against common bacterial pathogens of horses. *American Journal of Veterinary Research*, **66**, 30–35.

40 Hewson, J., Johnson, R., Arroyo, L.G. *et al.* (2013) Comparison of continuous infusion with intermittent bolus administration of cefotaxime on blood and cavity fluid drug concentrations in neonatal foals. *Journal of Veterinary Pharmacology and Therapeutics*, **36**, 68–77.

41 Gardner, S.Y. & Papich, M.G. (2001) Comparison of cefepime pharmacokinetics in neonatal foals and adult dogs. *Journal of Veterinary Pharmacology and Therapeutics*, **24**, 187–192.

42 Rohdich, N., Zschiesche, E., Heckeroth, A., Wilhelm, C., Leendertse, I. & Thomas, E. (2009) Treatment of septicaemia and severe bacterial infections in foals with a new cefquinome formulation: A field study. *Deutsche Tierarztliche Wochenschrift*, **116**, 316–320.

43 Thomas, E., Thomas, V. & Wilhelm, C. (2006) Antibacterial activity of cefquinome against equine bacterial pathogens. *Veterinary Microbiology*, **115**, 140–147.

44 Orsini, J.A., Moate, P.J., Boston, R.C. *et al.* (2005) Pharmacokinetics of imipenem-cilastatin following intravenous administration in healthy adult horses. *Journal of Veterinary Pharmacology and Therapeutics*, **28**, 355–361.

45 Davenport, C.L., Boston, R.C. & Richardson, D.W. (2001) Effects of enrofloxacin and magnesium deficiency on matrix metabolism in equine articular cartilage. *American Journal of Veterinary Research*, **62**, 160–166.

46 Vivrette, S., Bostian, A., Bermingham, E. & Papich, M.G. (2001) Quinolone-induced arthropathy in neonatal foals. *Proceedings of the American Association of Equine Practitioners*, **47**, 376–377.

47 Demmers, S., Johannisson, A., Grondahl, G. & Jensen-Waern, M. (2001) Neutrophil functions and serum IgG in growing foals. *Equine Veterinary Journal*, **33**, 676–680.

48 Hollis, A.R. & Corley, K.T. (2007) Practical guide to fluid therapy in neonatal foals. *In Practice*, **29**, 130–137.

49 Magdesian, K.G. & Madigan, J.E. (2003) Volume replacement in the neonatal ICU: Crystalloids and colloids. *Clinical Techniques in Equine Practice*, **2**, 20–30.

50 Buechner-Maxwell, V.A. (2005) Nutritional support for neonatal foals. *Veterinary Clinics of North America Equine Practice*, **21**, 487–510.

51 Hollis, A.R., Wilkins, P.A., Palmer, J.E. & Boston, R.C. (2008) Bacteremia in equine neonatal diarrhea: A retrospective study (1990–2007). *Journal of Veterinary Internal Medicine*, **22**, 1203–1209.

52 McKenzie, H.C., 3rd & Geor, R.J. (2009) Feeding management of sick neonatal foals. *Veterinary Clinics of North America Equine Practice*, **25**, 109–119, vii.

53 Palmer, J.E. (2004) Fluid therapy in the neonate: Not your mother's fluid space. *Veterinary Clinics of North America Equine Practice*, **20**, 63–75.

54 Peek, S.F., Semrad, S., McGuirk, S.M. *et al.* (2006) Prognostic value of clinicopathologic variables obtained at admission and effect of antiendotoxin plasma on survival in septic and critically ill foals. *Journal of Veterinary Internal Medicine*, **20**, 569–574.

55 Durando, M.M., MacKay, R.J., Linda, S. & Skelley, L.A. (1994) Effects of polymyxin B and Salmonella typhimurium antiserum on horses given endotoxin intravenously. *American Journal of Veterinary Research*, **55**, 921–927.

56 Semrad, S.D., Sams, R.A. & Ashcraft, S.M. (1993) Pharmacokinetics of and serum thromboxane suppression by flunixin meglumine in healthy foals during the first month of life. *American Journal of Veterinary Research*, **54**, 2083–2087.

57 Traub-Dargatz, J.L., Bertone, J.J., Gould, D.H., Wrigley, R.H., Weiser, M.G. & Forney, S.D. (1988) Chronic flunixin meglumine therapy in foals. *American Journal of Veterinary Research*, **49**, 7–12.

58 Semrad, S.D., Hardee, G.E., Hardee, M.M. & Moore, J.N. (1987) Low dose flunixin meglumine: Effects on eicosanoid production and clinical signs induced by experimental endotoxaemia in horses. *Equine Veterinary Journal*, **19**, 201–206.

59 Letendre, L.T., Tessman, R.K., McClure, S.R., Kvaternick, V.J., Fischer, J.B. & Hanson, P.D. (2008) Pharmacokinetics of firocoxib after administration of multiple consecutive

daily doses to horses. *American Journal of Veterinary Research*, **69**, 1399–1405.

60 Valverde, A., Giguere, S., Sanchez, L.C., Shih, A. & Ryan, C. (2006) Effects of dobutamine, norepinephrine, and vasopressin on cardiovascular function in anesthetized neonatal foals with induced hypotension. *American Journal of Veterinary Research*, **67**, 1730–1737.

61 Corley, K.T., Donaldson, L.L. & Furr, M.O. (2002) Comparison of lithium dilution and thermodilution cardiac output measurements in anaesthetised neonatal foals. *Equine Veterinary Journal*, **34**, 598–601.

62 Haggett, E.F., Magdesian, K.G. & Kass, P.H. (2011) Clinical implications of high liver enzyme activities in hospitalized neonatal foals. *Journal of the American Veterinary Medical Association*, **239**, 661–667.

63 Frederick, J., Giguere, S. & Sanchez, L.C. (2009) Infectious agents detected in the feces of diarrheic foals: A retrospective study of 233 cases (2003–2008). *Journal of Veterinary Internal Medicine*, **23**, 1254–1260.

64 Lawler, J.B., Hassel, D.M., Magnuson, R.J., Hill, A.E., McCue, P.M. & Traub-Dargatz, J.L. (2008) Adsorptive effects of di-tri- octahedral smectite on Clostridium perfringens alpha, beta, and beta-2 exotoxins and equine colostral antibodies. *American Journal of Veterinary Research*, **69**, 233–239.

65 Weese, J.S., Cote, N.M. & deGannes, R.V. (2003) Evaluation of in vitro properties of di-tri- octahedral smectite on clostridial toxins and growth. *Equine Veterinary Journal*, **35**, 638–641.

66 Musher, D.M., Logan, N., Hamill, R.J. *et al.* (2006) Nitazoxanide for the treatment of Clostridium difficile colitis. *Clinical Infectious Diseases*, **43**, 421–427.

67 Rossignol, J.F., Abu-Zekry, M., Hussein, A. & Santoro, M.G. (2006) Effect of nitazoxanide for treatment of severe rotavirus diarrhoea: Randomised double-blind placebo-controlled trial. *Lancet*, **368**, 124–129.

68 Weese, J.S., Parsons, D.A. & Staempfli, H.R. (1999) Association of Clostridium difficile with enterocolitis and lactose intolerance in a foal. *Journal of the American Veterinary Medical Association*, **214**, 229–232 205.

69 Furr, M., Cohen, N.D., Axon, J.E. *et al.* (2012) Treatment with histamine-type 2 receptor antagonists and omeprazole increase the risk of diarrhoea in neonatal foals treated in intensive care units. *Equine Veterinary Journal Supplement*, 80–86.

70 Murray, M.J. (1989) Endoscopic appearance of gastric lesions in foals: 94 cases (1987–1988). *Journal of the American Veterinary Medical Association*, **195**, 1135–1141.

71 Murray, M.J., Murray, C.M., Sweeney, H.J., Weld, J., Digby, N.J. & Stoneham, S.J. (1990) Prevalence of gastric lesions in foals without signs of gastric disease: An endoscopic survey. *Equine Veterinary Journal*, **22**, 6–8.

72 Videla, R., Sommardahl, C.S., Elliott, S.B., Vasili, A. & Andrews, F.M. (2011) Effects of intravenously administered esomeprazole sodium on gastric juice pH in adult female horses. *Journal of Veterinary Internal Medicine*, **25**, 558–562.

73 Ryan, C.A., Sanchez, L.C., Giguere, S. & Vickroy, T. (2005) Pharmacokinetics and pharmacodynamics of pantoprazole

in clinically normal neonatal foals. *Equine Veterinary Journal*, **37**, 336–341.

74 Sanchez, L.C., Murray, M.J. & Merritt, A.M. (2004) Effect of omeprazole paste on intragastric pH in clinically normal neonatal foals. *American Journal of Veterinary Research*, **65**, 1039–1041.

75 Sanchez, L.C., Lester, G.D. & Merritt, A.M. (2001) Intragastric pH in critically ill neonatal foals and the effect of ranitidine. *Journal of the American Veterinary Medical Association*, **218**, 907–911.

76 Geor, R.J., Petrie, L., Papich, M.G. & Rousseaux, C. (1989) The protective effects of sucralfate and ranitidine in foals experimentally intoxicated with phenylbutazone. *Canadian Journal of Veterinary Research*, **53**, 231–238.

77 Akman, M., Akbal, H., Emir, H., Oztürk, R., Erdogan, E. & Yeker, D. (2000) The effects of sucralfate and selective intestinal decontamination on bacterial translocation. *Pediatric Surgery International*, **16**, 91–93.

78 Lam, H.S. & Ng, P.C. (2011) Use of prokinetics in the preterm infant. *Current Opinion in Pediatrics*, **23**, 156–160.

79 Hoffman, A.M., Viel, L., Prescott, J.F., Rosendal, S. & Thorsen, J. (1993) Association of microbiologic flora with clinical, endoscopic, and pulmonary cytologic findings in foals with distal respiratory tract infection. *American Journal of Veterinary Research*, **54**, 1615–1622.

80 Clark-Price, S.C., Cox, J.H., Bartoe, J.T. & Davis, E.G. (2004) Use of dapsone in the treatment of Pneumocystis carinii pneumonia in a foal. *Journal of the American Veterinary Medical Association*, **224**, 407–410, 371.

81 Leclere, M., Magdesian, K.G., Kass, P.H., Pusterla, N. & Rhodes, D.M. (2011) Comparison of the clinical, microbiological, radiological and haematological features of foals with pneumonia caused by Rhodococcus equi and other bacteria. *Veterinary Journal*, **187**, 109–112.

82 Giguere, S., Hernandez, J., Gaskin, J., Miller, C. & Bowman, J.L. (2003) Evaluation of white blood cell concentration, plasma fibrinogen concentration, and an agar gel immunodiffusion test for early identification of foals with Rhodococcus equi pneumonia. *Journal of the American Veterinary Medical Association*, **222**, 775–781.

83 Giguere, S., Jacks, S., Roberts, G.D., Hernandez, J., Long, M.T. & Ellis, C. (2004) Retrospective comparison of azithromycin, clarithromycin, and erythromycin for the treatment of foals with Rhodococcus equi pneumonia. *Journal of Veterinary Internal Medicine*, **18**, 568–573.

84 Stratton-Phelps, M., Wilson, W.D. & Gardner, I.A. (2000) Risk of adverse effects in pneumonic foals treated with erythromycin versus other antibiotics: 143 cases (1986–1996). *Journal of the American Veterinary Medical Association*, **217**, 68–73.

85 Berghaus, L.J., Giguere, S., Sturgill, T.L., Bade, D., Malinski, T.J. & Huang, R. (2011) Plasma pharmacokinetics, pulmonary distribution, and in vitro activity of gamithromycin in foals. *Journal of Veterinary Pharmacology and Therapeutics*, **35**, 59–66.

86 Carlson, K.L., Kuskie, K.R., Chaffin, K.M. *et al.* (2010) Antimicrobial activity of tulathromycin and 14 other anti-

microbials against virulent Rhodococcus equi in vitro. *Veterinary Therapeutics*, **11**, E1–E9.

87 Womble, A., Giguere, S., Murthy, Y.V., Cox, C. & Obare, E. (2006) Pulmonary disposition of tilmicosin in foals and in vitro activity against Rhodococcus equi and other common equine bacterial pathogens. *Journal of Veterinary Pharmacology and Therapeutics*, **29**, 561–568.

88 Giguere, S., Lee, E., Williams, E. *et al.* (2010) Determination of the prevalence of antimicrobial resistance to macrolide antimicrobials or rifampin in Rhodococcus equi isolates and treatment outcome in foals infected with antimicrobial-resistant isolates of R. equi. *Journal of the American Veterinary Medical Association*, **237**, 74–81.

89 Garcia-Cantu, M.C.H.F., Brown, C.M. & Darien, B.J. (2000) Bordetella bronchiseptica and equine respiratory infections: A review of 30 cases. *Equine Veterinary Education*, **12**, 45–50.

90 McKenzie, H. (2006) Treating foal pneumonia. *Compendium Equine*, 47–53.

91 McKenzie, H.C. (2003) Characterization of antimicrobial aerosols for administration to horses. *Veterinary Therapeutics*, **4**, 110–119.

92 McKenzie, H.C., 3rd & Murray, M.J. (2000) Concentrations of gentamicin in serum and bronchial lavage fluid after intravenous and aerosol administration of gentamicin to horses. *American Journal of Veterinary Research*, **61**, 1185–1190.

93 Weber, A., Morlin, G., Cohen, M., Williams-Warren, J., Ramsey, B. & Smith, A. (1997) Effect of nebulizer type and antibiotic concentration on device performance. *Pediatric Pulmonology*, **23**, 249–260.

94 Giguere, S., Slade, J.K. & Sanchez, L.C. (2008) Retrospective comparison of caffeine and doxapram for the treatment of hypercapnia in foals with hypoxic-ischemic encephalopathy. *Journal of Veterinary Internal Medicine*, **22**, 401–405.

95 Giguere, S., Sanchez, L.C., Shih, A., Szabo, N.J., Womble, A.Y. & Robertson, S.A. (2007) Comparison of the effects of caffeine and doxapram on respiratory and cardiovascular function in foals with induced respiratory acidosis. *American Journal of Veterinary Research*, **68**, 1407–1416.

96 Raidal, S.L. & Edwards, S. (2008) Pharmacokinetics of potassium bromide in adult horses. *Australian Veterinary Journal*, **86**, 187–193.

97 Fielding, C.L., Magdesian, K.G., Elliott, D.A., Craigmill, A.L., Wilson, W.D. & Carlson, G.P. (2003) Pharmacokinetics and clinical utility of sodium bromide (NaBr) as an estimator of extracellular fluid volume in horses. *Journal of Veterinary Internal Medicine*, **17**, 213–217.

CHAPTER 8

Fluids and electrolytes for the equine clinician

Brett Tennent-Brown

The University of Melbourne, Hawthorn, Victoria, Australia

Principles of fluid therapy

In equine practice, fluids are most often administered to horses with inadequate vascular volume in an effort to restore tissue perfusion and oxygen delivery. Early fluid resuscitation in emergent situations limits tissue hypoxia, prevents organ dysfunction, and is expected to improve outcome. Additional indications for fluid administration in equine practice include provision of maintenance fluid and electrolyte requirements, correction of electrolyte abnormalities, and management of hypoproteinemia and renal disease.

Formulating a fluid therapy plan

A fluid therapy plan should include volume of fluids to be administered, rate of fluid administration, and type of fluid to be employed. The route of fluid administration should also be considered; intravenous (IV) administration is preferred in emergent situations, but oral administration might be more appropriate in some cases [1, 2]. A complete plan must also include a monitoring regimen to ensure that therapeutic goals are achieved within an appropriate time frame and to guide modifications to the fluid plan as the patient's condition changes.

Traditionally, fluid therapy plans have been formulated from estimates of (i) the initial fluid deficit based on physical examination findings and the results of laboratory tests, (ii) maintenance fluid requirements, and (iii) ongoing losses. This approach has some merit in the management of horses with chronic fluid deficits. However, it is less useful in the treatment of horses with severe, acute volume losses because accurate estimation of both the initial fluid deficit and ongoing losses is difficult if not impossible for many patients [3, 4]. A modification of the traditional approach better addresses the key goals of fluid therapy and is more appropriate for the critically ill patient requiring rapid volume replacement. This modified approach includes (i) a resuscitation phase that rapidly restores vascular volume and organ perfusion, (ii) a rehydration phase that restores interstitial and intracellular fluid volume over a longer time period, and (iii) a maintenance phase that provides for maintenance fluid requirements and ongoing losses [5]. For critically ill horses, the clinician should concentrate on restoring vascular volume and tissue perfusion as quickly as possible; formulating a comprehensive fluid plan that accounts for rehydration, maintenance requirements, and ongoing losses can be postponed until the patient is stabilized. Regardless of the approach used, it is essential to recognize that an initial fluid therapy plan is just a starting point that will require constant modification as the patient's condition changes during treatment.

Identifying patients requiring fluid therapy

Although they occur simultaneously in many horses that require fluid therapy, it is important to distinguish hypovolemia from dehydration. Hypovolemia is a loss of vascular or effective circulating volume, while dehydration occurs when fluid is lost from the interstitial and intracellular spaces. Clinical signs and laboratory tests used to evaluate fluid status (Table 8.1) typically assess aspects of both but provide only a very crude estimate of a patient's actual fluid deficit [3, 6, 7].

Equine Pharmacology, First Edition. Edited by Cynthia Cole, Bradford Bentz and Lara Maxwell.
© 2015 John Wiley & Sons, Inc. Published 2015 by John Wiley & Sons, Inc.

Table 8.1 Summary of clinical signs associated with hypovolemia and dehydration in adult horses.

	Dehydration (%)	Mucous membranes	Capillary refill time (s)	Heart rate (/min)	Other clinical signs
Mild	5–8	Normal to slightly tacky	Normal (<2)	Normal	Decreased urine production
Moderate	8–10	Tacky	Variable (often 2–3)	40–60	Decreased arterial blood pressure
Severe	10–12	Dry	Variable (often prolonged >4)	>60	Jugular fill slow, peripheral pulses weak, sunken eyes

Note that not all signs are consistently present in all horses.

Assessment of heart rate, jugular fill, pulse character, skin tent duration, extremity temperature, and mucous membrane character provides a practical starting point in developing a fluid plan and is critical in monitoring the response to fluid therapy. Immediate laboratory assessment of hydration status will not be available to many ambulatory practitioners; however, information generated by inexpensive point-of-care meters (e.g., handheld lactate meters) can be useful. For practitioners with access to hematology and plasma chemistry analyzers, measurement of packed cell volume (PCV) and albumin, total protein, creatinine, and lactate concentrations can be invaluable. Unfortunately, there is great individual variation in PCV, and it is affected by splenic contraction. Total protein (or albumin) concentration can also be misleading as many of the diseases in horses requiring fluid therapy are accompanied by protein loss. Despite these short comings, measurement of both PCV and protein concentrations can provide valuable patient information quickly and inexpensively. In the absence of renal disease, measurement of plasma or serum creatinine concentrations can be useful. A creatinine concentration at the high end of the reference range might suggest a mild fluid deficit. Creatinine concentrations above the reference range, but below 4–5 mg/dl and accompanied by a urine-specific gravity greater than 1.035, indicate prerenal azotemia and decreased renal perfusion. Renal dysfunction should be considered when creatinine concentrations exceed 5 mg/dl. Hyperlactatemia in equine patients is most commonly the result of decreased tissue perfusion and oxygen delivery (DO_2) with subsequent anaerobic metabolism. Blood lactate concentrations greater than 1.5 mmol/l in adult horses suggest a significant fluid deficit. Blood lactate concentrations in healthy, euhydrated foals exceed

adult concentrations at birth but decrease to adult concentrations over the first 1–3 days of life [8].

Volume of fluids to administer

As discussed previously, traditional approaches to fluid therapy provide for correction of a fluid deficit if present, maintenance requirements, and ongoing loses. In the critically ill patient, the clinician's first goal should be volume resuscitation (detailed in the following); however, estimates of maintenance requirements and ongoing losses will be required once resuscitation is complete.

Deficit

Combinations of clinical examination findings and results of basic laboratory tests are commonly used to estimate the fluid deficit (Table 8.1). The volume (in liters) required to correct an estimated deficit is calculated as the product of the percentage deficit and body weight (in kilograms). For example, if a 450 kg horse is judged to be 5–8% (mildly) dehydrated, the estimated deficit is approximately 22–36 l (i.e., 450×0.05 to $450 \times 0.08 = 22.5$–36 l). As noted previously, these estimates provide only a very crude indication of an animal's actual fluid status [3, 6, 7].

Maintenance

Maintenance water (and electrolyte) requirements in horses account for normal urinary and fecal losses and losses from the respiratory tract and skin. The value most commonly used for maintenance requirements is 60 ml/kg/day [9]. However, maintenance fluid requirements reflect metabolic rate, rather than being directly related to body weight, which is are more closely related to body surface area [10]. For example, larger animals (with a relatively smaller surface area) tend to have lower metabolic rates (and maintenance fluid requirements) when compared to smaller animals. In addition, metabolic rate and fluid requirements are influenced by age, physiologic status, and environmental conditions. Finally, most estimates of maintenance fluid requirements are based on studies in normal, nonanorexic animals; maintenance fluid requirements in sick animals are likely to be quite different. Despite these limitations, 50–60 ml/kg/day is a reasonable starting point for adult horses and is typically well tolerated. Foals have greater maintenance fluid requirements than adult horses; with 80–100 ml/kg/day being a good initial maintenance rate for equine neonates. Daily maintenance fluid requirements for an adult horse weighing 450 kg are therefore approximately 23–27 l (or ~1 l/h). A 50 kg foal will require approximately 4–5 l/day (or 170–200 ml/h). Note that healthy, growing foals will often consume 20–25% of their body weight daily in milk (~10–12.5 l for a 50 kg foal), but it is not necessary to provide this much fluid to sick neonates to meet maintenance requirements.

Losses

Considerable losses can occur in horses with diarrhea, persistent gastric reflux, polyuric renal failure, profuse sweating, or sequestration of fluid within a body cavity. In some cases, it might be possible to measure ongoing losses (e.g., horses with gastric reflux or polyuria); however, in most cases, it is difficult to determine ongoing losses with any accuracy. Horses with severe diarrhea might lose 200 ml/kg (i.e., ~90–100 l) or more daily [4]. In most cases, an approximation of ongoing losses must be made and the fluid rate titrated based on clinical response.

Correcting hypovolemia

In horses with clinically significant hypovolemia, restoration of vascular volume and organ perfusion is the priority. A commonly employed means of fluid resuscitation is to administer 20 ml/kg (i.e., 1 l for a 50 kg foal or 10 l for a 500 kg adult) as a rapid IV fluid bolus over 15–20 min. This approximates the "shock" fluid rates used in small animal medicine. This rate of fluid administration is easily achieved in foals but is very difficult and often impossible to achieve in adult horses.

Therefore by necessity, volume resuscitation in adult horses often occurs over a longer time period than ideal. Bolus administration is repeated until resuscitation is complete or 60–80 ml/kg (i.e., 3–4 boluses) has been administered. At this point, the patient is carefully reevaluated, and if vascular volume is inadequate, additional fluid boluses are administered. If vascular volume is adequate, but tissue perfusion remains poor, inotrope or vasopressor therapy should be considered.

Rate of fluid administration

The rate at which fluids are administered depends on the patient, severity of the deficit, and practical limitations of fluid administration. As discussed, rapid (over 15–20 min) IV administration of 20 ml/kg fluid boluses, with reassessment between boluses, is indicated for treatment of hypovolemia. Following resuscitation, fluid rate is determined by the need to complete rehydration, meet maintenance requirements, and account for ongoing losses. Using the traditional approach, half the calculated fluid deficit is typically administered over the first 2–6 h of therapy for horses with moderate to severe deficits. The remainder of the fluid deficit is then administered over the subsequent 18–22 h along with calculated volumes for maintenance requirements and ongoing losses. For horses with a mild estimated fluid deficit, the deficit volume can be combined with calculated volumes for maintenance requirements and ongoing losses and administered over 24 h. In reality, these two schemes often result in similar administration rates.

Currently, recommended fluid rates for resuscitation are much higher than those suggested historically. Concerns of producing pulmonary edema prompted recommendations of lower rates in early texts describing fluid therapy. However, rapid restoration of vascular volume is critical in hypovolemic patients and pulmonary edema is generally of little concern at the fluid rates that can be achieved in adult horses. Although it is certainly possible to cause pulmonary edema in neonates, fluid rates of at least 60 ml/kg/h (i.e., 3×20 ml/kg boluses administered over an hour) are typically well tolerated by critically ill foals. However, careful monitoring of pulmonary function in neonates is mandatory, and clinicians should be particularly cautious when administering fluids to neonates suspected to have acute lung injury (ALI) or acute respiratory distress syndrome (ARDS).

Choosing the type of fluid to be administered

Fluids can be classified as either "crystalloid" or "colloid." Crystalloids are solutions containing electrolyte and nonelectrolyte solutes that are distributed widely across the body's fluid compartments. Colloids contain substances of large molecular weight that are confined to the vascular space.

Crystalloids

Crystalloid fluids consist primarily of electrolytes with some nonelectrolyte solutes (e.g., dextrose and buffering agents) in water. They are widely available, relatively inexpensive, and safe for use under a wide range of situations. The major disadvantage of the crystalloids is that they rapidly equilibrate with the body's other fluid spaces and are consequently retained within the vascular space for only a short time. The effect of crystalloids in restoring vascular volume is, therefore, generally short lived. Within 30 min of infusion, 25% or less of an administered isotonic crystalloid might remain within the vascular space [5, 11]. The movement of crystalloid fluids into the interstitial space can lead to or exacerbate edema formation that, in turn, impairs oxygen delivery, although as discussed previously this is of less concern in adult horses than other smaller species.

Crystalloid fluids are commonly classified as either "replacement" or "maintenance." Replacement-type fluids are approximately isotonic and have a sodium concentration similar to plasma (i.e., 130–140 mmol/l). However, horses have a low daily sodium requirement (~3 mEq/kg/day), which, for a horse weighing 450 kg, is supplied by approximately 10 l of a replacement-type fluid (i.e., slightly less than half the volume of maintenance fluid requirements). For a 50 kg foal, the daily sodium requirement is met by a single bag of replacement-type fluids. Horses receiving fluids even at just maintenance rates, therefore, receive far more sodium than they require. In most cases, the kidneys are able to excrete the surplus sodium. However, some critically ill patients, particularly neonates, are unable to do so, leading to hypernatremia fluid retention and edema formation. In contrast, equine diets contain high concentrations of potassium, such that potassium depletion and hypokalemia commonly occur in anorectic horses receiving replacement-type fluids, as they typically contain little or no potassium. To address these issues, maintenance-type

fluids have been developed that contain lower sodium and chloride and higher potassium concentrations. Based on their electrolyte concentrations, maintenance-type fluids are hypotonic, but dextrose is typically added so that they are isotonic for administration. Unfortunately, maintenance-type fluids are usually only available in 1 l bags and are really only practical when treating smaller equine patients. When using replacement-type fluids to meet maintenance requirements, it is important to monitor electrolyte concentrations, as potassium supplementation (10–20 mmol/l) is often necessary. Calcium and magnesium might also need to be supplemented.

Balanced polyionic fluids

The term "balanced" refers to crystalloid solutions that have sodium, chloride, and potassium concentrations similar to that of plasma (Table 8.2). Rapid administration of balanced polyionic fluids is less likely to cause deleterious electrolyte derangements (or exacerbate existing electrolyte derangements). Therefore, this type of fluid is most appropriate during the resuscitation phase of fluid therapy particularly when the patient's electrolyte concentrations are unknown. Most of the polyionic fluids contain lactate, acetate, or gluconate as a buffering agent. Following administration, these compounds are metabolized to bicarbonate, carbon dioxide, and water, but the site of metabolism differs for each. Lactate is metabolized by the liver and acetate within the muscles, and gluconate is metabolized by a range of tissues. Because buffering agents are supplied as an anion, administration of lactate-containing fluids will not exacerbate a lactic acidosis due to hypoperfusion [12]. Some authorities have suggested that lactate-containing fluids should be avoided in patients with liver disease; however, in most cases, this precaution is unnecessary. Some polyionic fluids are supplemented with calcium, while others contain magnesium. The addition of calcium makes those fluids incompatible with bicarbonate-containing solutions, and they should not be mixed with anticoagulated whole blood.

Saline solutions

Physiological or normal (0.9%) saline has an osmolarity of 308 mosmol/l and is approximately isotonic with plasma (Table 8.2). The sodium concentration (154 mmol/l) slightly exceeds that of equine plasma, but the chloride concentration (154 mmol/l) is much higher and far from physiological! Normal saline solutions have been

Table 8.2 Composition of some commercially available fluids.

	Na⁺ (mmol/l)	K⁺ (mmol/l)	Ca²⁺ (mmol/l)	Mg²⁺ (mmol/l)	Cl⁻ (mmol/l)	Buffer (mmol/l)	Glucose (mmol/l)	pH
5% dextrose	0	0	0	0	0	0	276	4.0
0.9% NaCl	154	0	0	0	154	0	0	5.0
7.0% NaCl	1200	0	0	0	1200	0	0	
1.3% NaHCO₃	155	0	0	0	0	Bicarbonate (155)	0	
8.4% NaHCO₃	1000	0	0	0	0	Bicarbonate (1000)	0	
Hartmann's solution	131	5	2	0	112	Lactate (28)	0	6.3
Normosol-R	140	5	0	1.5	98	Acetate (27) Gluconate (23)	0	5.7
Normosol-M	40	13	0	3	40	Acetate (16)	276	5.5

recommended for resuscitation of patients with renal disease to avoid causing or exacerbating hyperkalemia; however, in most cases, this precaution is unnecessary. Although widely used as a resuscitation fluid in human medicine, rapid administration of large volumes of 0.9% saline in horses can cause acidosis and might cause or exacerbate electrolyte abnormalities [13, 14]. Normal saline might be indicated in a few specific equine cases (e.g., hyperkalemic periodic paralysis [HYPP] and foals with ruptured bladders), but the balanced polyionic fluids are a better choice in most situations.

Hypertonic saline solutions

A range of hypertonic saline solutions are available, but those used most often are 7.0–7.5% (i.e., 70–75 g/l) NaCl solutions with sodium (and chloride) concentrations of approximately 1200–1285 mmol/l. Intravenous administration of hypertonic solutions draws fluid from the intracellular fluid space into the extracellular fluid space, rapidly increasing vascular volume at the expense of tissue hydration. Hypertonic saline solutions reduce endothelial cell and erythrocyte swelling, which improves tissue perfusion and oxygen delivery [15, 16]. Hypertonic saline solutions are also reported to have immunomodulatory properties that could be beneficial in the treatment of inflammatory conditions [15, 16]. Small volume resuscitation, as it is called, with hypertonic solutions has been widely used to rapidly restore the circulating volume of human trauma patients. The combination of hypertonic saline with a colloid appears to be particularly effective. It is important to recognize that these patients are presumably euhydrated at the time of trauma and are expected to have a normal intracellular volume that can be drawn upon to replenish vascular volume. In contrast, equine patients requiring rapid volume resuscitation (e.g., severe colic or colitis cases) are often both hypovolemic and dehydrated. Because their interstitial and intracellular fluid volumes might already be depleted, it has been suggested that hypertonic solutions might not be appropriate in these cases. In human medicine, it has been argued that cells become edematous in shock states, so hypertonic resuscitation of shock tends to normalize cell volume rather than reduce it below normal [15]. Whether this same rationale can be applied to severely hypovolemic and dehydrated horses is not known. If hypertonic solutions are used, they must be followed by large volumes of isotonic crystalloids (at least five times the administered volume of hypertonic saline) within 2–3 h of hypertonic saline administration.

Bicarbonate solutions

Bicarbonate solutions at 1.3% (13 g/l) are approximately isotonic with plasma. Bicarbonate solutions have historically been recommended for treatment of metabolic acidosis, when the pH falls below 7.2 or the bicarbonate concentration below 12 mmol/l. In equine practice, metabolic acidosis is usually a consequence of hypovolemia and decreased tissue perfusion with subsequent anaerobic metabolism and lactate production. As such, restoration of vascular volume and tissue perfusion with a balanced polyionic solution should be the primary objective. Bicarbonate administration often improves the demeanor of acidotic patients and is indicated in the treatment of renal tubular acidosis and, perhaps, acidemia caused by hyponatremia or hyperchloremia. However, treatment with bicarbonate generally does not address the underlying cause of an acidemia, and concerns that a low pH is detrimental to cellular function might be incorrect. Furthermore, bicarbonate administration is not necessarily benign; overzealous administration of sodium bicarbonate can cause a range of disturbances including hypernatremia, hypokalemia, a decrease in the ionized calcium concentration, and paradoxical central nervous system acidosis.

Dextrose solutions

Dextrose solutions at 5% (50 g/l) are approximately isotonic, but because the dextrose is rapidly metabolized after IV administration, these solutions are effectively hypotonic. Dextrose solutions are indicated to replace a pure water loss or when water losses exceed electrolyte losses. The addition of dextrose prevents the erythrolysis that would otherwise occur with pure water administration. Because free water rapidly equilibrates across the entire volume of body water, dextrose solutions maintain vascular volume poorly. Dextrose is often added to polyionic solutions to decrease the sodium and chloride concentrations (i.e., in the creation of maintenance fluids). However, because of the relatively low caloric content of dextrose (~4 cal/g [17 kJ/g]), it is difficult to meet energy requirements with dextrose solutions alone. Many critically ill animals will not tolerate even relatively low dextrose infusion rates, and initially, blood glucose concentrations should be checked frequently (e.g., every 3–6 h). Glucose concentrations exceeding the renal threshold (~180 mg/dl [10 mmol/l]) can induce an osmotic diuresis, and persistent hyperglycemia above this level should be treated by either reducing the rate of dextrose infusion or administration of insulin.

Colloids

Colloid solutions contain large sugar or protein molecules that are maintained within the vascular space, thereby increasing intravascular oncotic pressure. Oncotic pressure is the osmotic pressure exerted by molecules that do not cross the vascular endothelium; oncotic pressure acts to retain water within the vascular space. As colloid solutions remain within the vasculature longer than crystalloid solutions, lower volumes of colloid solutions are required to restore and maintain circulation.

A bewildering array of natural and synthetic colloidal solutions is available with various types and sizes of colloidal molecules. Although albumin solutions have been used in human medicine for years, stored or fresh frozen plasma is the predominant form of natural colloid used in equine medicine. Three types of synthetic colloids are commonly described: the hydroxyethyl starches are polymers of modified amylopectin (a plant starch); the dextrans are glucose polymers synthesized by bacterial fermentation; and the gelatins are derived from hydrolysis of bovine collagen. In equine medicine, the hydroxyethyl starches have been most commonly employed [17–19].

Synthetic colloids are described on the basis of their average molecular weight; however, they are polydisperse solutions containing molecules of widely variable weights. Individual molecules within a colloid solution might range from a few thousand to a few million Daltons in weight. The hydroxyethyl starches are further characterized in terms of the extent to which the hydroxyl groups on constituent glucose molecules have been replaced with hydroxyethyl groups and the location within the glucose molecule of those substitutions. Substitution of a hydroxyl with a hydroxyethyl group increases the polymer's resistance to degradation by serum α-amylases and, therefore, prolongs intravascular persistence. The highly substituted hydroxyethyl starches (e.g., hetastarch with a molar substitution ratio of 0.7) are therefore more resistant to enzymatic degradation than the minimally substituted hydroxyethyl starches (e.g., tetrastarch with a molar substitution ratio of 0.4) and should have a greater duration of effect. Similarly, a high (>8) C2:C6 compared to a low (<8) C2:C6 substitution ratio more effectively slows polymer degradation.

The extent and duration of plasma volume expansion following administration of a colloid is highly variable and depends on the specific colloid formulation, the dose administered, as well as the volume status of the patient and the permeability of their microvascular. As a general rule, higher molecular weight molecules persist longer within the vascular space; however, it is the number of molecules rather than their size that determines oncotic effect. For the same concentration (i.e., grams of colloid per liter), colloids with a smaller average molecular weight contain more molecules and therefore generate greater oncotic pressure, but they tend to have a shorter duration of action. At a concentration of 6 g/dl (i.e., 6% solution), hetastarch is slightly (30–35 mmHg) and dextran 70 is markedly (60–75 mmHg) hyperoncotic. Hetastarch is expected to expand plasma volume by a volume equal to that infused and dextran 70 by 20–50% more than the infused volume. The half-life of hetastarch at the commonly used dose of 10 ml/kg is approximately 7 h in normal horses, but the half-life will increase with the dose [20]. Colloidal molecules are primarily eliminated by renal excretion, extravasation, or metabolism by the reticuloendothelial system. Molecules weighing less than 50–55 kDa are freely filtered by the glomerulus; larger molecules are more slowly removed from the circulation by cells of the RE system. Depending on the integrity of the vascular endothelium, a portion of colloid molecules will also be lost to the interstitial space. The behavior of colloid solutions in healthy animals can differ considerably from that in sick animals, in which the extent and duration of effect tends to be reduced [18].

Suggested indications for colloid administration include treatment of hypoproteinemia and maintenance of oncotic pressure, treatment of capillary leak syndrome (i.e., large colloid molecules are thought to plug gaps in injured capillaries), and acute fluid resuscitation. Plasma is not used for colloidal support in human medicine because of the risk of disease transmission and anaphylaxis and the higher cost when compared with synthetic colloids. Plasma is occasionally used, however, for colloidal support in hypoproteinemic horses. The volume of plasma required to increase a patient's plasma protein concentration (and therefore oncotic pressure) can be estimated from the following:

$$\text{Volume (l)} = \frac{\left(\left[\text{TP}_{\text{Target}} - \text{TP}_{\text{Patient}}\right] \times 0.05 \times \text{Body weight}\right)}{\text{TP}_{\text{Donor}}}$$

where TP is total protein concentration and body weight is measured in kilograms. At least 4–5 l of plasma is typically required to increase the plasma protein concentration of an average-sized horse by 1 g/dl; however, the actual increase in protein concentration is almost always disappointing. Since at least 80% of plasma's oncotic pressure is provided by albumin, plasma administration to patients with a protein-losing disease

process is of questionable value, because the administered albumin is expected to be lost at a rate similar to endogenous albumin. In general, colloidal support for adult horses is usually better and more economically provided by administration of a synthetic colloid with a large average molecular weight. Using plasma as a colloid in foals may be reasonable, as their smaller body size reduces the volume of plasma required to increase oncotic pressure. Care is required, however, to avoid volume overload in hypoproteinemic but euvolemic foals.

The benefits of colloid compared to crystalloid solutions in acute volume resuscitation have been debated for decades. Because they are better retained within the vascular space, it is expected that a smaller volume of colloid solutions will be required to restore and maintain vascular volume when compared to crystalloids. Edema formation should also be less likely following colloid administration. Some studies have shown improved outcomes in human patients resuscitated with colloid solutions particularly those combined with hypertonic saline; however, this has been far from a universal finding. In a large study comparing iso-oncotic (4%) albumin to 0.9% saline in resuscitation, there was no difference in overall survival between the two treatment groups [21]. However, there might be some benefit of colloids or crystalloids in select patient groups. Patients with sepsis might have better outcomes when resuscitated with albumin, while survival might improve in patients with head trauma resuscitated with 0.9% saline [22, 23]. In light of the additional cost of colloid solutions and the lack of clear benefits for their use, crystalloids should remain the fluid of choice for resuscitation in equine medicine.

In addition, administration of colloid solutions is not without side effects. For example, most will cause some degree of coagulopathy, particularly at higher doses, and some have been associated with acute renal injury. Although large colloid molecules might plug gaps in the vascular endothelium in patients with increased microvascular permeability, smaller colloidal molecules will enter the interstitial space where they can contribute to edema formation [24, 25].

Route of fluid administration

Intravenous administration is preferred for most horses requiring fluid therapy; however, in some situations, enteral fluids might be more practical, efficacious, and economical. Colon impactions are often more effectively treated with enteral rather than IV fluids, and horses with a functional gastrointestinal tracts and relatively low fluid requirements might also be good candidates for enteral fluids [1]. The relatively small volume of the equine stomach means that enteral fluids must be administered frequently. Small diameter (12–18 French [4–6 mm internal diameter] 108–250 cm length) feeding tubes are available (MILA International Inc., Erlanger, KY 41018) that can be left in place so that enteral fluids can be administered either continuously or as frequent, small boluses. Bolus administration of enteral fluids might be more efficacious than boluses of IV fluids in some cases because the colon might act as a fluid "reservoir."

Intraosseous fluid administration can be useful in neonates in which placement of an IV catheter has been impossible. A steel 14 gauge needle (or purpose-designed bone screw) is placed in the proximal one-third of the tibia medially where there is no muscle coverage. The radius can also be used although placement of the needle is more difficult. Fluids (and drugs) can be rapidly administered via this route until venous access is achieved.

Practical aspects of fluid therapy

The jugular vein is most commonly used when administering IV fluids to horses. Its large diameter and high blood flow allows high fluid rates and the administration of hypertonic solutions. Catheterization of the jugular vein is straightforward in all but the most hypovolemic animals, and jugular vein catheters are well tolerated and easily maintained. In horses requiring very rapid fluid administration rates, both jugular veins can be catheterized, although the second catheter should be removed once resuscitation is complete to reduce the risk of thrombosis. In horses with one thrombosed jugular vein, it is usually prudent to use either the cephalic or lateral thoracic vein rather than risking bilateral jugular vein thrombosis. Catheterization of the cephalic or lateral thoracic veins is technically more demanding, and the maximum achievable fluid rate is lower than for the jugular vein. However, the consequences of thrombosis of a cephalic or lateral thoracic vein are less serious. Good restraint or sedation is typically required for catheterization of the cephalic vein.

The lateral thoracic vein can be difficult to identify, but it is usually easily located with the aid of an ultrasound. Maintenance of catheters in the cephalic or lateral thoracic vein can be difficult, and they tend to require replacement more frequently than those in the jugular vein. In foals, the saphenous vein can also be catheterized.

Polyurethane, polytetrafluoroethylene (Teflon), and silicon elastomers (sometimes referred to as Silastics) are the materials most commonly used to manufacture IV catheters. Because they are inexpensive and easy to place, polyurethane and Teflon catheters are used most commonly in equine medicine. Teflon catheters are relatively rigid, which increases mechanical irritation to the vessel lumen, and they are more prone to kinking and cracking. Teflon catheters are also associated with a greater incidence of thrombophlebitis, when compared to those constructed from polyurethane or silicon [26]. Therefore, Teflon catheters should only be used for short-term venous access and removed after 72 h. Polyurethane catheters are more flexible, are less likely to cause thrombophlebitis, and are preferred for horses likely to require long-term catheterization. If properly maintained, polyurethane catheters can be left in place for at least 14 days and should only be removed if there are signs of a problem [26]. Achievable fluid flow rates increase with increasing catheter diameter but are inversely proportional to catheter length. Twelve- to fourteen-gauge catheters are appropriate for most adult horses; however, 10 gauge and/or multiple catheters should be used in severely hypovolemic horses requiring very high fluid rates [27]. When using very-large-gauge catheters, a stab incision through the skin aids placement. Sixteen gauge catheters are suitable for most equine neonates [27]. In human medicine, large-gauge catheters are associated with an increased risk of thrombophlebitis when compared to small-gauge catheters possibly due to the physical trauma caused by the insertion of a large-gauge catheter into the vein [28]. If very-large-gauge catheters are used for resuscitation, they should be removed as soon as possible. Because flow is inversely proportional to catheter length, longer catheters will reduce the achievable fluid rate. The length of catheter does not appear to affect the incidence of thrombophlebitis in human studies, but longer catheters are less likely to become dislodged and the risk of extravasation of medications is probably reduced [28].

Although relatively expensive, large-bore coiled administration sets (e.g., STAT Large Animal IV Set, International WIN Limited, Kennett Square, PA 19348) are ideal for rapid administration of large volumes of fluids to adult horses. In addition to allowing high fluid rates, these coiled sets enable the patient to move about the stall and lie down without dislodging the catheter. Smaller coiled sets with smaller lumens are available for foals and smaller patients. Noncoiled administration sets are inexpensive and more practical when administering intermittent fluid boluses. Based on human studies, fluid administration sets that have not been used to administer lipids, blood, or blood products can be safely left in place for up to 96 h [29]. While hospital barns are obviously less sanitary than human hospital wards, similar recommendations are probably appropriate in equine medicine although special care must be taken if fluid lines are repeatedly disconnected (e.g., between fluid boluses). However, administration sets that have been used to administer whole blood or blood products should be discarded after use.

Practical aspects of fluid therapy for the ambulatory veterinarian

For horses that are to be transported to a referral hospital, the benefits of fluid resuscitation must be balanced against those of getting to the referral institution as quickly as possible. Rapid administration of the large volume of fluids often required by adult horses can be difficult to achieve, and even administration of relatively small volumes can be time consuming. Large-bore administration sets and multiple catheters are usually required to administer fluids at rates faster than 5 l/h. However, if there is time and the hospital is some hours away, it can be worthwhile to at least begin resuscitation.

For horses requiring long-term fluid administration, continuous infusion is preferred as it allows the clinician to more closely match fluid administration with requirements. In addition, because crystalloids rapidly move out of the vascular space and excess fluids are rapidly excreted or extravasated, bolus fluid administration is generally less effective. However, continuous fluid administration requires that the horse is confined to a stall and monitored around the clock, both of which can be difficult for veterinarians treating horses in the field or with limited technical staff. Many veterinarians must, by necessity, administer fluids as boluses throughout the day. Although not always optimal, effective fluid

therapy is possible outside of the hospital setting with careful patient selection and planning.

Horses that are to be administered fluids in the field should have a large-gauge (e.g., 12 gauge), long-term jugular catheter placed and connected to a short extension set. A large-bore needle can be attached to the end of the fluid administration set, and the needle inserted through the injection cap of the extension set. After bolus administration, the fluid line can be disconnected, and the catheter flushed and extension set clamped. Clients can be trained or support staff utilized to manage the practical parts of fluid administration. The important aspects to consider when training laypersons to manage fluid administration include:

1 "Catheter maintenance and monitoring": Catheter-related problems are common, and thorough training on appropriate handling and maintenance of the catheter is paramount. Clients or staff should be instructed to always wear examination gloves when handling the catheter. Injection caps should be carefully cleaned with alcohol prior to injection and replaced frequently (at least every 24 h). The importance of regularly (e.g., every 6 h) flushing the catheter with heparinized saline (5 U/ml) to maintain patency should be emphasized. The risks of air embolism and how to avoid them (i.e., careful clamping of lines when fluids are not running) should be explained. The catheter site and vein must be closely inspected at least twice daily and preferably at least once daily by a veterinarian. Signs of catheter site infections and thrombophlebitis must be carefully explained so that infections are quickly recognized.

2 "Care of fluid administration sets": Following fluid administration, the end of the fluid administration set should be capped with a new sterile needle (and needle cap) immediately after disconnection from the patient. Some clinicians might prefer to keep fluid lines attached to the horse between boluses; if this is the case, it is obviously important to ensure the lines are completely clamped off and that the catheter is flushed regularly to maintain patency. It is also important to emphasize that fluids should not be allowed to completely run out so that fluid lines do not become filled with blood.

3 "Appropriate techniques for changing fluid bags": If possible, the timing of bolus administration should be arranged so that the veterinarian can assess the patient and determine if additional fluids are required.

The veterinarian is then able to change the fluid bags and prime the administration set so that air is not introduced into the fluid lines. If a layperson is changing fluid bags, the importance of asepsis and avoiding the introduction of air into fluid lines must be emphasized. Gloves should be worn and priming of the fluid lines demonstrated.

Monitoring fluid therapy

Monitoring begins with clinical assessment and careful physical examination. Assessment of heart rate, pulse pressure, extremity temperature, and mucous membrane character can be extremely useful in evaluating the effectiveness of fluid therapy. Clinical pathologic markers enable quantification of clinical findings, but results might not be immediately available to make real-time decisions. Cardiovascular monitoring equipment (e.g., blood pressure monitors) can provide valuable information in select cases but are often not available outside the hospital setting. Selection of monitoring techniques should be based on reliability, expense, practicality, and the value of information they provide. The choice of monitoring techniques should also reflect the original goals of fluid therapy and will differ between patients (e.g., compare horses requiring acute volume resuscitation with those receiving treatment of acute renal failure). Regardless of the technique used, measurements should be performed repeatedly because trends are generally more informative than values obtained at a single time point. The frequency with which measurements are repeated will depend on the stability of the patient, ease of the monitoring technique, expected rate of change of a monitored variable, and cost. Clinical examination parameters will be checked after each fluid bolus in critically ill horses requiring fluid resuscitation. Basic clinical pathologic parameters (e.g., PCV and total solids and blood lactate concentrations) might be checked every 6–12 h initially. Patients with severe electrolyte abnormalities, particularly sodium and potassium derangements, should have the concentrations of these electrolytes checked as frequently as possible (e.g., every 6–12 h) to allow timely changes in management.

Additional monitoring techniques that can be used to help guide fluid therapy include measurement of urine production (subjective or quantitative), urine-specific gravity, central venous pressure, direct or indirect blood pressure, and oxygen extraction ratios or venous hemoglobin saturation. Unfortunately, no single monitoring technique will be sufficient for all patients, and a combination of methods is usually required. Fortunately, relatively simple monitoring is generally sufficient for most patients with only the most critically ill requiring more sophisticated techniques.

Complications of fluid therapy

Resuscitation fluid rates recommended in the past were lower than current recommendations. These were based on concerns of pulmonary edema; however, it is generally difficult to administer fluids fast enough to cause pulmonary edema in adult horses, and fluid rates of at least 60 ml/kg/h (i.e., 20 ml/kg administered over 20 min) are well tolerated by most foals. Exceptions to this might include patients with marked hypoproteinemia, marked systemic inflammatory response and increased vascular permeability, or with heart failure. Patients receiving fluids at very high rates should be monitored closely for signs of pulmonary edema, particularly if any of these predisposing factors are present. Many critically ill neonates are hypoproteinemic, have increased vascular permeability, and might have depressed myocardial function; these patients require particular attention while receiving rapid fluid boluses. Pulmonary edema has obvious implications for gas exchange, but edema of other tissues is also deleterious. Edema impairs tissue oxygen delivery by increasing the diffusion distance between capillaries and cells and by compressing capillaries within tissue beds.

Volume resuscitation is a critical component in the management of severe blood loss. However, caution is required in patients with uncontrolled hemorrhage as the increase in blood pressure with aggressive volume resuscitation can disrupt newly formed blood clots. In addition, a dilutional coagulopathy can occur following fluid resuscitation, which will exacerbate bleeding. These concerns have led to the concept of permissive hypotension during resuscitation in human patients with severe hemorrhage in which mean arterial pressures (MAP) below the standard 65 mmHg are targeted. The use of a target MAP of 50 mmHg has shown some promise in human trauma patients [30]. It is currently unknown whether a target MAP of 50 mmHg is an optimal and appropriate resuscitation target for horses with severe hemorrhage.

Electrolyte derangements are common in horses receiving IV fluids. As mentioned, horses administered replacement-type fluids receive far more sodium than required; most are able to excrete the excess, but some, particularly sick neonates, are unable to do so. Sodium retention leads to either hypernatremia or fluid retention and edema. In contrast, many horses receiving IV fluids become hypokalemic particularly if anorectic. Additional electrolyte abnormalities that can occur include derangements in calcium, magnesium, and phosphorus. To avoid adverse consequences of electrolyte derangements, critical patients at least initially should have electrolyte concentrations checked daily. Critical patients with marked electrolyte disturbances might require more frequent assessment. When supplementing potassium, the maximum rate of replacement should not exceed 0.5 mmol/kg/h. Overly rapid administration of calcium and magnesium also has severe cardiovascular effects. Calcium can be empirically supplemented by addition of concentrated calcium solutions (e.g., 250 ml of 23% calcium borogluconate for a full size adult horse) to fluid bags to ensure slow infusion once or twice daily. Magnesium can also be empirically supplemented as magnesium sulfate administered at a rate of 1 g/min up to a maximum dose of 25 g as indicated by laboratory results.

Overly rapid correction of chronic (i.e., >3 days in duration) hyponatremia or hypernatremia can have severe adverse neurologic consequences in humans. Whether this is a concern in equine medicine is unclear; however, it would seem prudent to follow human recommendations that sodium concentrations are not changed by more than 10–12 mmol/l over a 24 h period (i.e., ~0.5 mmol/l/h). Hyponatremia is the more common derangement and most often encountered in horses with severe diarrhea of several days' duration. In practical terms, appropriate correction of sodium derangements is difficult because the equations used to calculate sodium deficits are relatively crude and none account for the ongoing electrolyte and water losses. The preferred approach in these patients is to use a balanced polyionic fluid (i.e., with a sodium concentration close to that of normal plasma) for resuscitation. When volume resuscitation is complete, the sodium content of the administered fluid is adjusted based on frequent checks (i.e., every 6 h) of the patient's sodium concentration. Solutions

with a higher than expected sodium concentration are often required to increase serum sodium concentrations in severe hyponatremia.

Catheter site infections and thrombophlebitis are probably the most common catheter-related complications. While rarely life threatening, they can be costly and time consuming to treat and will occasionally cause serious problems. Catheter characteristics and the conditions under which the catheter is placed play important roles in catheter-related problems; however, the duration of catheterization and patient characteristics are at least as important [31, 32]. To reduce the likelihood of catheter-related problems, strict attention to asepsis and care to reduce venous trauma during catheter placement are required. The catheter site and catheterized vein should be checked closely twice daily especially in patients known to be at risk for thrombophlebitis [31]. Ultrasonography has been suggested as a sensitive means to detect early changes in catheterized veins [33]. Swelling, heat, or pain at the catheter site or changes to the vein should prompt removal of the catheter and, ideally, culture of the catheter tip. Most catheter site infections and cases of thrombophlebitis will respond to symptomatic treatment with hot-packing and topical anti-inflammatories. More severe cases will require systemic antimicrobials and anti-inflammatories, and in very severe cases, the affected vein may need to be removed surgically. Salicylic acid (10 mg/kg orally every 48 h) has been recommended to limit thrombus progression. Catheterization of the contralateral jugular vein should be avoided in horses with acute or chronic jugular vein thrombophlebitis or thrombosis.

Conclusions

A fluid therapy plan will include the volume to be administered, rate of administration, and type of fluid to be employed. Continuous IV fluid administration is preferred for most patients. However, enteral fluids might be more appropriate in select cases, and bolus administration is necessary in some situations. Horses requiring volume resuscitation should receive rapid 20 ml/kg fluid boluses to effect to restore vascular volume and tissue perfusion. Tissue rehydration can occur over a longer period along with provision of maintenance requirements and replacement of ongoing losses. In most cases, a balanced, polyionic fluid that resembles plasma in its electrolyte concentrations should be used particularly if the patient's electrolyte concentrations are unknown. A monitoring regimen that allows appropriate and timely changes in response to changes in the patient's condition must be included in any fluid plan. The realities of ambulatory practice often limit the ability to administer fluids for reasons other than emergency resuscitation; however, with careful planning, it can be possible to administer effective fluid therapy in the field. Fluid administration is not without complications, but with careful planning and monitoring, most serious complications can be avoided. Catheter-related problems are probably most commonly encountered but can usually be managed symptomatically if detected promptly.

References

1 Lopes, M.A., Walker, B.L., White, N.A., 2nd & Ward, D.L. (2002) Treatments to promote colonic hydration: Enteral fluid therapy versus intravenous fluid therapy and magnesium sulphate. *Equine Veterinary Journal*, **34**, 505–509.

2 Lopes, M.A., White, N.A., 2nd, Donaldson, L., Crisman, M.V. & Ward, D.L. (2004) Effects of enteral and intravenous fluid therapy, magnesium sulfate, and sodium sulfate on colonic contents and feces in horses. *American Journal of Veterinary Research*, **65**, 695–704.

3 Pritchard, J.C., Burn, C.C., Barr, A.R. & Whay, H.R. (2008) Validity of indicators of dehydration in working horses: A longitudinal study of changes in skin tent duration, mucous membrane dryness and drinking behaviour. *Equine Veterinary Journal*, **40**, 558–564.

4 Rose, R.J. (1981) A physiological approach to fluid and electrolyte therapy in the horse. *Equine Veterinary Journal*, **13**, 7–14.

5 Corley, K.T.T. (2004) Fluid therapy. In: J.J. Bertone & L.J.I. Horspool (eds), *Equine Clinical Pharmacology*, 1st edn, pp. 327–364. Saunders, London.

6 Constable, P.D., Walker, P.G., Morin, D.E. & Foreman, J.H. (1998) Clinical and laboratory assessment of hydration status of neonatal calves with diarrhea. *Journal of the American Veterinary Medical Association*, **212**, 991–996.

7 Hansen, B. & DeFrancesco, T. (2002) Relationship between hydration estimate and body weight change after fluid therapy in critically ill dogs and cats. *Journal of Veterinary Emergency and Critical Care*, **12**, 235–243.

8 Magdesian, G.K. (2003) *Blood lactate levels in neonatal foals: Normal values and temporal effects in the post-partum period.* International Veterinary Emergency and Critical Care Symposium, New Orleans, LA, p. 174.

9 Groenendyk, S., English, P.B. & Abetz, I. (1988) External balance of water and electrolytes in the horse. *Equine Veterinary Journal*, **20**, 189–193.

10 Holliday, M.A. & Segar, W.E. (1957) The maintenance need for water in parenteral fluid therapy. *Pediatrics*, **19**, 823–832.

11 Hughes, D. & Boag, A. (2012) Fluid therapy with macromolecular plasma volume expanders. In: S.P. DiBartola (ed), *Fluid, Electrolyte, and Acid-Base Disorders in Small Animal Practice*, 4th edn, pp. 647–664. Elsevier, St. Louis.

12 Didwania, A., Miller, J., Kassel, D., Jackson, E.V., Jr & Chernow, B. (1997) Effect of intravenous lactated Ringer's solution infusion on the circulating lactate concentration: Part 3. Results of a prospective, randomized, double-blind, placebo-controlled trial. *Critical Care Medicine*, **25**, 1851–1854.

13 Reid, F., Lobo, D.N., Williams, R.N., Rowlands, B.J. & Allison, S.P. (2003) (Ab)normal saline and physiological Hartmann's solution: A randomized double-blind crossover study. *Clinical Science*, **104**, 17–24.

14 Scheingraber, S., Rehm, M., Sehmisch, C. & Finsterer, U. (1999) Rapid saline infusion produces hyperchloremic acidosis in patients undergoing gynecologic surgery. *Anesthesiology*, **90**, 1265–1270.

15 Kramer, G.C. (2003) Hypertonic resuscitation: Physiologic mechanisms and recommendations for trauma care. *Journal of Trauma*, **54**, S89–S99.

16 Pascual, J.L., Khwaja, K.A., Chaudhury, P. & Christou, N.V. (2003) Hypertonic saline and the microcirculation. *Journal of Trauma*, **54**, S133–S140.

17 Hallowell, G.D. & Corley, K.T. (2006) Preoperative administration of hydroxyethyl starch or hypertonic saline to horses with colic. *Journal of Veterinary Internal Medicine*, **20**, 980–986.

18 Jones, P.A., Bain, F.T., Byars, T.D., David, J.B. & Boston, R.C. (2001) Effect of hydroxyethyl starch infusion on colloid oncotic pressure in hypoproteinemic horses. *Journal of the American Veterinary Medical Association*, **218**, 1130–1135.

19 Wendt-Hornickle, E.L., Snyder, L.B., Tang, R. & Johnson, R.A. (2011) The effects of lactated Ringer's solution (LRS) or LRS and 6% hetastarch on the colloid osmotic pressure, total protein and osmolality in healthy horses under general anesthesia. *Veterinary Anaesthesia and Analgesia*, **38**, 336–343.

20 Schusser, G.F., Rieckhoff, K., Ungemach, F.R., Huskamp, N.H. & Scheidemann, W. (2007) Effect of hydroxyethyl starch solution in normal horses and horses with colic or acute colitis. *Journal of Veterinary Medicine A*, **54**, 592–598.

21 Finfer, S., Bellomo, R., Boyce, N., French, J., Myburgh, J. & Norton, R. (2004) A comparison of albumin and saline for fluid resuscitation in the intensive care unit. *New England Journal of Medicine*, **350**, 2247–2256.

22 Finfer, S., McEvoy, S., Bellomo, R., McArthur, C., Myburgh, J. & Norton, R. (2011) Impact of albumin compared to saline on organ function and mortality of patients with severe sepsis. *Intensive Care Medicine*, **37**, 86–96.

23 Myburgh, J., Cooper, D.J., Finfer, S. *et al.* (2007) Saline or albumin for fluid resuscitation in patients with traumatic brain injury. *New England Journal of Medicine*, **357**, 874–884.

24 Zikria, B.A., Subbarao, C., Oz, M.C. *et al.* (1989) Macromolecules reduce abnormal microvascular permeability in rat limb ischemia-reperfusion injury. *Critical Care Medicine*, **17**, 1306–1309.

25 Zikria, B.A., King, T.C., Stanford, J. & Freeman, H.P. (1989) A biophysical approach to capillary permeability. *Surgery*, **105**, 625–631.

26 Spurlock, S.L., Spurlock, G.H., Parker, G. & Ward, M.V. (1990) Long-term jugular vein catheterization in horses. *Journal of the American Veterinary Medical Association*, **196**, 425–430.

27 Tan, R.H., Dart, A.J. & Dowling, B.A. (2003) Catheters: A review of the selection, utilisation and complications of catheters for peripheral venous access. *Australian Veterinary Journal*, **81**, 136–139.

28 Tagalakis, V., Kahn, S.R., Libman, M. & Blostein, M. (2002) The epidemiology of peripheral vein infusion thrombophlebitis: A critical review. *American Journal of Medicine*, **113**, 146–151.

29 Webster, J., Osborne, S., Rickard, C. & Hall, J. (2010) Clinically-indicated replacement versus routine replacement of peripheral venous catheters. *Cochrane Database of Systematic Reviews*, 3, CD007798.

30 Morrison, C.A., Carrick, M.M., Norman, M.A. *et al.* (2011) Hypotensive resuscitation strategy reduces transfusion requirements and severe postoperative coagulopathy in trauma patients with hemorrhagic shock: Preliminary results of a randomized controlled trial. *Journal of Trauma*, **70**, 652–663.

31 Dolente, B.A., Beech, J., Lindborg, S. & Smith, G. (2005) Evaluation of risk factors for development of catheter-associated jugular thrombophlebitis in horses: 50 cases (1993–1998). *Journal of the American Veterinary Medical Association*, **227**, 1134–1141.

32 Lankveld, D.P., Ensink, J.M., van Dijk, P. & Klein, W.R. (2001) Factors influencing the occurrence of thrombophlebitis after post-surgical long-term intravenous catheterization of colic horses: A study of 38 cases. *Journal of Veterinary Medicine A*, **48**, 545–552.

33 Geraghty, T.E., Love, S., Taylor, D.J., Heller, J., Mellor, D.J. & Hughes, K.J. (2009) Assessment of subclinical venous catheter-related diseases in horses and associated risk factors. *Veterinary Record*, **164**, 227–231.

CHAPTER 9

Drug and medication control programs in equine athletes

Scot Waterman[1] and Jennifer Durenburger[2]

[1] *Arizona Department of Racing, Tucson, AZ, USA*
[2] *Massachusetts Gaming Commission, Boston, MA, USA*

Introduction

As the popularity of equine sports grows, many practitioners will see client-owned horses that participate in regulated competitions. The regulatory bodies of the various disciplines may prohibit or restrict certain veterinary practices, stipulate how medications may be administered to participants, and conduct drug testing on selected competitors. For some disciplines, particularly where pari-mutuel wagering is involved, special licensure requirements may also exist for the equine practitioner.

Where a regulatory body has determined that a violation of its rules has occurred and a veterinarian is responsible, the consequences may be significant. The veterinarian's client may be fined or suspended or the client's horse may be disqualified from an event. The veterinarian may also be fined or suspended, and violations may be reported to the state veterinary medical board for further action. In rare instances, criminal charges may even be filed. Any disciplinary action taken against a veterinarian must be reported at the time of license renewal in all jurisdictions, as well as at the time of membership renewal for most veterinary affiliated organizations. Practicing in a regulated environment may also raise ethical concerns.

Organizations such as the American Association of Equine Practitioners (AAEP) and American Veterinary Medical Association (AVMA) have established codes of ethics by which their members agree to abide and have published position statements and white papers addressing the practitioner's role in specific equine sports. The challenges of practicing on equine athletes can be both professionally rewarding and demanding. Developing an understanding of the regulatory framework that governs equine sport can help the practitioner succeed in this challenging and unique environment.

Regulation of equine sport

Why are equine sports and competitions regulated? The answer, in a nutshell, is to level the playing field. But the term "level playing field" actually means several things. It means that anyone who enters the competition is assured that if they bring the best horse or the best horse and rider (or driver) combination to the event, they have a reasonable chance of winning. It means that when a breeder makes a decision about which champion to breed to, that decision can be made with the confidence that the horse's lifetime record is accurate and reflects his or her true athletic capabilities. It means that the health and safety of all participants—both equine and human—is not jeopardized for the sake of winning the competition. And, finally in the pari-mutuel environment, it means that the betting public is wagering on a reasonably consistent product.

The practitioner's role vis-à-vis the equine athlete is to attend to the health and welfare of the horse. The regulatory body's role is to enforce the rules that have been agreed upon by the sport's participants. In most equine sports, committees that consist of representatives

Equine Pharmacology, First Edition. Edited by Cynthia Cole, Bradford Bentz and Lara Maxwell.
© 2015 John Wiley & Sons, Inc. Published 2015 by John Wiley & Sons, Inc.

from each of the various stakeholder groups, such as owners and trainers, adopt rules under which the sport will be conducted. In the pari-mutuel environment, a public comment period is almost always required before a regulation may be added or changed, and in some instances, a rule change must go through the entire legislative process like any other law.

By deriving income by practicing on a client's horse that competes at regulated events, the veterinarian, at a minimum, has implicitly agreed to abide by the governing body's rules and regulations. In the pari-mutuel wagering environment, the veterinarian may also have to comply with specific conditions of special licensure. Such conditions may include written waivers permitting the governing authority to search the veterinarian's practice vehicle and medical records. In order to be compliant, it is important that the practitioner is knowledgeable regarding the rules and regulations, particularly those pertaining to medication and veterinary practices. Relying on a client's interpretation of the rules, or even that of a practicing colleague's, can be a recipe for disaster. In addition, most governing bodies provide an official veterinarian who should be contacted immediately if there is any question of how best to comply with the rules.

Governing authorities

Racing

The pari-mutuel racing industry is undoubtedly the most closely regulated of the equine sports due primarily to the legal wagering component. Pari-mutuel wagering in the USA is an approximately $12 billion/year industry, and the authority to regulate this industry lies entirely with an administrative agency within each individual state [1]. This is largely due to the fact that the decision to allow legal wagering has always been considered a state decision, as opposed to federal. A state that wishes to conduct pari-mutuel wagering must have legislative and executive approval. The state legislature passes enabling language that establishes an agency within the government to regulate the activity. The enabling language typically includes a mandate that the agency protect the health and welfare of participants and the interests of the wagering public. It also establishes the composition of the agency. In most cases, the agency is comprised of commissioners that are appointed

by the governor with an executive staff, but there are a few exceptions to this model. It is worthwhile for the clinician to understand the rulemaking process and composition of the state regulatory agency or agencies in each state in which they practice, if their case load includes racehorses.

In recent years, there has been a national effort underway to standardize both the rules relating to medication and the methodologies employed in postrace testing to assure compliance with those rules. This effort has been led primarily by the Racing Medication & Testing Consortium (RMTC) and the Association of Racing Commissioners International (ARCI). Both are essentially racing industry trade associations with no power to mandate change at the state racing commission level. Although significant progress has been made by these organizations, the goal of truly uniform regulations across state lines remains elusive in US racing. Both organizations make a host of resources available to the practitioner on their respective websites. The RMTC (www.rmtcnet.com) offers a state-by-state database of withdrawal times (the time period before a race when a medication should be discontinued in order to allow the drug to clear the horse's system and avoid a positive drug test) and a collection of recently published journal articles on medication and racing. The ARCI (www.arci.com) has made its model rules available for download and also offers the most recent version of the "Uniform Classification Guidelines for Foreign Substances and Recommended Penalties and Model Rules" (https://ua-rtip.org/industry_service/download_model_rules). This document, which most racing commission personnel rely upon, classifies over 1000 substances by their respective pharmacology into five distinct classes. The classifications range from class 1 substances, which have no therapeutic value and a high potential to influence athletic performance, to class 5 substances, which are therapeutic in nature and thought to have little potential to affect athletic performance. When a violation of the medication rule has been determined to have occurred, the classification of that drug or medication is one of the determining factors of the penalty issued.

Medication use and veterinary practice for racehorses are regulated differently in Canada. Like the USA, there is a provincial commission that regulates racing in a given province including the practice of veterinary medicine on the racetrack. Unlike the USA, however, the use of and postrace testing for medications and nonpermitted substances are regulated by the federal government through the Canadian Pari-Mutuel Agency (CPMA). Also unlike the USA, there is a single laboratory contracted by the CPMA that performs the testing for all racing samples collected in Canada. The CPMA also publishes a "Schedule of Drugs," which contains withdrawal guidelines for over 50 therapeutic medications. Through the use of this schedule, it is much easier for the practitioner to determine how to comply with the rules in Canada, no matter the province. The schedule is available for download at the CPMA website (http://www.equin-ecanada.ca/index.php?option=com_docman&task=doc_view&gid=5588&Itemid=88&lang=en) and further information is available at http://www.agr.gc.ca/eng/about-us/partners-and-agencies/canadian-pari-mutuel-agency/equine-drug-control-program/?id=1204670391600.

The regulation of medication and veterinary practice in racing outside the USA and Canada is typically performed by a single nongovernmental organization established by the racing industry, such as the British Horseracing Authority, the France Galop, and the Hong Kong Jockey Club. Similar to efforts in the USA to foster uniformity between states, there have been recent efforts to harmonize the detection of therapeutic medications between the various racing countries. This approach has focused on the adoption of screening limits and determination of detection times by European laboratories and regulatory authorities, respectively. A list of detection times can be found on the European Horserace Scientific Liaison Committee website at www.ehslc.com. North American practitioners with clients that will be racing in European countries should check the detection times available on the website well in advance of travel, as some of the listed detection times in Europe are significantly longer in duration than those typically found for the same medication in the USA or Canada.

Show horse

As opposed to the entirely governmental regulation of racing in the USA, medication rules in show horse competitions are typically administered by nongovernmental organizations. The United States Equestrian Federation (USEF) is the largest oversight body, and it has established its own medication rules and administers its own drug testing program. Samples collected under the program are tested at the USEF laboratory in Lexington, Kentucky. USEF is also the recognized US affiliate of the Fédération Equestre Internationale (FEI), which is the governing body for international competitions recognized by the International Olympic Committee and the World Anti-Doping Association (WADA).

According to USEF regulations, every competition sanctioned by the organization is conducted under one of two sets of rules, and the Division Committee of each breed and/or discipline makes the determination under which rule they will compete. The No Foreign Substance Rule is exceptionally strict and considers a prohibited substance as any agent capable at any time of acting on one or more of the following mammalian body systems: the nervous system, the cardiovascular system, the urinary system, the reproductive system, the musculoskeletal system, the blood system, the endocrine system, the immune system (other than licensed vaccines against infectious agents), the digestive system (other than orally administered antiulcer medications), and the skin. The No Foreign Substance Rule is equivalent to the FEI medication rule. The list of medications allowed under the FEI rules as permitted substances is short and includes antibiotics (except procaine penicillin), antiparasitic compounds (except levamisole), and the antiulcer medications omeprazole, ranitidine, and cimetidine.

The second USEF rule is the Therapeutic Substance Rule. Under this rule, a prohibited substance is defined as any stimulant, depressant, tranquilizer, local anesthetic, or psychotropic agent and/or drug, which might affect the performance of a horse and/or pony or any metabolite and/or analog of any such substance, except where expressly permitted. With certain limitations, the rule allows practitioners to administer medications they deem necessary for the diagnosis or treatment of a horse with an existing illness or injury. As part of the Therapeutic Substance Rule, the USEF has also adopted thresholds for a number of therapeutic substances including nonsteroidal anti-inflammatory drugs (NSAIDs), corticosteroids, and methocarbamol. More information can be obtained at the USEF Drugs & Medications page of their website (http://www.usef.org).

Practicing within a regulated environment

There are two approaches that are commonly used to enforce drug and medication rules. First, the administration of medications and the performing of certain veterinary practices are often restricted for some period of time before the competition. Second, a testing program carried out on samples collected from participants, usually immediately after the competition, is often conducting concurrently to ensure that the drug and medication rule has been followed. For example, in the ARCI Model Rule, administration of the nonsteroidal anti-inflammatory agent phenylbutazone is prohibited within 24 h of the race in which the horse is entered. To enforce that rule, blood samples are collected after the race and the concentration of phenylbutazone in serum from that sample cannot be higher than 2 µg/ml. If the concentration of phenylbutazone exceeds that limit, it is a violation of the rule regardless of time the phenylbutazone was administered (https://ua-rtip.org/industry_service/download_model_rules).

By adhering to the restrictions on when medications can be administered and certain veterinary practices can be performed, the practitioner can avoid many rule violations. Nevertheless, some medications can be detected for long periods of time following administration of therapeutic doses, and therefore, one of most important pieces of information for the practitioner to know for any medication administered to a horse is the recommended withdrawal time. Unfortunately, generating accurate withdrawal times is exceptionally difficult due to the numerous factors affecting the time period after a drug has been discontinued that it remains detectable by a laboratory.

The length of the withdrawal time needed to avoid a positive test is based on a number of factors. The characteristics of the drug itself are extremely critical and include the dose administered and the frequency and route of administration. For instance, typically, the larger the dose administered, the longer a drug will remain detectable. In addition, intravenous routes of administration generally have the shortest detection periods. The practitioner also needs to remember that some drugs when administered over a period of time may bioaccumulate in the body, which can result in very long detection periods, particularly if the drug is eliminated by the kidney and testing is performed on urine samples. The formulation of the drug product can also affect the withdrawal time. For example, compounded medications can vary tremendously from batch to batch in their potency, as well as the rate and extent that they are absorbed, and therefore, the withdrawal time can vary accordingly. A second factor

affecting the withdrawal time is the methodology employed by the laboratory to analyze the samples collected in a drug testing program. The lowest concentration of a drug that an analytical method can reliably differentiate from a sample that does not contain any drug is termed the lower limit of detection (LLOD). In general, the lower the LLOD is for a particular drug, the longer that substance will be detectable in a sample collected after that drug has been administered and, therefore, the longer the withdrawal period for the drug. A third factor affecting withdrawal times is the horse itself. There can be significant horse-to-horse variation in the rate and extent to which they absorb, distribute, metabolize, and eliminate any given drug, and that is always out of the control of the practitioner.

Altogether, these factors demonstrate why it is so difficult to determine accurate withdrawal times. Practitioners may give different dosages for variable periods of time, laboratories may use different testing methods with different LLODs, and horses may eliminate the same drug at very different rates. This variation is why many regulatory bodies in the USA are reluctant to produce withdrawal time recommendations fearing that the advice will be used against them if a positive test is reported. Some regulatory bodies have included hold harmless language in their recommendations and clearly stipulate in their guidance documents that the trainer is ultimately responsible for assuring that the horse does not have an overage of a permitted medication or the presence of a nonpermitted substance in his system at the time of a race.

Compounded medications

Increasingly, compounded medications are aggressively marketed and available to equine practitioners. Compounding is the practice of combining, manipulating, or otherwise altering a drug substance or substances in order to produce a medication, which will meet the needs of a specific patient. The Center for Veterinary Medicine within the Food and Drug Administration (FDA) considers that with a few minor exceptions, only approved finished drug products should be used to produce compounded medications. In contrast, many pharmacies that specialize in producing compounded medications argue that the use of bulk drug substances in the production of compounded medications is legal, ethical, and safe. The resolution of the disagreement is currently being argued in the US courts, but it is unlikely to be resolved any time soon. Both the AVMA and the AAEP provide excellent resources to help the practitioner understand the legal and ethical issues surrounding the prescription and use of compounded medications. The veterinarian practicing in a regulated environment must be cognizant of the fact that compounded medications are not subject to the same bioequivalence tests or quality control/good manufacturing (cGMP) practices required of FDA-approved pioneer and generic drugs and that medication overages have been traced to compounded medications.

Over-the-counter products and herbal remedies and supplements

Practitioners are often asked by their clients to comment on whether or not an over-the-counter product or herbal supplement will "test" or result in a positive drug test. While it is easy to spot nonpermitted substances when they are included on a label, not all of these products are labeled clearly or completely. Medication positives have also resulted from products and feeds that were inadvertently contaminated with nonpermitted substances. An additional consideration is the product's indication for use. Even a permitted substance may violate a treatment regulation if it is being given for strictly performance-enhancing reasons.

The drug testing process

While security and investigatory techniques play an important role in the enforcement of drug and medication rules, the lynchpin of the system is the collection of blood and/or urine samples for analysis at a forensic laboratory. From a regulatory and legal standpoint, the process begins when the horse is identified for testing. At that point, steps are taken to ensure that the sample is being collected from the correct horse and that no one has an opportunity to administer anything to the horse. Once the sample is collected, it is sealed, labeled, and stored in a secure site until it is shipped to the analytical laboratory. The process of collection, storage, shipment, and analysis is all documented to produce a chain of custody that ensures that the regulatory body had

complete control over the sample throughout the process. In addition, procedures and policies are typically put in place by regulatory bodies in order to prevent any contamination from substances that could otherwise be present in the facility in which samples are collected. For example, food and drink are typically prohibited from the testing facility for this reason. The samples are secured in locked containers or coolers prior to shipment to the laboratory. Depending on the specific situation, samples are either held at a collection site for a short time frozen or they may be immediately shipped chilled overnight to ensure there is no degradation of the sample.

Recently, there has been a moderate shift in the primary fluid used for testing. For years, urine was the primary matrix used for postcompetition testing. This was largely due to the fact that most drugs are eliminated via the urine and the resulting concentrations tend to be much higher than in blood, making detection easier for less sensitive methodologies. With the advent of new, more sensitive testing methodologies however, serum is being used more and more as the preferred matrix. There are several advantages to testing for substances in serum. Firstly, it is usually easier to collect and typically there is a more direct correlation between the drug concentration in serum and its pharmacological activity. In addition, serum contains fewer substances than urine that could interfere with the testing process.

Once at the laboratory, the samples are unpacked and examined to ensure that the containers and seals are intact and free from evidence of tampering. Samples are logged into a computer system by the unique sample number on the label or, more typically, by a bar code reader. It is important to note that the laboratory is provided no information that would allow it to identify the horse from which the sample was collected or its human connections. Typically, the laboratory knows only the day the sample was collected, the track from where it was collected, and the sample number.

All of the test samples are subjected to a screening analysis, which involves testing the samples for a wide array of substances in a rapid, sensitive, and inexpensive manner. In this stage of the process, it is not critical that the methods employed by the laboratory be specific because a violation is not reported based on the screening results alone. In most equine sport laboratories, some combinations of thin-layer chromatography (TLC), enzyme-linked immunosorbent assays (ELISAs), and instrumental techniques using mass spectrometry (MS) are used to screen samples. Each methodology has advantages and disadvantages, and the menu employed by a particular laboratory is often driven by the overall testing budget.

If all of the screening tests return negative results, the sample is considered negative and either frozen for future testing or discarded. If, however, the results of one or more of the screening tests suggest the presence of a drug, the sample will undergo a second analysis designed to confirm and specifically identify the suspicious finding of first analysis. Because the confirmation method determines whether a violation is reported, the results must be able to withstand significant scientific and legal scrutiny. For this reason, the gold standard for confirmatory testing is MS. MS works by fragmenting molecules and then identifying the resulting ions by molecular weight. The fragmentation pattern of every molecule is unique, which has led to the identification of a substance by MS referred to as a "molecular fingerprint." Most forensic laboratories use a high-performance liquid chromatography as a means of separating analytes within the sample, prior to mass spectral identification, and the combined instrument is referred to as an LC/MS. Gas chromatography (GC)/MS, once the gold standard, is also used for confirmation procedures for select drugs, but not as commonly as LC/MS.

The selection by the regulatory authority or laboratory of the methodology used to screen the samples for a particular drug can have enormous implications to the practitioner because the different methodologies can have very different LLODs. If the concentration of a drug in a sample is below the screening method's limit of detection, the laboratory will declare that sample to be negative for the presence of that drug. The difference in LLODs between the various screening methodologies is significant. TLC, which is the oldest of the current screening methods, typically cannot detect a substance in a sample below 100 ng/ml. ELISAs are generally capable of detecting concentrations down to around 1 ng/ml. Meanwhile, the newer mass spectral methods, depending on the analyte, are capable of detecting low picogram (parts per trillion) to even subpicogram concentrations. All other variables being equal, the selection of one screening methodology over another can potentially make a 30-day difference in the length of time a drug can be detected.

Conclusion

Most equine clinicians at some point in their career will practice on horses that are subject to drug and medication rules. As previously discussed, those rules can vary significantly depending on what state or country the horse is competing in, what sport the horse is participating in, and the caliber of the competition. While no program is perfect, the analytical laboratories are constantly improving their ability to detect and identify nonpermitted medications. Finally, the ramifications for violating a medication rule can be substantial for everyone involved with the horse, even if the violation was not intentional. Therefore, it behooves the veterinarian to take the time to understand and comply with applicable medication rules and they ignore those rules at their peril.

Reference

1 The Jockey Club. (2011) *The jockey club factbook*. http://www.jockeyclub.com/factbook/StateFactBook/Kentucky.pdf [accessed on May 16, 2003].

CHAPTER 10

Clinical pharmacology of the respiratory system

Melissa R. Mazan[1] and Michelle L. Ceresia[2]

[1] Tufts University, North Grafton, MA, USA

[2] MCPHS University, Boston, MA, USA

Respiratory anatomy as it pertains to clinical pharmacology

The respiratory system is commonly divided into two sections, the upper respiratory tract (URT) and the lower respiratory tract (LRT). The lung has the privilege of having an extremely large surface area and, in fact, contacts more of the outside environment than does any other epithelial surface of the body. Although the respiratory system has other important functions, such as producing sounds, the vital functions of the respiratory system include the conduction of air, the exchange of oxygen and carbon dioxide, and protecting the respiratory surfaces from infection and exposure to noxious elements.

Upper respiratory tract (URT)

The horse, being an obligate nose breather, lacks an oropharyngeal component, and therefore, the URT is composed of the nasopharynx and the larynx. Cell types found in the URT include pseudostratified epithelium at the proximal portion, progressing to columnar, ciliated, and goblet cells in the more distal portions. Deposition of systemically administered drugs to the URT is not complex, resembling the delivery of such medications to any other simple tissue.

Lower respiratory tract (LRT)

The LRT consists of a conducting system, comprised of the trachea, bronchi, and bronchioles, and the respiratory portion, comprised of the respiratory bronchioles, alveolar ducts, and alveoli. The cells of the LRT change to reflect the functional needs of the respiratory system as air traverses from the trachea to the alveoli. More proximal portions of the LRT, including the trachea and the bronchi, are well endowed with goblet cells to produce mucus and ciliated cells to move the mucus and its entrapped particulates along the well-named mucociliary escalator. This epithelium gives way to a simple squamous epithelium in the alveoli—the type I and type II alveolar epithelium. The alveolar type I cells are thin and simple, ideally suited for the exchange of gases. The alveolar type II cells are much larger and specialize in producing surfactant. The gas exchange surface also includes the endothelial cells lining the capillaries that accompany the alveoli and the basement membrane in which the basal lamina is shared between the epithelium and the endothelium.

Anatomy of the pleura

Each lung occupies a pleural cavity lined by a serous membrane that folds back upon itself to envelope the lung. The external layer is termed the parietal pleura, and the layer that adheres to the lung is called the visceral pleura. The production of a small amount of pleural fluid prevents friction between the two layers.

Respiratory tract defense system

The respiratory tract defense system is comprised of anatomical barriers, as well as the innate and adaptive immune systems. The horse's nose provides the first

Equine Pharmacology, First Edition. Edited by Cynthia Cole, Bradford Bentz and Lara Maxwell.
© 2015 John Wiley & Sons, Inc. Published 2015 by John Wiley & Sons, Inc.

obstacle to foreign particles. The ornate scrollwork of the turbinates, as well as hairs that line the proximal portion of the nasal passages, physically removes large particulates. Moving more distally, there are mucus production and the cilia that serve to sweep the mucus and its engulfed debris proximally until it is ejected from the respiratory system. The innate immune system includes such nonspecific defenses as antimicrobial peptides, complement, and reactive oxygen species that are produced by phagocytic cells. Macrophages, located in the alveoli and within the interstitium, can phagocytize foreign material, including bacteria, to remove it from the body. Another important component of the lung's defense system is the cough. Triggered by irritants, such as chemical vapors, high air flows, and particulates, it helps the lungs expel noxious material. As with other organs, the lung mounts both cellular and humoral adaptive immune responses with lymphoid tissue distributed throughout the system and foci in the nares, larynx, and bronchioles. The nasopharynx, for example, is responsible for the production of IgA, one of the first lines of defense against an inhaled pathogen.

Considerations for distribution of drugs to the respiratory system

The anatomy of the respiratory system becomes important when we consider which drugs to use in targeting a particular infection or disease. Many studies in humans and other animals and now a series of studies in horses have shown that serum antimicrobial concentrations are not good indicators of drug concentrations in the lung [1, 2]. Moreover, drug concentrations in one section of the lung, for instance, the pulmonary epithelial lining fluid (PELF), may not reflect concentrations achieved in the parenchyma or even the bronchial epithelium. Nevertheless, the PELF concentration is the best indicator of a drug's penetration into the respiratory system. Beyond the anatomy of the respiratory system, drug-specific factors, including protein binding and tissue penetration, also affect the disposition of drugs to the lungs.

The means by which the horse has acquired a respiratory tract infection has important implications for treatment. Many infections are acquired by inhalation, for example, pneumonia secondary to esophageal obstruction or "shipping fever" pneumonia associated with high levels of particulates and microbes in the air during long-distance transport. Blood-borne pneumonia is less common in adult horses but relatively frequent in foals with septicemia. These distinctions help to determine if the infection is systemic, making it is necessary to consider drug distribution to the rest of the body, or if the infection is localized to the lung, and therefore, the lung is the primary target.

When treating infections of the LRT, it is important to consider where the infection is located—in the airway, in the interstitium, or in the alveolar space itself, as these spaces are anatomically and physiologically very different. Somewhat counterintuitively, distribution of systemically administered drugs is actually greater to the airways than to the alveolar space. This is because delivery of an antimicrobial to the airway is a relatively simple process of diffusion from the capillaries to the bronchial mucosa. In contrast, although the capillary endothelium is quite permeable, the alveolar epithelium is well supplied with zonula occludens, which prevent many substances, including many antimicrobials, from crossing the alveolar barrier. This is commonly termed the blood–bronchial barrier.

The disease state itself also strongly affects drug penetration into the respiratory system. Inflammation, which routinely accompanies infection, causes vasodilation that enhances drug delivery. However, inflammation can also increase the thickness of important barriers, such as the alveolar epithelium that will impair drug delivery. Other factors that enhance the penetration of drugs to the lung include high lipophilicity, low protein binding and ionization, and a relatively basic pKa. These characteristics improve passive diffusion through any membrane, but are particularly important in the face of the tight junctions that predominate in the lung [3].

Infectious diseases of the LRT

Bacterial pneumonia

There are two major presentations of bacterial infections in the lungs: juvenile bronchopneumonia and adult pneumonia/pleuropneumonia; the latter is also known as "shipping fever" pleuropneumonia. Juvenile bronchopneumonia is quite common in foals less than 8 months old, whereas pneumonia/pleuropneumonia occurs with much less frequency in adult horses. Nevertheless, both the juvenile and adult forms share important similarities: they are most common secondary to physiologic stressors, such as shipping in adults and weaning in foals, viral URT infections, and/or crowded housing. Other risk factors in adult horses include racing and general anesthesia. In both juveniles and adults, the bacterial population is frequently mixed; however, *Streptococcus equi* subsp. *zooepidemicus* (*Strep. zoo.*) will almost always be present. When we consider that risk factors, such as long-distance transport, strenuous exercise, and viral respiratory diseases, all suppress the immune system and that *Strep. zoo.* is resistant to phagocytosis by both macrophages and neutrophils and causes alveolar macrophage dysfunction and death, the combination of the presence of the bacterium and those risk factors often creates a perfect storm for the development of disease.

Epidemiology and etiology

Adult pneumonia most commonly occurs after an incident that impairs airway defenses, such as long-distance travel, anesthesia, and racing, or that provokes aspiration of oropharyngeal contents, such as esophageal obstruction. Prior viral infection is also an important risk factor. Pleuropneumonia is most often an extension of pneumonia that was either untreated or inadequately treated. In the USA, pleuropneumonia is more common in the late winter and spring in the northeast, when horses are returning from winter stays in Florida, and in the autumn in the south, when horses are making the reverse trip [4]. Juvenile pneumonia is most likely also a result of inhaled microbes or aspiration of oropharyngeal contents but is seen most commonly in the 3–6-month age group, when maternal antibodies are waning and the foal does not yet have its own full complement of antibodies. Adult and juvenile pneumonia and pleuropneumonia in adults all have moderate to good prognoses with prompt and appropriate treatment but moderate to poor prognoses when treatment is delayed.

Pathogenesis

The bacteria that are commonly seen in these diseases are normal commensals of the oropharynx and nasopharynx. The most common route of entry for the microorganism to the LRT is by aspiration of oropharyngeal contents. Inhalation is less common, and blood-borne infection even less so, other than in neonatal foals with septicemia. URT infections also prime the lower airway for infectious disease, as they denude the respiratory epithelium, interfere with the mucociliary apparatus, and suppress the

activity of alveolar macrophages. Severe nonseptic inflammatory diseases are uncommonly associated with secondary pneumonia, although excessive mucus production can interfere with airway clearance and thus contribute to LRT bacterial infections.

The most common pathogen isolated in cases of pneumonia is *Strep. zoo.* Pleuropneumonia arises most commonly secondary to primary pneumonia, with extension of the infection to visceral pleura, rupture of the pleural surface, and inoculation of parietal pleura, resulting in rapid effusion and exudation. Rarely cases of pleuropneumonia may result from other stressors, such as enterocolitis or secondary to septic emboli from infected jugular veins (septic thrombophlebitis). Other bacteria commonly isolated in cases of pneumonia include a variety of Gram-negative organisms, such as *Bordetella bronchiseptica*, *Actinobacillus* spp., *Klebsiella* spp., and *Escherichia coli*. The isolation of *Pseudomonas* spp. usually indicates a severe airway clearance problem, such as bronchiectasis, or contamination of the endoscope used to collect respiratory secretions. Anaerobic bacteria are more commonly isolated from cases of pleuropneumonia or severe pneumonia. Although viral infection is a common risk factor for bacterial pneumonia, viral pneumonia per se appears to be quite uncommon in equines.

Clinical presentation

Juvenile pneumonia and adult pneumonia have many similarities, although the clinical signs may be more severe in foals. Depending on the severity of disease, both groups will show fever, nasal discharge, cough, tachypnea, and dyspnea. It is far more common to see overt cyanosis in foals, but both groups are often hypoxic. Adult horses in which pneumonia has progressed to pleuropneumonia may be very painful, exhibiting a characteristic elbows-out posture. Foals may be recumbent, which only increases their work of breathing. Abnormal lung sounds are easier to auscultate in foals, as their smaller and more compliant chests cause less attenuation of lung sounds. Nonetheless, it is a good rule of thumb in both foals and adults that if crackles and wheezes are auscultable, it is a strong indication of disease, but the absence of such sounds does not, conversely, rule out disease. In horses with pleuropneumonia, there is often an absence of lung sounds in the ventral lung fields and bronchovesicular sounds in the dorsal lung fields. Clinical examination and history will give a strong suspicion of pneumonia; however, thoracic radiographs are confirmatory in uncomplicated pneumonia; ultrasound will be of most benefit in cases of suspected pleuropneumonia. Although it is safe to assume that the infectious organisms will comprise a combination of *Strep. zoo.* and other Gram-positive and Gram-negative organisms, a transtracheal aspirate for culture and sensitivity (C&S) testing is important for formulating the best treatment plan. Bronchoalveolar lavage (BAL) is inappropriate in this case, as it is impossible to acquire a sterile sample, and if disease is isolated to a particular segment of the lung, it can be missed on BAL. It is important to remember that BAL is not appropriate in horses that are in any respiratory distress. Thoracocentesis can be both diagnostic and therapeutic in cases of pleuropneumonia; however, cultures of the fluid retrieved are frequently negative, and transtracheal aspirates often deliver more rewarding samples. The leukogram will often show leukocytosis with hyperfibrinogenemia.

Treatment

The primary goal is eradication of the infectious organism through appropriate use of antimicrobials. Because of the horse's status as a hindgut fermenter, the second very important goal must be to avoid comorbidity due to antibiotic-induced colitis.

General Approach to Treatment: It is important to assess the severity of the infection when designing the treatment plan. Pneumonia can present as a disease primarily located in the respiratory system, with little effect on oxygenation or well-being at rest, or as a respiratory disease with systemic involvement, which may be life threatening. In the case of severe, life-threatening disease, supplemental treatment with oxygen, antiendotoxin medication such as polymyxin B, intravenous (IV) fluids, anti-inflammatories, frog support for potential laminitis, and other adjunctive therapies may be necessary but are beyond the scope of this chapter.

Pharmacologic Therapy: Selection of Appropriate Antimicrobial Agents. Designing an appropriate broad-spectrum antimicrobial therapy is critical for successful treatment of pneumonia, although good supportive care is also extremely important. In the case of pleuropneumonia, thoracentesis is also often necessary to remove the effusion. Although C&S testing of tracheal aspirates is an important guide to appropriate antimicrobial therapy, the clinician must use good

judgment and knowledge of the most likely bacteria present in pneumonia/pleuropneumonia, while these results are pending. The clinician should assume a mixed infection that includes streptococcal and Gram-negative species unless and until C&S results prove otherwise. In addition, anaerobic bacteria are frequently present in pleuropneumonia. Fetid nasal breath is often a good indicator of an anaerobic bacterial infection, but it may not always be present. In addition, anaerobic cultures are notoriously problematic, so negative culture results will not rule out their presence. Thus, broad-spectrum coverage with a beta-lactam (penicillin or cephalosporin) in conjunction with an aminoglycoside or enrofloxacin is usually a good start. Although penicillin is a reasonable choice for most anaerobic bacteria, the *Bacteroides* spp. are often resistant, and therefore, metronidazole is commonly included if anaerobic infections are suspected. Depending on the clinical picture, as discussed in the following text, other antimicrobials may be better options.

Whether the antimicrobial is a bacteriostatic or bactericidal agent is an important consideration in drug selection. In general, bactericidal drugs are usually thought of as superior to bacteriostatic, but it is important to remember, especially in horses, which are particularly sensitive to endotoxin, that bactericidal antimicrobials can increase the release of endotoxin. It should also be kept in mind that many bacteriostatic antimicrobials are bactericidal at high concentrations and that many bactericidal antimicrobials will only be bacteriostatic if appropriate concentrations cannot be achieved or maintained as required. Regardless of bactericidal versus bacteriostatic nature of the antimicrobial, it must be able to reach the site of infection to be effective. For instance, aminoglycosides will not penetrate a pulmonary abscess to any clinically significant degree and will therefore be ineffective *in vivo*, although *in vitro* C&S testing may suggest good efficacy. Therefore, in situations where pulmonary abscessation is suspected, a fluoroquinolone would be a better choice than an aminoglycoside, because it would penetrate any abscess more readily.

Precautions: Although broad-spectrum therapy is mandatory in the face of severe illness, it is preferable eventually to tailor treatment to culture results, especially with the known danger of antibiotic-induced colitis in horses. It is very important to remember that fluoroquinolones adversely affect the cartilage in growing foals, so this drug class is contraindicated in this population unless there is no other choice, and the disease is life threatening. The use of marbofloxacin, a newer fluoroquinolone, has anecdotally been noted to be somewhat less prone to these side effects, however, because it belongs to the same class as enrofloxacin, it should be reserved only for those cases in which all other reasonable alternatives have failed, or can be predicted to fail based on results of culture and sensitivity. Even in adults, enrofloxacin has been noted rarely to cause severe tendinopathies, so caution should be exercised with long-term use. Although macrolides form an essential cornerstone of *Rhodococcus equi* treatment in foals and weanlings (see following text), they have a strong propensity to cause fulminant colitis in adult horses, so they should be avoided in this population. There is some evidence that the newer macrolides, such as azithromycin, may have improved safety profiles in adult horses, but additional studies are needed before their use in client-owned animals can be recommended [5].

Duration of Therapy and Mode of Administration: Although mild septic bronchitis or bronchopneumonia may require only 7–10 days of antimicrobial therapy, more severe disease often requires several weeks to even months of treatment. In the case of a critically ill horse with pleuropneumonia or severe bronchopneumonia, it is preferable, when possible, to hospitalize the horse for the first 5–7 days for IV antibiotic therapy, especially when other ancillary treatments, such as drainage of pleural effusion and placement of indwelling drains, may be necessary. IV administrations of antimicrobials provide the most reliable and predictable pharmacokinetic profiles. In milder cases, intramuscular (IM) or even oral administration may be efficacious. The practitioner frequently has many competing reasons for choosing one mode of administration over another. One may be expense, and another may be practicality. Although IM injection frequently achieves good blood and tissue concentrations, in the thin or fractious horse, it may not be a realistic approach. IV injections, when administered chronically, require an indwelling IV catheter, which is impractical for all but the most skilled and dedicated of horse owners or barn managers, thus the earlier recommendation for hospitalization when possible. Once it is clear that the horse is responding favorably to treatment, a transition to IM or oral administration of antimicrobials is often possible (Table 10.1).

Drugs administered by IV or IM injection

Ampicillin: One of the more time-honored drugs used to treat equine pneumonia is the beta-lactam ampicillin. Numerous studies have shown that many respiratory pathogens are susceptible to ampicillin, especially streptococci, and it has been shown to actually accumulate in the PELF over time, which may be partially due to its low serum protein binding. For most streptococcal infections of the LRT, ampicillin administered IV at doses of 15 mg/kg bwt should produce concentrations in the PELF above MIC for 12 h [6]. As previously discussed, however, as most pneumonias are mixed infections and may involve bacteria less sensitive than streptococci, it might be necessary to increase the frequency of administration of ampicillin to every 6–8 h to achieve higher PELF concentrations for longer periods of time. Penicillin has a similar pharmacokinetic profile to ampicillin, but less activity against Gram-negative aerobic microbes.

Cephalosporins: A 3rd-generation cephalosporin, ceftiofur is metabolized to the active moiety desfuroyl-ceftiofur and was first marketed for respiratory infections in cattle. It is now approved for use in the horse for treatment of LRT infections with susceptible microorganisms and is highly efficacious against *Strep. zoo* [7]. Early studies indicated that 12 h after administration, concentrations of ceftiofur and its metabolites in lung homogenate were only slightly lower than plasma concentrations [8]. The original sodium salt formulation is reconstituted with sterile water, and the label indicates it is to be administered IM at a dosage of 2.2–4.4 mg/kg bwt once a day. It has been shown to have very similar pharmacokinetics when administered IV. Ceftiofur has recently been formulated as a sustained-release product that is labeled to be administered twice, IM, 4 days apart. A recent clinical trial demonstrated that the sustained-release formulation is effective in treating naturally acquired LRT infections due to *Strep. zoo* [9]. It is important for the practitioner to be certain of the etiology of the LRT infection before using a sustained-release antibiotic, as its use cannot be retracted and it commits the practitioner to that therapeutic approach for at least 4 days. Although ceftiofur is the most commonly used cephalosporin in horses, recent information suggests that cefquinome may be efficacious against many bacterial respiratory pathogens in horses. As a 4th-generation cephalosporin, it has greater activity against Gram-negative bacteria and is more resistant to

Table 10.1 Common antibiotics administered to adult horses with respiratory infections.

Aminoglycosides (amikacin (AMIK), gentamicin (GENT))—mechanism, irreversibly bind to 30S ribosomal subunit and inhibit protein synthesis; bactericidal; concentration-dependent killing; O_2 and alkaline pH required for efficacy; synergy with cell wall inhibitors (penicillins, vancomycin)

Spectrum of coverage[1-7]	Absorption	Distribution penetration	Elimination	Adverse effects	Dosing[8-10]	Cost/ day	Comments
Gram(+):	Minimal PO absorption	• Distribute primarily in the ECF[11,12]	Renal	Nephrotoxic	AMIK	AMIK $$$$	• Aminoglycoside activity ↓ with low pH (e.g., endobronchial pH), possibly a result of pH effect on porin channels and drugs ↓ ability to enter the bacterial cell[11,18–20]
• R. equi		• IV administration → low lung []; GENT (dosed QD) estimated to be effective for about 8 h based on the time bronchial drug [] > MIC and postantibiotic effect (PAE)[13,14]		Ototoxic	• 20–25 mg/kg IV q24 h	GENT $	• Limited efficacy in abscesses; drug requires O_2-dependent transport[18]
• Corynebacterium pseudotuberculosis GENT				• Vestibular	GENT		• Phenylbutazone ↓ GENT distribution and half-life; monitor GENT trough [][21]
• Coag(+) Staphylococcus GENT				• Auditory	• 6.6 mg/kg IV or IM q24 h		• Penicillin beta-lactam ring PLUS amino group from aminoglycoside form an inactive amide; occurs with ↑ contact time and higher []; well documented with extended-spectrum penicillins.[22–27] Avoid mixing both drugs in same IV bag[28]; Serum aminoglycoside samples should be assayed as early as possible or frozen at 70°C[25]; monitor aminoglycoside [] in renal failure; coadministration may be a concern because drug [] will be the highest, that is, before distribution and both drugs will be primarily in the central compartment (intravascular); however, no significant aminoglycoside inactivation occurred after 1 h incubation with extended-spectrum penicillins[24–26]
• Staphylococcus aureus GENT				Neuromuscular blockade (rare)	• Pleuropneumonia 8 mg/kg IV and then adjust dose based on serum []		
Covers primarily Gram(−) bacteria:		• Aerosolized GENT obtained higher bronchial lining fluid [] versus IV and was well tolerated (1 g q24 h)[14,15]		• ↑ risk with botulism and neuromuscular blocking agents	Drug serum []		
• Actinobacillus sp.				• Monitor $[Mg^{2+}]$[16,17]	• Target peak drawn ½ h postadministration; at least 8–10 times the MIC for efficacy		
• Enterobacter sp. AMIK		• Protein binding <30%		IM injection → muscle irritation	• Target trough drawn before dose; <2 µg/ ml GENT and <8 µg/ ml AMIK		
• Escherichia coli AMIK							
• Klebsiella							
• Pasteurella sp. GENT							
• Salmonella AMIK							

Cephalosporins (3rd generation, ceftiofur (CEFT))—mechanism, inhibit the peptidoglycan cross-linking within the bacterial cell wall or membrane; bactericidal; time-dependent killing

Spectrum of coverage[1,3–5,7,29–32]	Absorption	Distribution penetration	Elimination	Adverse effects	Dosing[8–10]	Cost/day	Comments
Gram(+):		Desfuroyl-CEFT	Rapid liver hydrolysis ↓	Swelling injection site (Excede®)	CEFT Crystalline Free Acid (Excede)	$$	
• S. equi		• High protein binding		Diarrhea	• 6.6 mg/kg IM; repeat in 4 days		
• Strep. zoo.		Good lung penetration	Desfuroyl-CEFT, an equally active metabolite	Hypersensitivity reaction	CEFT Na⁺ (Naxcel®)		
Covers Gram(−) but slightly resistant:					• Strangles: 2.2 mg/kg IM q12–24 h		
• E. coli					• 2.2–4.4 mg/kg IM q24 h		
• Klebsiella					• Gram(−) infections require higher dose or more frequent administration		
• Pasteurella							
Anaerobes:							
• Fusobacterium necrophorum							
• Peptostreptococcus anaerobius							

Chloramphenicol (CHLOR)—mechanism, reversibly binds to the 50S subunit of the bacterial ribosomes inhibiting protein synthesis; broad spectrum; bacteriostatic; bactericidal for some pathogens

Spectrum of coverage	Absorption	Distribution penetration	Elimination	Adverse effects	Dosing	Cost/day	Comments
• Mycoplasma	PO route Rapid absorption peak of 2–3 h (humans)	Good tissue penetration	Sodium succinate (prodrug) 30% renal elimination ↓	Bone marrow suppression (dose related and reversible)	• 45–60 mg/kg PO q8 h	$$	• CHLOR ↓ the clearance of drugs cleared by CYP enzymes (e.g., phenylbutazone, xylazine, pentobarbital)[33,34]
Gram(+):		Protein binding 50%	Hydrolyzed		• 46–60 mg/kg IM, SC, or IV q6–8 h		
• C. pseudotuberculosis							
• Beta-hemolytic Streptococcus spp.	Sodium succinate (IV form) up to 30% ↓ bioavailability		CYP450				• Rifampin (potent enzyme inducer) may ↓ CHLOR half-life resulting in subtherapeutic [][35]
• S. equi			Metabolism inactive metabolite				
• Strep. zoo.							
• S. aureus							
Gram(−):							
• Actinobacillus suis-like							
• Pasteurella sp.							
Anaerobes:							
• Bacteroides							
• Clostridium							

(Continued)

Table 10.1 (*Continued*)

Spectrum of coverage[4,5,7]	Absorption	Distribution penetration	Elimination	Adverse effects	Dosing[8-10]	Cost/day	Comments
Fluoroquinolones (enrofloxacin (ENRO))—mechanism, inhibit bacterial DNA gyrase or topoisomerase IV preventing DNA supercoiling and replication; concentration-dependent killing							
Gram(+): • *Staph.* sp. Primarily Gram(−): • *Klebsiella* • *Pasteurella* sp. • *S. enterica* • *E. coli*	Oral bioavailability 65%	Excellent tissue penetration Protein binding 22%	ENRO De-ethylate ↓ Ciprofloxacin Excreted by glomerular filtration and tubular excretion	Tendinopathy CNS stimulation (higher concentrations)	• 5 mg/kg IV q24 h • 7.5 mg/kg PO q24 h	$$	• Tendonitis and spontaneous tendon rupture in humans; risks—older adults, concurrent steroids, strenuous physical activity, renal failure, previous tendon disorders; occurs during and up to several months after therapy[23] • ENRO effects on adult equine tendon cells → morphological changes and inhibition of cell proliferation; use ENRO cautiously in horses[36]
Nitroimidazoles (metronidazole (METRO))—mechanism, disrupt DNA and inhibit nucleic acid synthesis; concentration-dependent killing; narrow therapeutic index							
Anaerobes	Oral • Rapid absorption • Bioavailability 74–97% Rectal route 30% bioavailability	Penetrate tissue well Protein binding 20% in humans	Hepatic metabolism	• GI upset, diarrhea, anorexia • Dose of 30 mg/kg → ↓ appetite, hepatotoxic lesions, and peripheral neuropathy[37] • Neurotoxicity—depression, ataxia, seizures • Disulfiram-like reaction	Oral • Colitis 20–25 mg/kg PO q8–12 h or 15 mg/kg PO q6 h Rectal • 25 mg/kg **PR** q6–12 h IV • 20 mg/kg IV q8–12 h	$	• 5% injectable formulation is expensive, and because drug is poorly soluble, dose is administered in large volume of fluid[9] • Commercial product METRO Base is bitter tasting; compounded product is often formulated with METRO Benzoate, which is tasteless; note: 1 g METRO Base=1.6 g METRO benzoate • Enzyme inducers (e.g., phenobarbital, rifampin (RIF)) may ↑ METRO metabolism resulting in subtherapeutic [][23]

Macrolides (azithromycin (AZM), clarithromycin (CLR), erythromycin (ERY))—mechanism, inhibit protein synthesis by binding reversibly to 50S ribosomal subunits; bacteriostatic; bactericidal high doses; time-dependent killing; synergy with RIF

Spectrum of coverage[4,9,38]	Absorption[9,39,40]	Distribution penetration[9,39,40]	Elimination	Adverse effects[9]	Dosing[8–10]	Cost/day	Comments
Gram(+):	Bioavailability ERY freebase or phosphate salt 10–40%; AZM 39–56%; CLR 57%	High lipid solubility	ERY stearate hydrolyzed in the intestine →	• Foals (ERY + RIF): bruxism, anorexia, mild colitis, and diarrhea[41]	*R. equi* pneumonia in foals	Price for Foals	• RIF ↓ the bioavailability of CLR (>70%) → serum [] below the MIC$_{90}$ of *R. equi*; the interaction is thought to occur by inhibition of an
• *R. equi* (ERY and CLR activity > AZM)		Excellent penetration into cells			Combination therapy:	AZM $	unknown intestinal uptake transporter; despite the
• Beta-hemolytic Streptococcus sp.		Phagocyte[] very high versus serum [] and persists for a longer time	ERY base	• Severe hyperthermia and tachypnea (ERY) occur usually between 2nd and 4th day of therapy; although can occur anytime; can result in death; ↓	• CLR 7.5 mg/kg PO q12 h "or"	CLR $	drug interaction, the combination of a macrolide with RIF is recommended to
• Staphylococcus sp.	Better bioavailability in foals with ERY estolate and microencapsulated base versus other dosage forms				• AZM 10 mg/kg PO QD×5 day and then QOD "or"	ERY $	treat *R. equi* pneumonia in foals since the drugs achieve
• Actinomyces pyogenes		Active intracellularly and at acidic pH	ERY esters (estolate and ethyl succinate) absorbed →	temperature with cold water or alcohol baths, cold water enemas and fans[9,41]	• ERY 25 mg/kg PO q6 h "plus"		higher [] and persist longer in BAL cells versus plasma and epithelial lining fluid
• Bacillus sp.		Protein binding 18–30%			• RIF 5 mg/kg PO q12 h OR 10 mg/kg PO QD		and have a relatively long postantibiotic effect[42–45].
• Corynebacterium sp.	Better absorption when food withheld		hydrolyzed ↓ ERY base	• Hepatotoxicity			Also, the combination has been shown to ↑ survival in foals afflicted *R. equi*
• Listeria sp.				• Epigastric distress (ERY > CLR/AZM), mild colic; diarrhea— severe in adult horses	Do not crush enteric-coated ERY tablets; the drug will get destroyed by stomach acid		pneumonia[46,47], staggering the doses may be of benefit
• Erysipelothrix rhusiopathiae			Metabolism by hepatic microsomal enzymes	• Pseudomembranous colitis			• Macrolides inhibit CYP3A4 potentiating the effects of drugs such as theophylline,
Gram(−):				• Cardiac arrhythmias—rare			warfarin, carbamazepine, digoxin, triazolam
• Actinobacillus sp.				• Allergic reaction			
• Brucella spp.							
• Campylobacter sp.							
• Leptospira sp.							
• Pasteurella sp.							
Anaerobes:							
• Actinomyces sp.							
• Bacteroides sp. (except *Bacteroides fragilis*)							
• Clostridium							
• Fusobacterium sp.							

(Continued)

Table 10.1 (*Continued*)

Spectrum of coverage[48,49]	Absorption	Distribution penetration	Elimination	Adverse effects	Dosing[8-10]	Cost/day	Comments
Penicillins (ampicillin (AMP), penicillin G (PEN))—mechanism, inhibit the peptidoglycan cross-linking within the bacterial cell wall or membrane; bactericidal; time-dependent killing							
Gram(+): • *Beta-hemolytic Streptococcus* spp. • *S. equi* • *S. equisimilis* • *Strep. zoo.* Gram(−): • *Pasteurella* sp. • *Proteus mirabilis* (AMP) • *E. coli* (AMP) • *Listeria* • *Salmonella* spp. (AMP) Anaerobes: • *Peptococcus* (PEN) • *Peptostreptococcus* (PEN) • *Clostridium* (PEN) • *Fusobacterium* • *Bacteroides* spp. (except *B. fragilis*)	Poor oral absorption	AUC_{PELF}/AUC_{plasma} ratio$_{0-12\,h}$ = 0.40 after IV AMP injection (i.e., pulmonary [] achieved adequate to treat equine respiratory infections, e.g., *Streptococcus*, up to 12 h)[50]	Hydrolyzed to inactive metabolites Excreted by tubular secretion	Anaphylactic reaction	AMP Na⁺ • 20–50 mg/kg IV or IM TID AMP trihydrate depot injection • 5–20 mg/kg IM BID PEN K⁺ or Na⁺ • 10,000–20,000 U/kg IV or IM q6 h Serious infections: 22,000–44,000 U/kg IV q6 h • Strangles: 22,000 U/kg IM, IV, or SC q6 h Procaine PEN depot injection • 22,000 U/kg IM or SC q12 h	AMP $$$$ PEN $$ to $$$	• AMP trihydrate IM injection is irritating and stings; the spectrum of activity is limited by low serum concentrations[9] • See aminoglycosides for drug interaction • Bacteriostatic antibiotics (e.g., CHLOR, TETRA, macrolides) combined with bactericidal antibiotics (e.g., beta-lactam antibiotics) → *in vitro* antagonism; however, clinical relevance is not clear
Rifampins (RIF)—mechanism, inhibit RNA polymerase; bactericidal; concentration-dependent killing (*M. tuberculosis*); time-dependent killing (*R. equi*); postantibiotic effect median 4.7 h, range 4.0–7.8 h; synergy with macrolides; resistance develops quickly (monotherapy) → indicated for use in combination therapy; enzyme inducer							
Gram(+): • *S. aureus* • *R. equi* • *Mycobacterium* sp. • *Corynebacterium* sp. • *Streptococcus* sp.	Bioavailability 70% Food reduces absorption	• High tissue penetration • Penetrate phagocytes and active intracellularly at acidic pH[9] • Protein binding 78%	Hepatic metabolism CYP3A	• Rusty orange urine, mucous membranes, and secretions • RIF bad taste → anorexia; rinse mouth before eating • Diarrhea • False ↑ LFTs	*R. equi* pneumonia in foals: • CLR 7.5 mg/kg PO q12 h "plus" RIF 5 mg/kg PO q12 h Administer RIF far back on tongue and make sure horse swallows	Price for foal$	• Effective in abscesses • RIF, an enzyme inducer, can ↓ serum [] of drugs (theophylline, warfarin, diazepam, phenobarbital, digoxin, phenylbutazone, CHLOR, ciprofloxacin, azole antifungals, beta-blockers, trimethoprim, corticosteroids) • RIF is an autoinducer

Sulfonamide/diaminopyrimidine combination (sulfamethoxazole (SMZ)/trimethoprim (TMP), sulfadiazine (SDZ/TMP)—inhibit dihydrofolate reductase; broad spectrum; bacteriostatic (each agent alone); bactericidal (together) for some pathogens

Spectrum of coverage[2,51,52]	Absorption	Distribution penetration	Elimination[52]	Adverse effects[9]	Dosing[8-10]	Cost/day	Comments
Gram(+): • *S. equisimilis* • *Listeria monocytogenes* • *A. pyogenes* • *Bacillus* sp. • *E. rhusiopathiae* Gram(–): • *Brucella abortus* • *Chlamydia* spp. Protozoa: • *Pneumocystis carinii*	Good oral absorption Bioavailability in fed horses • SDZ 74% • TMP 46% Food → delays absorption	• Penetrates tissues well (lipophilic) • SDZ/TMP AUC$_{PELF}$/AUC$_{Plasma}$ ratio = 0.92 SDZ and 0.46 TMP after PO administration • TMP rapidly cleared from PELF [53,54] • PELF → difficult to maintain TMP • Protein binding TMP 50%	Metabolism Metabolites ↓ Efficacy ↓ Hydroxyl metabolite or inactive	• Transient pruritus (IV) • Reversible neutropenia associated with prolong therapy Treatment: supplement with folinic acid, for example, Brewer's yeast • Diarrhea • Pseudomembranous colitis • Rapid IV administration → tremors, excitement, ataxia, collapse, and rare deaths • Crystalluria	Adult horses • 15–30 mg/kg PO q12 h • Give 30 min prior to food Foals • 15 mg/kg IV q12 h; administer slowly • 15–30 mg/kg PO q12 h Note: mg/kg dose is based on the addition of both drug components, that is, 30 mg/kg dose = 25 mg sulfonamide plus 5 mg trimethoprim (5:1 ratio) • Products (five parts sulfonamide to one part trimethoprim) Human products SMZ/TMP: tablets 400/80 mg and 800/160 mg; oral suspension 40 mg/8 mg/ml; injection 80 mg/16 mg/ml Veterinary products SDZ/TMP: oral paste and powder 333/67 mg; injection 400 mg/80 mg/ml	$	• Reports of death after IV administration, possibly a result of vagal stimulation leading to bradycardia and vasodilation; pharmaceutical formulation (e.g., excipients, solvents) maybe the cause[55] • IV TMP/sulfonamide–detomidine interaction; associated with dysrhythmias, hypotension, and death; avoid combination[9]

(Continued)

Table 10.1 (*Continued*)

Tetracyclines (doxycycline (DOX), minocycline (MINO), oxytetracycline (OXY), tetracycline (TET))—mechanism, bind reversibly to receptors of the 30S ribosomal subunit inhibiting protein synthesis; broad spectrum

Spectrum of coverage[7,56]	Absorption[57]	Distribution penetration[56]	Elimination[56]	Adverse effects[56]	Dosing[8-10]	Cost/day	Comments
Gram(+): • *R. equi* (DOX) • *C. pseudotuberculosis* • *S. equi* • *L. monocytogenes* • *E. rhusiopathiae* • Some streptococci Gram(−): • *Actinobacillus* • *Pasteurella* spp. • *Brucella* spp. • *Campylobacter fetus* • *Haemophilus parasuis* • *Mycoplasma* Spirochetes: • *Borrelia burgdorferi* • *Leptospira*	Bioavailability DOX in nonfasted horses • 17% intragastric administration • 6% mixed in feed[58] Food ↓ absorption (OXY and TET)	DOX and MINO have great tissue and intracellular penetration; MINO is more lipophilic than DOXY[59] AUC_{PELF}/AUC_{plasma} ratio = 0.87 after intragastric DOX administration[58] Protein binding • DOX 81% • MINO 68% • OXY 50%[59]	TET eliminated • Urine via glomerular filtration (60%) • Feces (40%) Excreted primarily in the large intestines/feces (DOX) TET excreted in the bile	Esophagitis: ↑ prevalence with DOX hyclate Bone and teeth discoloration Nephrotoxic renal tubular necrosis • High doses • Prolonged administration • Outdated drugs Photosensitivity Hypersensitivity reactions	Oral formulations: • DOX hyclate • DOX monohydrate DOX • 10–20 mg/kg PO q12 h[56] MINO • 4 mg/kg PO q12 h OXY • 6.6 mg/kg IV q12–24 h	DOX Oral $ MINO Oral $ OXY $	• IV DOX administration related to cardiovascular adverse effects and death[60] • Oral TET chelate divalent and trivalent cations (e.g., antacids) resulting in ↓ antibiotic [] • DOXY and MINO have anti-inflammatory effects • Microsomal enzyme inducers (e.g., barbiturates) ↑ elimination of DOX → ↓ DOX serum []; adjustment of DOX dosage or substitute with another TET[57,61]

$, inexpensive; $$, relatively inexpensive; $$$, expensive; $$$$, extremely expensive.

The authors have tried to include the clinically relevant drug interactions and/or problems associated with the drugs listed in this chart; thus, the drug interactions covered are not an inclusive list.

1 Adamson, P.J., Wilson, W.D., Hirsh, D.C., Baggot, J.D. & Martin, L.D. (1985) Susceptibility of equine bacterial isolates to antimicrobial agents. *American Journal of Veterinary Research*, **46** (2), 447–450.

2 Erol, E., Locke, S.J., Donahoe, J.K., Mackin, M.A. & Carter, C.N. (2012) Antimicrobic susceptibility of bacterial pathogens from horses. *Veterinary Clinics of North America Equine Practice*, **3** (1), 181–190.

3 Hirsh, D.C. & Jang, S.S. (1987) Antimicrobic susceptibility of bacterial pathogens from horses. *Veterinary Clinics of North America Equine Practice*, **3** (1), 181–190.

4 Jacks, S.S., Giguère, S. & Nguyen, A. (2003) In vitro susceptibilities of *Rhodococcus equi* and other common equine pathogens to azithromycin, clarithromycin, and 20 other antimicrobials. *Antimicrobial Agents and Chemotherapy*, **47** (5), 1742–1745.

5 Rubin, J.E., Ball, K.R. & Chirino-Trejo, M. (2011) Antimicrobial susceptibility of *Staphylococcus aureus* and *Staphylococcus pseudintermedius* isolated from various animals. *Canadian Veterinary Journal*, **52** (2), 153–157.

6 Sweeney, C.R., Holcombe, S.J., Barningham, S.C. & Beech, J. (1991) Aerobic and anaerobic bacterial isolates from horses with pneumonia or pleuropneumonia and antimicrobial susceptibility patterns of the aerobes. *Journal of the American Veterinary Medical Association*, **198** (5), 839–842.

7 Giguere, S., Prescott, J.F., Baggot, J.D., Walker, R.D. & Dowling, P.M. (eds) (2006) *Antimicrobial Therapy in Veterinary Medicine*, 4th edn. Blackwell Publishing, Ames.

8 Plumb, D.C. (2011) *Plumb's Veterinary Drug Handbook*, 7th edn. Wiley-Blackwell, Ames.

9 Wilson, W.D. (2001) Rational selection of antimicrobials for use in horses. *AAEP Proceedings*, **47**, 75–93.

10 Riviere, J.E. & Papich, M.G. (eds) (2009) *Veterinary Pharmacology and Therapeutics*, 9th edn. Wiley-Blackwell, Ames.

11 Edson, R.S. & Terrell, C.L. (1999) Symposium of antimicrobial agents, part VIII. The aminoglycosides. *Mayo Clinic Proceedings*, **74 (5)**, 519–528.

12 USP, AAVPT Veterinary Drug Expert Committee (2007) *Aminoglycosides (Veterinary—Systemic)*. The United States Pharmacopeial Convention.

13 Godber, L.M., Walker, R.D., Stein, G.E., Hauptman, J.G. & Derksen, F.J. (1995) Pharmacokinetics, nephrotoxicosis, and in vitro antibacterial activity associated with single versus multiple (three times) daily gentamicin treatments in horses. *American Journal of Veterinary Research*, **56 (5)**, 613–618.

14 McKenzie, H.C., 3rd & Murray, M.J. (2000) Concentrations of gentamicin in serum and bronchial lavage fluid after intravenous and aerosol administration of gentamicin to horses. *American Journal of Veterinary Research*, **61**, 1185–1190.

15 McKenzie, H.C., 3rd & Murray, M.J. (2004) Concentrations of gentamicin in serum and bronchial lavage fluid after once-daily aerosol administration to horses for seven days. *American Journal of Veterinary Research*, **65**, 173–178.

16 L'Hommedieu, C.S., Nicholas, D., Armes, D.A., Jones, P., Nelson, T. & Pickering, L.K. (1983) Potentiation of magnesium sulfate-induced neuromuscular weakness by gentamicin, tobramycin, and amikacin. *Journal of Pediatrics*, **102 (4)**, 629–631.

17 MacDougall, C. & Chambers, H.F. (2011) Aminoglycosides. In: L.L. Brunton, B.A. Chabner & B.C. Knollman (eds), *Goodman & Gilman's the Pharmacological Basis of Therapeutics*, 12th edn, pp. 1505–1520. McGraw-Hill Medical, New York.

18 Vaudaux, P. (1981) Peripheral inactivation of gentamicin. *Journal of Antimicrobial Chemotherapy*, **8** (Suppl. A), 17–25.

19 Todt, J.C., Rocque, W.J. & McGroarty, J. (1992) Effects of pH on bacterial porin function. *Biochemistry*, **31**, 10471–10478.

20 Bodem, C.R., Lampton, L.M., Miller, D.P., Tarka, E.F. & Everett, E.D. (1983) Endobronchial pH. Relevance to aminoglycoside activity in gram-negative bacillary pneumonia. *American Review of Respiratory Disease*, **127 (1)**, 39–41.

21 Whittem, T., Firth, E.C., Hodge, H. & Turner, K. (1996) Pharmacokinetic interactions between repeated dose phenylbutazone and gentamicin in the horse. *Journal of Veterinary Pharmacology and Therapeutics*, **19 (6)**, 454–459.

22 Susla, J.M. (2011) Miscellaneous antibiotics. In: S.C. Piscitelli, R.A. Rodvold & M.P. Pai (eds), *Drug Interactions in Infectious Diseases*, 3rd edn, p. 392. Humana Press, New York.

23 American Society of Health-System Pharmacists (ASHP) (2012) *AHFS Drug Information 2012*. ASHP, Bethesda.

24 Shwed, J.A., Ceresia, M.L., Taylor, A.J. & Bosso, J.A. (1995) Lack of effect of clavulanic acid on aminoglycoside inactivation by ticarcillin. *Journal of Infectious Disease Pharmacotherapy*, **2**, 35–43.

25 Pickering, L.K. & Rutherford, I. (1981) Effect of concentration and time upon inactivation of tobramycin, gentamicin, netilmicin and amikacin by azlocillin, carbenicillin, mecillinam, mezlocillin and piperacillin. *Journal of Pharmacology and Experimental Therapeutics*, **217 (2)**, 345–349.

26 Halstenson, C.E., Wong, M.O., Herman, C.S. et al. (1992) Effect of concomitant administration of piperacillin on the dispositions of isepamicin and gentamicin in patients with end-stage renal disease. *Antimicrobial Agents and Chemotherapy*, **36 (9)**, 1832–1836.

27 Walterspiel, J.N., Feldman, S., Van, R. & Ravis, W.R. (1991) Comparative inactivation of isepamicin, amikacin, and gentamicin by nine β-lactams and two β-lactamase inhibitors, cilastatin and heparin. *Antimicrobial Agents and Chemotherapy*, **35 (9)**, 1875–1878.

28 Gilbert, D.N. & Leggett, J.E. (2010) Aminoglycosides. In: G.L. Mandell, G.E. Bennett & R. Dolin (eds), *Mandell, Douglas, and Bennett's Principles and Practice of Infectious Diseases*, 7th edn, pp. 359–384. Churchill Livingstone/Elsevier, Philadelphia.

29 Samitz, E.M., Jang, S.S. & Hirsh, D.C. (1996) In vitro susceptibilities of selected obligate anaerobic bacteria obtained from bovine and equine sources to ceftiofur. *Journal of Veterinary Diagnostic Investigation*, **8 (1)**, 121–123.

30 Jacks, S.S., Giguère, S. & Nguyen, A. (2003) In vitro susceptibilities of Rhodococcus equi and other common equine pathogens to azithromycin, clarithromycin, and 20 other antimicrobials. *Antimicrobial Agents and Chemotherapy*, **47 (5)**, 1742–1745.

31 Salmon, S.A., Watts, J.L., Yancey, R.J., Jr. (1996) In vitro activity of ceftiofur and its primary metabolite, desfuroylceftiofur, against organisms of veterinary importance. *Journal of Veterinary Diagnostic Investigation*, **8 (3)**, 332–336.

32 Bade, D.J., Sibert, G.J., Hallberg, J., Portis, E.S., Boucher, J. & Bryson, L. (2009) Ceftiofur susceptibility of Streptococcus equi subsp zooepidemicus isolated from horses in North America between 1989 and 2008. *Veterinary Therapeutics*, **10**, E1–E7.

33 Burrows, G.E., MacAllister, C.G., Tripp, P. & Black, J. (1989) Interactions between chloramphenicol, acepromazine, phenylbutazone, rifampin and thiamylal in the horse. *Equine Veterinary Journal*, **21 (1)**, 34–38.

34 Grubb, T.L., Muir, W.W., III, Bertone, A.L., Beluche, L.A. & Garcia-Calderon, M. (1997) Use of yohimbine to reverse prolonged effects of xylazine hydrochloride in a horse being treated with chloramphenicol. *Journal of the American Veterinary Medical Association*, **210 (12)**, 1771–1773.

35 MacDougall, C. & Chambers, H.F. (2011) Protein synthesis inhibitors and miscellaneous antibacterial agents. In: L.L. Brunton, B.A. Chabner & B.C. Knollman (eds), *Goodman & Gilman's the Pharmacological Basis of Therapeutics*, 12th edn, pp. 1521–1547. McGraw-Hill Medical, New York.

(Continued)

Table 10.1 (*Continued*)

36 Yoon, J.H., Brooks, R.L., Jr, Khan, A. et al. (2004) The effect of enrofloxacin on cell proliferation and proteoglycans in horse tendon cells. *Cell Biology and Toxicology*, **20 (1)**, 41–54.

37 White, G.W., Hamm, D., Turchi, P., Jones, W. & Beasley, J. (1996) Toxicity of an orally administered formulation of metronidazole in healthy horses. *AAEP Proceedings*, **42**, 303–305.

38 Giguère, S. (2006) Macrolides, azalides, and ketolides. In: S. Giguère, J.F. Prescott, J.D. Baggot, R.D. Walker & P.M. Dowling (eds), *Antimicrobial Therapy in Veterinary Medicine*, 4th edn, pp. 191–205. Blackwell Publishing, Ames.

39 USP, AAVPT Veterinary Drug Expert Committee (2007) *Macrolides (Veterinary—Systemic)*. The United States Pharmacopeial Convention.

40 Papich, M.G. & Riviere, J.E. (2009) Chloramphenicol and derivatives, macrolides, lincosamides, and miscellaneous antimicrobials. In: J.E. Riviere & M.G. Papich (eds), *Veterinary Pharmacology and Therapeutics*, 9th edn, pp. 945–982. Wiley-Blackwell, Ames.

41 Muscatello, G. (2012) Rhodococcus equi pneumonia in the foal, part 2. Diagnostics, treatment and disease management. *Veterinary Journal*, **192**, 27–33.

42 Villarino, N. & Martin-Jimenez, T. (2013) Pharmacokinetics of macrolides in foals. *Journal of Veterinary Pharmacology and Therapeutics*, **36 (1)**, 1–13.

43 Peters, J., Block, W., Oswald, S. et al. (2011) Oral absorption of clarithromycin is nearly abolished by chronic comedication of rifampicin in foals. *Drug Metabolism and Disposition*, **39 (9)**, 1643–1649.

44 Giguère, S., Lee, E.A., Guldbech, K.M. & Berghaus, L.J. (2012) In vitro synergy, pharmacodynamics, and postantibiotic effect of 11 antimicrobial agents against Rhodococcus equi. *Veterinary Microbiology*, **160 (1–2)**, 207–213.

45 Peters, J., Eggers, K., Oswald, S. et al. (2012) Clarithromycin is absorbed by an intestinal uptake mechanism that is sensitive to major inhibition by rifampicin: Results of a short-term drug interaction study in foals. *Drug Metabolism and Disposition*, **40 (3)**, 522–528.

46 Hillidge, C.J. (1987) Use of erythromycin–rifampin combination in treatment of Rhodococcus equi pneumonia. *Veterinary Microbiology*, **14**, 337–342.

47 Sweeney, C.R., Sweeney, R.W. & Divers, T.J. (1987) Rhodococcus equi pneumonia in 48 foals: Response to antimicrobial therapy. *Veterinary Microbiology*, **14**, 329–336.

48 Papich, M.G. & Riviere, J.E. (2009) Beta lactam antibiotics: Penicillins, cephalosporins, and related drugs. In: J.E. Riviere & M.G. Papich (eds), *Veterinary Pharmacology and Therapeutics*, 9th edn, pp. 865–893. Wiley-Blackwell, Ames.

49 Chambers, H.F. (2010) Penicillins and beta-lactam inhibitors. In: G.L. Mandell, J.E. Bennett & R. Dolin (eds), *Mandell, Douglas and Bennett's Principles and Practice of Infectious Diseases*, 7th edn, pp. 309–321. Churchill Livingstone/Elsevier, Philadelphia.

50 Winther, L., Baptiste, K.E. & Friis, C. (2012) Pharmacokinetics in pulmonary epithelial lining fluid and plasma of ampicillin and pivampicillin administered to horses. *Research in Veterinary Science*, **92**, 111–115.

51 Prescott, J.F. (2006) Sulfonamides, diaminopyrimidines, and their combinations. In: S. Giguère, J.F. Prescott, J.D. Baggot, R.D. Walker & P.M. Dowling (eds), *Antimicrobial Therapy in Veterinary Medicine*, 4th edn, pp. 249–262. Blackwell Publishing, Ames.

52 Papich, M.G. & Riviere, J.E. (2009) Sulfonamides and potentiated sulfonamides. In: J.E. Riviere & M.G. Papich (eds), *Veterinary Pharmacology and Therapeutics*, 9th edn, pp. 835–864. Wiley-Blackwell, Ames.

53 Winther, L. (2012) Antimicrobial drug concentrations and sampling techniques in the equine lung. *Veterinary Journal*, **193 (2)**, 326–335.

54 Winther, L., Guardabassi, L., Baptiste, K.E. & Friis, C. (2011) Antimicrobial disposition in pulmonary epithelial lining fluid of horses, part I. Sulfadiazine and trimethoprim. *Journal of Veterinary Pharmacology and Therapeutics*, **34**, 277–284.

55 Van Duijkeren, E., Vulto, A.G. & Van Miert, A.S. (1994) Trimethoprim/sulfonamide combinations in the horse: A review. *Journal of Veterinary Pharmacology and Therapeutics*, **17 (1)**, 64–73.

56 Papich, M.G. & Riviere, J.E. (2009) Tetracycline antibiotics. In: J.E. Riviere & M.G. Papich (eds), *Veterinary Pharmacology and Therapeutics*, 9th edn, pp. 895–913. Wiley-Blackwell, Ames.

57 USP, AAVPT Veterinary Drug Expert Committee (2003) *Tetracyclines (Veterinary—Systemic)*. The United States Pharmacopeial Convention.

58 Winther, L., Honore Hansen, S., Baptiste, K.E. & Friis, C. (2011) Antimicrobial disposition in pulmonary epithelial lining fluid of horses, part II. Doxycycline. *Journal of Veterinary Pharmacology and Therapeutics*, **34**, 285–289.

59 Schnabel, L.V., Papich, M.G., Divers, T.J. et al. (2012) Pharmacokinetics and distribution of minocycline in mature horses after oral administration of multiple doses and comparison with minimum inhibitory concentrations. *Equine Veterinary Journal*, **44 (4)**, 453–458.

60 Riond, J.L., Riviere, J.E., Duckett, W.M. et al. (1992) Cardiovascular effects and fatalities associated with intravenous administration of doxycycline to horses and ponies. *Equine Veterinary Journal*, **24 (1)**, 41–45.

61 Neuvonen, P.J. & Penttila, O. (1974) Interaction between doxycycline and barbiturates. *British Medical Journal*, **1**, 535–536.

plasmid-mediated cephalosporinases than earlier-generation cephalosporins. In addition, it has a very low MIC for *Strep. zoo* [10]. Pharmacokinetic studies suggest that twice-daily IV administration at a dosage of 1 mg/kg bwt will produce optimal concentrations in the lung [11]. Cefquinome is approved in the UK for use in the horse, but not currently in the USA. Although the fluoroquinolone enrofloxacin can be administered IV and orally (PO), the latter is more common, and so it is discussed in the section on PO administered drugs.

Drugs administered orally

Potentiated Sulfonamides: Although the potentiated sulfonamide combinations trimethoprim–sulfadiazine and trimethoprim–sulfamethoxazole (TMS) have the benefits of being quite inexpensive and easy to administer PO, pharmacokinetic studies in horses have shown that it is difficult to maintain clinically relevant concentrations of trimethoprim in the lung. This is partially because the oral bioavailability of trimethoprim is significantly lower than that of sulfadiazine or sulfamethoxazole but also because it is much more rapidly eliminated from the body than either sulfonamide. Protein binding of trimethoprim is also higher in the PELF than in the plasma, which further decreases the amount of active drug at that site [12]. Finally, TMS has poor efficacy in pus and necrotic material, the very environment that is present in severe lung disease. For these reasons, even when C&S results indicate the presence of sensitive microbes, TMS is not a drug of choice for severe lower airway infections.

Doxycycline: Like TMS, doxycycline has the benefit of being inexpensive and easy to administer PO. Moreover, it has a rapid distribution into the PELF and is relatively slowly eliminated, which gives it a good profile as a drug targeting the lower respiratory system. The presence of ingesta can dramatically decrease the bioavailability of doxycycline in horses, however, so it should ideally be administered 8 h after and 2 h before feeding [13, 14].

Chloramphenicol: A highly lipophilic drug, chloramphenicol has relatively good penetration into the lung; however, there are serious, although rare, human health risks, specifically aplastic anemia, associated with its use. In addition, there is some evidence that due to poor bioavailability and rapid elimination, chloramphenicol is unlikely to be efficacious in the horse, although anecdotal reports of its efficacy are common

[1, 15, 16]. Its best use may be in treatment of chronic infections and lung abscesses, where long-term therapy and good penetration are required.

Rifampin: Although it is quite lipophilic and demonstrates good penetration into tissues, rifampin is seldom used in adult horses because it is quite expensive. Nevertheless, it can be very useful when the practitioner is faced with an infection that fails to respond to more typical antimicrobial therapy. It must always be used in combination with another antimicrobial, such as macrolides in foals, because resistance develops quite rapidly if used a single agent. It has a very narrow spectrum of activity of Gram-positive aerobes, so if broad-spectrum coverage is required, antimicrobials with good Gram-negative coverage, such as an aminoglycoside or a fluoroquinolone, should also be included.

Fluoroquinolones: Although fluoroquinolones have a broad spectrum of activity and good penetration into the respiratory system, it is very important to remember that their efficacy against streptococcal species is less than it is for other Gram-positive aerobes such as *Staph* spp. Enrofloxacin is the most commonly used fluoroquinolone in horses. Recently, the pharmacokinetics of marbofloxacin in horses have been explored, with 93% of diseased horses achieving what would be an effective concentrations in plasma at a dose of 2 mg/kg bwt when administered IV or PO [17]. Although anecdotally there seems to be a much lower risk of cartilage damage for marbofloxacin in growing horses than with enrofloxacin, there is no scientific data to support this conclusion, and so as with foals, this drug should be reserved for cases that are refractory to other treatment.

Drugs administered by aerosol

The use of aerosolized antimicrobials to treat pulmonary infections is intuitively attractive. In the best of circumstances, the clinician can achieve a very high concentration at the site of infection without risking systemic toxicity. As previously discussed, because of the blood–bronchial barrier, some drugs when administered systemically do not penetrate into the PELF sufficient to achieve clinically relevant concentrations. On the other hand, delivery of drug by the aerosol route requires that the airways are patent and that the primary infection is within the PELF and not within the parenchyma or in cells, such as alveolar macrophages or neutrophils. In these latter cases, systemic administration of antimicrobials will also be required. It is also possible that the combination of aerosolized therapy with systemic administration will produce a synergistic effect.

There are large gaps in our knowledge, however, about the best practices that should be followed when administering antimicrobials by the aerosolized route. Selecting an antimicrobial to which the identified organisms should be or are known to be sensitive is just the beginning of the process. For example, the disease itself may hinder drug delivery. Factors that are known to inhibit aerosol delivery to the lung include atelectasis, bronchoconstriction, excessive mucus production, and inflammation, and many of these are present to some degree in most pneumonic lungs. The clinician must be sure that the nebulizer is actually capable of delivering the appropriate particle size and that the drug will actually reach the site of infection and will stay in the appropriate site for a clinically relevant period of time. Some drugs when administered by nebulization are so rapidly cleared by the blood that they do not stay in the lung long enough to be therapeutically useful [18]. Hydrophobic drugs especially those with extra polycationic charges, such as tobramycin, can bind to lung tissue and thus have a much longer half-life. Even in human medicine, only tobramycin and aztreonam have been formulated specifically for use as aerosolized drugs.

The most common type of nebulizer used in veterinary medicine is the jet nebulizer, as it is the least expensive. Jet nebulizers, however, are slow, highly affected by flow rate, and can produce variable particle sizes. In addition, because jet nebulizers require a very large volume of solution to nebulize effectively, they are not cost effective when an expensive antibiotic is used. Ultrasonic nebulizers are faster, but they are considerably more expensive. They can also lead to degradation of the medication, because the high frequencies generate considerable heat.

With these caveats in mind, what evidence is there for using aerosolized antibiotics in horses? McKenzie and coworkers evaluated the use of gentamicin sulfate and ceftiofur sodium using an ultrasonic nebulizer. They found that the concentration of the antimicrobial affected the particle size distribution and aerosol density, and they determined that the optimum concentrations for nebulization were gentamicin at 50 mg/ml and ceftiofur at 25 mg/ml [19]. The same group went on to evaluate serum and bronchial lavage fluid concentrations of gentamicin in BAL samples collected from horses that had been administered the antimicrobial by aerosolization once daily at the recommended dose [20]. They found

low serum concentrations with high concentrations in the BAL fluid, but unfortunately, gentamicin caused coughing when administered by aerosol. Although cefquinome was well tolerated and concentrations were high in the PELF after administration of 225 mg using a jet nebulizer, it was rapidly cleared from the lung, remaining above the limit of detection of the assay used in the study for only 4 h after administration [11]. Similarly, the use of aerosolized marbofloxacin has been explored in horses at a dose of 300 mg nebulized at a concentration of 25 mg/ml [21]. Aerosolization produced mean concentrations of marbofloxacin in BAL samples of 0.17 µg/ml 15 min after dosing. In contrast when the same total dose of marbofloxacin was administered IV, mean BAL sample concentrations were 0.03 µg/ml 15 min after dosing [17, 22]. Following aerosol administrations, plasma concentrations were extremely low from 15 min to 24 h after administration. Importantly, the authors reported no significant changes in pulmonary function after either route of administration.

In summary, when faced with a case of pneumonia or pleuropneumonia, the clinician must begin treatment before receiving the results of microbial culture and sensitivity but may be guided by the results once they are received. It is important to remember that the most common pathogen in equine pneumonia is *Streptococcus equi* subspp. *equi* (*Strep. equi*), and it is therefore mandatory to make sure that the chosen antibiotic therapy is likely to be efficacious against this microbe. It is also important to remember that if the drug cannot penetrate the environment of the infected lung, it is not likely to be efficacious even if it has *in vitro* efficacy against the microbial milieu. Finally, if the bacteria have developed resistance to the drug, neither sensitivity nor penetration is of any use clinically. In most cases, for uncomplicated pneumonia, a broad-spectrum drug with good lung penetration, such as ceftiofur, would be an appropriate starting point. If the clinician suspects that there is a mixed bacterial infection, then the addition of enrofloxacin or gentamicin might be appropriate. If an anaerobic infection is suspected, then metronidazole should be added to the mix. It is important to remember that severe or chronic infections, especially pleuropneumonia, may require weeks to even months of treatment for full resolution; thus, the owner should be warned that treatment may be long and expensive. It is also important to warn the owner that it will be important to give the horse weeks to months of rest even after apparent clinical resolution.

Viral infections
Epidemiology
Viral infections of the respiratory tract are extremely common, the most important being equine influenza, equine herpesvirus 1 and 4, rhinovirus, adenovirus, and equine viral arteritis. Although viral disease is most common in young horses and is usually seen as an outbreak, all age groups are susceptible.

Clinical presentation
Horses with viral respiratory disease present with high fever, cough, serous nasal discharge that may change to a mucopurulent, and occasionally myalgia. Viral respiratory infections can be very difficult to distinguish from strangles, and it is quite difficult to distinguish one viral infection from another without evaluating serum antibody titer responses. Typically, fever abates by the 5th day of infection, unless a secondary bacterial infection has developed.

Diagnosis
Virus isolation and acute and convalescent serum antibody titers are used for diagnosis.

Treatment
The most important treatment is excellent supportive nursing care, ensuring that sick horses drink and eat sufficiently, as well as judicious use of nonsteroidal anti-inflammatory drugs (NSAIDs) to control fever and inflammation and afford pain relief.

Antiviral drugs may be useful for herpesvirus infections. Although oral acyclovir has been used in the past, it has been established that it is not absorbed to any significant degree from the equine gastrointestinal (GI) tract. The recommended dosage of valacyclovir is 30 mg/kg bwt, PO, q8 h for 2 days and then 20 mg/kg bwt, PO, q12 h for 1–2 weeks. Unfortunately, the use of valacyclovir can be financially crippling for many owners. Ganciclovir is even more expensive but, given IV, is thought to be the drug of choice for horses with established disease. The recommended dosage is 2.5 mg/kg bwt, IV, q8 h for 1 day and then 2.5 mg/kg bwt, IV, q12 h for 1 week [23]. For financial reasons, these drugs are rarely used for the respiratory manifestation of herpesvirus, which has low mortality rates, and are reserved for use in the neurological manifestation, which has much higher mortality rates. Although the use of amantadine has been described in horses, the combination

of adverse side effects and cost prevents their use for influenza infections in this species [24].

Parasitic pneumonia
Epidemiology
Parasitic pneumonia is most common in young horses exposed to *Parascaris equorum* and any age of horse exposed to pastures shared with donkeys carrying *Dictyocaulus arnfieldi*.

Pathogenesis: Lungworms of all varieties cause bronchitis, which may cause obstruction of the large and smaller airways. In addition, a secondary bacterial component may also develop.

Clinical presentation
Coughing is the most common clinical sign during the acute stage of the disease. As the condition progresses, interstitial emphysema and pulmonary edema can ensue. In severe infections, respiratory embarrassment may lead to anorexia and subsequent weight loss.

Treatment
Therapeutic Goal: Treatment is aimed at eradication of the parasite and any secondary bacterial component while avoiding excessive inflammation due to parasite die-off.

General Approach: Successful treatment requires anthelmintic therapy, with both benzimidazoles, particularly fenbendazole, and macrocyclic lactones, such as ivermectin and moxidectin (see Chapter 6, for more details).

Antimicrobial Selection: Secondary bacterial infections often clear with eradication of the primary offending parasite; however, further antibiotic therapy may be necessary and should be based on C&S results of tracheal aspirates.

Evaluation of Therapeutic Outcome: Successful therapy should result in resolution of cough, normalization of the leukogram, and normalization of chest radiographs if they were initially taken.

Fungal pneumonia
Epidemiology
Although the horse's environment is rife with fungi, and indeed, mold spores from hay may be routinely found engulfed by alveolar macrophages on examination of BAL fluid, fungal pneumonia is rare in horses. Opportunistic infections, however, may arise in horses that have been treated extensively with antimicrobials or that have severe GI disease allowing translocation of fungi.

Pathogenesis

Fungal infections may begin as low-grade inflammatory disease that does not effectively eliminate the causative agent. Chronic inflammation may result in nodules throughout the lung, and both necrosis and purulent exudation may be seen. Erosion of the vasculature can occur with *Aspergillus* spp. infections.

Clinical presentation

Horses frequently have other comorbidities. Pneumonia will present with tachypnea, fever, malaise, and cough, as well as weight loss in the chronically affected animal. Diagnosis relies on radiographs, as well as tracheal aspirate or BAL.

Treatment

Therapeutic Goals: Desired outcome includes resolution of signs, return to function, and prevention of relapse when drug therapy is withdrawn.

General Approach: It is important to recognize the contributing factors in development of fungal pneumonia. Resolution of primary GI disease is important, as is discontinuation, when possible, of antibiotics that have disrupted the normal flora and allowed invasion of the fungus. Horses with GI disease may benefit from so-called cecal cocktails, similar to transfaunation of ruminants, to repopulate the denuded bacterial biome of the GI system.

Antifungal Selection: Ideally, antifungals would be chosen on the basis of C&S results, but these can be difficult to obtain, and treatment is usually needed long before results of these tests are known. Cytological examination of tracheal aspirates or BAL samples can often start the process of speciation of the fungus, providing a general guide to antifungal selection. Aspergillus is the most commonly identified pathogenic fungus in horses, so it is important to use an antifungal that is effective against this agent. There are questions about the relationship between *in vitro* and *in vivo* susceptibilities of antifungals. In addition, some animals may fail to respond to what appears to be an appropriate antifungal therapy, because their immune system is not capable of clearing the infection or because the fungus is resistant to the antimicrobial selected (Table 10.2).

Amphotericin B: A polyene antimicrobial, amphotericin B combines with ergosterol in the fungal membrane, resulting in an increase in cell membrane permeability and eventually cell death. Because of toxicity concerns

in human medicine, amphotericin B is slowly being replaced by either newer, safer antifungals for the treatment of aspergillus infections or the more costly liposomal formulation is being used [25]. Despite its toxicity, it remains, however, the drug of choice for treatment of systemic aspergillus infections in horses. Successful use of amphotericin B for treatment of cryptococcal pneumonia in the horse has also been reported [26].

Azoles: Benzimidazole derivatives, the azoles inhibit a sterol demethylase, which prevents the formation of ergosterol, thereby compromising the integrity of the fungal cell membrane. Although itraconazole is reported to have high oral bioavailability in the horse, this does "not" apply to the compounded formulation but only to the Sporanox® solution (Janssen Pharmaceutica NV, Olen, Belgium). If the Sporanox solution is used, a dose of 5 mg/kg bwt, PO, once a day should produce plasma concentrations that are likely to be inhibitory against fungi known to infect horses [27]. Fluconazole has good penetration into equine plasma; however, its penetration into respiratory secretions and tissues has not been determined in horses [28]. A recent study determined that voriconazole is well distributed to multiple body fluids, including the PELF, after a daily oral dose of 4 mg/kg bwt, and it has been reported to have been used in the successful treatment of invasive pulmonary aspergillosis in a foal [29, 30]. Voriconazole has an extremely broad spectrum, with activity against *Candida* spp., *Cryptococcus neoformans*, *Aspergillus*, and *Fusarium*. Unfortunately, voriconazole is prohibitively expensive, which limits its use in horses.

Noninfectious LRT disease

Nonseptic inflammatory diseases of the lower airways
Epidemiology

The devastating disease heaves, also known as recurrent airway obstruction (RAO), was described more than 2000 years ago and is seen most commonly in middle-aged to older horses. In contrast, it is only within the past few decades that low-grade inflammation of the small airways (inflammatory airway disease (IAD)) has been recognized as a common cause of poor performance in young to middle-aged athletic horses. Both RAO and IAD are seen most commonly in stabled horses, and

Table 10.2 Common antifungals administered to adult horses with respiratory infections.

Azoles—mechanism, inhibit fungal cell membrane (P450-mediated sterol synthesis); drug interactions, potent inhibitor of CYP3A4 isoenzyme system, which should be used with caution when drugs relying on this system are administered; contraindications, with quinidine or cisapride administration[1–3]

Note: Injectable ITRA and VORI contain the cyclodextrin vehicle—therapy should be limited to 2 weeks due to the potential for nephrotoxicity from cyclodextrin accumulation[2,4,5]

	Spectrum of coverage	Absorption	Distribution penetration	Elimination	Adverse effects	Dosing	Cost/day	Comments
Fluconazole (FLUC)	• Blastomyces[6] • Candida[6] • Coccidioides[6] • Cryptococcus[6] • Histoplasma[6] • Many aspergillus resistant to this drug	PO administration • 90% absorbed[6] • Polar molecule; water soluble[7]	• Penetrates the CSF, eye, saliva, and peritoneal fluid well[6,7] • Low protein binding[7] (10% in humans)[8]	• Renal; >80% unchanged in urine (humans)[4,6] • Adjust dose if renal compromise[6]	• Primarily GI disturbance[6] • Exfoliative disorders and thrombocytopenia (humans)[6] • Dose-dependent hepatotoxicity (humans)[9]	• 14 mg/kg loading dose and then 5 mg/ kg PO q12 h[9] • Same dose may be given q24 h[6]	$$ generic	• Pregnant mares have been successfully treated with FLUC without complications; however, treatment should be based on risks versus benefits since FLUC has been shown to be teratogenic[9] • FLUC has better absorption versus ketoconazole and ITRA[10]
Voriconazole (VORI)	• Broad spectrum includes Aspergillus and Fusarium[11]	• 95–100% oral bioavailability[12] • Fasting ↑ absorption (humans)[5,13]	• Highly lipid soluble[11] • Excellent penetration includes BAL[11] • Protein binding 31%[6]	• Metabolized via CYP2C19, CYP3A4, and CYP2C9 (humans)[4]	• Possible urticaria • Visual disturbance incidence is low (humans)[14,15] • Hepatotoxicity: ↑ incidence at higher[] (humans)[14,15]	• 4 mg/kg PO q24 h; this dose achieves plasma [] adequate to treat fungi with MIC ≤1 µg/ ml[11,16]	$$$ $$	• Injectable voriconazole (Vfend®) is formulated with cyclodextrin

(Continued)

Table 10.2 (Continued)

	Spectrum of coverage	Absorption	Distribution penetration	Elimination	Adverse effects	Dosing	Cost/day	Comments
Azoles—mechanism, inhibit fungal cell membrane (P450-mediated sterol synthesis); drug interactions, potent inhibitor of CYP3A4 isoenzyme system, which should be used with caution when drugs relying on this system are administered; contraindications, with quinidine or cisapride administration[1-3]								
Note: Injectable ITRA and VORI contain the cyclodextrin vehicle—therapy should be limited to 2 weeks due to the potential for nephrotoxicity from cyclodextrin accumulation[2,4,5]								
Itraconazole (ITRA)	• Broad-spectrum antifungal • Covers aspergillus • *Conidiobolus* reported to be resistant in a horse[10]	• ↓ oral absorption • Large molecular weight (705); note: drugs larger than GI phospholipid molecules (>750 daltons) → ↑ absorption[17] • Very lipophilic ITRA must go into solution before it can be absorbed • Weak base (pK$_a$ 3.7); ionization of ITRA in acidic pH required for solubility[14]	• Good tissue penetration → exception CSF (drug [] achieved <1%)[8] • High protein binding (ITRA 99.8% and hydroxy-ITRA 99.5)[1]	• Metabolized ↓ Hydroxy-ITRA[8] (active metabolite)	• GI disturbance[6] • Hepatotoxicity[6] • Rash (humans)	• 5 mg/kg PO once daily[6,18]	$$	• Avoid proton pump inhibitors, H$_2$ blockers, and antacids[1] • Cyclodextrin delivery system (found in commercial product Sporanox® oral solution and injectable) enhances ITRA solubility; Sporanox capsules are not formulated with cyclodextrin; therefore, Sporanox oral solution has greater bioavailability compared to the capsule[1] • Due to ITRA properties (low solubility in water and the requirement for a low pH for ionization to ↑ solubility), compounded ITRA products may → ↓ absorption versus the commercial Sporanox formulation[6,14,19] • Note: Oral cyclodextrin is not absorbed[2,4]

Topical azole antifungals (clotrimazole, enilconazole, miconazole) for treatment of GPM—spectrum, broad includes *Aspergillus* spp.[7]; **topical absorption, poor**[7,20,21]; **dosing, clotrimazole,** 0.08% emulsion irrigated daily for 14 days[21]; **enilconazole,** 60 ml of aqueous enilconazole 33.3 mg/ml solution sprayed directly on fungal lesion via endoscopic guidance daily[18]; **miconazole** (under endoscopic guidance), 1 treatment (70 mg of injectable miconazole diluted in isotonic solution to a volume of 10 ml) administered in the affected pouch daily for 1 week and then QOD for the next 2 weeks OR for guttural pouch with neurological signs; administer gynecological preparation of miconazole (400 mg/treatment) via catheter in the affected pouch daily × 1 week and then QOD × 2 weeks followed by twice a week × 3 weeks[22]

Note: Labor-intensive treatment but cost-effective compared to systemic administration of antifungals

	Spectrum of coverage	Absorption	Distribution penetration	Elimination	Adverse effects	Dosing	Cost/day	Comments
Polyenes—mechanism, bind to ergosterol in fungal cell membrane, thus altering permeability resulting in leakage of intracellular contents								
Amphotericin B (AMP-B)	• Broad spectrum • Covers *Aspergillus*	• Poor oral absorption	• Highly protein bound ~90%[15] • Very large V_d	• Unclear, excretion in urine negligible • Azotemia and hepatic failure have little effect on plasma []'[10]	• Acute infusion reactions: fever, ↑ RR, chills, ↓ BP, headache, anorexia, nausea, vomiting[15] • Nephrotoxicity (dose related): (1) AMP-B binds to cholesterol in tubular cells → renal tubular acidosis; (2) AMP-B → renal vasoconstriction[14] • ↓ K^+, ↓ Mg^{2+}	There are many dosing regimens; below are a few examples: (1) AMP-B:[23] • 0.3 mg/kg IV on day 1 • Increase dose by 0.1 mg/kg each subsequent day • Every 4th day no treatment • Treatment is continued for at least 21–35 days (2) AMP-B:[14] • 0.3–0.6 mg/kg IV in 1 l D_5W QD or QOD	$$	To ↓ side effects: • Administer AMP-B "slowly" (2–6 h)[14] • Pretreat with IV normal saline[14] (↓ azotemia) • If infusion reaction occurs for subsequent doses, pretreat with acetaminophen, diphenhydramine, corticosteroids, and meperidine (↓ shaking and chills)[15] Traditional formulation: • AMP-B deoxycholate (Fungizone®) Lipid formulations—developed to ↓ incidence of nephrotoxicity: • AMB-B cholesteryl sulfate complex (Amphotec®) • AMB-B lipid complex (Abelcet®) • AMB-B liposomal (AmBisome®) • Avoid administering with other nephrotoxic drugs
Sodium iodide (NaI) and potassium iodide (KI)—mechanism, unknown[14]								
Iodide	• Narrow spectrum of activity • Sporotrichosis • *Basidiobolus* • *Conidiobolus* • *Pseudallescheria*[14] • NaI and KI should be used in conjunction with other antifungals[14]	• Good oral absorption[24]	• Primarily in extracellular fluid[24] • Trapped in thyroid	• Renal[25]	Iodism[14,23] • Cough • Tachycardia • Lacrimation • Dry scruffy coat with hair loss • Salivation • Anorexia • Dry scaly skin	NaI 20% solution • 125 ml IV q24 h for 3 days and then 30 g PO q24h; continue treatment for 30 days after clinical signs resolve[14] • Administer slowly by the IV route[6] • Do not inject IM[6]	$	• Not recommended for use in pregnant or lactating mares or foals[6,14,23] • Not recommended in patients with hyperthyroidism, renal failure, or severe dehydration[6]

$, inexpensive; $$, relatively inexpensive; $$$, expensive.

1 Sporanox®. Janssen Pharmaceuticals, Titusville, NJ. http://www.janssenpharmaceuticalsinc.com/assets/sporanox.pdf [accessed on August 23, 2013].

2 Stevens, D.A. (1999) Itraconazole in cyclodextrin solution. *Pharmacotherapy*, **19**, 603–611.

3 Diflucan®. Pfizer Inc, New York. http://labeling.pfizer.com/ShowLabeling.aspx?id=575 [accessed on September 5, 2013].

4 Carver, P.L. (2011) Invasive fungal infections. In: J.T. DiPiro, R.L. Talbert, G.C. Yee, G.R. Matzke, B.G. Wells & L.M. Posey (eds), *Pharmacotherapy: A Pathophysiologic Approach*, 8th edn, pp. 2073–2104. McGraw-Hill, New York.

(Continued)

Table 10.2 (*Continued*)

5 Vfend®. Pfizer Inc, New York. http://labeling.pfizer.com/ShowLabeling.aspx?id=618 [accessed on September 5, 2013].

6 Plumb, D.C. (2011) *Plumb's Veterinary Drug Handbook*, 7th edn. Wiley-Blackwell, Ames.

7 Bossche, H.V., Engelen, M. & Rochette, F. (2003) Antifungal agents of use in animal health—chemical, biochemical and pharmacological aspects. *Journal of Veterinary Pharmacology and Therapeutics*, **26**, 5–29.

8 Kethireddy, S. & Andes, D. (2007) CNS pharmacokinetics of antifungal agents. *Expert Opinion on Drug Metabolism & Toxicology*, **3** (**4**), 573–581.

9 Taintor, J., Crowe, C., Hancock, S., Schumacher, J. & Livesey, L. (2004) Treatment of conidiobolomycosis with fluconazole in two pregnant mares. *Journal of Veterinary Internal Medicine*, **18**, 363–364.

10 Korenek, N.L., Legendre, A.M., Andrews, F.M. *et al.* (1994) Treatment of mycotic rhinitis with itraconazole in three horses. *Journal of Veterinary Internal Medicine*, **8** (**3**), 224–227.

11 Passler, N.H., Chan, H.M., Stewart, A.J. *et al.* (2010) Distribution of voriconazole in seven body fluids of adult horses after repeated oral dosing. *Journal of Veterinary Pharmacology and Therapeutics*, **33**, 35–41.

12 Colitz, C.M.H., Latimer, F.G., Cheng, H., Chan, K.K., Reed, S.M. & Pennick, G.J. (2007) Pharmacokinetics of voriconazole following intravenous and oral administration and body fluid concentrations of voriconazole following repeated oral administration in horses. *American Journal of Veterinary Research*, **68**, 1115–1121.

13 Purkins, L., Wood, N., Kleinermans, D., Greenhalgh, K. & Nichols, D. (2003) Effect of food on the pharmacokinetics of multiple-dose oral voriconazole. *British Journal of Clinical Pharmacology*, **56**, 17–23.

14 Davis, J.L., Papich, M.G. & Heit, M.C. (2009) Antifungal and antiviral drugs. In: J.E. Riviere & M.G. Papich (eds), *Veterinary Pharmacology and Therapeutics*, 9th edn, pp. 1013–1049. Wiley-Blackwell, Ames.

15 McEvoy, Gerald K. (ed) (2013) *AHFS Drug Information®*. American Society of Health-System Pharmacists, Inc, Bethesda. ISBN 978-1-58528-247-0. ISSN 8756-6028. STAT!Ref Online Electronic Medical Library. http://online.statref.com/Document.aspx?fxid=1&docid=134. 8/4/2013 7:00:19 PM CDT (UTC -05:00).

16 Davis, J.L., Salmon, J.H. & Papich, M.G. (2006) Pharmacokinetics of voriconazole after oral and intravenous administration to horses. *American Journal of Veterinary Research*, **67** (**6**), 1070–1075.

17 Pidgeon, C., Ong, S., Liu, H. *et al.* (1996) IAM chromatography: An in vitro screen for predicting drug membrane permeability. *Journal of Medicinal Chemistry*, **38** (**4**), 590–594.

18 Davis, E.W. & Legendre, A.M. (1994) Successful treatment of guttural pouch mycosis with itraconazole and topical enilconazole in a horse. *Journal of Veterinary Internal Medicine*, **8** (**4**), 304–305.

19 Smith, J.A., Papich, M.G., Russell, G. & Mitchell, M.A. (2010) Effects of compounding on pharmacokinetics of itraconazole in black-footed penguins (Spheniscus demersus). *Journal of Zoo and Wildlife Medicine*, **41** (**3**), 487–495.

20 European Medicines Agency (EMA) (1998) Committee for veterinary medicinal products enilconazole summary. EMEA/MRL/496/98-FINAL. European Medicines Agency, London. http://www.ema.europa.eu/docs/en_GB/document_library/Maximum_Residue_Limits_-_Report/2009/11/WC500014130.pdf [accessed on September 10, 2013].

21 Eichentopf, A., Snyder, A., Recknagel, S., Uhlig, A., Waltl, V. & Schusser, G.F. (2013) Dysphagia caused by focal guttural pouch mycosis: Mononeuropathy of the pharyngeal ramus of the vagal nerve in a 20-year-old pony mare. *Irish Veterinary Journal*, **66**, 13.

22 Giraudet, A.J. (2005) Medical treatment with miconazole in four cases. *Journal of Veterinary Internal Medicine*, **19**, 485.

23 Knottenbelt, D.C. (2002) Fungal airway diseases. In: P. Lekeux (ed), *Equine Respiratory Diseases*. International Veterinary Information Service, Ithaca, NY.

24 Yadav, M. (ed) (2008) Thyroid gland. In: *Mammalian Endocrinology*, p. 101. India Discovery Publishing House, New Delhi.

25 Greenbaum, R.F. & Raiziss, G.W. (1927) The elimination of iodine after oral or intravenous administration of various iodine compounds in single massive doses. *Journal of Pharmacology and Experimental Therapeutics*, **30** (**5**), 407–427.

there is a strong association with exposure to organic and inorganic particulates, as well as noxious gases that are commonly found in the stable environment. A subset of horses living in warm climates experiences the same respiratory complaint at pasture, likely due to exposure to outdoor molds and pollens.

Pathogenesis

Although clinical signs of RAO can be reliably induced in affected horses with exposure to moldy hay or organic dust, no single cause of IAD has been identified. There has been plentiful speculation about the role of environment, viral disease, bacterial infection, air pollution, and genetic predisposition in the development of both IAD and RAO. Dust levels in the horse's breathing zone can be so high as to be considered unacceptable in any human workplace. This alone can go far to explain the development of airway neutrophilia as a nonspecific response to high levels of particulates. It is also likely that increased levels of endotoxin in hay and grain dust contribute to the development of airway neutrophilia in both diseases. It is easy to understand why an environment high in organic particulates and endotoxin leads to airway inflammation in a large percentage of horses. What we do not understand is why some horses exposed to this environment develop the much more severe respiratory condition, heaves. Both the innate and adaptive immune systems appear to be involved in heaves, and both Th1 and Th2 cytokine responses have been detected in both IAD and heaves [31, 32]. It is most likely that there are multiple factors contributing to the likelihood of an individual horse developing IAD or RAO.

Clinical presentation

Horses with heaves have a history of pronounced respiratory effort after exposure to moldy hay or an environment with a high organic dust load. The horse affected with RAO is at first intermittently crippled by the ensuing respiratory embarrassment, and eventually, the respiratory impairment will become permanent. Owners also report paroxysmal coughing. Immediate relief is afforded by bronchodilators unless other comorbid conditions, such as bronchiectasis or bullae, exist. While horses with IAD also often have a history of coughing, they generally do not have episodes of difficulty breathing at rest and are usually athletic horses that fail to perform as well as expected.

Diagnosis

In both IAD and heaves, analysis of BAL samples reveals mild to moderate airway inflammation that may involve neutrophils, mast cells, eosinophils, and/or lymphocytes. Horses with IAD have variable clinical signs, including cough, nasal discharge, and abnormal lung sounds, and tracheobronchial mucus accumulation. Notably, they do not exhibit increased respiratory effort or abnormal lung function at rest, although airway hyperresponsiveness to nonspecific agents, such as histamine, is present. Horses with RAO have marked airway inflammation during exacerbations of the disease, with the predominant cell type being neutrophils. During remission, the high neutrophil percentage usually diminishes markedly or may even normalize. During exacerbation, horses with RAO have markedly increased respiratory resistance and decreased dynamic compliance, as well as marked airway hyperresponsiveness to histamine. Deficits in lung function and airway hyperresponsiveness improve, but do not completely resolve, during remission.

Treatment

Therapeutic Goals: Goals in treating RAO should include (i) immediate relief of the bronchospasm that causes cough and excessive respiratory effort, (ii) reduction of lower airway inflammation, (iii) long-term prevention of episodes of heaves by control of lower airway inflammation and airway obstruction, and (iv) return to limited or even full athletic potential. The goals for treatment of IAD are similar: (i) eliminate cough and bronchoconstriction that impair performance, (ii) reduce mucus production and airway plugging, (iii) reduce airway reactivity, and (iv) prevent recurrences.

General Approach: There must be a treatment strategy with recognizable and achievable goals in place that is approved by both the attending veterinarian and the owner or trainer in order for RAO or IAD to be treated successfully. Treatment of these diseases entails a team approach and an acceptance that this may be a lifelong problem that may be modified, but that is unlikely to "go away." One of the most important aspects to successful treatment is establishment of a reasonable definition of "return to athletic use." It is entirely reasonable to expect that a young racehorse would be able to return to racing after a short, targeted period of treatment. The owner of the older horse with heaves, however, must recognize that a much more modest return to light pleasure riding is a reasonable goal. The use of lung function testing to assess response to bronchodilator therapy can be very useful in identifying horses that are less likely to respond to therapy.

Although it is important to assess the horse's immediate clinical presentation, it is equally important for both RAO and IAD to take an in-depth history to try to document environmental triggers. A very thorough inspection and assessment of the horse's environment is also critical to develop a plan to achieve environmental remediation. For instance, if the history suggests that the horse is consistently worse in the spring, whereas clinical signs are abated in the barn in the winter, it suggests that the worst culprits for this horse are the molds and pollens associated with moist warm weather, and the clinician may prescribe clean indoor living for the horse during that period. It is very useful for the owner or trainer to keep a diary for the affected horse, noting when exacerbations occur.

There is good evidence for the use of glucocorticoids and bronchodilators in heaves, and this knowledge has been extrapolated to the treatment of IAD. For both, the mainstay of treatment has become a combination of environmental remediation, corticosteroid therapy, and bronchodilators.

Long-Term Control: Corticosteroid Therapy: Corticosteroids remain the cornerstone of successful treatment for both IAD and RAO. Inflammation underlies remodeling of the airways with accompanying airway hyperreactivity and consequent coughing and expiratory dyspnea. Bronchodilator drugs will help to relieve acute, debilitating bronchospasm, but only consistent anti-inflammatory therapy, in conjunction with avoidance of environmental triggers, will break the vicious cycle of inflammation, airway hyperreactivity, and bronchoconstriction. The anti-inflammatory effect of corticosteroids in both RAO and IAD is impressive. Corticosteroids activate glucocorticoid receptors, thus putting into motion a profound inhibition of the arachidonic acid cascade and limiting production of leukotrienes and other inflammatory molecules. Response to steroids can vary considerably from horse to horse.

Corticosteroids can be administered both systemically and via aerosolized delivery (Tables 10.3 and 10.4). Depending on the severity of disease, initial treatment may be systemic or a combination of systemic and aerosolized delivery and more chronic treatment may be aerosolized. The decision as to which delivery method

is preferable may be influenced by a number of factors, including financial, as aerosolized drugs and their delivery devices are quite expensive, as well as known and putative side effects. It is important to remember that corticosteroids can, among other things, adversely affect tissue growth and protein use, impair the barrier function of the intestinal mucosa, cause immune suppression, and suppress adrenal function.

Systemic Corticosteroids: Multiple studies have demonstrated the positive effects of corticosteroid drugs on horses with heaves, but the evidence for their use in IAD, despite good clinical response anecdotally, is less robust. Prednisolone and dexamethasone are the corticosteroids used most frequently in the treatment of RAO and IAD. Triamcinolone acetonide has also been shown to relieve airway obstruction in heaves [33]. Triamcinolone, however, is anecdotally more closely associated with the development of laminitis in horses than other corticosteroids. A recent study has shown profound and persistent hyperglycemia and hypertriglyceridemia (3–4 days) in horses after a single injection of triamcinolone, which may explain the anecdotal reports [34]. Thus, its use is discouraged in the treatment of noninfectious IAD. Prednisone was also frequently used in the past, but studies have shown therapeutic failures in heaves likely due to the horse's inability to absorb prednisone after oral administration [35]. In a study looking at heaves-affected horses treated with either oral prednisolone (1.0 mg/kg bwt) or IM dexamethasone (0.1 mg/kg bwt) in conjunction with environmental control, both drugs had similar positive effects on the clinical signs of heaves, endoscopic scores, and blood gases. However, dexamethasone had a more beneficial effect on BAL cytology [36]. In a different study, both prednisolone (2.0 mg/kg bwt, PO, once per day) and dexamethasone (0.05 mg/kg bwt, PO, once per day) improved pulmonary function, in spite of continuous antigen exposure. However, in that study, oral dexamethasone was more effective than oral prednisolone in improving lung function in the heavy horses [37]. A recent study also showed that horses suffering from heaves that were treated for 14 days with either isoflupredone acetate (0.03 mg/kg bwt, IM, once a day) or dexamethasone (0.04 mg/kg bwt, IV, once a day) all showed improvements in lung function, although BAL fluid samples were not assessed. Isoflupredone, however, resulted in hypokalemia, making it a less than optimal treatment.

Table 10.3 Inhaled medications used in RAO and IAD: anti-inflammatories.

Corticosteroid	Brand name	Concentration (μg/actuation)	Doses per canister	Receptor binding affinity[1,*]	Receptor binding $T_{1/2}$ (h)2,*	Dosing (450 kg horse)	Method of delivery	Cost	Comments
BDP HFA	QVAR[5]	40 and 80	50 (80 μg only), 100, and 120	0.4/13.5[†]	7.5	No data in horse (see text for case)	MDI	$$$$	• QVAR very fine particle size → ↑ lung disposition, for example, in asthmatic patients, 53% of QVAR dose deposited in the lungs versus 16.2% with CFC-BDP[8]; documentation in equines lacking • QVAR has been shown to control asthma at ½ the dose required of a CFC-BDP[9,10] • CFC-BDP, Vanceril® dose: 500 μg q12 h[11] "or" 2500–3750 μg q12–24 h[3]) • Inhaled BDP may ↓ serum cortisol → may be due to systemic effects of active metabolite[3]
	Beclazone[®6,‡]	50, 100, and 250	200						
	Beclotide[®7,‡]	50,100, and 250	200						
	Generic beclomethasone[‡]	100 and 200	200						
Flunisolide HFA	Aerospan[®12]	80	60 and 120	1.8	3.5	No data in horse (see text for case)	MDI	$$$	
Fluticasone propionate HFA	Flovent[®13]	44, 110, and 220	120	18	10.5	• 2000 μg q12 h[11] • 2000–2500 μg q12–24 h[3]	MDI	$$$$	• Fluticasone propionate ↑ potency, ↓ systemic deposition (humans)[1]
	Flixotide[®14,‡]	25 and (CFC-Free) Inhaler 50, 125, or 250	120						

Mechanism, binds to glucocorticoid receptors causing the release of NF-κB; this leads to the inhibition of synthesis of inflammatory cytokines and an inhibition of the downregulation of β-2 adrenoreceptors[3]; **dose,** high dose usually for initial 2 weeks and then taper[4]; **drug interaction,** reports of Cushing's syndrome, adrenal insufficiency, and death with the coadministration of inhaled corticosteroids and potent CYP3A4 inhibitors (e.g., ketoconazole, itraconazole)[1,4]; may take 3–7 days for clinical improvement[3]

Note: Deposition of inhaled medications is highly dependent upon the device used and the cooperation of the horse—see text

$$$, expensive; $$$$, moderately expensive.

Note: Corticosteroid products that have been discontinued from the US market include the following: Aerobid®, Azmacort®, Vanceril®, Beclovent®, and Pulmicort Turbuhaler®. Many products discontinued contained propellants and chlorofluorocarbons that deplete the ozone and were withdrawn from the market to comply with the Montreal Protocol. Pulmicort Turbuhaler was removed because of complex manufacturing issues.[8,9,10]

CFC, chlorofluorocarbon; HFA, hydrofluoroalkane.

*Relative to dexamethasone with a value of 1.

†Beclomethasone dipropionate is a prodrug that is converted in the lung to the active metabolite, beclomethasone 17-monopropionate.

(Continued)

Table 10.3 (*Continued*)

ᵃNot available on the US market; although these drugs cannot be purchased legally in the USA, international readers may be able to purchase them locally.

1 Kelly, H.W. (2009) Comparison of inhaled corticosteroids: An update. *Annals of Pharmacotherapy*, **43**, 519–527.

2 Dubois, E.F.L. (2005) Clinical potencies of glucocorticoids: What do we really measure? *Current Respiratory Medicine Reviews*, **1**, 103–108.

3 Le'guillette, R. (2003) Recurrent airway obstruction—heaves. *Veterinary Clinical Equine*, **19**, 63–86.

4 Raissy, H.H., Kelly, H.W., Harkins, M. & Szefler, S.J. (2013) Inhaled corticosteroids in lung diseases. *American Journal of Respiratory and Critical Care Medicine*, **187** (**8**), 798–803.

5 QVAR®. QVAR (beclomethasone dipropionate HFA) Inhalation Aerosol. http://www.qvar.com/library/docs/prescribing-information.pdf [accessed on July 21, 2013].

6 New Zealand Data Sheet Beclazone® CFC-Free Inhaler. Norton Healthcare Limited, Fielding. http://www.medsafe.govt.nz/profs/datasheet/b/BeclazoneCFCinh.pdf [accessed on July 25, 2013].

7 Becotide Evohaler®. GlaxoSmithKline (Ireland) Ltd, Dublin. http://hcp.gsk.ie/products/becotide.html [accessed on July 25, 2013].

8 Labiris, N.R. & Dolovich, M.B. (2003) Pulmonary drug delivery, part II. The role of inhalant delivery devices and drug formulations in therapeutic effectiveness of aerosolized medications. *British Journal of Clinical Pharmacology*, **56**, 600–612.

9 Vanden Burgt, J.A., Busse, W.W., Martin, R.J., Szefler, S.J. & Donnell, D. (2000) Efficacy and safety overview of a new inhaled corticosteroid, QVAR (hydrofluoroalkane-beclomethasone extrafine inhalation aerosol), in asthma. *Journal of the American Academy of Allergy, Asthma and Immunology*, **106** (**6**), 1209–1226.

10 Davies, R.J., Stampone, P. & O'Connor, B.J. (1998) Hydrofluoroalkane-134a beclomethasone dipropionate extrafine aerosol provides equivalent asthma control to chlorofluorocarbon beclomethasone dipropionate at approximately half the total daily dose. *Respiratory Medicine*, **92** (Suppl A), 23–31.

11 Robinson, N.E. (2002) Recurrent airway obstruction (heaves). In: P. Lekeux (ed), *Equine Respiratory Diseases*. International Veterinary Information Service, Ithaca, NY.

12 Aerospan®. Aerospan (flunisolide HFA, 80 µg) Inhalation Aerosol. http://www.actonpharmaceuticals.com/pdf/AerospanLabelNov12Approval.pdf [accessed on July 21, 2013].

13 Flovent HFA®. Flovent HFA (fluticasone propionate) Inhalation Aerosol. https://www.gsksource.com/gskprm/en/US/adirect/gskprm?cmd=ProductDetailPage&product_id=1244169108743 &featureKey=600580#nlmhighlights [accessed on July 21, 2013].

14 Flixotide Inhaler. GlaxoSmithKline NZ Ltd, Auckland. http://www.medsafe.govt.nz/consumers/cmi/f/flixotideinhaler.pdf [accessed on July 22, 2013].

15 FDA, HHS (2005) Use of ozone-depleting substances; removal of essential use designations. *Federal Register*, **70** (**63**), 17167–17192.

16 AstraZeneca (2012) AstraZeneca to discontinue production of PULMICORT® pMDI, other respiratory medicines not affected, March 7. http://www.astrazeneca.com/Media/Press-releases/Article/20100703-AstraZeneca-to-discontinue-production-of-PULMICORT [accessed on July 22, 2013].

17 FDA (2010) Asthma and COPD inhalers that contain ozone-depleting CFCs to be phased out; alternative treatments. *FDA News Release*. http://www.fda.gov/NewsEvents/Newsroom/PressAnnouncements/ucm208302.htm [accessed on July 22, 2013].

Table 10.4 Systemic medications used in RAO and IAD.

Anti-inflammatories

Corticosteroids—mechanism, bind to glucocorticoid receptors causing the downregulation of β-2 adrenoreceptors[4]; adverse effects, [4] hypokalemia, hyperglycemia, sodium and water retention, HPA suppression, impaired wound healing, inhibition of leukocyte and monocyte function, redistribution of fat, glaucoma, cataracts, osteoporosis, GI irritation/ulceration (high doses, long-term administration), mental status changes, laminitis (relatively rare → a result of glucocorticoid-induced insulin resistance, vascular dysfunction, negative effects on keratinocyte proliferation and differentiation, and matrix integrity. Systemic glucocorticoids should be used with caution in horses that are overweight, are insulin resistant, and/or have recently been treated for laminitis)[5]; dosing, glucocorticoids are often administered until the disease is controlled and then tapered to avoid adrenal suppression; for example, steroid therapy may be administered daily for a week or two (2–4 weeks for IAD) followed by a decrease in dose for 2 weeks and then alternate-day therapy[4,6,7]; drug interaction, coadministration of glucocorticoids with CYP3A4 inducers (e.g., barbiturates, rifampin) and/or inhibitors (e.g., macrolides, ketoconazole) affects glucocorticoid clearance → ↓ efficacy and/or ↑ adverse effects[8]

Drug	Brand name	Glucocorticoid potency[1,2,*]	Mineralocorticoid potency[1,2,*]	Equivalent dose (mg)[3]	Biologic T½ (h)[1]	Dosing[4]	Cost	Comments
Dexamethasone	• Azium®	25–30	+/−	0.15	36–54	0.03–0.1 mg/kg PO, IV, IM q24 h	$	• Oral bioavailability was 42–61% in nonfed horses; feeding ↓ bioavailability; after IV and PO dexamethasone administration, serum cortisol [] was reported to be significantly lesser than baseline in fed (1–72 h) and nonfed (2–48 h) horses[9–11] • ADRs: risk of injection site infection after IM administration, laminitis[4]
Dexamethasone 21-isonicotinate	• Voren®	25–30	+/−	0.15	36–54	0.04 mg/kg IM q3 days	$	• Long-acting form of dexamethasone
Isoflupredone acetate	• Predef 2X®	17	No data	No data	No data	0.03 mg/kg IM q24 h	$	
Prednisolone		4	0.25–0.8	1	18–36	0.8–1 mg/kg PO q12 h	$	• Oral bioavailability 50%[6] • Prednisone is ineffective in treating RAO; lack of efficacy may be due to ↓ absorption or horse inability to convert prednisone to the active form, prednisolone[4,6]
Triamcinolone acetonide	• Vetalog®	3–5	+/−	0.8	18–36	0.05–0.09 mg/kg IM q4–8 weeks	$	• ADR: laminitis[6]

(Continued)

Table 10.4 (*Continued*)

Bronchodilators

Drug	Brand name[12]	Onset of action	Duration of effect	Elimination[12]	Dose[4,12,13]	Cost	Comments
β-2 adrenergic agonists—mechanism, direct effect (cause receptor-mediated airway smooth muscle relaxation and bronchodilation) and indirect effect (enhance mucociliary clearance and inhibit mediators from inflammatory cell) (anti-inflammatory is effect controversial it may modify acute inflammation; however, it does not have a significant effect on chronic inflammation)[14]; **adverse effects,** (acutely) after IV injection ↓ BP followed by reflex ↑ HR and PAP (lasts 2 min)[15]; (high doses) tremor, restlessness, and sweating[4,15]; (other side effects) tachycardia, hypokalemia, V/Q mismatch, and metabolic effects[14]; **tolerance,** may develop with long-term therapy due to downregulation of β-2 receptors; combination therapy with corticosteroids reduces tolerance[16,17]							
Clenbuterol	Oral syrup • Ventipulmin® • Aeropulmin® • Parenteral formulation not available commercially in the USA	PO administration • C_{peak} occurs at 2 h[12] • Significant difference occurred between clenbuterol and placebo at 90 min for FEV_1 and at 120 min for $FEF_{25–75}$[18]	6–8 h[12]	• Urinary elimination prolonged and irregular[15] • $T_{1/2}$ 10–13 h[12]	• 0.8–3.2 µg/kg PO, IV q12–24 h • If therapeutic effect is not seen at 0.8 µg/kg PO, then ↑ dose by increments of 25%[19]	$	• Oral bioavailability 83%[20] • Monitor plasma concentrations (as opposed to urinary concentrations) in racehorses[15] • β-2/β-1 ratio is four for clenbuterol; at low doses, the drug predominately activates the β-2 receptor, and at high doses, it starts to activate the β-1 receptor[15] • ↑ lipophilicity versus other β-2 agonist; crosses blood–brain barrier and accumulates in fat[15]

Drug	Brand name[12]	Onset of action	Duration of effect	Elimination[12]	Dose[4,12,13]	Cost	Comments
Muscarinic cholinergic antagonist (parasympatholytic drugs)—mechanism, competitive antagonist of acetylcholine binding to muscarinic receptors resulting in direct blocking of bronchial smooth muscle constriction[14]; **adverse effects (related to anticholinergic properties),** dry secretions, mydriasis, blurred vision, tachycardia, and urinary retention; inhibits GI motility[12,21]							
Note: The following antimuscarinic drugs are reserved for rescue therapy for severe life-threatening airway obstruction when all other options have either failed or are not available[18]							
Atropine	• Atrolect® • Atropine SA® • Generic available	• Bronchodilation within 15 min[6]	• Short duration of action (2 h)[21]	• Metabolism • 30–50% excreted unchanged in urine	• 0.01–0.025 mg/kg IV once	$	• Distributes throughout body • Additional ADRs: ileus, abdominal pain, CNS toxicity, thickening airway secretions, impaired mucociliary clearance, ↑ HR[17,19], large doses cause excitement and delirium[22]
Glycopyrrolate	• Robinul® • Generic available	• Maximum bronchodilator effect occurred at 2 h post-IV injection[23]	• Bronchodilation effect stable for 3 h in guinea pigs[24] and >4 h in humans[23]	• Majority eliminated unchanged in urine and feces • Metabolism (minor route)[12] • Median $T_{1/2}$ ~8 h[25]	• Based on a 450 kg horse → initial dose of 2–3 mg IM BID–TID[12] • 0.005–0.007 mg/kg IV, IM[6,26]	$	• ADRs: may cause colic[19]; in humans, maximum ↑ HR (32% above control versus atropine 60% above control) occurs 30 min post-IV injection[23] • Poor lipid solubility • Polar nitrogen moiety → ↓ CNS penetration; ↓ CNS side effects[22]
N-butylscopolammonium bromide (hyoscine butylbromide)[12]	• Buscopan®	• Maximum effect within 10 min[13]	• <1 h[13]	• Eliminated in urine and feces • Estimated $T_{1/2}$ ~6 h	• 0.3 mg/kg via slow IV infusion one time	$	• ADRs: large doses cause excitement and delirium[22]

Phosphodiesterase inhibitors (methylxanthines)—mechanism, increase intracellular concentrations of cAMP to cause bronchodilation and inhibit mast cell degranulation[19], anti-inflammatory action reported at low doses (takes several weeks of oral therapy to occur)[27]; **adverse effects (dose dependent),** tachycardia, excitement, tremors, nausea, vomiting (high serum concentrations), cardiac arrhythmias, and seizures[27,28], narrow therapeutic index

Note: Theophylline is not commonly used to treat horses with RAO and is not considered a first-line agent

Drug	Brand name[12]	Onset of action	Duration of effect	Elimination[12]	Dose[4,12,13]	Cost	Comments
Theophylline	• Multiple brand name and generic theophylline products available in controlled- and immediate-release oral forms; also available as injectable in D_5W[12] • Generic aminophylline available[12] • Note: Aminophylline (hydrus) contains ~79% theophylline (anhydrous); aminophylline (anhydrous) contains ~86% theophylline (anhydrous)[12]	• Average onset 2–4 h[29]	• Duration variable, up to 24 h for sustained-release product[30]	• Metabolism primarily by the liver via CYP450 enzymes[28] • 10% eliminated unchanged in urine[28] • $T_{1/2}$ 12–15 h[28]	Theophylline dosing: • 0.5–1 mg/kg PO q8 h[4,6] • 5 mg/kg PO q12 h[28] Aminophylline dosing: • 5–10 mg/kg PO or IV BID[12] "or" • 4–6 mg/kg PO TID[12] • Dilute in 100 ml D_5W or NS and do not exceed administration rate of 25 mg/min[12] • Therapeutic bronchodilator [] in humans 5–15 µg/ml[31,32], in horses [] >15 µg/ml → adverse effects[28] • Anti-inflammatory [] 5–10 µg/ml[28] • Serum theophylline [] should be checked 1–2 h postdose; steady state occurs at ~3 days[33]	$	• Theophylline bioavailability 100%[28] • In the therapeutic range (5–15 µg/ml), theophylline commonly follows 1st-order pharmacokinetics; it can follow nonlinear or Michaelis–Menten pharmacokinetics in this range; however, most often this occurs in [] >15 µg/ml[32] • Erythromycin and enrofloxacin may inhibit the metabolism of theophylline[28] • Enzyme inducers rifampin and phenobarbital may ↑ the clearance of theophylline[28]

$, inexpensive.

*Relative milligram comparisons to cortisol as 1. +/− indicates mineralocorticoid activity (i.e., sodium retention) is negligible with the administration of common doses of dexamethasone and triamcinolone.

1 Dubois, E.F.L. (2005) Clinical potencies of glucocorticoids: What do we really measure? *Current Respiratory Medicine Reviews,* **1**, 103–108.

2 USP, AAVPT Veterinary Drug Expert Committee (2008) *Corticosteroids-Glucocorticoid Effects (Veterinary—Systemic).* The United States Pharmacopeial Convention. http://aavpt. affiniscape.com/associations/12658/files/corticosteroids2008.pdf [accessed on July 4, 2013].

3 Behrend, E.N. & Kemppainen, R.J. (1997) Glucocorticoid therapy: Pharmacology, indications and complications. *Veterinary Clinics of North America Small Animal Practice,* **27 (2)**, 187–213.

4 Le guillette, R. (2003) Recurrent airway obstruction—heaves. *Veterinary Clinical Equine,* **19**, 63–86.

5 McEvoy, Gerald K. (ed) (2013) *AHFS Drug Information®.* American Society of Health-System Pharmacists, Inc, Bethesda. ISBN 978-1-58528-247-0. ISSN 8756-6028. STATIRef Online Electronic Medical Library. http://online.statref.com/document.aspx?fxid=1&docid=1160. 7/26/2013 2:55:22 PM CDT (UTC -05:00).

6 Cornelisse, C.J. & Robinson, N.E. (2013) Glucocorticoid therapy and the risk of equine laminitis. *Equine Veterinary Education,* **25 (1)**, 39–46.

7 Robinson, N.E. (2002) Recurrent airway obstruction (heaves). In: P. Lekeux (ed), *Equine Respiratory Diseases.* International Veterinary Information Service, Ithaca, NY.

8 Couetil, L.L., Hoffman, A.M., Hodgson, J. *et al.* (2007) Inflammatory airway disease of horses. *Journal of Veterinary Internal Medicine,* **21**, 356–361.

9 Cornelisse, C.J., Robinson, N.E., Berney, C.E., Kobe, C.A., Boruta, D.T. & Derksen, F.J. (2004) Efficacy of oral and intravenous dexamethasone in horses with recurrent airway obstruction. *Equine Veterinary Journal,* **36 (5)**, 426–430.

10 Grady, J.A., Davis, E.G., Kukanich, B. & Sherck, A.B. (2010) Pharmacokinetics and pharmacodynamics of dexamethasone after oral administration in apparently healthy horses. *American Journal of Veterinary Research,* **71 (7)**, 831–839.

11 Soma, L.R., Uboh, C.E., Liu, Y. et al. (2012) Pharmacokinetics of dexamethasone following intra-articular, intravenous, intramuscular, and oral administration in horses and its effects on endogenous hydrocortisone. Journal of Veterinary Pharmacology and Therapeutics, 36, 181–191.

(Continued)

Table 10.4 (*Continued*)

12 Plumb, D.C. (2011) *Plumb's Veterinary Drug Handbook*, 7th edn. Wiley-Blackwell, Ames.

13 Couetil, L., Hammer, J., Miskovic Feutz, M., Nogradi, N., Perez-Moreno, C. & Ivester, K. (2012) Effects of N-butylscopolammonium bromide on lung function in horses with recurrent airway obstruction. *Journal of Veterinary Internal Medicine*, **26 (6)**, 1433–1438.

14 Barnes, P.J. (2011) Pulmonary pharmacology. In: L.L. Brunton, B.A. Chabner & B.C. Knollman (eds), *Goodman & Gilman's the Pharmacological Basis of Therapeutics*, 12th edn, pp. 1031–1065. McGraw-Hill Medical, New York.

15 Robinson, N.E. (2000) Clenbuterol and the horse. *AAEP Proceedings*, **46**, 229–232.

16 Adams, H.R. (2009) Adrenergic agonists and antagonist. In: J.E. Riviere & M.G. Papich (eds), *Veterinary Pharmacology and Therapeutics*, 9th edn, pp. 125–155. Wiley-Blackwell, Ames.

17 Davis, E. & Rush, B.R. (2002) Equine recurrent airway obstruction: Pathogenesis, diagnosis and patient management. *Veterinary Clinical Equine*, **18**, 453–467.

18 Boner, A.L., Sette, L., Castellani, C. & Schiassi, M. (1987) Oral clenbuterol and procaterol: A double-blind comparison of bronchodilator effects in children and chronic asthma. *Journal of Asthma*, **24 (6)**, 347–353.

19 Ainsworth, D.M. & Cheetham, J. (2010) Disorders of the respiratory system. In: S.M. Reed, W.M. Bayley & D.C. Sellon (eds), *Equine Internal Medicine*, 3rd edn, pp. 290–371. Saunders-Elsevier, St. Louis.

20 Soma, L.R., Uboh, C.E., Guan, F. *et al.* (2004) Pharmacokinetics and disposition of clenbuterol in the horse. *Journal of Veterinary Pharmacology and Therapeutics*, **27**, 71–77.

21 Williams, D.M. & Bourdet, S.V. (2011) Chronic obstructive pulmonary disease. In: J.T. DiPiro, R.L. Talbert, G.C. Yee, G.R. Matzke, B.G. Wells & L.M. Posey (eds), *Pharmacotherapy: A Pathophysiologic Approach*, 8th edn, pp. 471–496. McGraw-Hill, New York.

22 Adams, H.R. (2009) Cholinergic pharmacology: Autonomic drugs. In: J.E. Riviere & M.G. Papich (eds), *Veterinary Pharmacology and Therapeutics*, 9th edn, pp. 157–179. Wiley-Blackwell, Ames.

23 Gal, T.J. & Suratt, P.M. (1981) Atropine and glycopyrrolate effects on lung mechanics in normal man. *Anesthesia & Analgesia*, **60**, 85–90.

24 Villetti, G., Bergamaschi, M., Bassani, F. *et al.* (2006) Pharmacological assessment of the duration of action of glycopyrrolate vs tiotropium and ipratropium in guinea-pig and human airways. *British Journal of Pharmacology*, **148 (3)**, 291–298.

25 Rumpler, M.J., Sams, R.A. & Colahan, P. (2011) Pharmacokinetics of glycopyrrolate following intravenous administration in the horse. *Journal of Veterinary Pharmacology and Therapeutics*, **34**, 605–608.

26 Ainsworth, D.M. (2010) Review of recurrent airway obstruction (RAO, heaves): Diagnosis and treatment options. *Proceedings of the AAEP Focus on Upper and Lower Respiratory Diseases*. Salt Lake City, pp. 93–99. http://www.ivis.org/proceedings/aaepfocus/2010/Ainsworth3.pdf [accessed on July 13, 2013].

27 Cunningham, F.M. & Dunkel, B. (2008) Equine recurrent airway obstruction and insect bite hypersensitivity: Understanding the diseases and uncovering possible new therapeutic approaches. *Veterinary Journal*, **177**, 334–344.

28 Papich, M.G. (2009) Drugs that affect the respiratory system. In: J.E. Riviere & M.G. Papich (eds), *Veterinary Pharmacology and Therapeutics*, 9th edn, pp. 1295–1311. Wiley-Blackwell, Ames.

29 Kelloway, J.S., Wyatt, R.A. & Adlis, S.A. (1994) Comparison of patients' compliance with prescribed oral and inhaled asthma medications. *Archives of Internal Medicine*, **154 (12)**, 1349–1352.

30 GOLD (2013) *Global Initiative for Chronic Obstructive Lung Disease*. http://www.goldcopd.org/uploads/users/files/GOLD_Report_2013_Feb20.pdf [accessed on July 16, 2013].

31 Whelan, G.J. & Szefler, S.J. (2006) Asthma management. In: M.E. Burton, L.M. Shaw, J.J. Schentag & W.E. Evans (eds), *Applied Pharmacokinetics and Pharmacodynamics: Principles of Therapeutic Drug Monitoring*, 4th edn, pp. 259–284. Lippincott Williams & Wilkins, Baltimore.

32 DiPiro, Joseph T., Spruill, William J., Wade, William E., Blouin, Robert A. & Pruemer, Jane M. (2005) *Concepts in Clinical Pharmacokinetics*, 5th edn. American Society of Health-System Pharmacists, Bethesda.

33 Dowling, P.M. (2010) Pharmacologic principles. In: S.M. Reed, W.M. Bayley & D.C. Sellon (eds), *Equine Internal Medicine*, 3rd edn, pp. 148–204. Saunders-Elsevier, St. Louis.

Inhaled Corticosteroids: The use of inhaled corticosteroids has truly revolutionized the treatment of RAO and IAD. While initial systemic tapered corticosteroid therapy is often necessary with all but very mild IAD, regular inhaled therapy is essential for long-term success in most cases. The most important factor that limits regular use of inhaled corticosteroids is cost, because drugs such as fluticasone and beclomethasone are very expensive. When assessing the effects of corticosteroids on horses with airway disease, it is important to note what delivery device and drug formulation were used because certain devices deliver more drugs to the lower airways, and certain drug formulations, such as QVAR®, a proprietary formulation of beclomethasone, have been shown at least in humans to reach the lower airways more reliably. For this reason, it is very difficult to make comparisons of drugs across studies that used different delivery devices. Moreover, the FDA has phased out the use of chlorofluorocarbon (CFC) propellants in metered-dose inhalers (MDIs) in accordance with the Montreal Protocol in order to protect the ozone layer; thus, studies employing CFC inhalers are not directly comparable to those using the currently available hydrofluoroalkane (HFA) inhalers.

Delivery Devices: Devices currently on the market for use in horses include the AeroMask (AeroHippus, Trudell, Ontario, Canada) and the Equine Haler (Equine HealthCare, Horsholm, Denmark). The choice as to which to use is largely determined by cost and which device will best suit the particular horse in question. A recent study compared the AeroHippus and the Equine Haler using a pressurized MDI and HFA albuterol to elicit bronchodilation in horses with bronchospasm associated with exacerbation of heaves [38]. There was no statistical difference in the decrease in pulmonary resistance produced by albuterol administered using the two different devices. Regardless of the type of mask/spacer device used, actual delivery of particles to the lower airways is poor in the horse, as indeed it is even in humans, and the least efficacious means of delivering aerosolized drugs is by nebulization [39–41]. Unfortunately, strategies that we know improve lung deposition of aerosolized drugs in humans, such as slow deep breathing and breath holding, are not practical in the horse.

Side Effects: Aerosolized corticosteroids are frequently preferred over systemic in order to decrease potential side effects. This is well documented in humans, but while this is a rational approach in horses, there is little

documentation to support it. However, using the AeroMask and fluticasone propionate at a dose of 2000 µg twice daily, heaves-affected horses were shown to have significant improvement in clinical signs, and lung function and immune responses were still intact [42]. In contrast, a single 0.025 mg/kg bwt dose of dexamethasone given IV decreased total lymphocyte counts in horses. Although there is evidence of hypothalamic–pituitary–adrenal (HPA) suppression with all clinically relevant doses of beclomethasone, this does not seem to pose a risk of chronic HPA suppression or rebound Addisonian crisis [40]. Likewise, inhaled fluticasone propionate (1500 µg q12 h) caused significant decreases in serum cortisol after 7 days [43]. Thus, inhaled corticosteroids certainly have systemic effects; the hope is that these effects will be less profound than with systemic therapy.

Efficacy of Inhaled Corticosteroids in Horses: When comparing the potency of inhaled corticosteroid, we are obliged to look at our favorite lab animal, the human, as no real comparative studies have been done in horses. Fluticasone propionate is thought to be the most potent, has the longest pulmonary residence time, and causes the least adrenal suppression. On the other hand, newer formulations of beclomethasone dipropionate (BDP) that incorporate HPA as the propellant have more uniform particle size and are more uniformly mixed, requiring little to no agitation or waiting before actuation of the inhaler. Fluticasone propionate resulted in complete resolution of clinical signs in horses with exacerbation of heaves, as well as normalization of pulmonary function tests (PFTs) and significant decrease in BAL neutrophilia. In humans, there is less systemic absorption of fluticasone, but it is not known whether this is true in horses. In our clinic, we use both QVAR and Flovent, and the deciding factor as to which one is used is often the cost. For reasons that are not well understood, some horses seem to do better on one drug versus the other, and the clinician must maintain a certain flexibility in choosing drugs.

In our clinic, we frequently treat with an initial course of parenteral corticosteroids, typically, a 4-week, decreasing course of prednisolone, followed by inhaled corticosteroids.

Bronchodilator Therapy: As with corticosteroids, bronchodilators can be administered both systemically and via aerosol; however, aerosolization is by far the preferred method (Table 10.4). Bronchodilators generally fall into one of two categories, either beta-2 agonists (B2-ARs) (sympathomimetics) or parasympatholytics. Of the B2-ARs commonly used in equine medicine, albuterol, which known as salbutamol everywhere but in the USA, is primarily administered by inhalation, and clenbuterol is administered PO. For the parasympatholytic agents, ipratropium is administered by inhalation, and atropine and Buscopan are administered parenterally.

Mechanism of Action of B2-ARs: When B2-ARs bind to their receptor, they activate adenyl cyclase, which subsequently causes an increase in cyclic adenosine monophosphate (cAMP) and protein kinase A. cAMP inhibits smooth muscle contraction by decreasing intra-cellular Ca^{2+} stores, and protein kinase A inhibits smooth muscle contraction by decreasing the activity of myosin light chain kinase. Together, these actions result in bron-chodilation in horses experiencing bronchoconstriction. In addition, airway ciliated epithelium possesses B-2 receptors that, when activated, increase cilia beat frequency. There is also some evidence that B2-ARs sup-press airway mucus production. A lesser but potentially useful action of B2-ARs is inhibition of release of inflammatory mediators from cells, such as neutrophils.

Mechanism of Action of Parasympatholytics: When the neurotransmitter acetylcholine binds to muscarinic receptors on bronchial smooth muscle, it produces an increase in the intracellular concentration of cyclic guanosine monophosphate that leads to an increase in intracellular Ca^{2+} release and ultimately bronchocon-striction. Ipratropium blocks muscarinic acetylcholine receptors, thereby preventing bronchoconstriction.

Systemic Bronchodilator Therapy: Clenbuterol is a B2-AR that was approved for use in horses in the USA in 1998 under the brand name Ventipulmin® (Boehringer Ingelheim Vetmedica, Inc., St Joseph, MO). In addition to its use as a bronchodilator, clenbuterol has tocolytic effects in both women and animals and has a profound repartitioning effect in muscle, although the mechanism of this latter effect is poorly understood. Practitioners should be aware that reports of severe toxicity in horses given improperly compounded formulations of clenbuterol have emerged [44]. The safety and efficacy of chronic administration of even the FDA-approved formulation of clenbuterol is controver-sial. Chronic administration of clenbuterol at 2.4 µg/kg (5 days on, 2 days off, for 8 weeks) was reported to have a negative impact on aerobic performance in horses; however, a recent study reported that no negative

effects on equine cardiac or skeletal muscle were seen when clenbuterol was administered at up to 3.2 µg/kg bwt, PO, daily for 14 days [45, 46]. Tachyphylaxis also appears to be a problem with chronic administration of clenbuterol. For example, a recent study demonstrated that after 3 weeks of clenbuterol administration at 0.8 µg/kg bwt, PO, q12 h, increased airway reactivity was evident and the horses were refractory to the broncho-dilatory effects of clenbuterol [47].

Reports of the efficacy of clenbuterol are also conflicting. A large study by Erichsen *et al.* showed that 25% of horses had a decrease in clinical signs of heaves when treated with clenbuterol at dose of 0.8 µg/kg bwt, but a second study failed to show any benefit on clinical signs when a much larger dose of 4.0 µg/kg bwt was administered [48, 49]. Most horses appear to tolerate the lower doses of clenbuterol well, but with higher doses, horses may have, among other signs, tremors, tachycardia, sweating, and an appearance of anxious-ness. Together, these findings suggest that the practice of administering clenbuterol to horses in order to enhance performance is probably misguided at best and harmful at worst. It is also important to recognize that the recommended duration of treatment is 30 days. Clenbuterol is not appropriate and should not be used as a chronic therapy.

Cautions: Clenbuterol should be avoided in horses with cardiac disease, as it can cause tachycardia and in pregnant mares, as it antagonizes the effects of oxytocin and $PGF_2\alpha$.

Short-Acting Inhaled B2-AR Therapy: These agents, such as albuterol and fenoterol, are of vital importance in treatment of acute exacerbations of RAO (Table 10.5). Albuterol is recognized universally as a rescue drug for both human asthmatics and horses with IAD/RAO. Horses with current exacerbations of RAO labor to breathe and experience paroxysmal coughing; within 15–30 min after aerosolized delivery of albuterol, they will experience significant relief. However, the effect wears off within 3–4 h. It is important to remember that the inflammatory condition will persist despite apparent improvement due to transient bronchodilation, and the disease will worsen. Regular use of B-2 agonists in the absence of anti-inflammatory medication may mask symptoms that would otherwise indicate progressive worsening of the disease, in particular further airway obstruction with mucus. Albuterol is the most afford-able of the short-acting B-2 agonists; however,

Table 10.5 Inhaled medications used in RAO and IAD: bronchodilators and mast cell stabilizers.

Bronchodilator	Brand name[1-5]	Concentration (µg/actuation)[1-5]	Doses per canister[1-5]	Dosing	Method of delivery	Cost	Comments
β-2 adrenergic agonists—mechanism, direct effect (cause receptor-mediated airway smooth muscle relaxation and bronchodilation) and indirect effect (enhance mucociliary clearance and inhibit mediators from inflammatory cell) (anti-inflammatory is effect controversial it may modify acute inflammation; however, it does not have a significant effect on chronic inflammation)[6]; adverse effects, tremor, CNS stimulation, tachycardia, and hypokalemia							
Short-acting β-2 adrenergic agonists; rescue drugs; onset, rapid within 15 min; duration, 2–4 h							
Albuterol	• Proventil® HFA[1] • Ventolin® HFA[2] • ProAir® HFA[3] • Generic albuterol*	• 90 µg albuterol freebase delivered from the mouthpiece[1-3]	200[1-3]	450 µg (5 puffs)	MDI	$$	• Albuterol is in racemic form; S-enantiomer may exacerbate bronchospasm in some individuals → evidence inconclusive[7] • Humans become refractory to chronic administration of albuterol without concomitant corticosteroid administration
Levalbuterol tartrate	• Xopenex® HFA[4]	• 45 µg levalbuterol freebase delivered from the mouthpiece	80 and 200	200–250 µg	MDI	$$	• Levalbuterol tartrate is the generic name for R-albuterol[4]; (theorized) ↓ chance of paradoxical bronchospasm
Long-acting β-2 adrenergic drugs; controller drugs not rescue drugs; onset, 20–30 min; peak, 3 h; duration, 12 h							
Salmeterol xinafoate	• Serevent® CFC-Free[5],*	• 25 µg	120	125–210 µg	MDI	$$	• Significant concerns over development of tachyphylaxis in humans. May be associated with sudden death in human asthmatics • In humans, it is strongly advised that long-acting β-2 agonists should "not" be used as a monotherapy and should only be used in conjunction with corticosteroid therapy; no data in horses

(Continued)

Table 10.5 (Continued)

Bronchodilator	Brand name[8-10]	Concentration (µg/actuation)[8-10]	Doses per canister[8-10]	Dosing[8-10]	Method of delivery	Cost	Comments
Muscarinic cholinergic antagonist (parasympatholytic drugs)—mechanism, competitive antagonist of acetylcholine binding to muscarinic receptors resulting in direct blocking of bronchial smooth muscle constriction[6]; adverse effects (related to anticholinergic properties), dry mouth; onset, slow 30–60 min; duration, 4–6 h							
Ipratropium	• Atrovent® HFA[8]	• 17 µg ipratropium bromide delivered from the mouthpiece	200	500–2,000 µg	MDI	$$	• No apparent systemic absorption in humans; inhaled drug not known to result in ileus in horses[11] • No development of tolerance in humans
Mast cell stabilizers (cromones)—mechanism, inhibit mast cell degranulation and release of inflammatory mediators; adverse effects, none reported in horses and bad taste and nausea reported in humans; onset, slow; duration: 4–6 h							
Nedocromil sodium	• Tilade® CFC-Free[9,*]	• 2000 µg (2 mg)	112	7–14 mg (7,000–14,000 µg)	MDI	$$	• Frequently poor owner compliance, as drug must be given consistently before onset of signs
Sodium cromoglycate	• Intal® CFC-Free[10,*]	• 5000 µg (5 mg)	112	8–12 mg QD–BID[12,13]	MDI		

$$, relatively inexpensive.

Note: Asthma products (bronchodilators and mast cell stabilizers) that have been withdrawn from the US market include the following: Alupent® Inhalation Aerosol (metaproterenol), Intal® Inhaler (cromolyn), Tilade® Inhaler (nedocromil), Maxair® Autohaler (pirbuterol), and Combivent® Inhalation Aerosol (albuterol and ipratropium in combination); withdrawal date is December 31, 2013. These discontinued products contained propellants and chlorofluorocarbons that deplete the ozone and were withdrawn from the market to comply with the Montreal Protocol.[14]

*Not available on the US market; although these drugs cannot be purchased legally in the USA, international readers may be able to purchase them locally.

1 Proventil® HFA Inhaler. Merck & Co., Inc, Whitehouse Station, NJ. http://www.merck.com/product/usa/pi_circulars/p/proventil_hfa/proventil_hfa_pi.pdf [accessed on July 31, 2013].

2 Ventolin® HFA Inhaler. GlaxoSmithKline, Research Triangle Park, NC. http://us.gsk.com/products/assets/us_ventolin_hfa.pdf [accessed on July 31, 2013].

3 ProAir® HFA Inhaler. IVAX Pharmaceuticals, Dublin. http://proairhfa.com/library/docs/ProAirDoseCounter-Prescribing-Information-PA0512G-PE2557.pdf [accessed on July 31, 2013].

4 Xopenex® HFA Inhaler. Sunovion Pharmaceuticals Inc. Marlborough, MA. http://www.xopenex.com/files/XOPENEX-HFA-Prescribing-Information.pdf [accessed on July 31, 2013].

5 Serevent® CFC-Free Inhaler. GlaxoSmithKline NZ Limited, Auckland. http://www.medsafe.govt.nz/profs/datasheet/s/SereventCFC-freeinh.pdf [accessed on July 31, 2013].

6 Barnes, P.J. (2011) Pulmonary pharmacology. In: L.L. Brunton, B.A. Chabner & B.C. Knollman (eds), Goodman & Gilman's the Pharmacological Basis of Therapeutics, 12th edn, pp. 1031–1065. McGraw-Hill Medical, New York.

7 Ameredes, B.T. & Calhoun, W.J. (2009) Levalbuterol vs albuterol. Current Allergy and Asthma Reports, **9**, 401–409.

8 Atrovent® HFA Inhalation Aerosol. Boehringer Ingelheim Pharmaceuticals, Inc., Ridgefield, CT. http://idocs.boehringer-ingelheim.com/BIWebAccess/ViewServlet.ser?docBase=renetnt&folderPath=/Prescribing+Information/Pis/Atrovent+HFA/10003001_US_1.pdf [accessed on June 5, 2014].

9 Tilade® CFC-Free Inhaler. Sanofi-Aventis New Zealand Limited, Auckland. http://www.medsafe.govt.nz/profs/datasheet/t/Tiladecfcfreeinh.pdf [accessed on June 5, 2014].

10 Intal® CFC-Free Inhaler. Drugs.com. http://www.drugs.com/mtm/intal-inhaler-inhalation.html [accessed on June 5, 2014].

11 Robinson, N.E. (2002) Recurrent airway obstruction (heaves). In: P. Lekeux (ed), Equine Respiratory Diseases. International Veterinary Information Service, Ithaca, NY.

12 Mazan, M. (2003) Use of Aerosolized bronchodilators and corticosteroids. In: N.E. Robinson (ed), Current Therapy in Equine Medicine, 5th edn, pp. 440–445. Saunders, Philadelphia.

13 Plumb, D.C. (2011) Plumb's Veterinary Drug Handbook, 7th edn. Wiley-Blackwell, Ames.

14 FDA (2010) Asthma and COPD inhalers that contain ozone-depleting CFCs to be phased out; alternative treatments. FDA News Release. http://www.fda.gov/NewsEvents/Newsroom/PressAnnouncements/ucm208302.htm [accessed on July 22, 2013].

levalbuterol, the R-enantiomer of albuterol, has recently become more affordable (Xopenex HFA, Sunovion Pharmaceuticals, Marlboro, MA). Albuterol is thought to cause bronchoconstriction in some asthmatics, and there are *in vitro* reports to suggest that it may do so in horse airways as well; this adverse event may be avoided with the use of levalbuterol.

The preponderance of evidence shows that short-acting B-2 agonists are not performance enhancing in humans; there is no evidence to indicate that they are performance enhancing in horses. Nonetheless, all equine sporting events ban albuterol, and due care should be taken to stop drug administration before competition, noting that albuterol can be detected in urine for at least 48 h after administration via MDI. Short-acting B-2 agonists can be useful in horses with RAO and underlying airway obstruction to improve the return to training. Short-acting bronchodilators are also useful during lung function testing to assess the reversibility of airway obstruction in horses with RAO. No more than 450 µg of albuterol by inhalation is necessary to bronchodilate most horses, irrespective of the delivery device chosen.

Although aerosolized B-2 agonists have a relatively low incidence of side effects, systemic effects such as trembling, anxiety, and cardiac arrhythmias have been observed in individuals particularly sensitive to their effects or those using high doses. The author has noted all these in individuals treated with 900 µg of albuterol, whereas other individuals show no signs of intolerance. Repeated use of the drug tends to decrease side effects as the body downregulates receptors. Very occasionally, horses may exhibit signs of bronchoconstriction following administration of B-2 agonists. This paradoxical response is likely due to the effects of the drug vehicle on airways and is usually transient.

Long-Acting Inhaled B2-AR Therapy: We treat selected cases of RAO and moderate IAD with long-acting B2-AR therapy in addition to inhaled corticosteroids, with the initial impression of enhanced performance and quality of life. It cannot be emphasized enough, however, that regular use of long-acting B2-ARs must be accompanied with regular use of inhaled corticosteroids. The most commonly used long-acting B2-ARs are salmeterol and formoterol, whose basic mechanism of action is the familiar cAMP pathway. Their duration of action in horses is 6–8 h.

Inhaled Parasympatholytic Therapy: The most commonly used inhaled parasympatholytic drug is ipratropium, a quaternary ammonium derivative of atropine, which produces bronchodilation lasting approximately 6 h, which is at least 2 h longer than albuterol [50]. Although adverse side effects such as thickened mucus, tachycardia, and decreased ciliary beat frequency are possible with parasympatholytics, no such side effects have been reported in horses administered doses up to 1200 µg. Ipratropium cannot be considered a rescue drug, unlike atropine, because it has much longer onset of action; however, the effect may last somewhat longer than atropine. In severely affected RAO horses, the combination of albuterol and ipratropium may be beneficial.

Mast Cell Stabilizers: These agents are cromones that block calcium channels preventing the release of histamine and tryptase and the subsequent downstream cascade of prostaglandin and leukotriene formulation that eventually cause bronchoconstriction. Sodium cromoglycate can be efficacious in treating known mast cell-mediated IAD, but will not be of use for treating the majority of horses with neutrophil-mediated disease, and therefore, they are less useful for RAO [51]. Their use, however, requires considerable owner compliance, as the maximum response to this drug occurs at 1–2 weeks after beginning treatment.

Environmental Remediation: It is important to note that a recent study demonstrated that environmental control was by far the most important means of treating airway inflammation and dysfunction in horses with heaves, and that, indeed, antigen avoidance decreases smooth muscle mass [52, 53]. The barn environment is replete with organic particulate matter, respirable endotoxin, molds, and volatile gases such as ammonia. The worst offenders appear to be hay and straw. Multiple studies have shown that significant improvements can be made by replacing dusty substrates and feed with less dusty substitutes. For instance, pelleted hay and wood shavings are often better than regular hay and straw bedding [54, 55]. Indoor arenas present another high dust challenge to the horse, with respirable particulate levels 20 times that which has been recognized to cause respiratory dysfunction in humans [56]. In addition to changing to low dust feeds and beddings, the following recommendations to owners should be made:

Feed hay from the ground, not from a hay net.

Soak hay well before feeding or use ensiled or baked hay products.

Wet any dusty grain (e.g., pellets) before feeding.

Sprinkle aisleways with water before sweeping.

Avoid storing hay overhead. If unavoidable, lay a tarp under the hay to avoid dust raining down on the horses.

Use a humectant or hygroscopic agent to reduce dust in the indoor and outdoor arenas.

Remove horses from the barn while cleaning stalls or moving hay.

Do not use blowers to clean aisles.

Remove cobwebs and other dust collectors routinely when horses are out of the barn.

An overarching principle that can be derived from the OSHA Dust Control Handbook is that prevention is better than cure. In addition to the well-known presentation of summer pasture-associated RAO in hot, humid southern states, it is important to remember that horses in New England can also have disease that presents primarily in the spring and summer and that seems to improve when horses are kept temporarily in clean, nondusty indoor environments.

Evaluation of Therapeutic Outcome: It is important to have a baseline assessment of the horse prior to initiating therapy. Ideally, this would include auscultation with and without a rebreathing bag, careful physical examination, observation during exercise, BAL, and baseline pulmonary function testing for horses with IAD and RAO and measurement of airway reactivity for horses suffering from IAD or, in the case of horses with RAO, postbronchodilator PFTs. Although historically pulmonary function testing was available only at a few specialized veterinary pulmonology clinics, user-friendly systems for field testing are now available, making objective baseline assessments possible for practitioners. The goal of a thorough baseline assessment is to facilitate a treatment regimen tailored to the individual horse and to monitor response to therapy. Horses should then be evaluated 1–2 months after initiation of therapy to assess response and guide therapy for the upcoming months. If there is poor response to therapy, it is important to do some detective work to determine why treatment has been unsuccessful. For example, it is essential to check the client's technique for using the drug delivery device. Failure to modify the environment may, in some horses, negate any attempts at drug therapy. Some horses with chronic, severe pathology may be resistant to corticosteroids or may have irreversible changes in the lungs that prevent response to bronchodilators. Finally, lack of response to therapy may be due to underlying infectious disease and may indicate the need for further diagnostics

and perhaps an entirely different approach or concomitant antibiotic use.

Exercise-induced pulmonary hemorrhage (EIPH)

Epidemiology

Exercise-induced pulmonary hemorrhage (EIPH) is seen in all horses that perform at a sufficiently high metabolic intensity, and thus, it is most common in racehorses. The risk of EIPH increases with age and exercise intensity [57].

Pathogenesis

EIPH is a disease of physiology in that exercise causes a large increase in the stress across the pulmonary capillaries. As the horse breathes in at the high frequencies and tidal volumes associated with intense exercise, there is an increased hydrostatic pressure in the vasculature along with greatly increased, more negative, pleural pressures. This increase in transmural stress causes rupture of the capillaries and subsequent bleeding [58].

Clinical presentation

Although it does occur, few horses experience overt epistaxis, and the primary complaint is usually poor performance.

Treatment
Therapeutic goals

To restore performance and prevent chronic episodes of bleeding and subsequent fibrosis and aberrant vascularization.

General approach

Any comorbidity, such as upper airway obstruction or lower airway inflammation should first be addressed. The efficacies of other treatments for EIPH are not clear. Although rest is recommended and even required by many racing jurisdictions, there is no evidence that this will ameliorate future episodes of bleeding. In the USA, furosemide is the most frequently used pharmaceutical for the treatment of EIPH, although its effects on the disease and the horse's performance are the subjects of much debate. There is evidence that it reduces the severity of bleeding, but there is also some evidence that it enhances a horse's racing performance independent of its effects on the disease [59–62].

Infectious diseases of the URT

Streptococcus equi infections
Epidemiology
Strep. equi known eponymously as strangles, was first described in 1251 by Jordanus Ruffus as a highly contagious disease spread by the use of communal water buckets. It is still considered one of the most important contagious equine diseases worldwide. It is spread easily by horse-to-horse contact, as well as by contact with nasal discharge or discharge from abscesses. Strangles can be transmitted by clinically sick horses and by carrier horses that do not demonstrate any outward signs of disease.

Clinical presentation
Classically affected horses have fever, profuse mucopurulent nasal discharge, and lymphadenopathy primarily of the retropharyngeal and submandibular lymph nodes. Horses that have previously been exposed to strangles or who have partial vaccinal immunity may present with high fever alone.

Pathogenesis
The strangles bacterium employs typical streptococcal strategies, including use of a hyaluronic capsule and secretion of exotoxins, to evade immune surveillance and damage the epithelium of the respiratory tract. The defining characteristic of most strangles infections is abscess formation, especially of the submandibular and retropharyngeal lymph nodes. *S. equi* preferentially adheres to the upper respiratory epithelium, although the means by which it achieves this is incompletely understood. Infrequently, disease can disseminate to other areas of the body referred to as metastatic or bastard strangles. Although rare, an immune complex-mediated syndrome, purpura hemorrhagica, can also ensue, causing severe vasculitis.

Diagnosis
Both culture and polymerase chain reaction (PCR) are used for diagnosis.

Treatment
Desired Outcome: Management of an outbreak must be the primary consideration for any practitioner facing an initial case of strangles on a premise. A good isolation policy is paramount to accomplishing this, but is beyond the discussion of this chapter. There are multiple objectives to the actual treatment of strangles, and pharmacologic therapy is not primary among them. With or without antibiotic therapy, the desired outcome for any affected horse is the eradication of the offending organism and avoidance of the carrier state.

General Approach to Treatment: Supportive care is the basis of treatment for the individual horse infected with *Strep. equi*. Pharmacologically, this often involves the judicious use of NSAIDs to control fever and inflammation and provide analgesia. Although antibiotics can be effective for treatment of *S. equi* abscesses, the duration of treatment for eventual success is many weeks to months, and morbidity from antibiotic use will frequently outweigh morbidity from the actual disease. Whether antibiotic use prolongs the disease, promotes abscessation, or increases the risk of metastatic disease, however, is unknown [63]. The general rule is that antibiotics should not be used for horses with abscesses; instead, abscesses should be allowed to develop and the disease allowed to take its natural course. Antibiotic therapy should be instituted in foals having difficulty breathing or nursing or in cases in adult that present with severe respiratory obstruction. Antibiotic therapy may also be considered in horses that have been exposed to known cases, but that do not yet have clinical signs. In addition, miniature horses, donkeys, and ponies at risk of hepatic lipidosis and pregnant mares for which inappetence may be a risk factor for other comorbidities should be considered candidates for antimicrobial therapy.

Selection of Antimicrobial Agent: The drug of choice for treatment of *S. equi* is penicillin, despite several obvious drawbacks, including poor antibiotic penetration into the abscess cavity and ineffectiveness in an acidic environment. These drawbacks, however, are countered by the exquisite sensitivity of the *S. equi* organism to penicillin. Nevertheless, IV administration at the high end of the dose range is recommended to maximize efficacy. IM procaine penicillin G (PPG) is effective, yet the goodwill of even the kindest horse is strained by twice-daily administrations of PPG for more than a few days. Other antimicrobials that have been reported to be efficacious include tetracyclines, cephalosporins, and fluoroquinolones, although the increasing emergence of fluoroquinolone-resistant streptococci makes the latter choice problematic [64]. Although TMS is often termed inappropriate for treatment of abscesses because of the high concentrations of folic acid in pus, the potentiated sulfas achieve very high concentrations in abscesses, which may negate that effect.

A rare but important complication of strangles is purpura hemorrhagica, an immune-mediated vasculitis, which requires treatment with corticosteroids, as well as concurrent penicillin therapy. Appropriate corticosteroids include dexamethasone and prednisolone (Table 10.4).

Guttural pouch mycosis
Epidemiology
Guttural pouch mycosis (GPM) is found in all breeds and ages of horses. There is an association with stabled horses in colder weather, which may coincide with increased levels of fungus-bearing particulates in the air.

Pathology
Although it is well accepted that GPM is an opportunistic infection, most commonly with *Aspergillus* spp., which colonize the mucosa of the guttural pouch, our understanding of why this happens, and why most lesions are on the roof of the medial compartment overlying the internal carotid, remains a mystery.

Clinical signs
The most obvious signs of GPM are epistaxis and neurologic abnormalities referable to the nerves that run through the guttural pouch: cranial nerves IX, X, and XI.

Treatment
Desired Outcome: The first goal in treatment of GPM must be to avoid fatal exsanguination due to erosion into one of the major arteries. Although various hemostatic agents have been recommended, there is no good evidence to support the efficacy of these drugs in horses with hemorrhage. As long as the travel time in the range of an hour, it is often better to transport the patient to a tertiary care facility that can stabilize and treat the primary problem.

Once bleeding is controlled or if GPM has been diagnosed before erosion into an artery has occurred, eradication of the fungal infection needs to be addressed. This goal is usually achieved with surgical therapy, although in early cases, pharmacologic therapy may be of use.

Antifungal Agents: Antifungal agents are generally unsuccessful for topical therapy of GPM, for many reasons. Firstly, the clot, when first established, is fragile, and physical application of antifungals may disrupt it. Secondly, there is no good method for maintaining high concentration of antifungal medication at the site.

Nonetheless, the author has, very rarely, had success in treating very small fungal lesions in the guttural pouch with ketoconazole applied topically every other day for several weeks.

Sinusitis
Epidemiology
Both primary sinusitis and secondary sinusitis are seen in horses, although primary sinusitis is far less common. Primary sinusitis can be due to viral respiratory pathogens or due to obstruction of the sinuses with resulting infection of the poorly draining space. Secondary sinusitis most commonly occurs in older horses with tooth root infections.

Pathogenesis
It is important to remember that the sinuses are lined with ciliated pseudostratified columnar epithelium and are thus susceptible to the same viral and bacterial pathogens that plague the rest of the respiratory tree. While C&S are pending, it is wise to assume that *Strep. zoo.* is present. A variety of other Gram-positive, Gram-negative, and anaerobic bacteria may also be present. In older horses, tooth root fractures or other infections of the caudal maxillary teeth often result in secondary sinusitis, as the roots of the teeth project into the maxillary sinuses.

Clinical presentation
The horse with a primary infection is more likely to present with a purulent, but not particularly smelly, nasal discharge [65]. In contrast, the malodorous discharge in a horse with a secondary, dental-associated sinusitis can be quite distinctive. If the infection is long standing, there may be bony involvement and the facial structure may be deformed. Radiographs are useful for demonstrating the presence of fluid in the sinuses.

Treatment
Therapeutic Goals: The therapeutic goals are to resolve the infection and relieve any predisposing causes of the infection.

General Approach: If there is blocked drainage of the sinuses, then treatment success will only be temporary unless the blockage is relieved. The same is true for dental involvement, which may necessitate surgery to ensure permanent resolution of the problem. At the same time, if there are financial concerns or there is the anticipation of significant comorbidity with surgery, flushing of the sinuses may afford considerable relief and delay the need for more invasive treatment. Concurrent treatment with antibiotics is usually necessary only when there is evidence of bony involvement.

Antimicrobial Selection: Antimicrobial use should be based on C&S results, however, and empirical choice would include a drug with a good spectrum against Gram-positive bacteria, especially streptococci, as well as anaerobes. A second requirement would be good penetration into bone if that tissue is involved.

Evaluation of Therapeutic Outcome: Successful treatment is signified by resolution of nasal discharge and absence of fluid lines or osteomyelitis on radiographs.

Fungal rhinitis
Epidemiology
Fungal rhinitis appears to be most common in horses in which an indwelling nasogastric tube has been placed, especially horses undergoing frequent reflux, such as those suffering from proximal duodenitis/jejunitis, secondary to pressure necrosis or trauma induced by the tube. Other trauma may also predispose to development of this disease. It has been suggested that fungal rhinitis is more common in stabled horses, which is logical given the high concentration of fungal spore particulates in the air due to hay feeding in confined spaces.

Pathogenesis
It appears that the fungal organisms, most frequently *Aspergillus* species, are secondary invaders in the presence of damaged mucosa. Tissues often appear necrotic, and hyphae may invade tissues.

Clinical presentation
Typically, horses have a history of a serous-to-mucoid nasal discharge. If the infection becomes more chronic, the horse may develop a foul-smelling purulent nasal discharge. The discharge may sometimes be hemorrhagic. Fungal spores are almost always present in equine airways, so diagnosis can be challenging, and endoscopy with biopsy is the best diagnostic option.

Treatment
It is important to try to remove the causative agent, such as the nasogastric tube, for resolution. In some cases, the infection may resolve spontaneously with removal of the predisposing cause.

Therapeutic Goals: The therapeutic goal should be to resolve the infection before it becomes chronic and before bone necrosis occurs.

General Approach: Treatment may be both local and systemic, and a combination may be most effective. It is often useful to debride the affected areas endoscopically before topical application of antifungal agents. If the horse is tolerant to having a topical solution applied to the nasal passages every day for several weeks, then the topical approach may be effective. Success with both enilconazole and itraconazole applied topically for fungal rhinitis has been reported [66]. Many horses will not tolerate this therapy, and systemic antifungals must then be used. The owner should be made aware that the treatment period may last many weeks to months.

Antimicrobial Selection: It is important to choose an antifungal to which aspergillus is sensitive. Although *Aspergillus* spp. have historically been sensitive to itraconazole, resistance is emerging to that active, and most aspergilli are currently resistant to fluconazole [67].

Evaluation of Therapeutic Outcome: Endoscopic evaluation of affected area is the best method of assessing resolution.

Noninfectious diseases of the URT

Ethmoid hematoma
Epidemiology
Ethmoid hematoma is a relatively rare disease that has been reported in all breeds except, interestingly, the standardbred. It is rare for horses less than 3 years of age to be affected.

Pathogenesis
The cause of ethmoid hematoma is poorly understood at best. It usually arises from the mucosa of the ethmoids but is also seen in the paranasal sinuses. It is best thought of as a hemangiomatous mass that can cause deformity, but is never neoplastic.

Clinical presentation
Horses may present with a chronic, low-grade hemorrhagic, purulent, or frankly bloody nasal discharge. If the lesion occupies enough space, they may have noisy breathing or may develop a facial deformity. Rarely, the lesion may occupy enough of the nasal passages that the animal shows respiratory embarrassment.

SAMPLE CASES: TREATMENT FOR NONINFECTIOUS INFLAMMATORY AIRWAY DISEASES (RECURRENT AIRWAY OBSTRUCTION, INFLAMMATORY AIRWAY DISEASE)

Case 10.1. A 14-year-old thoroughbred used for trail riding presents with a 4-year history of increasing nasal discharge, cough, and exercise intolerance. Recently, the owner has noted that the horse has intermittent episodes of apparent difficulty breathing even at rest. The horse lives in a modern barn with hay stored overhead and with an attached indoor arena. No dust suppressants are used on the arena. The horse is turned out for 4 h/day, in addition to trail riding three times per week. An inspection of the stall reveals a large dust buildup on the windows. Physical examination shows a moderately thin horse with bilateral mucoid nasal discharge. Although the horse is bright and interactive, obvious expiratory effort is noted. Fluidy sounds are heard on auscultation of the trachea, and crackles and wheezes are heard bilaterally. Lung function testing reveals an elevated baseline respiratory resistance and marked airway hyperreactivity. Cytology on BAL fluid reveals large amounts of mucus and 80% neutrophils. Hay spores and small particulates (dust) are found engulfed in macrophages; no bacteria are seen. You diagnose RAO or heaves as it is commonly referred to. You recommend environmental remediation for reduction of dust and hay spores in the environment. An initial pharmacologic treatment plan includes a 4-week tapering dose of prednisolone (Table 10.4). In addition, inhaled albuterol is administered at a dose of 5 puffs (90 µg/puff) four times a day during the first week, using a spacer/delivery device. During the second week, albuterol is continued, and fluticasone propionate HFA (220 µg/puff) is administered at a dose of 10 puffs twice daily. Because the horse is moderately intolerant of the inhaled drugs, you instruct the owner to give the fluticasone propionate HFA before the albuterol, as it is the most expensive drug and will help to control inflammation. During the third and fourth weeks of treatment with prednisolone, albuterol is continued, and fluticasone propionate HFA is decreased to once daily. At this time, you recommend a recheck of lung function and airway reactivity in order to plan for future treatment. The client is counseled that improvement should be noticed by the second week, but that the best outcome may not be seen for several months. Treatment may be continually or intermittently required on a long-term basis unless rigorous environmental management is instituted.

Case 10.2. A 6-year-old Quarter Horse used for show is presented with a 2-month history of nasal discharge after exercise and cough at the onset of exercise. The horse lives in an attractive, but old, converted cow barn. The ventilation is poor, the shavings in the stall are somewhat dusty, and hay, while stored in a separate building, is similarly dusty. The owners have only recently purchased the horse, and while it formerly lived outside year-round in a 100 acre pasture, it now spends 12–18 h a day indoors. The owner knows the former owner well and knew the horse previously: there was no history of previous respiratory disease. Lung function testing reveals a normal baseline and mild airway hyperreactivity. On endoscopy, there are occasional globs of mucus in the trachea, but they are nonconfluent. BAL cytology reveals a neutrophilia of 10%, with some mucus. An initial treatment plan includes environmental remediation of the dusty environment and pharmacological therapy with inhaled drugs only. During the first week, albuterol is administered at a dose of 5 puffs twice daily, followed 5 min later by administration of beclomethasone dipropionate HFA at 10 puffs twice daily (80 µg/puff). The owner was able to get the best price on the brand name QVAR product, so that was used for therapy. Over the next 3 weeks, the beclomethasone dipropionate HFA dose will be tapered to 10 puffs once daily, with an eventual goal of every other day administration. After the first week, albuterol will only be administered prior to exercise, ideally 20 min before, or if the horse is noted to have any difficulty breathing. You caution the owner that, depending on the show governing body, these drugs will need to be declared or they may be considered nonpermitted medications. If they are not permitted, a withdrawal time of at least 3 days is recommended, and more time may be necessary. The owners decide to look for an outdoor housing situation for this horse, as the onset of disease appears to be so clearly associated with indoor living, and this is a young horse with many productive years ahead.

Case 10.3. You are asked to give a second opinion on a 3-year-old thoroughbred racehorse with a recent history of poor performance. There is no history of cough or wheeze; however, the horse seems to "hit the wall," tiring very quickly and severely, at the ¾ pole. Physical examination reveals no abnormalities. You note, however, that the horse has a high respiratory rate after breezing (i.e., running at high speed for a short period of time). Baseline lung function testing reveals no abnormalities; however, the horse is markedly reactive to histamine bronchoprovocation. The BAL shows 6% mast cells and small amounts of mucus. The horse has previously been treated with beclomethasone dipropionate HFA and albuterol at appropriate doses. Although there has been some improvement, the horse continues to be slow. Because of the high percentage of mast cells present in the BAL, you suggest adding Tilade (nedocromil sodium) to the treatment regimen, starting with 13 puffs (2 mg/puff) four times a day. You warn the trainer that, because Tilade works by stabilizing mast cells, and thus preventing inflammation, the drug will need to be on board for up to several weeks before the best effect is seen. As with any competition horse, these may not be used during competition, and you advise the trainer to discuss appropriate withdrawal times with the appropriate regulatory authorities.

The diagnosis is made on endoscopic examination of the upper airways, radiography, or both.

Treatment

Therapeutic Goals: To remove the mass, restore normal respiratory ability, and prevent the mass from recurring.

General Approach: The approach to the ethmoid hematoma may involve surgical or laser ablation, cryotherapy, or a combination of these. A chemical approach has also been used.

Chemical Selection: 10% formalin can be injected into the ethmoid using a catheter extension needle and endoscopic guidance, or the ethmoid hematoma can be injected directly as part of the surgical ablation. It is often necessary to repeat the injection every 3–4 weeks for two to four repetitions. Care must be taken to ensure that the cribriform plate is intact before performing chemical ablation to avoid accidental migration of formalin to the brain, as has been reported [68, 69].

Evaluation of Therapeutic Outcome: Resolution of the problem is determined by clinical signs, endoscopy, and radiography.

References

1 Gronwall, R., Brown, M.P., Merritt, A.M. & Stone, H.W. (1986) Body fluid concentrations and pharmacokinetics of chloramphenicol given to mares intravenously or by repeated gavage. *American Journal of Veterinary Research*, **47**, 2591–2595.

2 Sisodia, C.S., Kramer, L.L., Gupta, V.S., Lerner, D.J. & Taksas, L. (1975) A pharmacological study of chloramphenicol in horses. *Canadian Journal of Comparative Medicine*, **39**, 216–223.

3 Rodvold, K.A., Yoo, L. & George, J.M. (2011) Penetration of anti-infective agents into pulmonary epithelial lining fluid: Focus on antifungal, antitubercular and miscellaneous anti-infective agents. *Clinical Pharmacokinetics*, **50**, 689–704.

4 Oikawa, M., Takagi, S., Anzai, R., Yoshikawa, H. & Yoshikawa, T. (1995) Pathology of equine respiratory disease occurring in association with transport. *Journal of Comparative Pathology*, **113**, 29–43.

5 Leclere, M., Magdesian, K.G., Cole, C.A. *et al.* (2012) Pharmacokinetics and preliminary safety evaluation of azithromycin in adult horses. *Journal of Veterinary Pharmacology and Therapeutics*, **35**, 541–549.

6 Winther, L., Baptiste, K.E. & Friis, C. (2012) Pharmacokinetics in pulmonary epithelial lining fluid and plasma of ampicillin and pivampicillin administered to horses. *Research in Veterinary Science*, **92**, 111–115.

7 Bade, D.J., Sibert, G.J., Hallberg, J., Portis, E.S., Boucher, J. & Bryson, L. (2009) Ceftiofur susceptibility of Streptococcus equi subsp zooepidemicus isolated from horses in North America between 1989 and 2008. *Veterinary Therapeutics*, **10**, E1–E7.

8 Jaglan, P.S., Roof, R.D., Yein, F.S., Arnold, T.S., Brown, S.A. & Gilbertson, T.J. (1994) Concentration of ceftiofur metabolites in the plasma and lungs of horses following intramuscular treatment. *Journal of Veterinary Pharmacology and Therapeutics*, **17**, 24–30.

9 McClure, S., Sibert, G., Hallberg, J. & Bade, D. (2011) Efficacy of a 2-dose regimen of a sustained release ceftiofur suspension in horses with Streptococcus equi subsp. zooepidemicus bronchopneumonia. *Journal of Veterinary Pharmacology and Therapeutics*, **34**, 442–447.

10 Thomas, E., Thomas, V. & Wilhelm, C. (2006) Antibacterial activity of cefquinome against equine bacterial pathogens. *Veterinary Microbiology*, **115**, 140–147.

11 Winther, L., Baptiste, K.E. & Friis, C. (2011) Antimicrobial disposition in pulmonary epithelial lining fluid of horses, part III. Cefquinome. *Journal of Veterinary Pharmacology and Therapeutics*, **34**, 482–486.

12 Winther, L., Guardabassi, L., Baptiste, K.E. & Friis, C. (2011) Antimicrobial disposition in pulmonary epithelial lining fluid of horses, part I. Sulfadiazine and trimethoprim. *Journal of Veterinary Pharmacology and Therapeutics*, **34**, 277–284.

13 Davis, J.L., Salmon, J.H. & Papich, M.G. (2006) Pharmacokinetics and tissue distribution of doxycycline after oral administration of single and multiple doses in horses. *American Journal of Veterinary Research*, **67**, 310–316.

14 Winther, L., Honore Hansen, S., Baptiste, K.E. & Friis, C. (2011) Antimicrobial disposition in pulmonary epithelial lining fluid of horses, part II. Doxycycline. *Journal of Veterinary Pharmacology and Therapeutics*, **34**, 285–289.

15 Brown, M.P., Kelly, R.H., Gronwall, R.R. & Stover, S.M. (1984) Chloramphenicol sodium succinate in the horse: Serum, synovial, peritoneal, and urine concentrations after single-dose intravenous administration. *American Journal of Veterinary Research*, **45**, 578–580.

16 De Corte-Baeten, K. & Debackere, M. (1975) Chloramphenicol plasma levels in horses, cattle and sheep after oral and intramuscular administration. *Zentralblatt fur Veterinarmedizin Reihe B*, **22**, 704–712.

17 Peyrou, M., Doucet, M.Y., Vrins, A., Concordet, D., Schneider, M. & Bousquet-Mélou, A. (2004) Population pharmacokinetics of marbofloxacin in horses: Preliminary analysis. *Journal of Veterinary Pharmacology and Therapeutics*, **27**, 283–288.

18 Olsson, B., Bondesson, W., Borgstrom, L. *et al.* (2011) Pulmonary drug metabolism, clearance, and absorption. In: H.D.C. Smyth & A.J. Hickey (eds), *Controlled Pulmonary Drug Delivery*, pp. 21–50. Springer, New York.

19 McKenzie, H.C., 3rd & Murray, M.J. (2000) Concentrations of gentamicin in serum and bronchial lavage fluid after

intravenous and aerosol administration of gentamicin to horses. *American Journal of Veterinary Research,* **61**, 1185–1190.

20 McKenzie, H.C., 3rd & Murray, M.J. (2004) Concentrations of gentamicin in serum and bronchial lavage fluid after once-daily aerosol administration to horses for seven days. *American Journal of Veterinary Research,* **65**, 173–178.

21 Art, T., de Moffarts, B., Bedoret, D., van Erck, E. & Lekeux, P. (2007) Pulmonary function and antimicrobial concentration after marbofloxacin inhalation in horses. *Veterinary Record,* **161**, 348–350.

22 Carretero, M., Rodriguez, C., San Andres, M.I. *et al.* (2002) Pharmacokinetics of marbofloxacin in mature horses after single intravenous and intramuscular administration. *Equine Veterinary Journal,* **34**, 360–365.

23 Maes, A., Garre, B., Desmet, N. *et al.* (2009) Determination of acyclovir in horse plasma and body fluids by high-performance liquid chromatography combined with fluorescence detection and heated electrospray ionization tandem mass spectrometry. *Biomedical Chromatography,* **23**, 132–140.

24 Rees, W.A., Harkins, J.D., Woods, W.E. *et al.* (1997) Amantadine and equine influenza: Pharmacology, pharmacokinetics and neurological effects in the horse. *Equine Veterinary Journal,* **29**, 104–110.

25 Moen, M.D., Lyseng-Williamson, K.A. & Scott, L.J. (2009) Liposomal amphotericin B: A review of its use as empirical therapy in febrile neutropenia and in the treatment of invasive fungal infections. *Drugs,* **69**, 361–392.

26 Begg, L.M., Hughes, K.J., Kessell, A., Krockenberger, M.B., Wigney, D.I. & Malik, R. (2004) Successful treatment of cryptococcal pneumonia in a pony mare. *Australian Veterinary Journal,* **82**, 686–692.

27 Davis, J.L., Salmon, J.H. & Papich, M.G. (2005) Pharmacokinetics and tissue distribution of itraconazole after oral and intravenous administration to horses. *American Journal of Veterinary Research,* **66**, 1694–1701.

28 Latimer, F.G., Colitz, C.M., Campbell, N.B. & Papich, M.G. (2001) Pharmacokinetics of fluconazole following intravenous and oral administration and body fluid concentrations of fluconazole following repeated oral dosing in horses. *American Journal of Veterinary Research,* **62**, 1606–1611.

29 Hilton, H., Galuppo, L., Puchalski, S.M. *et al.* (2009) Successful treatment of invasive pulmonary aspergillosis in a neonatal foal. *Journal of Veterinary Internal Medicine,* **23**, 375–378.

30 Passler, N.H., Chan, H.M., Stewart, A.J. *et al.* (2010) Distribution of voriconazole in seven body fluids of adult horses after repeated oral dosing. *Journal of Veterinary Pharmacology and Therapeutics,* **33**, 35–41.

31 Horohov, D.W., Beadle, R.E., Mouch, S. & Pourciau, S.S. (2005) Temporal regulation of cytokine mRNA expression in equine recurrent airway obstruction. *Veterinary Immunology and Immunopathology,* **108**, 237–245.

32 Joubert, P., Cordeau, M.E. & Lavoie, J.P. (2011) Cytokine mRNA expression of pulmonary macrophages varies with challenge but not with disease state in horses with heaves or in controls. *Veterinary Immunology and Immunopathology,* **142**, 236–242.

33 Lapointe, J.M., Lavoie, J.P. & Vrins, A.A. (1993) Effects of triamcinolone acetonide on pulmonary function and bronchoalveolar lavage cytologic features in horses with chronic obstructive pulmonary disease. *American Journal of Veterinary Research,* **54**, 1310–1316.

34 French, K., Pollitt, C.C. & Pass, M.A. (2000) Pharmacokinetics and metabolic effects of triamcinolone acetonide and their possible relationships to glucocorticoid-induced laminitis in horses. *Journal of Veterinary Pharmacology and Therapeutics,* **23**, 287–292.

35 Jackson, C.A., Berney, C., Jefcoat, A.M. & Robinson, N.E. (2000) Environment and prednisone interactions in the treatment of recurrent airway obstruction (heaves). *Equine Veterinary Journal,* **32**, 432–438.

36 Courouce-Malblanc, A., Fortier, G., Pronost, S., Siliart, B. & Brachet, G. (2008) Comparison of prednisolone and dexamethasone effects in the presence of environmental control in heaves-affected horses. *Veterinary Journal,* **175**, 227–233.

37 Leclere, M., Lefebvre-Lavoie, J., Beauchamp, G. & Lavoie, J.P. (2010) Efficacy of oral prednisolone and dexamethasone in horses with recurrent airway obstruction in the presence of continuous antigen exposure. *Equine Veterinary Journal,* **42**, 316–321.

38 Bertin, F.R., Ivester, K.M. & Couetil, L.L. (2011) Comparative efficacy of inhaled albuterol between two hand-held delivery devices in horses with recurrent airway obstruction. *Equine Veterinary Journal,* **43**, 393–398.

39 Leach, C.L., Davidson, P.J., Hasselquist, B.E. & Boudreau, R.J. (2005) Influence of particle size and patient dosing technique on lung deposition of HFA-beclomethasone from a metered dose inhaler. *Journal of Aerosol Medicine,* **18**, 379–385.

40 Rush, B.R., Trevino, I.C., Matson, C.J. & Hakala, J.E. (1999) Serum cortisol concentrations in response to incremental doses of inhaled beclomethasone dipropionate. *Equine Veterinary Journal,* **31**, 258–261.

41 Votion, D., Ghafir, Y., Munsters, K., Duvivier, D.H., Art, T. & Lekeux, P. (1997) Aerosol deposition in equine lungs following ultrasonic nebulisation versus jet aerosol delivery system. *Equine Veterinary Journal,* **29**, 388–393.

42 Dauvillier, J., Felippe, M.J., Lunn, D.P. *et al.* (2011) Effect of long-term fluticasone treatment on immune function in horses with heaves. *Journal of Veterinary Internal Medicine,* **25**, 549–557.

43 Laan, T.T., Westermann, C.M., Dijkstra, A.V., van Nieuwstadt, R.A. & Fink-Gremmels, J. (2004) Biological availability of inhaled fluticasone propionate in horses. *Veterinary Record,* **155**, 361–364.

44 Thompson, J.A., Mirza, M.H., Barker, S.A., Morgan, T.W., Bauer, R.W. & McConnico, R.S. (2011) Clenbuterol toxicosis in three Quarter Horse racehorses after administration of a compounded product. *Journal of the American Veterinary Medical Association*, **239**, 842–849.

45 Kearns, C.F. & McKeever, K.H. (2002) Clenbuterol diminishes aerobic performance in horses. *Medicine and Science in Sports and Exercise*, **34**, 1976–1985.

46 Thompson, J.A., Eades, S.C., Chapman, A.M., Paulsen, D.B., Barker, S.A. & McConnico, R.S. (2012) Effects of clenbuterol administration on serum biochemical, histologic, and echocardiographic measurements of muscle injury in exercising horses. *American Journal of Veterinary Research*, **73**, 875–883.

47 Read, J.R., Boston, R.C., Abraham, G., Bauquier, S.H., Soma, L.R. & Nolen-Walston, R.D. (2012) Effect of prolonged administration of clenbuterol on airway reactivity and sweating in horses with inflammatory airway disease. *American Journal of Veterinary Research*, **73**, 140–145.

48 Erichsen, D.F., Aviad, A.D., Schultz, R.H. & Kennedy, T.J. (1994) Clinical efficacy and safety of clenbuterol HCl when administered to effect in horses with chronic obstructive pulmonary disease (COPD). *Equine Veterinary Journal*, **26**, 331–336.

49 Traub-Dargatz, J.L., McKinnon, A.O., Thrall, M.A. *et al.* (1992) Evaluation of clinical signs of disease, bronchoalveolar and tracheal wash analysis, and arterial blood gas tensions in 13 horses with chronic obstructive pulmonary disease treated with prednisone, methyl sulfonmethane, and clenbuterol hydrochloride. *American Journal of Veterinary Research*, **53**, 1908–1916.

50 Robinson, N.E., Derksen, F.J., Berney, C. & Goossens, L. (1993) The airway response of horses with recurrent airway obstruction (heaves) to aerosol administration of ipratropium bromide. *Equine Veterinary Journal*, **25**, 299–303.

51 Hare, J.E., Viel, L., O'Byrne, P.M. & Conlon, P.D. (1994) Effect of sodium cromoglycate on light racehorses with elevated metachromatic cell numbers on bronchoalveolar lavage and reduced exercise tolerance. *Journal of Veterinary Pharmacology and Therapeutics*, **17**, 237–244.

52 Couetil, L.L., Chilcoat, C.D., DeNicola, D.B., Clark, S.P., Glickman, N.W. & Glickman, L.T. (2005) Randomized, controlled study of inhaled fluticasone propionate, oral administration of prednisone, and environmental management of horses with recurrent airway obstruction. *American Journal of Veterinary Research*, **66**, 1665–1674.

53 Lavoie-Lamoureux, A., Beauchamp, G., Quessy, S., Martin, J.G. & Lavoie, J.P. (2012) Systemic inflammation and priming of peripheral blood leukocytes persist during clinical remission in horses with heaves. *Veterinary Immunology and Immunopathology*, **146**, 35–45.

54 Kirschvink, N., Di Silvestro, F., Sbai, I. *et al.* (2002) The use of cardboard bedding material as part of an environmental control regime for heaves-affected horses: In vitro assessment of airborne dust and aeroallergen concentration and in vivo effects on lung function. *Veterinary Journal*, **163**, 319–325.

55 Woods, P.S., Robinson, N.E., Swanson, M.C., Reed, C.E., Broadstone, R.V. & Derksen, F.J. (1993) Airborne dust and aeroallergen concentration in a horse stable under two different management systems. *Equine Veterinary Journal*, **25**, 208–213.

56 May, M. & Robinson, N.E. (2004) Indoor air quality in a riding stable. *Proceedings of the 22nd Symposium of the Veterinary Comparative Respiratory Society*. Montreal, Quebec, pp. 42–44.

57 Pascoe, J.R., Ferraro, G.L., Cannon, J.H., Arthur, R.M. & Wheat, J.D. (1981) Exercise-induced pulmonary hemorrhage in racing thoroughbreds: A preliminary study. *American Journal of Veterinary Research*, **42**, 703–707.

58 West, J.B. & Mathieu-Costello, O. (1994) Stress failure of pulmonary capillaries as a mechanism for exercise induced pulmonary haemorrhage in the horse. *Equine Veterinary Journal*, **26**, 441–447.

59 Birks, E.K., Durando, M.M. & McBride, S. (2003) Exercise-induced pulmonary hemorrhage. *Veterinary Clinics of North America Equine Practice*, **19**, 87–100.

60 Hinchcliff, K.W., Jackson, M.A., Morley, P.S. *et al.* (2005) Association between exercise-induced pulmonary hemorrhage and performance in thoroughbred racehorses. *Journal of the American Veterinary Medical Association*, **227**, 768–774.

61 Hinchcliff, K.W., Morley, P.S. & Guthrie, A.J. (2011) Use of furosemide for exercise-induced pulmonary hemorrhage in racehorses. *Journal of the American Veterinary Medical Association*, **239**, 1407.

62 Hinchcliff, K.W., Morley, P.S. & Guthrie, A.J. (2009) Efficacy of furosemide for prevention of exercise-induced pulmonary hemorrhage in thoroughbred racehorses. *Journal of the American Veterinary Medical Association*, **235**, 76–82.

63 Sweeney, C.R., Timoney, J.F., Newton, J.R. & Hines, M.T. (2005) Streptococcus equi infections in horses: Guidelines for treatment, control, and prevention of strangles. *Journal of Veterinary Internal Medicine*, **19**, 123–134.

64 Arai, K., Hirakata, Y., Yano, H. *et al.* (2011) Emergence of fluoroquinolone-resistant Streptococcus pyogenes in Japan by a point mutation leading to a new amino acid substitution. *Journal of Antimicrobial Chemotherapy*, **66**, 494–498.

65 Dixon, P.M., Parkin, T.D., Collins, N. *et al.* (2011) Historical and clinical features of 200 cases of equine sinus disease. *Veterinary Record*, **169**, 439.

66 Kendall, A., Brojer, J., Karlstam, E. & Pringle, J. (2008) Enilconazole treatment of horses with superficial Aspergillus

spp. rhinitis. *Journal of Veterinary Internal Medicine*, **22**, 1239–1242.

67 Bueid, A., Howard, S.J., Moore, C.B. *et al.* (2010) Azole antifungal resistance in Aspergillus fumigatus: 2008 and 2009. *Journal of Antimicrobial Chemotherapy*, **65**, 2116–2118.

68 Dixon, P.M., Parkin, T.D., Collins, N. *et al.* (2011) Equine paranasal sinus disease: A long-term study of 200 cases (1997–2009): Ancillary diagnostic findings and involvement of the various sinus compartments. *Equine Veterinary Journal*, **44**, 267–271.

69 Frees, K.E., Gaughan, E.M., Lillich, J.D. *et al.* (2001) Severe complication after administration of formalin for treatment of progressive ethmoidal hematoma in a horse. *Journal of the American Veterinary Medical Association*, **219**, 950–952, 939.

SECTION 2
Therapeutics: A Systems Approach

CHAPTER 11

Clinical application of gastrointestinal therapeutics

L. Chris Sanchez

Large Animal Internal Medicine, University of Florida College of Veterinary Medicine, Gainesville, FL, USA

This chapter addresses agents commonly used for the treatment of gastrointestinal (GI) disorders. Treatment of abdominal pain and inflammation are not discussed in this chapter, as analgesic therapy and nonsteroidal anti-inflammatory drugs (NSAID) are discussed in detail in Chapter 4, and treatment of endotoxemia, which is frequently associated with GI disorders, is discussed in Chapter 7.

Therapy for the equine gastric ulcer syndrome

The term "equine gastric ulcer syndrome (EGUS)" applies to all forms of gastric ulceration, though they can be divided clinically into ulceration of the nonglandular gastric mucosa, ulceration of the glandular gastric mucosa, and inflammation and ulceration of the proximal duodenum and stomach in foals (gastroduodenal ulcer disease, GDUD). Clinically, these forms are typically treated similarly.

In general, antiulcer therapy is focused on decreasing gastric acid production. The principal drug classes used to accomplish this goal include proton pump inhibitors (PPIs), histamine type 2 receptor antagonists (H2RA), mucosal adherents, prostaglandin analogs, and antacids. As of this writing, the only PPI approved by the Food and Drug Administration (FDA) for treatment of EGUS in horses in the USA is omeprazole (GASTROGARD®, Merial Limited, Duluth, Georgia).

Proton pump inhibitors

PPIs block secretion of H^+ at the parietal cell membrane by irreversibly binding to the H^+, K^+-ATPase proton pump of the cell. These agents have a prolonged antisecretory effect that allows for once-daily dosing. Oral omeprazole is safe in foals and adult horses and has been shown to result in healing of NSAID-induced and naturally occurring ulcers in horses, including those maintained in race training [1–5]. Treatment with omeprazole at 1, 2, or 4 mg/kg bwt, orally (PO), q24 h has been shown to decrease or prevent disease and the recurrence of disease in animals maintained in training, whereas 4 mg/kg bwt was more likely to result in ulcer healing. Omeprazole appears more effective for ulcer healing than either ranitidine or cimetidine, including for animals maintained in race training [6–11]. Omeprazole administered at 4 mg/kg bwt will also result in increased intragastric pH in healthy or critically ill foals and ulcer healing in foals [3, 12, 13].

Compounded omeprazole preparations appear substantially inferior to the proprietary formulation in pharmacodynamic and clinical trials [14–16]. This is likely associated with rapid degradation of the omeprazole molecule in an acidic environment. Treatment of horses with an intravenous (IV) formulation of compounded omeprazole at a dose of 0.5 mg/kg bwt resulted in increased gastric pH and a decreased number of nonglandular lesions [17]. At a dose of 4 mg/kg bwt, PO, q2 h, omeprazole did not appear to have a performance-enhancing effect in standardbred racehorses [18].

Equine Pharmacology, First Edition. Edited by Cynthia Cole, Bradford Bentz and Lara Maxwell.
© 2015 John Wiley & Sons, Inc. Published 2015 by John Wiley & Sons, Inc.

Although other PPIs have been evaluated extensively in humans, they have not undergone much evaluation in horses. Pantoprazole, administered either IV or intragastrically at 1.5 mg/kg bwt, was shown to increase intragastric pH in healthy foals [19].

Histamine-2 receptor antagonists (H2RA)

The histamine-2 antagonists suppress hydrochloric acid secretion through competitive inhibition of H2 receptors in the parietal cell [20]. H2 antagonist therapy has been shown to increase gastric pH and improve or heal ulceration in foals and adult horses [21–23]. Dosage recommendations represent those necessary to increase pH and promote healing in the majority of horses, as the response varies tremendously among individual horses [24]. Recommended dosages in adult horses are as follows: cimetidine 20–30 mg/kg bwt, PO, q8 h or 6.6 mg/kg bwt, IV, q6 h and ranitidine 6.6 mg/kg bwt, PO, q8 h or 2 mg/kg bwt, IV, q6 h. Although clinically normal foals respond predictably to ranitidine, sick foals appear to respond less reliably [21, 25]. If clinical EGUS is confirmed or suspected, omeprazole is preferred, as H2RA therapy will likely result in less effective ulcer healing [10, 11].

Other therapies

In humans, sucralfate provides protection against stress-induced ulcers and decreases the risk of pathogenic gastric colonization [26]. The mechanism of action likely involves adherence to ulcerated mucosa, stimulation of mucus secretion, enhanced prostaglandin E synthesis, and/or concentration of growth factor at the site of ulceration [27]. The efficacy of sucralfate for prevention or healing of ulcers in horses has not been determined. In one trial, sucralfate did not promote subclinical ulcer healing in foals, compared to corn syrup [28]. In an experimental trial of phenylbutazone-induced disease in foals, simultaneous sucralfate administration reduced oral ulceration and gastric epithelial necrosis, but not squamous or glandular ulceration [29]. The currently recommended dose of sucralfate is 10–20 mg/kg bwt, PO, q6–8 h. Contrary to some reports, sucralfate does not appear to require an acidic environment to remain effective [30–32]. Hence, alternating the timing of sucralfate and antacid drugs appears unnecessary.

Due to the very large volume and frequent dosing schedule (i.e., 200 ml, PO, q2–4 h) necessary to alter intragastric pH, antacids do not provide a practical alternative for ulcer therapy in the horse [33].

The synthetic prostaglandin E1 analog misoprostol, which acts by inhibiting acid secretion and enhancing mucosal cytoprotection, has proven useful in the treatment of gastric and duodenal ulcers in humans [34]. In horses, misoprostol administered at a dose of 5 µg/kg bwt, PO, increased gastric pH [35]. Misoprostol has also been shown to ameliorate the adverse effects of flunixin on mucosal recovery after ischemic injury *in vitro* [36]. Misoprostol should not be used in pregnant mares due to the risk of abortion.

In foals with GDUD and evidence of delayed gastric emptying, it is important to determine whether or not a physical obstruction is present. If not, prokinetic therapy with either erythromycin or bethanechol (discussed later in this chapter) should be considered. If significant pyloric or duodenal stricture is present, surgical therapy is warranted.

Therapy for diarrhea and infectious causes of GI disease

In most cases of acute colitis, therapy consists primarily of crystalloid and/or colloid fluid therapy, anti-inflammatory and antiendotoxic therapy, and supportive care, including laminitis prevention. In foals less than 1 month of age with diarrhea, broad-spectrum antimicrobial therapy is strongly indicated due to the high likelihood of bacteremia [37, 38]. Based upon likely pathogens, initial therapy with ampicillin and amikacin is typically recommended. In adult horses, broad-spectrum antimicrobial therapy is not typically indicated in cases of acute or undifferentiated colitis and did not improve outcome in one retrospective report [39]. Some consider broad-spectrum bactericidal therapy indicated with clinical or laboratory evidence of bacteremia or severe immunosuppression (e.g., segmented neutrophil count <500 µl). Prolonged antimicrobial therapy should be avoided, however, as it can cause or exacerbate existing colitis. Some antimicrobials seem to predispose the horse to the development of colitis. For example, therapy with trimethoprim–sulfa or ceftiofur for as little as 1 week has been shown to disrupt the normal fecal microflora and allow proliferation of *Salmonella* and *Clostridium difficile* in healthy horses [40]. Despite that, the incidence of antimicrobial-associated diarrhea appears very low in referral private practices [41].

Loperamide, a phenylpiperidine derivative, has a similar structure to opiate receptor agonists, but poor bioavailability and no blood–brain barrier permeability [42]. Thus, it primarily has local effects upon the GI tract, and it has been shown in the horse to decrease fecal weight, fecal water, and sodium transport [43, 44]. Documentation of the clinical efficacy of loperamide in adult horses with diarrhea is lacking, but anecdotally, it has been effective in some diarrheic foals when administered at doses of 0.04–0.16 mg/kg bwt, PO, q6 h. Initially, there was some concern regarding the use of loperamide in cases of confirmed or potential infectious diarrhea, but it has been shown to be safe and effective in many randomized, placebo-controlled trials of traveler's diarrhea and children with acute diarrhea [45, 46]. In a meta-analysis of loperamide use in children, some serious adverse events were reported in those less than 3 years of age, especially with severe systemic illness or bloody diarrhea [46]. Thus, care should be taken when using loperamide in neonatal foals or those with suspected clostridial enteritis.

Di-tri-octahedral smectite (DTOS) has been shown to bind *C. difficile* toxins A, B, and C, as well as *Clostridium perfringens* enterotoxin (CPE); thus, it is recommended for antibiotic-associated or other clostridial diarrhea [47, 48]. Activated charcoal administered at a dose of 1–3 g/kg bwt, via a nasogastric tube as a slurry 1–2 times per day, may also be beneficial, especially following ingestion of a known toxin. Bismuth subsalicylate administered at a dose of 4–8 ml/kg bwt, PO, q4–8 h has antidiarrheal properties in other species. It has been shown less effective than DTOS for binding clostridial toxin *in vitro* and does not have documented efficacy in adult horses or foals [47].

Probiotics are frequently recommended as they are thought to potentially help, but not do harm. This theory may not be true, as demonstrated in the results of one study where a strain of *Lactobacillus pentosus* actually increased, rather than prevented, diarrhea in foals [49]. Another report demonstrated no apparent efficacy, but also no adverse effects, of *Saccharomyces boulardii* in the treatment of antimicrobial-associated diarrhea in adult horses [50]. A prior report, however, demonstrated potential efficacy of *S. boulardii* in the treatment of horses with acute colitis [51]. Thus, despite widespread use, the role of probiotics, in general, and many bacteria, specifically, for the treatment and prevention of diarrhea in horses warrants further study.

In certain geographic regions, sand enteropathy is associated with colic and/or diarrhea. Although most practitioners recommend therapy with psyllium, results in experimental trials have produced conflicting results as to its efficacy in increasing sand excretion. One early report found no significant effect of psyllium administration, while another found significantly increased sand elimination after therapy with psyllium in combination with mineral oil [52, 53]. Most recommendations for the treatment of sand enteropathy include psyllium mucilloid at a dose of 500 g in 2–4 l of mineral oil administered via nasogastric tube q24 h for 3–5 days.

Antimicrobial therapy is indicated for some specific infectious causes of GI disease in horses. Though salmonellosis is one of the most common infectious GI diseases in horses, directed antimicrobial therapy is rarely indicated, and it can increase *Salmonella* shedding [40]. In foals with documented salmonellosis, therapy with enrofloxacin is reserved for cases of localized infection, especially orthopedic infection, with documented resistance to aminoglycosides and 3rd-/4th-generation cephalosporins due to concerns for the development of arthropathy [54].

Therapy with metronidazole is typically recommended for clostridial enteritis in foals, though metronidazole use may also predispose to *C. difficile* diarrhea in adult horses [55]. Oxytetracycline administered at a dose of 6.6 mg/kg bwt, IV, q12–24 h for 3–5 days is the treatment of choice for Potomac horse fever. Affected horses typically begin to show improvement within 24 h after initiation of therapy, with reduction of fever and improvement in attitude and appetite [56]. Several antimicrobial options have been recommended for weanlings with suspected or confirmed equine proliferative enteropathy (EPE) caused by *Lawsonia intracellularis*. Typical choices include macrolides, chloramphenicol, oxytetracycline, doxycycline, or minocycline, depending upon the systemic status of the foal [57]. Drugs with significant potential for renal toxicity should be avoided in foals with hypovolemia or preexisting azotemia. In the rare instance of an adult horse with EPE, macrolides should be avoided due to the very significant risk of severe to fatal colitis. Antimicrobial therapy should continue for 2–3 weeks, as spontaneous resolution of clinically affected foals has not been documented. Clinical improvement usually precedes resolution of hypoproteinemia. Directed therapy is not indicated in viral causes of diarrhea in foals, as affected animals typically respond to supportive care alone, including broad-spectrum antimicrobial therapy in foals less than 1 month of age.

Therapy for ileus

Motility-modifying drugs play an important role in the treatment of GI ileus. Most motility-modifying drugs require a healthy intestinal wall in order to enhance intestinal contraction; thus, their effectiveness after intestinal manipulation or with primary inflammatory diseases, such as proximal enteritis, remains speculative. For cases of proximal enteritis, gastric decompression, anti-inflammatory and antiendotoxic therapy, laminitis prevention, and maintenance of plasma volume comprise the cornerstone of therapy. Specific prokinetic therapy has not demonstrated clinical benefit, but lidocaine, which has potential anti-inflammatory properties as well, may be useful [58]. Prokinetic drugs are typically used to prevent or treat postoperative ileus (POI) or cecal emptying dysfunction and are unlikely to be harmful, assuming the absence of a physical obstruction.

Lidocaine, an aminoamide local anesthetic, has been reported to be the most commonly used putative prokinetic agent [59]. When administered IV, lidocaine may suppress primary afferent neurons, thereby limiting reflex efferent inhibition of motility, or it may block the inhibitory effect of nonadrenergic, noncholinergic (NANC) neurotransmitters on smooth muscle [60]. Lidocaine also has significant anti-inflammatory properties, including amelioration of the lipopolysaccharide (LPS)-induced cytokine response, decreased neutrophil free-radical production, impaired leukocyte phagocytic function, and inhibition of leukocyte migration through suppression of chemokines [61, 62]. Lidocaine also decreased clinical scores after experimental LPS administration to healthy horses and ameliorated the inhibitory effects of flunixin meglumine on jejunal mucosal barrier recovery following ischemia. [62–64]

The most frequently recommended infusion rate of lidocaine is a loading dose of 1.3 mg/kg bwt administered over 15 min followed by a CRI at 0.05 mg/kg/min for 24 h. Target serum concentrations range from 1 to 2 mg/dl. In one prospective trial in horses following exploratory laparotomy for colic, lidocaine, relative to saline, had no significant effect on return of borborygmi,

time to first feces, or gastric reflux [65]. Unfortunately, very few horses in that trial had small intestinal strangulating lesions or POI, the primary conditions likely to benefit from lidocaine therapy. In other trials, lidocaine has been associated with reduced duration of reflux, time to first fecal passage, and hospital stay in horses with POI or duodenitis/proximal jejunitis (DPJ) and a reduced incidence of POI and increased short-term survival in horses undergoing surgery for small intestinal colic [60, 66].

Lidocaine infusions have been reported to be associated with muscle fasciculations, ataxia, and seizures; thus, close monitoring is warranted. These effects are dose dependent and reversible. They may also be more likely to occur in hypoproteinemic horses, for although the drug has a very short half-life, it is highly protein bound.

Bethanechol is a methyl derivate of carbachol and an acetylcholine receptor agonist. The drug acts both at the myenteric plexus and muscarinic receptors on intestinal smooth muscle cells, primarily at M_3 receptors, although M_2 receptors are involved to a lesser extent [67]. Bethanechol is not degraded by anticholinesterase. Potential adverse effects primarily relate to cholinergic activation and include abdominal discomfort, sweating, and salivation. Side effects are minimized by administering bethanechol at doses of 0.025–0.05 mg/kg bwt, SC. Although bethanechol stimulates motility throughout the GI tract, it is not used with any frequency in horses [59]. It is most commonly used in the management of delayed gastric emptying, as it has been shown to significantly increase gastric contractility and hasten both liquid- and solid-phase gastric emptying in healthy horses [68]. Bethanechol also increases the relative strength and duration of contractions in the cecum and right ventral colon, hastens cecal emptying, and increases large colon myoelectrical activity [69, 70].

Neostigmine, a cholinesterase inhibitor, has been shown to promote cecal and colonic contractile activity and enhance cecal emptying in normal ponies [69]. Neostigmine was also shown, however, to significantly delay gastric emptying in healthy adult horses [69, 70]. A survey of prokinetic use indicated that neostigmine was most commonly used in the management of large intestinal disease [59]. Recommended dosages of neostigmine range from 0.022 to 0.025 mg/kg bwt, IV.

Metoclopramide is a partial 5-hydroxytryptamine 4 (5HT-4) receptor agonist, a 5HT-3 receptor antagonist, and an antagonist of dopamine 1 (DA_1) and dopamine 2 (DA_2) receptors. Metoclopramide can cross the blood–brain barrier, and associated central DA_2 antagonism can cause extrapyramidal signs, including seizures [71]. For this reason, newer benzamides lack dopamine receptor antagonism activity. Metoclopramide administered IV at a dose of 0.125 mg/kg bwt partially ameliorated endotoxin-induced delayed gastric emptying, but adverse effects, including excitement, mild colic and diarrhea, muscle fasciculations, and elevated body temperatures, were reported in study horses [72]. In contrast, in a group of horses that had undergone colic surgery, metoclopramide administered during the immediate postoperative period as a CRI at a rate of 0.04 mg/kg/h was well tolerated and significantly decreased the volume and duration of gastric reflux, relative to control and intermittent infusions [73].

Mosapride, a selective 5HT-4 agonist, increased myoelectric activity of the small intestine and cecum of horses after oral administration, despite other reports that actions of 5HT on the equine jejunum were primarily mediated through 5HT-2 and 5HT-3 receptors [74]. Mosapride administered PO at a dose of 1.5–2 mg/kg bwt hastened gastric emptying and increased jejunal and cecal motility and the maximum amplitude of electrointestinography within the small intestine following jejunocecostomy in healthy horses [75, 76].

Tegaserod, a selective 5HT-4 agonist, is used in humans for the treatment of irritable bowel syndrome [77]. In horses, tegaserod has been shown to decrease total GI transit time and increase pelvic flexure contractile activity *in vitro* [78–80]. Tegaserod appears safe and therapeutic plasma concentrations were obtained after a single oral dose of 0.27 mg/kg bwt [79].

Domperidone acts as a competitive peripheral DA_2 receptor antagonist and has been used to manage gastroparesis in humans [81]. Due to drug-enhanced prolactin release from the anterior pituitary, domperidone has primarily been used at a dose of 1.1 mg/kg/day, PO, for management of agalactia in mares after grazing endophyte-infected tall fescue. A modest prokinetic effect was demonstrated in two ponies after IV administration of domperidone at a dose of 0.2 mg/kg bwt in a model of experimental ileus [82].

Erythromycin is a direct motilin receptor agonist that has been shown to enhance gastric emptying and hindgut motility [68, 83]. Despite a higher density of motilin receptors in the duodenum than the cecum or pelvic flexure,

the prokinetic effects appear more pronounced in the hindgut [63, 84]. Unfortunately, erythromycin has limited effectiveness clinically. Bethanechol is more effective for enhancing gastric emptying, although its effectiveness on cecal motility appears to be markedly reduced in the immediate postoperative period [68, 85]. High doses, constant infusion, or prolonged use of erythromycin also induces receptor tachyphylaxis and therefore reduced efficacy. In addition, the total number of motilin receptors and the amount of motilin receptor mRNA were significantly decreased after as little as 2 h of intraluminal distention [86]. Erythromycin can induce diarrhea in adult horses; thus, prolonged administration should be avoided.

Several opioid antagonists have potential for prokinetic activity. Naloxone administered at a dose of 0.05 mg/kg, IV, induced contractile activity in the cecum and left colon of horses, but was not beneficial for preventing POI in humans [87, 88]. Peripherally acting opioid antagonists, such as *N*-methylnaltrexone (MNTX), improved GI tract function in humans requiring opioids for pain management and had a similar effect—that of partially preventing morphine-associated alterations in GI transit—in healthy horses [89].

Alpha-2 adrenoreceptor antagonists, such as yohimbine and tolazoline, counteract increased sympathetic outflow in response to nociceptive stimulation. Yohimbine administered at a dose of 75 µg/kg bwt, slow IV, increased cecal motility and emptying in normal ponies and attenuated endotoxin-associated effects on motility [69, 90].

References

1 Plue, R.E., Wall, H.G., Daurio, C., Attebery, D.K., Cox, J.L. & Wallace, D.H. (1999) Safety of omeprazole paste in foals and mature horses. *Equine Veterinary Journal Supplement*, **31** (S29), 63–66.

2 Murray, M.J., Eichorn, E.S., Holste, J.E. *et al.* (1999) Safety, acceptability and endoscopic findings in foals and yearling horses treated with a paste formulation of omeprazole for twenty-eight days. *Equine Veterinary Journal Supplement*, **31** (S29), 67–70.

3 MacAllister, C.G., Sifferman, R.L., McClure, S.R. *et al.* (1999) Effects of omeprazole paste on healing of spontaneous gastric ulcers in horses and foals: A field trial. *Equine Veterinary Journal Supplement*, **31** (S29), 77–80.

4 Murray, M.J., Haven, M.L., Eichorn, E.S., Zhang, D., Eagleson, J. & Hickey, G.J. (1997) Effects of omeprazole on healing of naturally-occurring gastric ulcers in thoroughbred racehorses. *Equine Veterinary Journal*, **29**, 425–429.

5 Vatistas, N.J., Snyder, J.R., Nieto, J., Thompson, D., Pollmeier, M. & Holste, J. (1999) Acceptability of a paste formulation and efficacy of high dose omeprazole in healing gastric ulcers in horses maintained in race training. *Equine Veterinary Journal Supplement*, **31** (S29), 71–76.

6 Andrews, F.M., Sifferman, R.L., Bernard, W. *et al.* (1999) Efficacy of omeprazole paste in the treatment and prevention of gastric ulcers in horses. *Equine Veterinary Journal Supplement*, 81–86.

7 McClure, S.R., White, G.W., Sifferman, R.L. *et al.* (2005) Efficacy of omeprazole paste for prevention of recurrence of gastric ulcers in horses in race training. *Journal of the American Veterinary Medical Association*, **226**, 1685–1688.

8 McClure, S.R., White, G.W., Sifferman, R.L. *et al.* (2005) Efficacy of omeprazole paste for prevention of gastric ulcers in horses in race training. *Journal of the American Veterinary Medical Association*, **226**, 1681–1684.

9 White, G., McClure, S.R., Sifferman, R. *et al.* (2007) Effects of short-term light to heavy exercise on gastric ulcer development in horses and efficacy of omeprazole paste in preventing gastric ulceration. *Journal of the American Veterinary Medical Association*, **230**, 1680–1682.

10 Lester, G.D., Smith, R.L. & Robertson, I.D. (2005) Effects of treatment with omeprazole or ranitidine on gastric squamous ulceration in racing Thoroughbreds. *Journal of the American Veterinary Medical Association*, **227**, 1636–1639.

11 Nieto, J.E., Spier, S.J., Van Hoogmoed, L., Pipers, F., Timmerman, B. & Snyder, J.R. (2001) Comparison of omeprazole and cimetidine in healing of gastric ulcers and prevention of recurrence in horses. *Equine Veterinary Education*, **13**, 260–264.

12 Sanchez, L.C., Murray, M.J. & Merritt, A.M. (2004) Effect of omeprazole paste on intragastric pH in clinically normal neonatal foals. *American Journal of Veterinary Research*, **65**, 1039–1041.

13 Javsicas, L.H. & Sanchez, L.C. (2008) The effect of omeprazole paste on intragastric pH in clinically ill neonatal foals. *Equine Veterinary Journal*, **40**, 41–44.

14 Merritt, A.M., Sanchez, L.C., Burrow, J.A., Church, M. & Ludzia, S. (2003) Effect of GastroGard and three compounded oral omeprazole preparations on 24 h intragastric pH in gastrically cannulated mature horses. *Equine Veterinary Journal*, **35**, 691–695.

15 Nieto, J.E., Spier, S., Pipers, F.S. *et al.* (2002) Comparison of paste and suspension formulations of omeprazole in the healing of gastric ulcers in racehorses in active training. *Journal of the American Veterinary Medical Association*, **221**, 1139–1143.

16 Orsini, J.A., Haddock, M., Stine, L., Sullivan, E.K., Rabuffo, T.S. & Smith, G. (2003) Odds of moderate or severe gastric ulceration in racehorses receiving antiulcer medications. *Journal of the American Veterinary Medical Association*, **223**, 336–339.

17 Andrews, F.M., Frank, N., Sommardahl, C.S., Buchanan, B.R., Elliott, S.B. & Allen, V.A. (2006) Effects of intravenously administrated omeprazole on gastric juice pH and gastric ulcer scores in adult horses. *Journal of Veterinary Internal Medicine*, **20**, 1202–1206.

18 McKeever, J.M., McKeever, K.H., Albeirci, J.M., Gordon, M.E. & Manso Filho, H.C. (2006) Effect of omeprazole on markers of performance in gastric ulcer-free standardbred horses. *Equine Veterinary Journal Supplement*, **38** (S36), 668–671.

19 Ryan, C.A., Sanchez, L.C., Giguere, S. & Vickroy, T. (2005) Pharmacokinetics and pharmacodynamics of pantoprazole in clinically normal neonatal foals. *Equine Veterinary Journal*, **37**, 336–341.

20 Campbell-Thompson, M.L. & Merritt, A.M. (1987) Effect of ranitidine on gastric acid secretion in young male horses. *American Journal of Veterinary Research*, **48**, 1511–1515.

21 Sanchez, L.C., Lester, G.D. & Merritt, A.M. (1998) Effect of ranitidine on intragastric pH in clinically normal neonatal foals. *Journal of the American Veterinary Medical Association*, **212**, 1407–1412.

22 Becht, J.L. & Byars, T.D. (1986) Gastroduodenal ulceration in foals. *Equine Veterinary Journal*, **18**, 307–312.

23 Furr, M.O. & Murray, M.J. (1989) Treatment of gastric ulcers in horses with histamine type 2 receptor antagonists. *Equine Veterinary Journal Supplement*, 77–79.

24 Murray, M.J. & Grodinsky, C. (1992) The effects of famotidine, ranitidine and magnesium hydroxide/aluminium hydroxide on gastric fluid pH in adult horses. *Equine Veterinary Journal Supplement*, 52–55.

25 Sanchez, L.C., Lester, G.D. & Merritt, A.M. (2001) Intragastric pH in critically ill neonatal foals and the effect of ranitidine. *Journal of the American Veterinary Medical Association*, **218**, 907–911.

26 Ephgrave, K.S., Kleiman-Wexler, R., Pfaller, M. *et al.* (1998) Effects of sucralfate vs antacids on gastric pathogens: Results of a double-blind clinical trial. *Archives of Surgery*, **133**, 251–257.

27 Ogihara, Y. & Okabe, S. (1993) Effect and mechanism of sucralfate on healing of acetic acid-induced gastric ulcers in rats. *Journal of Physiology and Pharmacology*, **44**, 109–118.

28 Borne, A.T. & MacAllister, C.G. (1993) Effect of sucralfate on healing of subclinical gastric ulcers in foals. *Journal of the American Veterinary Medical Association*, **202**, 1465–1468.

29 Geor, R.J., Petrie, L., Papich, M.G. & Rousseaux, C. (1989) The protective effects of sucralfate and ranitidine in foals experimentally intoxicated with phenylbutazone. *Canadian Journal of Veterinary Research*, **53**, 231–238.

30 Danesh, B.J., Duncan, A. & Russell, R.I. (1987) Is an acid pH medium required for the protective effect of sucralfate against mucosal injury? *American Journal of Medicine*, **83**, 11–13.

31 Konturek, S.J., Brzozowski, T., Mach, T., Konturek, W.J., Bogdal, J. & Stachura, J. (1989) Importance of an acid milieu in the sucralfate-induced gastroprotection against ethanol damage. *Scandinavian Journal of Gastroenterology*, **24**, 807–812.

32 Danesh, J.Z., Duncan, A., Russell, R.I. & Mitchell, G. (1988) Effect of intragastric pH on mucosal protective action of sucralfate. *Gut*, **29**, 1379–1385.

33 Clark, C.K., Merritt, A.M., Burrow, J.A. & Steible, C.K. (1996) Effect of aluminum hydroxide/magnesium hydroxide antacid and bismuth subsalicylate on gastric pH in horses. *Journal of the American Veterinary Medical Association*, **208**, 1687–1691.

34 Leandro, G., Pilotto, A., Franceschi, M., Bertin, T., Lichino, E. & Di Mario, F. (2001) Prevention of acute NSAID-related gastroduodenal damage: A meta- analysis of controlled clinical trials. *Digestive Diseases and Sciences*, **46**, 1924–1936.

35 Sangiah, S., MacAllister, C.C. & Amouzadeh, H.R. (1989) Effects of misoprostol and omeprazole on basal gastric pH and free acid content in horses. *Research in Veterinary Science*, **47**, 350–354.

36 Tomlinson, J.E. & Blikslager, A.T. (2005) Effects of cyclooxygenase inhibitors flunixin and deracoxib on permeability of ischaemic-injured equine jejunum. *Equine Veterinary Journal*, **37**, 75–80.

37 Frederick, J., Giguere, S. & Sanchez, L.C. (2009) Infectious agents detected in the feces of diarrheic foals: A retrospective study of 233 cases (2003–2008). *Journal of Veterinary Internal Medicine*, **23**, 1254–1260.

38 Hollis, A.R., Wilkins, P.A., Palmer, J.E. & Boston, R.C. (2008) Bacteremia in equine neonatal diarrhea: A retrospective study (1990–2007). *Journal of Veterinary Internal Medicine*, **22**, 1203–1209.

39 Chilcoat, C.L., Glickman, L. & Glickman, N. (1998) Is antimicrobial therapy beneficial in the treatment of undifferentiated colitis in the horse? 6th Equine Colic Research Symposium, November 8–11, Georgia Center for Continuing Education, University of Georgia, Athens GA. p. 20.

40 Harlow, B.E., Lawrence, L.M. & Flythe, M.D. (2013) Diarrhea-associated pathogens, lactobacilli and cellulolytic bacteria in equine feces: Responses to antibiotic challenge. *Veterinary Microbiology*, **166**, 225–232.

41 Barr, B.S., Waldridge, B.M., Morresey, P.R. *et al.* (2013) Antimicrobial-associated diarrhoea in three equine referral practices. *Equine Veterinary Journal*, **45**, 154–158.

42 Baker, D.E. (2007) Loperamide: A pharmacological review. *Reviews in Gastroenterological Disorders*, **7** (Suppl 3), S11–S18.

43 Roberts, M.C. & Argenzio, A. (1986) Effects of amitraz, several opiate derivatives and anticholinergic agents on intestinal transit in ponies. *Equine Veterinary Journal*, **18**, 256–260.

44 Alexander, F. (1978) The effect of some anti-diarrhoeal drugs on intestinal transit and faecal excretion of water and electrolytes in the horse. *Equine Veterinary Journal*, **10**, 229–234.

45 Riddle, M.S., Arnold, S. & Tribble, D.R. (2008) Effect of adjunctive loperamide in combination with antibiotics on treatment outcomes in traveler's diarrhea: A systematic review and meta-analysis. *Clinical Infectious Diseases*, **47**, 1007–1014.

46 Li, S.T., Grossman, D.C. & Cummings, P. (2007) Loperamide therapy for acute diarrhea in children: Systematic review and meta-analysis. *PLoS Medicine*, **4**, e98.

47 Lawler, J.B., Hassel, D.M., Magnuson, R.J., Hill, A.E., McCue, P.M. & Traub-Dargatz, J.L. (2008) Adsorptive effects of di-tri-octahedral smectite on Clostridium perfringens alpha, beta, and beta-2 exotoxins and equine colostral antibodies. *American Journal of Veterinary Research*, **69**, 233–239.

48 Weese, J.S., Cote, N.M. & de Gannes, R.V. (2003) Evaluation of in vitro properties of di-tri-octahedral smectite on clostridial toxins and growth. *Equine Veterinary Journal*, **35**, 638–641.

49 Weese, J.S. & Rousseau, J. (2005) Evaluation of Lactobacillus pentosus WE7 for prevention of diarrhea in neonatal foals. *Journal of the American Veterinary Medical Association*, **226**, 2031–2034.

50 Boyle, A.G., Magdesian, K.G., Gallop, R., Gallop, R. & Sigdel, S. (2013) Saccharomyces boulardii viability and efficacy in horses with antimicrobial-induced diarrhoea. *Veterinary Record*, **172**, 128.

51 Desrochers, A.M., Dolente, B.A., Roy, M.F., Boston, R. & Carlisle, S. (2005) Efficacy of Saccharomyces boulardii for treatment of horses with acute enterocolitis. *Journal of the American Veterinary Medical Association*, **227**, 954–959.

52 Hotwagner, K. & Iben, C. (2008) Evacuation of sand from the equine intestine with mineral oil, with and without psyllium. *Journal of Animal Physiology and Animal Nutrition*, **92**, 86–91.

53 Hammock, P.D., Freeman, D.E. & Baker, G.J. (1998) Failure of psyllium mucilloid to hasten evaluation of sand from the equine large intestine. *Veterinary Surgery*, **27**, 547–554.

54 Vivrette, S.L., Bostian, A., Bermingham, E. & Papich, M.G. (2001) Quinolone-induced arthropathy in neonatal foals. *Proceedings of the American Association of Equine Practitioners*, **47**, 376–377.

55 Ruby, R., Magdesian, K.G. & Kass, P.H. (2009) Comparison of clinical, microbiologic, and clinicopathologic findings in horses positive and negative for Clostridium difficile infection. *Journal of the American Veterinary Medical Association*, **234**, 777–784.

56 Bartol, J.M. (2002) Potomac horse fever. In: T. Mair, T. Divers & N. Ducharme (eds), *Manual of Equine Gastroenterology*, pp. 412–415. W.B. Saunders, London.

57 Pusterla, N. & Gebhart, C. (2013) Lawsonia intracellularis infection and proliferative enteropathy in foals. *Veterinary Microbiology*, **167**, 34–41.

58 Cohen, N.D., Faber, N.A. & Brumbaugh, G.W. (1995) Use of bethanechol and metoclopramide in horses with duodenitis proximal jejunitis: 13 cases (1987–1993). *Journal of Equine Veterinary Science*, **15**, 492–494.

59 Van Hoogmoed, L.M., Nieto, J.E., Snyder, J.R. & Harmon, F.A. (2004) Survey of prokinetic use in horses with gastrointestinal injury. *Veterinary Surgery*, **33**, 279–285.

60 Malone, E., Ensink, J., Turner, T. *et al.* (2006) Intravenous continuous infusion of lidocaine for treatment of equine ileus. *Veterinary Surgery*, **35**, 60–66.

61 Li, C.Y., Tsai, C.S., Hsu, P.C., Chueh, S.H., Wong, C.S. & Ho, S.T. (2003) Lidocaine attenuates monocyte chemoattractant protein-1 production and chemotaxis in human

monocytes: Possible mechanisms for its effect on inflammation. *Anesthesia & Analgesia*, **97**, 1312–1316.

62 Peiro, J.R., Barnabe, P.A., Cadioli, F.A. *et al.* (2010) Effects of lidocaine infusion during experimental endotoxemia in horses. *Journal of Veterinary Internal Medicine*, **24**, 940–948.

63 Cook, V.L., Jones, S.J., McDowell, M., Campbell, N.B., Davis, J.L. & Blikslager, A.T. (2008) Attenuation of ischaemic injury in the equine jejunum by administration of systemic lidocaine. *Equine Veterinary Journal*, **40**, 353–357.

64 Cook, V.L., Jones Shults, J., McDowell, M.R. *et al.* (2009) Anti-inflammatory effects of intravenously administered lidocaine hydrochloride on ischemia-injured jejunum in horses. *American Journal of Veterinary Research*, **70**, 1259–1268.

65 Brianceau, P., Chevalier, H., Karas, A. *et al.* (2002) Intravenous lidocaine and small-intestinal size, abdominal fluid, and outcome after colic surgery in horses. *Journal of Veterinary Internal Medicine*, **16**, 736–741.

66 Torfs, S., Delesalle, C., Dewulf, J., Devisscher, L. & Deprez, P. (2009) Risk factors for equine postoperative ileus and effectiveness of prophylactic lidocaine. *Journal of Veterinary Internal Medicine*, **23**, 606–611.

67 Marti, M., Mevissen, M., Althaus, H. & Steiner, A. (2005) In vitro effects of bethanechol on equine gastrointestinal contractility and functional characterization of involved muscarinic receptor subtypes. *Journal of Veterinary Pharmacology and Therapeutics*, **28**, 565–574.

68 Ringger, N.C., Lester, G.D., Neuwirth, L., Merritt, A.M., Vetro, T. & Harrison, J. (1996) Effect of bethanechol or erythromycin on gastric emptying in horses. *American Journal of Veterinary Research*, **57**, 1771–1775.

69 Lester, G.D., Merritt, A.M., Neuwirth, L., Vetro-Widenhouse, T., Steible, C. & Rice, B. (1998) Effect of alpha 2-adrenergic, cholinergic, and nonsteroidal anti-inflammatory drugs on myoelectric activity of ileum, cecum, and right ventral colon and on cecal emptying of radiolabeled markers in clinically normal ponies. *American Journal of Veterinary Research*, **59**, 320–327.

70 Roger, T. & Ruckebusch, Y. (1987) Pharmacological modulation of postprandial colonic motor activity in the pony. *Journal of Veterinary Pharmacology and Therapeutics*, **10**, 273–282.

71 Gerring, E.E. & Hunt, J.M. (1986) Pathophysiology of equine postoperative ileus: Effect of adrenergic blockade, parasympathetic stimulation and metoclopramide in an experimental model. *Equine Veterinary Journal*, **18**, 249–255.

72 Doherty, T.J., Andrews, F.M., Abraha, T.W., Osborne, D. & Frazier, D.L. (1999) Metoclopramide ameliorates the effects of endotoxin on gastric emptying of acetaminophen in horses. *Canadian Journal of Veterinary Research*, **63**, 37–40.

73 Dart, A.J., Peauroi, J.R., Hodgson, D.R. & Pascoe, J.R. (1996) Efficacy of metoclopramide for treatment of ileus in horses following small intestinal surgery: 70 cases (1989–1992). *Australian Veterinary Journal*, **74**, 280–284.

74 Nieto, J.E., Snyder, J.R., Kollias-Baker, C. & Stanley, S. (2000) In vitro effects of 5-hydroxytryptamine and cisapride on the circular smooth muscle of the jejunum of horses. *American Journal of Veterinary Research*, **61**, 1561–1565.

75 Okamura, K., Sasaki, N., Yamada, M., Yamada, H. & Inokuma, H. (2009) Effects of mosapride citrate, metoclopramide hydrochloride, lidocaine hydrochloride, and cisapride citrate on equine gastric emptying, small intestinal and caecal motility. *Research in Veterinary Science*, **86**, 302–308.

76 Okamura, K., Sasaki, N., Kikuchi, T. *et al.* (2009) Effects of mosapride on motility of the small intestine and caecum in normal horses after jejunocaecostomy. *Journal of Veterinary Science*, **10**, 157–160.

77 Camilleri, M. (2001) Management of the irritable bowel syndrome. *Gastroenterology*, **120**, 652–668.

78 Lippold, B.S., Hildebrand, J. & Straub, R. (2004) Tegaserod (HTF 919) stimulates gut motility in normal horses. *Equine Veterinary Journal*, **36**, 622–627.

79 Delco, M.L., Nieto, J.E., Craigmill, A.L., Stanley, S.D. & Snyder, J.R. (2007) Pharmacokinetics and in vitro effects of tegaserod, a serotonin 5-hydroxytryptamine 4 (5-HT4) receptor agonist with prokinetic activity in horses. *Veterinary Therapeutics*, **8**, 77–87.

80 Weiss, R., Abel, D., Scholtysik, G., Straub, R. & Mevissen, M. (2002) 5-Hydroxytryptamine mediated contractions in isolated preparations of equine ileum and pelvic flexure: Pharmacological characterization of a new 5-HT(4) agonist. *Journal of Veterinary Pharmacology and Therapeutics*, **25**, 49–58.

81 Ahmad, N., Keith-Ferris, J., Gooden, E. & Abell, T. (2006) Making a case for domperidone in the treatment of gastrointestinal motility disorders. *Current Opinion in Pharmacology*, **6**, 571–576.

82 Gerring, E.L. (1989) Effects of pharmacological agents on gastrointestinal motility. *Veterinary Clinics of North America: Equine Practice*, **5**, 283–294.

83 Lester, G.D., Merritt, A.M., Neuwirth, L., Vetro-Widenhouse, T., Steible, C. & Rice, B. (1998) Effect of erythromycin lactobionate on myoelectric activity of ileum, cecum, and right ventral colon, and cecal emptying of radiolabeled markers in clinically normal ponies. *American Journal of Veterinary Research*, **59**, 328–334.

84 Koenig, J.B., Cote, N., LaMarre, J. *et al.* (2002) Binding of radiolabeled porcine motilin and erythromycin lactobionate to smooth muscle membranes in various segments of the equine gastrointestinal tract. *American Journal of Veterinary Research*, **63**, 1545–1550.

85 Roussel, A.J., Hooper, R.N., Cohen, N.D., Bye, A.D., Hicks, R.J. & Bohl, T.W. (2000) Prokinetic effects of erythromycin on the ileum, cecum, and pelvic flexure of horses during the postoperative period. *American Journal of Veterinary Research*, **61**, 420–424.

86 Koenig, J.B., Sawhney, S., Cote, N. & LaMarre, J. (2006) Effect of intraluminal distension or ischemic strangulation obstruction of the equine jejunum on jejunal motilin receptors and binding of erythromycin lactobionate. *American Journal of Veterinary Research*, **67**, 815–820.

87 Roger, T., Bardon, T. & Ruckebusch, Y. (1985) Colonic motor responses in the pony: Relevance of colonic stimulation by opiate antagonists. *American Journal of Veterinary Research*, **46**, 31–35.

88 Luckey, A., Livingston, E. & Tache, Y. (2003) Mechanisms and treatment of postoperative ileus. *Archives of Surgery*, **138**, 206–214.

89 Boscan, P., Van Hoogmoed, L.M., Pypendop, B.H., Farver, T.B. & Snyder, J.R. (2006) Pharmacokinetics of the opioid antagonist N-methylnaltrexone and evaluation of its effects on gastrointestinal tract function in horses treated or not treated with morphine. *American Journal of Veterinary Research*, **67**, 998–1004.

90 Eades, S.C. & Moore, J.N. (1993) Blockade of endotoxin-induced cecal hypoperfusion and ileus with an alpha 2 antagonist in horses. *American Journal of Veterinary Research*, **54**, 586–590.

CHAPTER 12

Treatment of equine nervous system disorders

Cynthia Cole[1] and Bradford Bentz[2]

[1] Mars Veterinary, Portland, OR, USA
[2] Equine Medicine and Surgery, Bossier City, LA, USA

Introduction

In terms of drug therapy, the nervous system presents unique challenges compared to most other organ systems. Chief among these are the blood–brain barrier (BBB) and blood–cerebral spinal fluid (CSF) barrier. Although structurally different, both of these barriers limit the diffusion of all but the smallest and most hydrophobic of molecules, such as O_2 and CO_2. These barriers are not, however, inactive. For example, the BBB actively transports metabolic products, such as glucose, and occasionally exogenous agents, such as drugs or toxins, across the barrier with the aid of specific proteins. These transport proteins within the barriers also actively move molecules from the brain parenchyma and the CSF back into the blood. The physical barriers and active transport systems make it difficult to achieve clinically significant concentrations of many therapeutic agents within the brain and CSF. Penetration of a drug into the brain and CSF is dependent upon its physiochemical properties, including its molecular weight, lipid solubility, and ionization, as well as the degree to which it is bound to plasma proteins [1]. While the presence of meningeal inflammation may decrease the integrity of the barriers, allowing more drugs to cross, it is hard to predict the significance of this effect in any individual case. Finally, clinicians need to be aware that drug concentrations in the brain and spinal cord tissue may be different from those in the CSF. For example, concentrations of the highly lipophilic antimicrobial agent chloramphenicol

are higher in brain tissue, but lower in the CSF, compared to those produced in serum [2].

Central nervous system trauma

Trauma is a major cause of neurologic disease in the horse, with the spinal cord affected more commonly than the brain [3]. Manifestations of injury can vary tremendously from coma and paralysis in severe cases to weakness and gait deficits in milder cases. Trauma is usually divided into brain injury and spinal cord injury (SCI). Although there are similarities in the mechanisms of cell injury and responses in both tissues, there are also significant differences. Studies on the pathophysiology of central nervous system (CNS) injury in horses are lacking, but there is a large body of evidence from human and laboratory animal studies from which comparisons can be drawn. Excellent reviews of this material and its applicability to horses are available elsewhere [4, 5]. One important aspect to traumatic injury in the brain and spinal cord is that the damage often occurs in two phases. Phase one occurs from the initial traumatic event itself. Phase two occurs hours, days, or even weeks later when a complex cascade of biochemical and cellular responses to the initial injury causes a second round of tissue damage. Treatment of traumatic injuries to the brain and/or spinal cord is complex and requires extensive monitoring. Therefore, transportation to a tertiary care center should be considered whenever possible. In most field situations, the goals of

---

Equine Pharmacology, First Edition. Edited by Cynthia Cole, Bradford Bentz and Lara Maxwell.
© 2015 John Wiley & Sons, Inc. Published 2015 by John Wiley & Sons, Inc.

therapy are to prevent additional damage and stabilize the horse for transportation.

Traumatic brain injury

Head trauma in horses is typically caused by collisions with solid objects, falling, or flipping over backward. The forces of any impact are transmitted through the skull to the soft tissues beneath. Although the site of impact usually suffers the worst damage, the contralateral tissue can also be damaged from impacting the inside of the skull on the opposing side. Of particular concern in cases of traumatic brain injury (TBI) are increases in intracranial pressure (ICP), which can cause significant additional damage to the brain or even death. Unlike most other tissues, the brain is enclosed in a nonexpandable case of bone. Because the brain parenchyma is not compressible, blood flow in and out of the brain must be closely regulated. Increases in ICP can ultimately lead to decreases in cerebral blood flow, causing ischemia and cell death.

Treatment of TBI

The primary goal of therapy is to optimize delivery of oxygen and metabolic substrates to the brain to preserve undamaged cells and stabilize reversibly damaged tissue [4]. This is accomplished by optimizing cerebral blood flow and blood hemoglobin concentration. Cerebral perfusion pressure (CPP) is the difference between the mean arterial pressure (MAP) and ICP. Normally, autoregulatory mechanisms maintain cerebral blood flow over a wide range of MAP, but with TBI, these mechanisms may be disturbed and cerebral blood flow can become linearly related to MAP [6]. In these situations, decreases in MAP or increases in ICP can decrease CPP and thus cerebral blood flow, leading to ischemia. To optimize cerebral blood flow, mean arterial blood pressure should be maintained within normal limits, which in humans is >90 mm Hg, and increases in ICP should be prevented or addressed. In most cases of TBI, the sympathetic nervous system remains functional, and therefore, normal homeostatic mechanisms will aid in maintaining normal blood pressure. Intravenous infusion of isotonic fluid solutions, however, may be necessary to maintain or expand blood volume. If volume resuscitation alone does not restore normal pressure, pressor agents and/or inotropic drugs may be necessary. (see Chapters 15, and 7, for more details.) Glucose-containing fluids should be avoided because the

carbohydrate suppresses ketogenesis and may increase lactic acid production [7]. In the presence of severe hemorrhage, blood transfusions may be necessary to ensure the oxygen delivering capacity of the blood, but this is rarely the case in adult horses. Hypoxemia, which in this setting would be a PaO_2 <90 mm Hg, should be addressed by establishing a patent airway, treating any underlying pulmonary disease, and beginning nasal or tracheal insufflation with oxygen at 10–15 l/min [8, 9]. Foals can be intubated and mechanically ventilated if necessary.

Unfortunately, the final component needed to optimize cerebral blood flow, assessment and correction of elevated ICP, is the most difficult to achieve. Although no controlled studies have been conducted, raising the horse's head by 10–30, assuming no cervical fractures are present, is one of the simplest methods to help decrease ICP [4, 8]. In human neurocritical care settings, hyperventilation has been advocated to decrease ICP. However, recent research has demonstrated that hyperventilation decreases PaCO2, leading to CNS vasoconstriction, lower cerebral blood flow, and neurologic tissue injury [10]. Other interventions used to treat humans with elevated ICP include drainage of CSF, sedation, barbiturates, hyperosmolar treatment, and surgical decompression.

In horses, hyperosmolar therapy, with either hypertonic saline or mannitol, is most commonly used to treat elevated ICP. Hypertonic saline (5–7% NaCl) is typically administered at a dose of 4–6 ml/kg bwt over 15 min [4]. Because the BBB is only slightly permeable to sodium, hypertonic saline creates a large osmotic gradient to pull fluid from the cerebral interstitial space into the vascular space, which can dramatically decrease ICP. It can also produce similar effects systemically, ultimately resulting in increases in CPP. It is contraindicated in cases of dehydration, renal failure, hyperkalemic periodic paralysis, hypothermia, and ongoing intracerebral hemorrhage. Side effects include coagulopathies, excessive intravascular volume, and electrolyte abnormalities. Ideally, monitoring of serum electrolytes and central venous pressure, maintaining a normal pressure of 5–7 cm H_2O, should be carried out concurrently with hypertonic saline administration. The alcohol sugar mannitol has been used for many years in human and veterinary medicine as an osmotherapeutic agent. In horses, a 20% solution of mannitol can be administered at a dose of 0.25–2.0 mg/kg bwt, IV, over 20 min [4]. Mannitol has also been shown to reduce CSF production by up to 50%, leading to a prolonged decrease in ICP [11]. The use of mannitol has several limitations including causing hypotension and the development of hyperosmolality, which is associated with adverse effects on the renal and nervous systems [12]. Although these adverse effects may occur less commonly with hypertonic saline therapy, they do still occur. In addition, the beneficial effects of osmotherapy on long-term outcomes in humans suffering from TBI have not been definitively demonstrated [13]. Nevertheless, because other interventions for elevated ICP in horses are limited, osmotherapy should be considered in horses with TBI, but its potential adverse effects should be remembered as well.

The loop diuretic furosemide has also been used to decrease elevated ICP, although its efficacy is not well documented. In animal models of closed head trauma, one study demonstrated no effect of furosemide, when used either alone or in combination with mannitol, while another study demonstrated that furosemide worked synergistically with hypertonic saline to decrease brain edema [14, 15]. Nevertheless, in nondehydrated horses, the adverse effects of furosemide administration are minimal. Therefore, in horses with suspected or confirmed elevated ICP, furosemide has been recommended to be administered at a dose of 1.0 mg/kg bwt IV or as a continuous rate infusion (CRI) of 0.5 mg/kg/h either alone or 45 min after mannitol administration [16].

In human patients, barbiturates are believed to reduce ICP by suppressing cerebral metabolism, thus reducing cerebral metabolic demands and cerebral blood volume. Barbiturates also reduce blood pressure, however, and may decrease CPP. A recent review of data from seven clinical trials involving 341 people concluded that there is no evidence that barbiturates reduce death secondary to head trauma [17]. Although barbiturates did reduce ICP, they also caused hypotension in one out of four patients, an adverse effect that would offset any advantage. Nevertheless, in refractory cases, general anesthesia induced with guaifenesin at a dose of 50 mg/kg bwt IV as a 5% solution to effect and thiopental at a dose of 5 mg/kg bwt IV, followed by a CRI at 0.05 mg/kg/min, has been recommended [18]. Prior administration of mannitol or furosemide can exacerbate hypotension caused by barbiturates.

Anti-inflammatory medications are commonly administered after horses suffer a TBI to provide analgesia and reduce fever, which is often present. Fever has been shown to negatively affect outcome, and therefore, even if the TBI patient does not present with a fever, an NSAID should be administered preemptively. In addition, NSAIDs inhibit the inflammatory cascade associated with the development of secondary injury. Flunixin meglumine at a dose of 1.1 mg/kg bwt IV q12 h has been used most commonly for horses suffering from a TBI [8]. Corticosteroids are commonly administered in cases of TBI, but their efficacy has not been well defined in any species, including the horse, although they have been shown to be beneficial in spinal cord trauma [19]. Based on the studies of SCI, methylprednisolone sodium succinate (MPSS) administered within the first 8 h of TBI has been recommended at an initial dose of 30 mg/kg bwt IV followed by a CRI at 5.4 mg/kg/h for 24–48 h. DMSO has also been recommended for its antioxidant properties [4]. A dose of 1 gm/kg bwt administered as a 10% solution either IV or via a nasogastric tube q12 h is commonly used for TBI [8]. Cerebral trauma can be associated with the development of seizures in any species and the horse is no exception. Controlling seizures is important because they significantly increase the cerebral metabolic rate, promoting secondary injury [4]. Benzodiazepines, such as diazepam and midazolam, are the drugs of choice to terminate seizure activity. If benzodiazepines are not available or the seizures are unresponsive, pentobarbital and phenobarbital have also been used. Finally, general anesthesia may be induced for the most recalcitrant seizures. Ketamine should be avoided as it increases ICP. (See Section "Seizure control and management in horses" for more information and dosage recommendations.) Adequate nutrition is important to facilitate recovery. If the horse is incapable of eating on its own or sustaining a feeding tube, parenteral nutritional support may be necessary.

Spinal cord injury

Like TBI, trauma to the spinal cord is usually associated with some type of collision or fall. Although the entire vertebral column is susceptible, the cervical area is the most commonly affected. Acute trauma is most obvious in the gray matter with hemorrhage and cell death. Within minutes to hours, however, secondary injury processes spread centripetally from the initial injury site causing necrosis, edema, and ischemic damage.

Treatment of SCI

Like TBI, SCI injuries have a primary and secondary component. The period of secondary injury, however, has been studied more extensively in SCI. The primary goal of therapy is to optimize delivery of oxygen and metabolic substrates to the spinal cord to preserve undamaged cells and stabilize reversibly damaged tissue. As in TBI, maintaining cardiovascular function is essential for accomplishing these goals, but unlike TBI, the cardiovascular system is often significantly impaired with SCI. Injuries cranial to C5, which affect the respiratory center, often result in hypoventilation, while lesions cranial to T2 impair the functioning of the sympathetic nervous system, resulting in bradycardia and hypotension [4].

How to prevent the secondary phase of injury characteristic of traumatic damage to the nervous system has been the focus of a great deal of research. The use of corticosteroids for this purpose remains controversial despite years of study. The primary benefits of corticosteroid therapy in CNS injury are anti-inflammatory effects, free-radical scavenging properties, and preservation of spinal cord blood flow [5]. MPSS has been evaluated in the treatment of SCI in humans and animals more than any other corticosteroid. Over the years, numerous clinical trials have been conducted in human medicine, and the results have been far from definitive [20–23]. Proponents of its use state that the preponderance of evidence indicates that high-dose MPSS given within 8 h of acute SCI is a safe and modestly effective therapy that may result in improved clinical recoveries for some patients [19]. This conclusion, however, is not universally shared, and many do not consider high-dose MPSS standard of care [5, 24]. It should also be remembered, however, that administering MPSS after 8 h resulted in worse clinical outcomes. In addition, other adverse effects of high-dose MPSS include gastrointestinal ulceration, immunosuppression, hyperglycemia, and acute adrenal insufficiency [5]. The dose of MPSS used in the majority of human clinical trials was 30 mg/kg bwt IV followed by a CRI at 5.4 mg/kg/h for 23 h. It is unclear whether this is an appropriate dose for the horse. Dexamethasone is used much more commonly in horses suffering from SCI. The recommended dose ranges from 0.1 to 0.25 mg/kg bwt, IV, q6–8 h for 24–48 h [4]. For prolonged therapy, oral prednisolone is often administered at a dose range of 0.5–1.0 mg/kg bwt q12–24 h. Once the patient is stable, the dose should be tapered to the minimum effective dose, ideally administered every other day in order to decrease the suppression of endogenous cortisol production.

Other medications and therapies are also commonly used in the treatment of spinal cord injuries. For example, in addition to corticosteroids, NSAIDs are often used to control inflammation, pain, and fever, if present. Care must be exercised, however, when both classes of drug are concurrently administered because the risk of gastrointestinal ulceration is substantially increased. As in cases of cerebral injury, DMSO has been proposed to be efficacious in the treatment of SCI by scavenging free radicals; reducing inflammation, edema, and platelet aggregation; and promoting vasodilation. For SCI, it is usually administered at a dose of 1 gm/kg bwt, IV as a 10% solution, q12 h for the first 72 h and then according to clinician preference. Although its use is common, the beneficial effects of DMSO on SCI have not been well documented.

Numerous adjunct therapies have been recommended for the treatment of SCI. Although in many cases they appear promising in experimental animal models of SCI, few have proven to be efficacious in clinical trials. For example, various antioxidants have been advocated based on the theory that they may reduce damage from free radicals. For example, both vitamin E and N-acetylcysteine have proven effective in experimental animal models of SCI, but no large-scale clinical studies have been conducted in any other species. Calcium channel blockers, 21-aminosteroids, opiate receptor antagonists, and thyrotrophin-releasing hormone are just a few of the agents that have been evaluated as potential therapies for SCI, but to date, none have withstood the test of time and they are not considered to be standard of care.

Supportive care is extremely critical to the long-term outcome of cases of SCI. Antimicrobial therapy may be indicated in many, if not most, cases of SCI in order to help prevent or treat infections of open wounds and other organ systems. Fluids and nutritional support may also be necessary.

Spinal cord injuries that occur above the cauda equina leave the S2–S4 levels of the spinal cord intact. As such, all the spinal and autonomic nerves located in these levels can still function in a reflexive manner, resulting in a spastic or upper motor neuron (UMN) bladder syndrome characterized by frequent, uncontrolled micturition. Generally, in this syndrome, the detrusor muscle tone is elevated, and occasionally, the external sphincter becomes spastic as well. The goal of therapy is to decrease urethral sphincter and detrusor muscle tone, and diazepam and dantrolene are commonly used to produce this outcome in the horse [25]. Diazepam is recommended at a dose of 0.2–0.5 mg/kg bwt IV, although this dose will frequently cause sedation. Dantrolene is administered at a loading dose of 10 mg/kg bwt orally (PO), followed by 2.5 mg/kg bwt, PO, q6 h. Prazosin, an alpha adrenergic antagonist, has been recommended for UMN bladder syndrome at an initial dose of 5 mg for an adult horse, PO, q8 h [25]. The dose may need to be increased to produce the desired effect, but the maximum dose should not exceed 10 mg due to concerns of systemic hypotension. Phenoxybenzamine, which is used in small animals suffering from UMN bladder syndrome, is prohibitively expensive to use in the horse, and its efficacy has not been determined. Urinary catheterization may be necessary acutely along with care to prevent urine scalding. (See Section "Cauda equina syndrome" for discussion of the treatment of atonic or lower motor neuron (LMN) bladder syndrome.)

Nonpharmacological therapies, such as physical therapy, can help the horse gain strength, reestablish proprioception, and facilitate development of compensatory pathways. Massage, hydrotherapy, and passive flexion and extension exercises may also be helpful to the recumbent horse.

Cervical vertebral stenotic myelopathy

Cervical vertebral myelopathy refers to a condition that causes compression in the cervical segment of the spinal cord. The condition has been more specifically referred to as cervical vertebral stenotic myelopathy (CVSM) and has recently been subdivided into two broad categories. One affects primarily young horses with compression resulting from developmental abnormalities of the cervical vertebral column, and the other affects older horses with compression resulting from osteoarthritis of the articular processes [26]. Cervical cord compression can be either static or dynamic. Static lesions cause compression of the cord regardless of head position or changes in neck flexion. In contrast, dynamic lesions may only cause cord compression when the neck is flexed or extended at a specific position, and therefore, clinical signs may not be consistently present. Diagnosis of CVSM is based on the presence of clinical signs of symmetric spinal ataxia and narrow cervical vertebrae on radiographs and contrast myelography, together with the elimination of other etiologies [26].

Medical therapy for horses with CVSM is aimed at reducing inflammation and edema, which should decrease the severity of the cord compression. Following an acute onset of the condition, treatment with NSAID and DMSO is often initiated. (See Section "Central nervous system trauma" for more detailed information and dosages.) When cervical vertebral myelopathy is diagnosed in horses less than 1 year of age, a program of restricted diet and exercise reduction along with alterations in the concentrations of trace minerals in the diet, such as copper and zinc, may be beneficial [26]. The theory behind this controlled or paced growth approach is that by slowing growth it allows the vertebral column to "catch up." [26] In these horses, supplementation of vitamin E and selenium is recommended because equine degenerative myelopathy (EDM) is an important differential diagnosis.

In adult horses, anti-inflammatory therapy can help stabilize the neurologic status. In addition, injecting the articular joints with corticosteroids with or without hyaluronate may decrease soft tissue swelling and help prevent additional bony proliferation [27]. Horses that benefit most from this approach have minimum to no neurologic deficits and significant degenerative joint changes on radiography. Surgical stabilization, which involves interbody fusion of the vertebral bodies, is an option for some horses, but it is expensive, requires extensive postoperative care, and is not without its own risks. The cost, practicality, and prognosis should be carefully weighed before surgery is recommended [26, 28].

Equine protozoal myeloencephalitis

Equine protozoal myeloencephalitis (EPM) is a CNS disease of horses caused by a protozoan parasite, *Sarcocystis neurona* or, less commonly, *Neospora hughesi*. The diagnosis of EPM is not straightforward. The clinical signs can be variable and sometimes subtle, and the available diagnostic tests are complex and rarely definitive. In-depth reviews of the diagnosis of EPM, including the strengths and weaknesses of the various diagnostic tests, are reviewed elsewhere [29–32]. A general criticism of all of the current tests, however, is that they detect antibody to the infectious organism, and therefore, they are an indication of exposure and not necessarily of an active infection. The incidence of exposure of horses to the causative agents of EPM varies with the geographic location, but on average, it is in the range of 30–40% [33].

There are several options for the treatment of EPM. The first treatment widely used was a combination of pyrimethamine and a sulfonamide antimicrobial, usually sulfadiazine. This drug combination works synergistically; the sulfa drug interferes with the synthesis of folate by competing with para-aminobenzoic acid, while pyrimethamine inhibits folate synthesis through competition with dihydrofolate reductase. For convenience, some practitioners have used pyrimethamine combined with the potentiated sulfonamide, trimethoprim–sulfamethoxazole. This combination, however, is less than ideal because sulfamethoxazole does not cross the BBB to the same extent as sulfadiazine. The recommended dose is 1 mg/kg bwt of pyrimethamine and 20 mg/kg bwt of the sulfadiazine administered PO once a day. Reported success rates are in the range of 60%, but duration of treatment is long, ranging from 90 to 270 days and relapses have been reported [34]. Long-term administration of this drug combination is also associated with anemia and the potential for fetal toxicity in pregnant mares. Originally only available through compounding pharmacies, a pyrimethamine–sulfadiazine formulation was approved by the FDA in 2004 (ReBalance™ Antiprotozoal Oral Suspension, IVX Animal Health Inc., St Joseph, MO). Although many practitioners prefer newer medications, such as ponazuril and diclazuril, with shorter durations of therapy, pyrimethamine–sulfadiazine should still be considered a viable treatment option for horses with EPM.

Of the newer EPM therapies, ponazuril (Marquis®, Bayer HealthCare LLC, Animal Health Division, Shawnee Mission, KS) has been the most extensively evaluated and was actually the first medication approved by the FDA for the treatment of the disease [35]. The dose of ponazuril is 5 mg/kg bwt, PO, daily for a minimum of 28 days. As a triazinone coccidiostat, ponazuril is selectively internalized by the apicoplast of *S. neurona*, where it disrupts the function of respiratory chain enzymes of the mitochondria and the apicoplast. Oral administration of ponazuril at 5 mg/kg bwt produced CSF concentrations of 0.16 ± 0.06 mg/l, which are likely to be therapeutic based on sensitivity data determined *in vitro* [36, 37]. Absorption of ponazuril can be enhanced by administration of 2 ounces of corn oil

immediately prior to dosing with resulting CSF ponazuril concentrations increased by up to 25% [32]. In a clinical field trial, ponazuril had an efficacy rate of approximately 60% with 28 days of a therapy at the recommended dose [35]. Adverse events reported in that study included two horses that developed blisters on their nose and mouth, three horses that showed skin rashes or hives for up to 18 days, one horse that had loose stools throughout treatment, one horse that had mild colic on one day, and one horse that seizured while on the medication. In a target animal safety study also submitted to FDA, administration of ponazuril at doses of 10 or 30 mg/kg bwt for 28 or 56 days produced transient episodes of loose feces, as well as changes in uterine tissues at the 30 mg/kg dose [35]. The conclusion of the study was that ponazuril administered as a 15% oral paste, at 10 and 30 mg/kg, equivalent to 2X and 6X the recommended dosage, was generally safe for adult horses. Treatment of both stallions and pregnant mare has been performed without apparent problems.

Another triazinone coccidiostat that is approved by the FDA for the treatment of EPM is diclazuril (Protazil® 1.56% diclazuril, Merck Animal Health, Summit, NJ). It is marketed as a top-dressing pellet for daily administration at a rate of 1 mg/kg bwt of diclazuril for 28 days [38]. When administered at the recommended label dose, the steady-state CSF diclazuril concentrations were predicted to be between 20 and 70 ng/ml, which significantly exceeds the *in vitro* IC95 concentration for inhibition of merozoite production of 1 ng/ml. In a clinical field trial, diclazuril had a success rate of 67%, based on seroconversion to negative Western blot and the number of horses classified as treatment successes [38]. It is important to note that there was no improvement in the success rate when horses in this trial were treated with a higher dose of 10 mg/kg bwt. The target animal safety study demonstrated that diclazuril was safe when administered to horses PO at the proposed dose of 1 mg/kg bwt daily for up to forty-two consecutive days.

Certain adjunctive therapies may also be helpful in the treatment of EPM. Anti-inflammatory therapy is recommended by some clinicians if the clinical signs worsen with the initiation of therapy. The etiology of this clinical phenomenon is proposed to be an increase in the inflammatory response due to rapid death of organisms in the CNS. NSAIDs are most commonly used for this purpose, but short-term administration of corticosteroids has also been advocated by some clinicians [32]. Although some clinicians advocate other adjunct therapies including vitamin E, homeopathic therapies, and acupuncture, there is no scientific literature to support their use. Immune stimulation has also been advocated, but the reports of its benefits are only anecdotal. Levamisole is purported to have immune stimulant activity when administered PO at a dose of 1 mg/kg bwt q24 h. In addition, Eq Stim® (Neogen Corporation, Lansing, MI) administered at a dose of 5 ml IM on days 1, 3, and 7 and then monthly and Equimune IV (Bioniche Animal Health USA, Inc., Bogart, GA) at a dose of 1.5 ml IV weekly for 3 weeks have also been recommended by some clinicians [32].

Viral disease of the equine nervous system

Most commonly, viral encephalitides are the result of a generalized viral infection that has spread to the CNS. Only two viruses have been shown to primarily infect the CNS: rabies and bornavirus. The diagnosis of viral encephalitis or myelitis is based on history, clinical examination, CSF analysis, medical imaging, and functional testing, as well as, unfortunately, postmortem examinations [39]. An accurate diagnosis is critical, because while most viral infections are treated only with supportive care, herpes viral infections have a specific therapy. In addition, the prognosis for recovery varies tremendously with the etiological agent. A number of the viruses that cause CNS infections in horses, including rabies, West Nile virus, and Eastern/Western and Venezuelan equine encephalitis virus, can be protected against by vaccination. The importance of vaccination for preventing these diseases cannot be overemphasized.

Nonspecific therapy for viral diseases of the CNS is primarily aimed at providing supportive care and curtailing the inflammatory cascade. Supportive care would include providing a well-padded and deeply bedded stall, ideally with the capacity to hoist the horse should slinging become necessary [39]. Depending on the horse's status, fluids and nutritional support may also be necessary. NSAIDs may help to minimize secondary damage caused by the inflammatory process. Flunixin meglumine at a dose of 0.5 mg/kg bwt, IV, q6–8 h is used most commonly for this purpose and has been proposed

to specifically inhibit equine herpes virus-1 (EHV-1) replication in endothelial cells [39]. Whether the treatment with osmotic diuretics, such as mannitol administered at a dose of 0.25–2.0 gm/kg bwt IV and/or DMSO administered at a dose of 1 gm/kg bwt IV as a 10% solution, would be beneficial should be made on a case-by-case basis. In a similar manner, no blanket recommendation can be made on the use of corticosteroids. While they are powerful anti-inflammatory agents, they can also suppress the immune system. Interferons are cytokines that stimulate the immune response to viruses and apoptosis of virally infected cells. Exogenous human alpha interferon has been used with apparent efficacy in the therapy of pulmonary infections in horses [40]. Alpha interferons have also been administered parenterally in the therapy of West Nile virus infections, but no controlled studies have evaluated the efficacy of interferon against CNS infections in horses. Although few side effects have been reported in horses, expected side effects include those associated with the inflammatory cytokines, such as lethargy and malaise.

Specific antiviral therapy for equine herpes Viruses 1 and 4

Herpes viruses are one of the few families of viruses for which specific and effective antiviral drugs exist. In humans, the viral DNA polymerase inhibitor acyclovir is commonly used for the treatment of sensitive herpes virus infections of the CNS [41]. Acyclovir is a synthetic purine nucleoside analog that selectively inhibits replication of herpes viruses by requiring drug activation by viral thymidine kinase enzymes. Acyclovir has been PO administered in the therapy of equine multinodular pulmonary fibrosis associated with EHV-5 and may be effective against highly sensitive herpes viruses [42]. However, oral acyclovir is not a viable option for the treatment of equine herpes myeloencephalopathy (EHM) due to its extremely poor bioavailability, resulting in failure to produce plasma concentrations effective against EHV-1 [43, 44]. The bioavailability of the prodrug valacyclovir, which is metabolized to acyclovir after absorption, was shown to be 30–40%, and it has been recommended to be administered at a dose of 27 mg/kg bwt, PO, q8 h for the first 48 h, followed by 18 mg/kg bwt, PO, q12 h [44, 45]. Alternative dosing recommendations include a dose rate of 40 mg/kg bwt, PO, q8 h [44]. However, the safety of the higher dosing rate has only been tested in foals over one week of administration, whereas the safety of the lower dosing regimen was tested over 2 weeks in geriatric horses. Although acyclovir and valacyclovir generally have a wide therapeutic index, high enough doses will result in toxicity. Oral valacyclovir dose rates of 240 mg/kg/day administered to cats resulted in bone marrow suppression and renal tubular necrosis, signs common to the toxicity of antiherpetic nucleoside analogs [46]. It is the maximal plasma concentrations of acyclovir that seem to be the most predicative of toxicity, since a dose rate of 10 mg/kg of acyclovir administered as a 15 min infusion produced trembling and muscle fasciculations in one of six horses, whereas the same dose administered as a one hour infusion was well tolerated in three subsequent studies involving 24 total horses [43–45]. Several studies have examined the ability of valacyclovir administration to protect horses from EHM and have yielded contradictory results. One study used the high valacyclovir dose rate cited earlier in weanling ponies, but did not find a substantial protective effect, whereas a second study in aged mares did indicate that either prophylactic administration or administration within the first 2 days of EHV-1 inoculation did protect horses from neurological disease [47, 48]. Although preliminary reports from *in vivo* challenge models are promising, valacyclovir efficacy has not been demonstrated in any type of clinical field trial. Nevertheless, valacyclovir has been used in several outbreaks of neurological herpes virus, and anecdotal reports of its efficacy are promising. The recent availability of generic formulations of valacyclovir has greatly decreased the cost of therapy, making early treatment of horses during an outbreak of EHV-1 more feasible. The pharmacokinetics of other antivirals, such as ganciclovir and famciclovir, have also been determined in the horse [49, 50]. These agents are very expensive, however, and their efficacy has not been determined in clinical filed trials. An experimental challenge model did find that IV ganciclovir administration rapidly decreased viral replication and ataxia when administered just before neurological signs were expected to develop, whereas valacyclovir administration was not effective when administered later in the course of disease [51]. IV administration of acyclovir has been evaluated in the horse [43, 44]. When acyclovir was administered at a single dose of 10 mg/kg bwt IV over 1 h, plasma concentrations likely to be efficacious against EHV-1 isolates were maintained for only 1–2 h [43, 44]. The disposition of PO administered valacyclovir is similar, with both

IV acyclovir and oral valacyclovir expected to accumulate with multiple doses and be associated with effective plasma concentrations. Injectable acyclovir is rarely selected over oral valacyclovir because it is more expensive and must be administered as a one hour infusion to avoid toxicity [43]. Only in select cases, such as when horses have anterior enteritis in conjunction with EHM, is therapy with IV acyclovir preferred to that of oral valacyclovir.

Equine degenerative myelopathy/neuroaxonal dystrophy

EDM is a breed-associated degenerative condition of the equine spinal cord. Neuroaxonal dystrophy (NAD) is similar to EDM. Both diseases lead to degenerative changes in the CNS, particularly the spinal cord, but they differ in what areas of the CNS are affected. A genetic basis is suspected for these diseases. Breeds that appear to be overrepresented include Appaloosas, Arabians, Quarter Horses, Paso Finos, Morgans, Paints, Norwegian Fjord horses, and Welsh ponies. Vitamin E deficiency is associated with both NAD and EDM, but detecting low vitamin E levels is not a reliable diagnostic confirmation as many affected horses have normal blood levels. Affected horses often present before 2 years of age. Vitamin E supplementation is currently the only known therapeutic approach that offers a potential for clinical benefit. Earlier recognition of an increased risk of EDM or NAD due to breed predilection may facilitate earlier vitamin E supplementation, but a positive clinical response to this therapy is not consistently observed. Suggested doses for vitamin E are variable and partially dependent on the formulation. They range from 5000 IU to over 10 000 IU/500 kg horse per day.

Equine motor neuron disease

Equine motor neuron disease (EMND) is classically divided into two forms: subacute and subclinical [46]. The signs of the subacute form of EMND include acute onset of trembling, muscle fasciculations, frequent recumbency, weight shifting in the rear legs, abnormal sweating, low head carriage, inability to lock the stifles, a characteristic "elephant on the ball" stance, and symmetrical loss of muscle mass. Some horses with prolonged vitamin E deficiency may be affected with a subclinical form and may not show the classic signs of EMND. Rather, the subclinical horse may exhibit subtle weakness that is only recognized by the owner. Additional clinical findings of EMND may include a vitamin E deficiency-induced retinopathy, characterized by a mosaic pattern of dark to yellow-brown pigmentation (lipofuscin-like pigment) of underlying the tapetum and dental tartar accumulation. Visual deficits may or may not be clinically evident. Horses at risk of developing EMND include those stabled with a horse with EMND and those being fed the same diet as an affected horse.

EMND is classified as an oxidative disorder. The disease results in preferential denervation atrophy of type 1 muscle fibers, whose parent motor neurons have higher oxidative activity. Horses deprived of pasture or green, high-quality hay and that are not supplemented with vitamin E for more than a year are reportedly at greatest risk for developing EMND. Normal vitamin E concentrations in blood are 1.5 µg/ml or higher. Definitive diagnosis involves histopathologic evaluation of a biopsy of the sacrocaudalis dorsalis muscle, where the muscle contains a relatively high percentage of type 1 muscle fibers. Vitamin E supplementation for treatment of EMND produces variable responses. Doses advocated range between 5000 IU and over 10 000 IU per day for an adult horse.

Headshaking

Headshaking is a clinical condition characterized by various unprovoked repetitive movements of the head and facial structures including flipping of the nose, nose rubbing, snorting, sneezing, and horses acting like a bee has flown up their nose [52]. Despite a fair amount of research, the etiology or etiologies have not been well described. For example, the clinical features have some commonality with trigeminal neuritis in humans, but other diseases associated with the condition in horses include tooth problems, allergies, ocular abnormalities, otitis, ear mites and other parasites, neck injury, cranial nerve dysfunction, and guttural pouch diseases. In most cases, a definitive etiology is rarely determined. Exercise and light have been proposed triggers, and the condition exhibits a seasonal occurrence in some horses.

Treatment of headshaking in horses depends a great deal on the etiology of the condition, if one can be determined. Firstly, any abnormalities found on physical examination that could be associated with the condition should be addressed. For example, tooth problems corrected, otitis treated, etc. If no obvious abnormalities are identified or if the headshaking persists when they have been addressed, a diagnosis of idiopathic headshaking is likely. No single therapeutic approach has been found to be effective in the majority of horses suffering from idiopathic headshaking. Therefore, the practitioner should council the owners that a process of trial and elimination will be necessary to determine what, if anything, will work best in any individual horse. One of the most benign therapies is application of a nose net. In one study, approximately 75% of owners reported some overall improvement with a nose net [53]. The nets significantly reduced the overall headshaking score, as well as a number of specific behaviors, but not all of the horses responded positively. If application of a nose net does not improve the condition, there are a number of pharmacologic therapies that have been advocated, if not thoroughly evaluated, although none are approved for use in the horse. Because of the similarities of the condition to trigeminal neuritis, some agents commonly used to treat neuropathic pain in humans have been used in horses with idiopathic headshaking. In one study, when the anticholinergic and serotonin antagonist cyproheptadine was concomitantly administered with carbamazepine, 80% of the horses demonstrated an 80–100% improvement [54]. Carbamazepine stabilizes the inactivated state of voltage-gated sodium channels and potentiates gamma-aminobutyric acid (GABA) receptors, making the neurons less excitable. Cyproheptadine was administered at a dose of 0.2–0.5 mg/kg bwt, PO, q12–24 h, and carbamazepine was administered at a dose of 4–8 mg/kg bwt, PO, q6–8 h [54]. The GABA analog gabapentin has also been used empirically, because of its efficacy in neuropathic pain in humans. Although no efficacy studies have been conducted on gabapentin, its kinetics in the horse have been evaluated. In one study, gabapentin was administered at a dose of 20 mg/kg bwt, once IV and once PO, to six horses [55]. The bioavailability of gabapentin following oral administration was poor at approximately 16%, resulting in low plasma concentrations. Following IV administration, gabapentin caused sedation for 1 h, but no other effects were noted. In another study, gabapentin was used in a pregnant mare diagnosed with neuropathic pain at a dose of 2.5 mg/kg bwt, PO, q12 h [56]. The horse appeared more comfortable shortly after therapy was initiated and the dose was tapered over the next 6 days. No adverse events were noted and the mare delivered a healthy foal. Medical therapy is not always successful, and because some horses have responded to local anesthesia of either the infraorbital or posterior ethmoidal branches of the trigeminal nerve, neurectomies of these nerves were evaluated for relief of the condition [54, 57]. These surgeries, however, have largely been abandoned due to lack of efficacy.

Cauda equina syndrome

The tapered caudal end of the spinal cord and the caudal extensions of the spinal nerve roots that extend within the spinal canal, actually beyond the termination of the cord, vaguely resemble a horse's tail, which has given rise to the name cauda equina. These spinal nerves actually exit the vertebral column at locations that are more caudal than the spinal cord segmental origins of the nerves. Therefore, the clinical signs that result from damage to the cauda equina can be attributed to damage to any or all of the sacrococcygeal nerve roots, which give rise to the pudendal, caudal rectal, pelvic, and coccygeal peripheral nerves and part of the sciatic and gluteal peripheral nerves [58]. As the term syndrome implies, the clinical signs can be caused by any number of pathological processes that damage the cauda equina.

The most common clinical signs of damage to the cauda equina are tail paralysis or weakness, anal hypotonia or atony, rectal and bladder weakness or paralysis, and penile prolapse or paralysis [58]. Other possible clinical signs include hypoalgesia or analgesia of the skin of the tail, anus, and perineum, as well as muscle atrophy of the coccygeal muscles. If the more cranial aspect of the cauda equina is damaged, hindlimb weakness, ataxia, or muscle atrophy may also be observed. Secondary clinical signs, such as urine scalding and rectal impactions, can occur secondary to the neuronal dysfunctions.

Potential causes of cauda equina syndrome are numerous and include trauma, toxicity, infections, inflammations, and causes related to development. Prognosis is dependent on the etiology, and therefore, a thorough history and physical examination including a complete neurologic examination are important to arrive at an accurate diagnosis. Ancillary testing, including routine clinical pathologic tests, CSF evaluation, and advanced imaging, may also be helpful. Symptomatic care must be provided as needed to prevent secondary complications, such as bacterial cystitis and impaction colic. In many cases, there may be no specific treatment of the underlying cause of the neurologic lesion, but even for conditions that are theoretically amenable to treatment, such as bacterial meningitis, it is difficult to predict the degree to which recovery will occur. Horses with cauda equina secondary to trauma are usually treated medically for 1–2 weeks with anti-inflammatory therapy, including corticosteroids, DMSO, and NSAID, as described in the section "Central nervous system trauma." In addition, surgical decompression and/or stabilization of fractures, if practical, may also be attempted. Complete resolution of cauda equina syndrome is likely in horses that survive EHV-1 myeloencephalitis and those that are successfully treated for EPM [58].

The urinary incontinence associated with cauda equine syndrome results from LMN damage to the parasympathetic supply to the detrusor muscle. The bladder is atonic and distended and can be easily expressed during transrectal examination. The parasympathomimetic bethanechol is often used to treat atonic bladder secondary to LMN damage. Bethanechol increases detrusor muscle tone and intravesicular pressure and decreases bladder capacity, but its efficacy is variable [25]. It should not be used in cases of urinary obstruction, however, because of the potential for bladder rupture. Oral doses of bethanechol range from 0.2 to 0.4 mg/kg bwt q6–8 h. Subcutaneous administration has also been recommended at doses of 0.025–0.075 mg/kg bwt q8 h [59]. Bethanechol should not be administered via the IV or IM routes, because of the risk of inducing colic and/or arrhythmias [25].

In addition to bethanechol, placement of an indwelling urinary catheter can help prevent bladder over distension and urine scalding, and it facilitates bladder lavage that can remove excessive sabulous material. It is believed that accumulation of large amounts of sabulous sediment in the bladder may cause myogenic bladder dysfunction, resulting in continued incontinence even if the neurogenic condition resolves [58]. Oral administration of antimicrobials, such as potentiated sulfonamides, is recommended to prevent the development of secondary bacterial cystitis.

Polyneuritis equi

Polyneuritis equi is a cause of cauda equina that can affect horses of any age and breed, although its incidence is quite low. Previously, it was referred to as "cauda equina neuritis"; however, as the nerves outside of the cauda equina are often involved, the more general term of polyneuritis equi is more accurate. Clinical signs are those classically described as cauda equina syndrome, but they are progressive and slow in their development. They include paralysis of the tail, anus, rectum, and bladder with symmetrical hindlimb weakness and ataxia [60]. Areas of hyperesthesia and hypalgesia around the perineal area are also common. Other reported signs include penile prolapse, muscle atrophy in the hind quarters, and occasionally cranial nerve dysfunction. The etiology of the condition is unknown; however, it has been proposed to be an allergic neuritis similar to Guillain–Barré syndrome in humans. For example, in both conditions, antibodies to the neuritogenic myelin protein P2 are present in the serum [61, 62]. Diagnosis of polyneuritis equi is based on the presence of clinical signs consistent with the condition and the exclusion of other possible diseases, such as EHV-1 myeloencephalitis, meningitis, EPM, etc. A definitive diagnosis is made on postmortem with histopathologic examination of the extradural and intradural nerve roots demonstrating gross thickening, demyelination and axonal degeneration, and the presence of inflammatory cellular infiltrates [60]. The primary treatment is palliative, addressing the urinary and fecal incontinences and providing other supportive care. Corticosteroid therapy, most commonly with dexamethasone at a dose of 0.05–0.1 mg/kg bwt, IV may be helpful in the short term, but in the long term, the prognosis is very poor [60].

Equine reflex hypertonia (stringhalt)

Stringhalt is characterized by a sudden, involuntary, exaggerated flexion of one or both hindlimbs during movement [63]. Varying degrees of hyperflexion occur, from mild to severe cases where the foot actually contacts the abdomen, thorax, or elbow. Two distinct syndromes are recognized, a plant-associated and a sporadic stringhalt.

Plant-associated stringhalt

Plant-associated stringhalt is also referred to as Australian stringhalt, although it has also been reported in many other countries. Usually, numerous horses within a herd will be affected. It is associated with ingestion of dandelion (*Taraxacum officinale*), flatweed (*Hypochoeris radicata*), and cheese weed (*Malva parviflora*), but the toxin has not been isolated. In addition, these plants are common the world over, but the disease occurs sporadically, which has led to the theory that the actual toxin is a soilborne fungus or mold. In severe cases, the thoracic limbs may also be affected. Most horses recover once they are removed from the affected pasture, although recovery may be prolonged if the exposure was high or chronic. Phenytoin administered at a dose of 15 mg/kg bwt, PO, q24 h for 2 weeks has been recommended to decrease the severity of the clinical signs [64].

Sporadic stringhalt

The sporadic form of stringhalt occurs worldwide and usually affects only a single horse in the herd and only one pelvic limb [63]. The etiology is unknown, but an injury damaging the reflex arc controlling muscle tone resulting in disruption in normal postural tone and coordination of muscle contraction has been proposed [65]. Rest and time will result in improvement or complete recovery in some cases. Tenectomy of a long section of the lateral digital extensor tendon and its musculotendinous junction has been advocated, but the results of the surgery have been inconsistent. Medical therapy may help decrease the severity of the clinical signs, but will not cure the condition. As with plant-associated stringhalt, phenytoin administered at 15–25 mg/kg bwt, PO, q24 h for 2 weeks has been advocated [65]. Baclofen, a GABA receptor agonist, administered at a dose of 1 mg/kg bwt, PO, q8 h has also reduced the severity of clinical signs during treatment, but most horses regressed once therapy was discontinued [65].

Seizure control and management in horses

A seizure is a paroxysmal event that arises due to excessive discharges of the cerebral cortical neurons [66]. The activity may originate in the cerebrum or result from rapid spread from other regions in the brain. While a seizure is a specific event, epilepsy, which occurs rarely in horses, is defined as a reoccurrence of seizures from a chronic underlying process [18]. Clinical signs of seizures in horses can vary from mild muscle fasciculations and subtle alterations in consciousness to recumbency with tonic–clonic struggling. It is important in the horse to differentiate between true seizures and disorders that may mimic seizures. Clinical conditions that can present with signs that can be confused with seizures include acute severe cardiovascular events; electrolyte abnormalities; muscle diseases, such as hyperkalemic periodic paralysis and myopathy; and toxicities, such as botulism and tetanus.

As in other species, seizures in horses can be classified as partial, generalized, or status epilepticus. Partial seizures arise from a discrete focus in the cerebral cortex and often the clinical signs will be limited to the area of the brain involved, such as facial or limb twitching. Generalized seizures arise from both cerebral hemispheres simultaneously. It can be difficult, however, to distinguish between true generalized seizures and partial seizures that spread rapidly to become generalized [18]. Status epilepticus, characterized by a rapid succession of seizures, is rare to uncommon in horses.

There are numerous causes of seizures in horses with trauma, hepatoencephalopathy, and toxicity being the most common etiologies in adult horses [67]. Therefore, the occurrence of a seizure in any horse necessitates a complete physical examination, including complete blood counts and chemistries, and ancillary testing, such as CSF analysis, skull radiographs, and blood gas analysis, depending on the findings of the physical examination.

Treatment of seizures

The primary goals of therapy are to stop the seizures if they are ongoing and prevent them from recurring. It is important to terminate the seizure activity as soon as possible to prevent neuronal hypoxia with subsequent necrosis, as well as increases in ICP.

Acute seizure control

Benzodiazepines are commonly used to terminate seizure activity acutely. They bind to GABA receptors potentiating GABA-mediated chloride channels, resulting in hyperpolarization of the neuronal cell membranes. In adult horses, diazepam is recommended to be administered at 0.05–0.2 mg/kg bwt IV. Although it is occasionally administered IM in emergencies, diazepam is poorly water soluble, so absorption may be erratic, and therefore, IV administration is preferred. Midazolam, which has been frequently used in foals, can also be administered to adult horses at doses of 0.05–0.1 mg/kg bwt either IV or IM, because unlike diazepam it is well absorbed following IM administration. The durations of effect of both diazepam and midazolam are short, usually 10–15 min, but they can be given repeatedly or as CRIs. Diazepam can be administered at a rate of 0.1 mg/kg/h. Midazolam has not been studied in adult horses, but in foals, a rate of 1–3 mg/h for a 50 kg foal has been recommended. Although they have wide safety margins, benzodiazepines do cause mild respiratory depression, which may be significant in foals or with repeated administrations. Midazolam and diazepam produce less respiratory depression, hypotension, and bradycardia than phenobarbital.

If the seizures prove refractory to benzodiazepines or those agents are not readily available, phenobarbital can be administered at a loading dose of 12 mg/kg bwt, IV, followed by 6.65 mg/kg bwt, IV, given over 20–30 min q12 h [68]. Once the seizures are adequately controlled, the horse can be transitioned to oral therapy for long-term treatment as described in the following section. Dose-related respiratory depression, sedation, bradycardia, and hypotension are associated with phenobarbital administration, and therefore, loading doses should be administered with care. Although pentobarbital is not a true anticonvulsant, it can terminate seizures due to its anesthetic effects [18]. Doses are 2–10 mg/kg bwt IV to effect, and it causes significant respiratory depression.

Many other common sedatives should be used with caution in seizuring horses. For example, acepromazine can cause hypotension that can lead to reduced cerebral perfusion and has been proposed to reduce the seizure threshold, although this last effect has not been proven. Xylazine reduces cerebral blood flow after transiently increasing ICP, and so its use should be avoided. The use of ketamine is also controversial. It has been reported to increase cerebral blood flow, but it also increases oxygen consumption and may exacerbate seizure-like activity. On the other hand, it is an NMDA receptor antagonist and was shown to control seizure activity in a rat model of status epilepticus [69]. Nevertheless, it is probably best avoided if at all possible.

Once the initial seizure episode has been controlled, it must be determined whether long-term anticonvulsant therapy is indicated. That decision should be based on the underlying cause and the type, severity, and frequency of the seizures. The owners need to understand that anticonvulsant therapy may not entirely eliminate the seizures and that it will need to be maintained for several months at a minimum. While phenobarbital is the most commonly used anticonvulsant therapy in the horse, other options include bromide, phenytoin, and primidone.

Long-term anticonvulsant therapy

Phenobarbital acts primarily by stabilizing neuronal membranes via GABA receptors, but it also inhibits glutamate-induced postsynaptic potentials and voltage-gated calcium channels. It is well absorbed following oral administration, but the rate and extent of its metabolism and elimination is variable. It is extensively metabolized by the liver and induces the hepatic cytochrome P450 enzyme system. Therefore, with chronic dosing, its elimination half-life can be expected to decrease, as will the half-life of other drugs that are metabolized by the P450 system, such as macrolide antimicrobials. The recommended dose of phenobarbital in adult horses is 1–4 mg/kg bwt, PO, q12 h. Given the variability in metabolism and elimination of phenobarbital, therapeutic drug monitoring is recommended. Four to five days after initiating oral therapy, serum samples should be collected approximately 2 h after dosing and then immediately before the next dose is administered. These will represent peak and trough concentrations, and based on extrapolation from other species, those concentrations should be between 15 and 45 µg/ml. The goal should be to achieve control of the seizures at the lowest possible dose. As previously discussed, phenobarbital induces hepatic metabolic enzymes, and therefore, serum concentrations should be determined on a regular basis and the dose adjusted as needed.

Bromide, either as a potassium or sodium salt, can also be used for long-term control of seizures in the horse [70]. The mechanism of action of bromide is not well understood, but it appears to hyperpolarize neuronal cell membranes by competing with chloride ions. Because its mechanism of action is unique among the anticonvulsants, it is also used in combination with other agents, such as phenobarbital in refractory cases. Although the elimination half-life of bromide at 3–5 days is significantly shorter in the horse than in many other species, several days are required to achieve therapeutic concentrations,

and therefore, its use is not suitable for an emergency situation. When used in combination with phenobarbital, an initial dose of 25–40 mg/kg/day, PO, has been recommended. When used as the sole anticonvulsant therapy, a loading dose of 120 mg/kg bwt, PO, daily for 5 days, followed by a maintenance dose of 40 mg/kg bwt daily, has been recommended [70]. Therapeutic serum concentrations in other species are reported to be between 1 and 3 mg/ml. When used in combination, the lower end of the therapeutic range should be targeted. Anecdotal reports are that bromide is generally well tolerated in horses, but it has not been thoroughly evaluated. In humans, respiratory and dermatological adverse events have been reported, but in dogs, reversible neurological signs have been reported more commonly [71].

Although not routinely used in horses, the pharmacokinetics of phenytoin have been determined [72]. Phenytoin acts by inactivating voltage-dependent sodium channels, preventing depolarization of excitatory neurons, and decreasing release of the stimulatory neurotransmitter glutamate. In the horse, however, the bioavailability is extremely variable, and therefore, therapeutic drug monitoring is needed to assure that therapeutic serum concentrations, which in humans are 5–20 µg/ml, are achieved. Side effects of phenytoin reported in foals include prolonged depression, mild atrioventricular block, and a decrease in blood pressure [73]. Phenytoin has not been used extensively enough in adult horses to determine an adverse event profile. Newer therapeutic options, such as topiramate, clorazepate, and gabapentin, are available, but they are expensive and have not been evaluated for controlling seizures in horses.

The long-term prognosis for horses with seizures depends on the etiology and their response to therapy. Horses should be seizure-free for 1–3 months before termination of anticonvulsant therapy is considered. In addition, doses should be slowly tapered, decreasing the dose by 20% every other day for 1–2 weeks before discontinuing therapy. Horses on anticonvulsant therapy should not be ridden and should be seizure-free without treatment for several months before being ridden again.

Narcolepsy

Two forms of equine narcolepsy have been recognized in horses. In the first form, foals are affected within a few days of birth, and in the second form, the horses are adults when clinical signs develop. These clinical signs include episodes of excessive sleepiness and cataplexy (i.e., muscle weakness and hypotonia) with horses appearing normal between the episodes [16]. Typically, the horse gradually lowers its head, and then the forelimbs buckle, but some horses will collapse suddenly. The pathogenesis of narcolepsy is not well understood, but there is evidence for a genetic component in dogs, humans, and miniature horse foals [74]. Usually, no organic brain disease is identified. Diagnosis of narcolepsy is based on the history, physical and neurological examination being consistent with the disease, and importantly exclusion of other causes. Basically, the physical and neurological examinations, including clinical pathology, should all be normal. Differential diagnoses include seizures, syncope, and diseases that prevent the horse from lying down to sleep, such as severe musculoskeletal disease. Physostigmine salicylate administered at a dose of 0.1 mg/kg bwt IV may elicit signs in affected individuals, but most animals do not respond [16]. Administration of the tricyclic antidepressant imipramine has been recommended at doses of 250 and 1000 mg/500 kg bwt, PO, q12 h, but the results have been inconsistent. Horses suffering from narcolepsy should not be ridden.

Antimicrobial therapy for CNS infections

Treatment of bacterial infections

Bacterial infections within the CNS, though rare in horses, present unique challenges for treatment. Effective antimicrobial therapy of the CNS depends on adequate penetration of the BBB in order to produce effective antimicrobial concentrations in this sequestered site. The ideal compound to treat CNS infections is of small molecular size, is moderately lipophilic, has a low level of plasma protein binding, has a volume of distribution of around 1 l/kg, and is not a strong ligand of an efflux pump at the BBB or blood–CSF barrier [75]. Based on these characteristics, few antimicrobials would be considered ideal. Nevertheless, many less than ideal antimicrobials can be effective against CNS infections, because of the significant changes in the integrity of the BBB that occurs with meningitis. Firstly, inflammation causes opening of the intercellular tight junctions of the

vessel walls. Secondly, CSF outflow resistance increases, which decreases the rate of CSF production and adsorption, and finally, *P*-glycoprotein efflux pump activity is inhibited by proinflammatory cytokines. These three mechanisms, when combined, result in a significant increase in the concentration of drugs in the CSF, particularly, drugs that would not readily enter the CSF in the absence of meningeal inflammation [75]. Nevertheless, it is difficult to determine the degree to which the BBB is compromised, and therefore, to the extent it is possible, the choice of an antimicrobial known to cross the BBB is preferred.

The selection of an appropriate antimicrobial agent is ideally guided by culture and sensitivity testing of the cerebrospinal fluid or a localized nidus of infection affecting or seeding the CNS, although evaluation of a Gram stain may be extremely helpful for initial drug selection. The bacteria types that cause CNS infections vary with the age of the horse. In foals, bacterial meningitis is most often secondary to Gram-negative bacterial septicemia. *E. coli* is most common, but *Salmonella* spp. are often reported as well [76]. In adult horses, *Streptococcus* spp. are most frequently identified, but a wide variety of Gram-positive and Gram-negative organisms have been reported, further emphasizing the need for culture and sensitivity testing [77].

Beta-lactams

Assuming the presence of a compromised BBB, penicillin and first-generation cephalosporins may be effective for bacterial meningitis caused by susceptible organisms including *Streptococcus* spp. and anaerobes, although there are better options that penetrate the CNS more reliably. If a Gram-negative infection is suspected, many of the third-generation cephalosporins are good choices, because they demonstrate excellent penetration of the BBB. Three that cross the BBB in other species and that have been preliminary evaluated in the horse or foal are ceftriaxone administered at a dose of 25–50 mg/kg bwt, IV, q12 h; cefotaxime administered at a dose of 40 mg/kg bwt, IV, q4–6 h; and cefepime administered at a dose of 11 mg/kg bwt, IV, q8 h [78–81]. Although it is considered a third-generation cephalosporin, ceftiofur is not recommended, because even in the presence of inflammation, it is unlikely to reach therapeutically significant concentrations.

Potentiated sulfonamides

The combination of trimethoprim with sulfadiazine or sulfamethoxazole (TMS/SMZ) can achieve concentrations that are clinically significant in the CSF, but resistance to these combinations is common. Therefore, they should be used only when culture and sensitivity testing indicate the presence of a sensitive organism. The recommended dose of TMS/SMZ is 2.4/12.4 mg/kg bwt, PO, q12 h [77].

Chloramphenicol

Chloramphenicol is a bacteriostatic, broad-spectrum antimicrobial with activity against many Gram-negative, Gram-positive, and anaerobic organisms. It is very lipophilic with low serum protein binding, and therefore, it distributes well into the CNS, achieving concentrations in the CSF that are approximately 50% of plasma concentrations under normal conditions. The recommended dose of chloramphenicol is 25–50 mg/kg bwt, PO, q12 h in foals less than 5 days of age and q6 h thereafter [78]. Its bacteriostatic activity has been proposed to be a positive attribute, because it does not cause the large acute release of endotoxin associated with bactericidal drugs in the case of Gram-negative infections [82]. Unfortunately, chloramphenicol can cause bone marrow suppression in humans, and although the reaction is rare, it can also be fatal. In addition, there is some concern regarding the efficacy of chloramphenicol based on the poor bioavailability and rapid clearance observed in the horse [83–85]. Despite the safety concerns and poor kinetic profile of chloramphenicol, clinicians continue to use it and anecdotal reports of its efficacy are common [77].

Fluoroquinolones

Fluoroquinolones have excellent activity against Gram-negative aerobes and good activity against many Gram-positive microbes, but they are not active against anaerobic bacteria and have variable activity against streptococci. In the presence of inflammation, fluoroquinolones penetrate well into the CNS, achieving concentrations in the CSF that are 20–50% of those in the plasma [82]. The recommended dose of enrofloxacin, which is the fluoroquinolone most studied in the horse, is 5.5 mg/kg bwt, IV, q24 h or 7.5 mg/kg bwt, PO, q24 h [78]. Fluoroquinolones should not be used in foals because they cause arthropathies.

Rifampin

Rifampin has excellent activity against Gram-positive and anaerobic bacteria. In addition, it is highly lipid soluble and achieves clinically significant concentrations in the CSF. Resistance to rifampin develops rapidly, however, so it should not be used as a sole agent. In combination with fluoroquinolones, it would provide broad coverage. The recommended dose of rifampin is 5–10 mg/kg bwt, PO, q12 h [77, 78].

Metronidazole

Metronidazole is extremely efficacious against anaerobic bacteria and is very lipophilic allowing it to achieve clinically significant concentrations in the CSF. The recommended dose of metronidazole is 15–25 mg/kg bwt, PO, q6–12 h.

Antifungal therapy

Although far from common in the horse, infections of the CNS by fungal organisms have been reported [86, 87]. Horses and foals that are immunosuppressed, undernourished, and/or undergoing therapy with broad-spectrum antimicrobials are particularly at risk for these infections. Identification of the infectious organism is important because there are only a limited number of antifungal agents suitable for systemic administration and some of these agents have very narrow spectrums of activity. Susceptibility testing can be performed, but it is more complex and expensive than bacterial susceptibility testing. Fortunately, acquired resistance to antifungal agents is less common and slower to develop in fungi than bacteria [88]. Therefore, if the fungi can be identified, drug selection can be made on an empirical basis.

To date, only two classes of antifungals have been used in the horse with any frequency: the azoles, which include itraconazole, ketoconazole, and voriconazole, and the polyenes, which include nystatin and amphotericin B. Amphotericin B is an amphoteric polyene macrolide that is poorly soluble in water and unstable at 37°C. The original formulation for IV administration was an amphotericin B sodium deoxycholate compound. In small animals and humans, however, newer lipid formulations that are less toxic have largely replaced the original formulation, but these have not been studied in the horse [88]. Amphotericin acts by binding to ergosterol, one of the primary components of the fungal cell membrane, which compromises the integrity of the membrane. Unfortunately, it also binds to cholesterol in mammalian cells, which is its mechanism of toxicity. It is a broad-spectrum antifungal with good fungicidal activity against most pathogenic fungi, although resistance has been reported [88]. For treatment of fungal meningitis in the horse, it must be administered IV, because oral absorption is very poor. Penetration into the CSF is also poor but increases in the presence of meningitis. Renal toxicity is a significant problem, and BUN and creatinine should be monitored during therapy. Generally, the damage is reversible, so if BUN and creatinine increase, the drug should be discontinued temporarily or the dose decreased. Other side effects include thrombophlebitis at the injection site, hypokalemia, sweating, and depression. The recommended dosage of amphotericin B is 0.3–0.9 mg/kg bwt, IV, q24–48 h [88]. The dose should be diluted to a concentration of 1 mg/ml in 5% dextrose and administered over 1–2 h.

The azoles inhibit cytochrome P450-dependent ergosterol synthesis, which leads to disruption of fungal membranes and membrane-bound enzymes. They are considered fungistatic, but at high concentrations, their effects may be fungicidal. There are several significant drug interactions that can occur with this class of antifungals. First, azoles are potent inhibitors of the mammalian cytochrome P450 3A4 (abbreviated CYP3A4) enzyme, a member of the cytochrome P450 mixed-function oxidase system, one of the most important enzymes involved in the metabolism of drugs in the body. Because they inhibit the functioning of CYP3A4, they can decrease the rate of elimination of other drugs that are metabolized by the CYP3A4 pathway, which include benzodiazepines, many macrolide antimicrobials, etc. Second, other drugs that induce the production of CYP3A4 enzymes, such as barbiturates and rifampin, may increase the rate of metabolism of the azole, resulting in lower than anticipated plasma concentrations. Therefore, the concurrent use of CYP3A4 inducers and inhibitors is strongly discouraged, because it is difficult to predict what the final outcome on plasma concentrations of both agents will be.

The azole ketoconazole is a poorly water-soluble, highly lipophilic compound that has broad fungistatic activity against a wide range of fungi. Based on the results of one study, it is difficult to recommend it for oral administration to horses, in general, but particularly for the treatment of CNS infections [89]. In that study, ketoconazole was administered to horses at a dose of 30 mg/kg bwt, via a nasogastric tube in 0.2N HCl at a concentration of 15.8 mg/ml [89]. The HCl solution was necessary to produce the acidic environment needed for adequate absorption of the molecule, and the nasogastric tube was used to prevent the acidic solution from injuring the esophagus. Although the dose produced adequate concentrations in many tissues, ketoconazole was only present in the CSF at detectable concentrations (i.e., 0.28 µg/ml) in only one of the 6 mares in the study 3 h after the fifth dose was administered. Although penetration into the CSF may be enhanced in the presence of meningitis, it is unlikely to produce clinically significant concentrations, and the necessity of intragastric administration makes the use of oral ketoconazole in horses extremely problematic. In that same study, a single IV dose of ketoconazole at 10 mg/kg bwt produced peak serum concentrations of 10 µg/ml, but corresponding CSF concentrations were not determined [89]. Ketoconazole undergoes extensive hepatic metabolism with biliary excretion, and adverse events commonly reported in other veterinary species include inappetence, pruritus, and alopecia, as well as increases in serum hepatic enzyme concentrations. Ketoconazole may be embryotoxic and teratogenic, so it should not be administered to pregnant mares. In summary, ketoconazole cannot be recommended for treatment of fungal CNS infections in the horse given the poor penetration of the molecule into the CSF under normal conditions.

The triazole itraconazole is a potent inhibitor of most fungal pathogens in animals with an improved safety margin, compared to ketoconazole, because of its greater selectivity for the fungal cytochrome system [88]. Itraconazole is well absorbed following oral administration and has a large volume of distribution, but its penetration into the CSF is poor. As with ketoconazole, an acidic environment will enhance absorption. In one study in horses when itraconazole solution was administered via a nasogastric tube and itraconazole capsules were administered PO, both at a dose of 5 mg/kg bwt, mean peak plasma concentrations were 0.41 ± 0.1 and 0.15 ± 0.12 µg/ml, respectively [90]. CSF concentrations were not determined in that study, but studies in other species indicate that penetration across the BBB is poor [91]. Nevertheless, itraconazole has been used successfully to treat cryptococcal meningitis in humans, although relapses were reported [92, 93]. In horses, the recommended dosage of itraconazole is

5 mg/kg bwt, PO, q12–24 h with treatment often lasting 60–90 days. Itraconazole is metabolized by the liver and eliminated, primarily, through the bile. Although there are reports in the literature regarding its use for ophthalmic and nasal mycotic infections, its efficacy for the treatment of CNS infections in horses has not been reported [94, 95].

The triazole fluconazole is a specific inhibitor of the fungal enzyme lanosterol 14α-demethylase, which prevents the conversion of lanosterol to ergosterol. Because it is highly selective for fungal enzymes, it has an improved safety profile over other azoles. Also different from the other azoles, fluconazole is water soluble and well absorbed following oral administration. In one study, when fluconazole was administered PO to horses at a loading dose of 14 mg/kg bwt, followed by a daily dose of 5 mg/kg bwt for 10 days, mean peak plasma and CSF concentrations were 30.5±23.9 and 15.0±1.9 μg/ml, respectively [96]. Based on this study, fluconazole should be considered a viable treatment for fungal CNS infections in the horse. Although it generally has broad antifungal activity, it is not effective against *Aspergillus* and has limited activity against *Blastomyces dermatitidis* and *Candida* spp. It is particularly effective at treating *Cryptococcus* infections in the CNS [88]. Although its metabolism and elimination have not been evaluated in the horse, in other species, it is primarily eliminated by the kidney in the urine.

Voriconazole is a second-generation triazole with a wide spectrum of antifungal activity. In contrast to fluconazole, it is active against *Candida* spp., but resistance has been reported. It also has good but slow activity against *Aspergillus*. It is available in both oral and IV formulations, but only the oral formulation has been used to any significant degree in veterinary medicine. It is well absorbed following oral administration, regardless of stomach pH, and it is extensively metabolized and eliminated by the liver. In one study in horses, the mean peak plasma concentration following a single oral administration of voriconazole at a dose of 4 mg/kg bwt was 2.43±0.40 μg/ml [97]. In a different study in horses, the mean plasma and CSF concentrations following administration of voriconazole at a dose of 3 mg/kg bwt, PO, q12 h were 5.163±1.594 and 2.508±1.616 μg/ml, respectively [98]. No adverse events were reported in either study and voriconazole is well tolerated in humans. Based on the results of these studies, voriconazole administered PO, once or twice a day, at a

dose of 3–4 mg/kg bwt may be effective for the treatment of sensitive fungal infections in the CSF in horses.

Flucytosine is a synthetic antimycotic that has no intrinsic antifungal activity. Rather, once taken up by susceptible fungal cells, it is converted into 5-fluorouracil, the metabolites of which inhibit fungal RNA and DNA synthesis [99]. Resistance is common, however, so it is most routinely used in combination with other antifungal agents, such as amphotericin B, to treat severe systemic fungal infections. Unfortunately, there are no published studies on flucytosine use in horses or foals.

Lyme disease/neuroborreliosis

Lyme disease is caused by the intracellular spirochete *Borrelia burgdorferi* and was first recognized in humans in Lyme, Connecticut, in 1975. It is the most common tick-borne disease in the northern hemisphere, and infections have been documented in many species including the horse. In 2000, 40% of the horses in the northeastern USA had been exposed to *B. burgdorferi* based on serological testing [100]. Diagnosing and treating Lyme disease, in general, remain difficult and controversial in both human and veterinary patients because exposure is fairly common as determined by serological testing and the common clinical signs are nonspecific and often wax and wane in their severity. Symptoms of Lyme disease in horses have been reported to include dermatitis, chronic weight loss, fever, swollen joints, uveitis, muscle pain, and sporadic and shifting leg lameness. On rare occasions, the infection can spread to the CNS, which is referred to as neuroborreliosis [101, 102]. Neuroborreliosis was confirmed in a 12-year-old Thoroughbred that presented with signs of depression, neck stiffness, poor performance, and a high antibody titer to *B. burgdorferi* [101]. Although the horse initially responded to treatment with doxycycline, it deteriorated when treatment was discontinued. On postmortem, leptomeningitis, lymphohistiocytic leptomeningeal vasculitis, cranial neuritis, and peripheral radiculoneuritis with Wallerian degeneration were observed, findings consistent with a diagnosis of neuroborreliosis. Immunodeficiency, which has been proposed to be a potential risk factor for the development of neuroborreliosis, was also present in this horse. The prevalence of Lyme disease and neuroborreliosis in horses has not been determined.

Effective antibiotic therapy for Lyme disease is problematic for a number of reasons. *B. burgdorferi* spirochetes utilize several mechanisms to resist antibiotic and immune destruction. *In vivo* antibiotic resistance is conferred by the ability to live intracellularly. In addition, since some antibiotics, such as beta-lactams, only kill actively dividing organisms, the well-documented slow division of this spirochete may also contribute to its ability to evade antimicrobial activity. *B. burgdorferi* also has the ability to form strains that lack cell walls, referred to as L-forms, which have been shown to specifically impact the ability of the bacteria to produce chronic infections. These L-forms of *B. burgdorferi* are also inherently resistant to many antimicrobials due to their lack of a cell wall and the loss of their ability to replicate.

Many horses diagnosed with Lyme disease based on the presence of persistent fevers and/or lameness are treated with tetracycline at a dose of 6.6 mg/kg bwt, IV, q24 h or doxycycline at a dose of 10 mg/kg bwt, PO, q12 h with reported positive clinical responses [103]. As the diagnosis of horses with Lyme disease, in general, remains controversial, it is therefore difficult to evaluate the true efficacy of these medications in its treatment. Nevertheless, for a horse diagnosed with neuroborreliosis, an inexpensive first approach would be to administer 2–4 weeks of IV tetracycline, followed by prolonged therapy of oral doxycycline. That said, neither of these agents cross the BBB to any significant degree, and it is unknown whether the inflammation produced in the presence of neuroborreliosis would increase their penetration. In human medicine, treatment of neuroborreliosis often begins with IV therapy using a third-generation cephalosporin, such as ceftriaxone or cefotaxime, which should be considered in horses with refractory infections [104].

Hepatic encephalopathy

Hepatic encephalopathy (HE) is characterized by an abnormal cerebral mental status associated with severe hepatic insufficiency, and it can affect any age or breed of horse [105]. Clinically, horses present with alterations in motor functions, as well as cognitive dysfunction that can progress to coma. In adult horses, the most common causes of liver disease that are associated with HE are acute and chronic hepatitis caused by pyrrolizidine alkaloid toxicity, cholelithiasis, and hemochromatosis [105]. The pathophysiology of HE is not well understood and numerous mechanisms have been proposed. For example, an augmentation of the GABAergic system, due to decreased GABA metabolism, and depression of the glutamine neuroexcitatory system have been hypothesized to be responsible for the cerebral dysfunction associated with HE [106, 107]. There is also evidence that accumulation of neurotoxins, primarily ammonia, and/or false neurotransmitters may also play significant roles in the development of HE [108].

Treatment of HE is controversial, perhaps due in large part to the still undetermined pathophysiology of the disease. Obviously, alleviation of the hepatic dysfunction would be an ideal therapeutic approach, but often, this is not possible. Good nursing and supportive care is critical to prevent factors, such as dehydration, infection, and electrolyte abnormalities, from complicating the clinical picture. Fluid supplementation may be necessary, either IV or via a nasogastric tube, as some horses with HE do not drink.

Lowering plasma ammonia concentrations is a common therapeutic approach to treat HE. Dietary protein restriction has been a mainstay of therapy since the 1950s; however, recent studies from the human scientific literature indicate that severe protein restriction can result in malnutrition and worsening of glutaminergic neurotransmission [107]. In human patients with mild HE, supplementation of their diet with branched-chain amino acids (BCAA) was shown to improve several neurophysiological test outcomes and preserve muscle mass [107]. Little is known regarding the effects of dietary protein on equine HE, but some feedstuffs typically included in a horse's diet, such as good quality grass hays, oats, barley, cracked corn, and softened beet pulp, are naturally relatively high in BCAA.

The disaccharide molecule lactulose has been shown to lower plasma ammonia concentrations and to improve clinical outcomes in humans suffering from HE [109]. In the colon, metabolism of lactulose decreases the pH, which favors the formation of the poorly soluble ammonium ion. In addition, lactulose results in formation of an osmotic gradient producing a laxative effect, which also increases ammonia losses. Although its effects in horses have not been well evaluated, it is commonly administered PO to horses with HE at a dose of 0.3–0.5 ml/kg bwt, PO, q6 h [105].

Antimicrobials have also been commonly used to reduce the ammonia-producing bacterial population in the colon, although they have not been shown to improve long-term clinical outcomes in humans with HE [107]. In veterinary medicine, neomycin at a dose of 10–50 mg/kg bwt PO, q6–12 h for 2 days and metronidazole at a dose of 15–25 mg/kg bwt, PO, q8 h have both been used for this purpose [105]. Other therapies including L-ornithine L-aspartate and acetyl L-carnitine have been shown to be effective in lowering serum ammonia concentrations and improving mental function in humans with HE, but neither has been studied in the horse.

If sedation is necessary in a horse suffering from HE either to facilitate diagnostic or therapeutic procedures or to manage maniacal behavior, xylazine administered at a dose of 0.25–1.0 mg/kg bwt IV is recommended over benzodiazepines, because the latter agents may exacerbate clinical signs by potentiating the GABAergic system. The benzodiazepine antagonist flumazenil has been used in humans and dogs with HE and temporarily improves some of the clinical signs of HE, but it has not been evaluated in horses [110].

Drugs used for behavioral modification

The use of drugs to modify equine behavior is a controversial subject. In most situations, nonpharmacological approaches should be tried initially, with medication reserved for refractory cases. In addition, the clinician needs to remember that most sporting horses compete under medication rules that prohibit the animal from participating in an event under the effects of agents that can alter its behavior. The use of medications during the training period may in some cases be appropriate, but the use of these agents during competition is unethical. More problematic are drugs that have legitimate medical uses, but that may also alter a horse's behavior as a side effect. For example, the administration of the corticosteroid dexamethasone to treat inflammatory or allergic disease is certainly appropriate, but its routine administration to produce mild sedation in show horses is not, regardless of how commonly it is done. Finally, the adverse events associated with some behavior-modifying agents can be extreme and represent a risk to the horse and its human handlers. The possibility of

these events also needs to be factored into the risk–benefit ratio for their use.

Stereotypical behaviors

Stereotypical behaviors can be defined as constant and repetitive actions, such as vocalization, grooming, walking, or weaving, that occur without any obvious external stimuli and that do not result from a pathological process. In the correct context, some or all of the behavior would be seen as normal, but either the context is lacking or the action so compulsive that the behavior is obviously abnormal. Common stereotypical behaviors in horses, including crib-biting, wind sucking, stall walking, pacing, pawing, and self-mutilation, have been well described elsewhere [111].

Because husbandry practices are believed to be critical to development of many stereotypical behaviors, changes in those practices can be extremely effective at decreasing their occurrence. The goal is to provide a calm, frustration-free environment, where the horse has ample opportunity to exhibit its natural behaviors. In most cases, when horses are turned out in relatively large pastures in a small herd situation (i.e., 25–30 horses) with their nutritional needs met primarily by forage, the stereotypical behaviors resolve [111]. Unfortunately, it is often difficult for owners to achieve this ideal situation. Nevertheless, the closer the horse's environment can be made to ideal, the more likely positive outcomes. For example, owners can increase the percentage of roughage that makes up the horse's diet, which will increase the amount of time spent eating. Depending on the age and workload of the horse, however, not all of its nutritional requirements may be able to be met by a total roughage diet. In these cases, the time spent eating can also be increased by limiting the accessibility of the forage, for example, using small holed hay nets [111]. There are a number of changes that can be made in most horses' environments, such as increasing their exercise and social interaction with other horses that can dramatically decrease the time spent exhibiting stereotypical behaviors. Nevertheless, not all horses will respond to changes in their environment or their improvement may not be enough to satisfy the owner. In these situations, pharmacological interventions may be attempted. No well-controlled clinical trials have been conducted on drugs used to modify behavior in horses; therefore, many recommendations are based on studies in other species or case reports and retrospective studies involving only a small number of horses.

Based on the theory that stereotypical behaviors induce the release of endogenous endorphins, the effects of opioid antagonists on the exhibition of those behaviors have been evaluated. For example, naloxone administered at doses ranging from 0.02 to 0.04 mg/kg bwt IM and IV reduced cribbing behavior for a matter of minutes, but doses only slightly higher (i.e., 0.75 mg/kg bwt IV) caused acute abdominal distress [112, 113]. Other opioid antagonists decreased cribbing behavior for longer periods of time. For example, nalmefene given IV, IM, or SC at doses ranging from 0.08 to 10.0 mg/kg bwt decreased cribbing for up to 7.5 days [112].

Other classes of compounds have also been used in horses exhibiting stereotypical behaviors. For example, the tricyclic antidepressants, such as imipramine and clomipramine, administered at doses ranging from 500 to 1000 mg, PO, q12 h for an average adult horse have been shown in one study to reduce self-mutilation in stallions, with the maximum effect observed after 8 days of treatment [114]. There is some evidence that the sedative acepromazine administered at doses of 0.1–0.4 mg/kg bwt IV or IM may also help reduce the exhibition of stereotypical behaviors [111]. Finally, supplementation of the amino acid tryptophan in the horse's diet at a dose rate of 1–3 gm q8–12 h was also reported to reduce some stereotypical behaviors [111].

Sedative agents

The use of sedatives in nonmedical situations by layman is an area of controversy in equine medicine. In many cases, these medications are used to facilitate common procedures, such as clipping the horse's ears and muzzle or cleaning his sheath, and their use can reduce or eliminate the need for physical restraint. In addition, farrier work on some horses with chronic osteoarthritic conditions may be much easier when mild sedation and analgesia is provided. For these purposes, alpha-2 adrenergic agonists, such as xylazine, romifidine, and detomidine, are used most commonly, because they produce dose-dependent sedation and analgesia. The recommended dose for xylazine is 0.2–1.1 mg/kg bwt IV or up to 2.2 mg/kg bwt IM. Romifidine is more potent than xylazine with a recommended dose ranging from 40 to 100 µg/kg bwt IV or up to 120 µg/kg bwt IM.

Finally, detomidine is the most potent of the alpha-2 agents commonly used in horses with a recommended dose ranging from 4 to 20 µg/kg bwt IV or up to 40 µg/kg bwt IM. These agents probably cause similar degrees of sedation and analgesia when administered in equipotent doses, although detomidine is generally considered to be the best analgesic with the longest duration of effect. Side effects include ataxia, transient hypertension followed by a more prolong period of hypotension, bradycardia, decreased gastric motility, and hyperglycemia. (see Chapters 3, and 4, for more details on their pharmacology.)

Although many owners and trainers may request doses of these agents be dispensed for lay administration at a later time, veterinarians need to consider the legal and ethical implications of dispensing them. Firstly, these sedatives can cause serious adverse events in horses, even when administered appropriately. Secondly, some state boards limit who can administer sedatives and tranquilizers in their veterinary practice acts. Finally, there is the human safety issue to consider. Serious injury or death can result from inadvertent or intentional administration of these sedatives to humans. Handlers are also at risk for injury should an adverse event occur in the horse following administration. In light of these concerns, a gel formulation of detomidine was developed for transmucosal absorption following administration under the tongue. The recommended dose is 0.040 mg/kg bwt under the tongue, and maximum sedation occurs in approximately 40 min. Duration of effect is considered to be 90–180 min. This formulation would seem to be an ideal product to dispense to layman; nevertheless, some veterinarians have expressed safety and liability concerns.

The phenothiazine tranquilizer acepromazine is also commonly used in horses at doses ranging from 0.01 to 0.5 mg/kg bwt, IV or IM, when only mild to moderate sedation is required. Clinicians need to remember that acepromazine does not provide any analgesia to the horse. Side effects include hypotension, which can be significant in geriatric horses, and penile prolapse in male horses. Classically, it has been taught that phenothiazines lower the seizure threshold and should not be used in a horse that has had a seizure. Although there is little in the scientific literature to substantiate this warning, it is best to avoid acepromazine in these horses if possible.

Long-acting sedatives

There are occasions when it is desirable to produce a long-term state of mild tranquilization in horses. The most common and legitimate situation would be when the horse has an injury and requires stall rest for an extended period of time. Some horses, particularly those that are very fit, may not adapt well, initially, to these "lay-ups" as they are referred to in the industry. In addition, tranquilization is used in fractious horses by some to facilitate training. While repeated administrations of short-acting agents are an option, the administration of long-acting agents that can be given once a month is preferred by some. Unfortunately, these long-acting agents have also been used in an unethical manner to produce tranquilization in show horses and racehorses. The two agents used most commonly for these purposes are fluphenazine and reserpine. They both produce a state that is characterized by many laymen and some veterinarians as sedation, although that is probably not a correct interpretation of the physiological response to them. The term neuroleptic syndrome is used in human medicine to describe the effects of these agents where spontaneous movements and complex behaviors are suppressed, but spinal reflexes and nociceptive avoidance behaviors remain intact [115]. In humans, these agents reduce initiative and interest in the environment as well, as manifestations of emotions and affect. As such, their effects are more profound and complex than simply sedation. It can be assumed that their effects in horses are also more complex than simple sedation or tranquilization, and the ethical implications of using antipsychotic agents to alter a nonpsychotic horse's behavior have not been addressed.

Fluphenazine

The phenothiazine agent fluphenazine is used in humans as an antipsychotic and it acts primarily by blocking dopamine receptors in the limbic system. In horses, it produces a state of decreased responsiveness to external stimuli and interest in the environment without apparently affecting motor coordination or athletic performance in most individuals. However, it can also block dopamine receptors in the striatum, resulting in an imbalance between the dopaminergic and cholinergic systems and causing the development of extrapyramidal motor signs in some individuals [116–119]. In horses, these signs include muscle rigidity,

involuntary muscle spasms of the cranial body, restlessness, intense pawing, and other bizarre behaviors. A slow-release decanoate formulation of fluphenazine is commonly used in horses, and IM administrations of 25 or 50 mg are thought to last approximately 4 weeks in the horse. Whether or not fluphenazine is an appropriate training aid is questionable, but it is commonly used for that purpose. It is considered a nonpermitted substance in most, if not all, racing jurisdictions and show horse medication rules. Because serum and urine concentrations of fluphenazine and its metabolites are quite low following administration, it presented a challenge for drug testing laboratories to detect its use in racing and show horses. Most laboratories, however, are currently capable of detecting fluphenazine quite readily in postadministration samples for an extended period of time. Therefore, adequate withdrawal times, generally considered to be at least 1 month, must be adhered to in order to prevent a positive finding in samples collected from treated horses.

The true incidence of adverse reactions following fluphenazine administrations is not known, but their occurrence is well documented [116–119]. Therefore, it is important for the practitioner to anticipate the potential for them to occur and plan accordingly. For example, in many horses exhibiting extrapyramidal signs, the administration of muscarinic antagonists reestablishes the balance in the dopaminergic and cholinergic systems, terminating the extrapyramidal signs. Diphenhydramine, which has antimuscarinic in addition to its primary antihistamine effects, has worked in some cases, but not all, at doses of 0.67–1.5 mg/kg bwt IV [116–118]. When effective, the response is quite striking, with the horse becoming bright, alert, and responsive in a matter of minutes following administration. Unfortunately, the effects can be short lived and doses may need to be repeated as frequently as every 4 h. Another antimuscarinic that is commonly used in humans that develop extrapyramidal signs associated with fluphenazine therapy is benztropine mesylate. In horses, doses of 0.018–0.035 mg/kg bwt, IV, q8 h have been effective at terminating extrapyramidal signs [116, 117]. In particularly refractory cases, horses can be sedated with sodium pentobarbital at a starting dose of 2 mg/kg bwt IV. Repeated doses or administration of pentobarbital as a CRI may be necessary. If the horses can be maintained for several days with antimuscarinics and/or sedatives, they usually recover with no permanent effects evident.

Reserpine

Reserpine is the principal alkaloid found in the roots of *Rauvolfia serpentina* plants that are native to India and Southeast Asia [120]. It acts by causing depletion of neuronal stores of neurotransmitters including norepinephrine, dopamine, and serotonin in the brain and peripheral nervous system [121, 122]. At one time, it was used to treat hypertension and psychosis in humans, although it has largely been replaced by agents that are safer and more efficacious. The recommended dose of reserpine ranges from 1 to 4 mg/500 kg horse administered PO or IM once daily. Adverse events observed with reserpine administration include severe depression, sweating, hypotension, penile prolapse, and colic. Diarrhea is also observed frequently, particularly with IM administration. Clinical signs generally resolve within several days, but supportive care may be necessary in severe cases. The hypotensive effects of reserpine may persist longer than the sedative effects, and they may be exacerbated by other agents that cause hypotension, such as the alpha-2 adrenergic agonists including xylazine and detomidine. Therefore, sedating or anesthetizing a horse that has been treated with reserpine can be extremely problematic.

References

1 Furr, M. (2008) Pharmaceutical considerations for treatment of central nervous system disease. In: M. Furr & S. Reed (eds), *Equine Neurology*, pp. 55–62. Blackwell Publishing, Ames.

2 Brewer, B.D. (1984) Therapeutic strategies involving antimicrobial treatment of the central nervous system in large animals. *Journal of the American Veterinary Medical Association*, **185**, 1217–1221.

3 Feige, K., Furst, A., Kaser-Hotz, B. & Ossent, P. (2000) Traumatic injury to the central nervous system in horses: Occurrence, diagnosis, and outcome. *Equine Veterinary Education*, **12**, 220–224.

4 Nout, Y. (2008) Central nervous system trauma. In: M. Furr & S. Reed (eds), *Equine Neurology*, pp. 305–328. Blackwell Publishing, Ames.

5 Park, E.H., White, G.A. & Tieber, L.M. (2012) Mechanisms of injury and emergency care of acute spinal cord injury in dogs and cats. *Journal of Veterinary Emergency and Critical Care*, **22**, 160–178.

6 Tsang, K.K. & Whitfield, P.C. (2012) Traumatic brain injury: Review of current management strategies. *British Journal of Oral and Maxillofacial Surgery*, **50**, 298–308.

7 Robertson, C.S., Goodman, J.C., Narayan, R.K., Contant, C.F. & Grossman, R.G. (1991) The effect of glucose administration on carbohydrate metabolism after head injury. *Journal of Neurosurgery*, **74**, 43–50.

8 MacKay, R.J. (2004) Brain injury after head trauma: Pathophysiology, diagnosis, and treatment. *Veterinary Clinics of North America: Equine Practice*, **20**, 199–216.

9 Wilson, D.V., Schott, H.C., 2nd, Robinson, N.E., Berney, C.E. & Eberhart, S.W. (2006) Response to nasopharyngeal oxygen administration in horses with lung disease. *Equine Veterinary Journal*, **38**, 219–223.

10 Gaither, J.B., Spaite, D.W., Bobrow, B.J. *et al.* (2012) Balancing the potential risks and benefits of out-of-hospital intubation in traumatic brain injury: The intubation/hyperventilation effect. *Annals of Emergency Medicine*, **60**, 732–736.

11 Paczynski, R.P. (1997) Osmotherapy. Basic concepts and controversies. *Critical Care Clinics*, **13**, 105–129.

12 Roberts, I., Schierhout, G. & Wakai, A. (2003) Mannitol for acute traumatic brain injury. *Cochrane Database of Systematic Reviews*, (4), CD001049.

13 Grande, P.O. & Romner, B. (2012) Osmotherapy in brain edema: A questionable therapy. *Journal of Neurosurgery and Anesthesiology*, **24**, 407–412.

14 Mayzler, O., Leon, A., Eilig, I. *et al.* (2006) The effect of hypertonic (3%) saline with and without furosemide on plasma osmolality, sodium concentration, and brain water content after closed head trauma in rats. *Journal of Neurosurgery and Anesthesiology*, **18**, 24–31.

15 Todd, M.M., Cutkomp, J. & Brian, J.E. (2006) Influence of mannitol and furosemide, alone and in combination, on brain water content after fluid percussion injury. *Anesthesiology*, **105**, 1176–1181.

16 Trogdon, H.M. (2003) Changes in mentation, seizures, and narcolepsy. In: N.E. Robinson (ed), *Current Therapy in Equine Medicine*, pp. 764–771. Saunders, St Louis.

17 Roberts, I. & Sydenham, E. (2012) Barbiturates for acute traumatic brain injury. *Cochrane Database of Systematic Reviews*, **12**, CD000033.

18 Lacombe, V. & Furr, M. (2008) Differential diagnosis and management of horses with seizures or alterations in consciousness. In: M. Furr & S. Reed (eds), *Equine Neurology*, pp. 77–93. Blackwell Publishing, Ames.

19 Bracken, M.B. (2002) Methylprednisolone and spinal cord injury. *Journal of Neurosurgery*, **96**, 140–141, author reply 142.

20 Bracken, M.B. (2001) Methylprednisolone and acute spinal cord injury: An update of the randomized evidence. *Spine*, **26**, S47–S54.

21 Bracken, M.B., Shepard, M.J., Collins, W.F. *et al.* (1990) A randomized, controlled trial of methylprednisolone or naloxone in the treatment of acute spinal-cord injury. Results of the Second National Acute Spinal Cord Injury Study. *New England Journal of Medicine*, **322**, 1405–1411.

22 Leake, G.C., Pascale, V.J., Alfano, S.L. & Bracken, M.B. (1990) Methylprednisolone for acute spinal cord injury. *American Journal of Hospital Pharmacy*, **47**, 1977–1978.

23 Shepard, M.J. & Bracken, M.B. (1994) The effect of methylprednisolone, naloxone, and spinal cord trauma on four liver enzymes: Observations from NASCIS 2. National Acute Spinal Cord Injury Study. *Paraplegia*, **32**, 236–245.

24 Sayer, F.T., Kronvall, E. & Nilsson, O.G. (2006) Methylprednisolone treatment in acute spinal cord injury: The myth challenged through a structured analysis of published literature. *Spine Journal*, **6**, 335–343.

25 Furr, M. & Sampieri, F. (2008) Differential diagnosis of urinary incontinence and cauda equina syndrome. In: M. Furr & S. Reed (eds), *Equine Neurology*, pp. 119–125. Blackwell Publishing, Ames.

26 Reed, S.K., Grant, B. & Nout, Y. (2008) Cervical vertebral stenotic myelopathy. In: M. Furr & S. Reed (eds), *Equine Neurology*, pp. 283–303. Blackwell Publishing, Ames.

27 Grisel, G.B., Grant, B.D. & Rantanen, N.W. (1996) Arthrocentesis of the equine cervical facets. 42nd Annual Convention of the American Association of Equine Practitioners, December 8–11, Denver, CO, pp. 197–198.

28 Levine, J.M., Adam, E., MacKay, R.J., Walker, M.A., Frederick, J.D. & Cohen, N.D. (2007) Confirmed and presumptive cervical vertebral compressive myelopathy in older horses: A retrospective study (1992–2004). *Journal of Veterinary Internal Medicine*, **21**, 812–819.

29 Furr, M., Howe, D., Reed, S. & Yeargan, M. (2011) Antibody coefficients for the diagnosis of equine protozoal myeloencephalitis. *Journal of Veterinary Internal Medicine*, **25**, 138–142.

30 Johnson, A.L., Morrow, J.K. & Sweeney, R.W. (2013) Indirect fluorescent antibody test and surface antigen ELISAs for antemortem diagnosis of equine protozoal myeloencephalitis. *Journal of Veterinary Internal Medicine*, **27**, 596–599.

31 Reed, S.M., Howe, D.K., Morrow, J.K. *et al.* (2013) Accurate antemortem diagnosis of equine protozoal myeloencephalitis (EPM) based on detecting intrathecal antibodies against Sarcocystis neurona using the SnSAG2 and SnSAG4/3 ELISAs. *Journal of Veterinary Internal Medicine*, **27**, 1193–1200.

32 Furr, M. (2008) Equine protozoal myeloencephalitis. In: M. Furr & S. Reed (eds), *Equine Neurology*, pp. 197–212. Blackwell Publishing, Ames.

33 Reed, S. (2008) Neurology is not a euphemism for necropsy: A review of selected neurological diseases affecting horses. Proceedings of the 54th Annual Convention of the American Association of Equine Practitioners, December 6-10, San Diego, CA, pp. 78–109.

34 Mackay, R.J. (2006) Equine Protozoal Myeloencephalitis: Treatment, prognosis, and prevention. *Clinical Techniques in Equine Practice*, **5**, 9–16.

35 Bayer Corporation (2001) *Freedom of information summary*. http://www.fda.gov/downloads/AnimalVeterinary/Products/

ApprovedAnimalDrugProducts/FOIADrugSummaries/ucm117581.pdf [accessed on May 16, 2014].

36 Furr, M. & Kennedy, T. (2001) Cerebrospinal fluid and serum concentrations of ponazuril in horses. *Veterinary Therapeutics*, **2**, 232–237.

37 Lindsay, D.S., Dubey, J. & Kennedy, T. (2000) Determination of the activity of ponazuril against Sarcocystis neurona in cell cultures. *Veterinary Parasitology*, **92**, 165–169.

38 Schering-Plough Animal Health Corporation. (2007) *Freedom of information summary*. http://www.fda.gov/downloads/Animal Veterinary/Products/ApprovedAnimalDrugProducts/FOIADrugSummaries/ucm062320.pdf [accessed on May 16, 2014].

39 Goehring, L. (2008) Viral diseases of the nervous system. In: M. Furr & S. Reed (eds), *Equine Neurology*, pp. 169–186. Blackwell Publishing, Ames.

40 Moore, I., Horney, B., Day, K., Lofstedt, J. & Cribb, A.E. (2004) Treatment of inflammatory airway disease in young standardbreds with interferon alpha. *Canadian Veterinary Journal*, **45**, 594–601.

41 Tyler, K.L. (2004) Herpes simplex virus infections of the central nervous system: Encephalitis and meningitis, including Mollaret's. *Herpes*, **11** (Suppl 2), 57A–64A.

42 Wong, D.M., Belgrave, R.L., Williams, K.J. *et al.* (2008) Multinodular pulmonary fibrosis in five horses. *Journal of the American Veterinary Medical Association*, **232**, 898–905.

43 Bentz, B.G., Maxwell, L.K., Erkert, R.S. *et al.* (2006) Pharmacokinetics of acyclovir after single intravenous and oral administration to adult horses. *Journal of Veterinary Internal Medicine*, **20**, 589–594.

44 Garre, B., Shebany, K., Gryspeerdt, A. *et al.* (2007) Pharmacokinetics of acyclovir after intravenous infusion of acyclovir and after oral administration of acyclovir and its prodrug valacyclovir in healthy adult horses. *Antimicrobial Agents and Chemotherapy*, **51**, 4308–4314.

45 Maxwell, L.K., Bentz, B.G., Bourne, D.W. & Erkert, R.S. (2008) Pharmacokinetics of valacyclovir in the adult horse. *Journal of Veterinary Pharmacology and Therapeutics*, **31**, 312–320.

46 Nasisse, M.P., Dorman, D.C., Jamison, K.C., Weigler, B.J., Hawkins, E.C. & Stevens, J.B. (1997) Effects of valacyclovir in cats infected with feline herpesvirus 1. *American Journal of Veterinary Research*, **58**, 1141–1144.

47 Garre, B., Gryspeerdt, A., Croubels, S., De Backer, P. & Nauwynck, H. (2009) Evaluation of orally administered valacyclovir in experimentally EHV1-infected ponies. *Veterinary Microbiology*, **135**, 214–221.

48 Maxwell, L., Bentz, B., Gilliam, L. *et al.* (2009) Efficacy of valacyclovir against disease following EHV-1 challenge. Proceedings of the American College of Veterinary Internal Medicine Forum, Montreal, Quebec Canada.

49 Carmichael, R.J., Whitfield, C. & Maxwell, L.K. (2013) Pharmacokinetics of ganciclovir and valganciclovir in the adult horse. *Journal of Veterinary Pharmacology and Therapeutics*, **36**, 441–449.

50 Tsujimura, K., Yamada, M., Nagata, S. *et al.* (2010) Pharmacokinetics of penciclovir after oral administration of its prodrug famciclovir to horses. *Journal of Veterinary Medical Science*, **72**, 357–361.

51 Maxwell, L., Gilliam, L., Pusterla, N. *et al.* (2011) Efficacy of delayed antiviral therapy against EHV-1 challenge. Proceedings of the American College of Veterinary Internal Medicine Forum. Denver, CO.

52 Madigan, J.E. & Bell, S.A. (1998) Characterisation of head-shaking syndrome-31 cases. *Equine Veterinary Journal Supplement*, **27**, 28–29.

53 Mills, D.S. & Taylor, K. (2003) Field study of the efficacy of three types of nose net for the treatment of headshaking in horses. *Veterinary Record*, **152**, 41–44.

54 Newton, S.A., Knottenbelt, D.C. & Eldridge, P.R. (2000) Headshaking in horses: Possible aetiopathogenesis suggested by the results of diagnostic tests and several treatment regimes used in 20 cases. *Equine Veterinary Journal*, **32**, 208–216.

55 Terry, R.L., McDonnell, S.M., Van Eps, A.W. *et al.* (2010) Pharmacokinetic profile and behavioral effects of gabapentin in the horse. *Journal of Veterinary Pharmacology and Therapeutics*, **33**, 485–494.

56 Davis, J.L., Posner, L.P. & Elce, Y. (2007) Gabapentin for the treatment of neuropathic pain in a pregnant horse. *Journal of the American Veterinary Medical Association*, **231**, 755–758.

57 Roberts, V. (2011) Idiopathic headshaking in horses: Understanding the pathophysiology. *Veterinary Record*, **168**, 17–18.

58 Pirie, R.S. (2003) Bladder, rectal, anal, tail paralysis; perineal hypalgesia; and other signs or cauda equina syndrome. In: N.E. Robinson (ed), *Current Therapy in Equine Medicine*, 5th edn, pp. 755–760. St. Louis, Saunders.

59 Jose-Cunilleras, E. & Hinchcliff, K.W. (1999) Renal pharmacology. *Veterinary Clinics of North America: Equine Practice*, **15**, 647–664 ix.

60 Furr, M. (2008) Disorders of the peripheral nervous system. In: M. Furr & S. Reed (eds), *Equine Neurology*, pp. 329–336. Blackwell Publishing, Ames.

61 Kadlubowski, M. & Ingram, P.L. (1981) Circulating antibodies to the neuritogenic myelin protein, P2, in neuritis of the cauda equina of the horse. *Nature*, **293**, 299–300.

62 Sheremata, W., Colby, S., Karkhanis, Y. & Eylar, E.H. (1975) Cellular hypersensitivity to basic myelin (P2) protein in the Guillain-Barre syndrome. *Canadian Journal of Neurological Sciences*, **2**, 87–90.

63 Hahn, C. (2008) Miscellaneous movement disorders. In: M. Furr & S. Reed (eds), *Equine Neurology*, pp. 365–372. Blackwell Publishing, Ames.

64 Huntington, P.J., Seneque, S., Slocombe, R.F., Jeffcott, L.B., McLean, A. & Luff, A.R. (1991) Use of phenytoin to treat horses with Australian stringhalt. *Australian Veterinary Journal*, **68**, 221–224.

65 Fintl, C. (2003) Idiopathic and rare neurologic diseases. In: N.E. Robinson (ed), *Current Therapy in Equine Medicine*, pp. 760–763. Saunders, St Louis.

66 Lowenstein, D.H. (2005) Seizures and epilepsy. In: D.L. Kasper, A. Fauci, D.L. Longo, E. Braunwald, S.L. Hauser & J.L. Jameson (eds), *Harrison's Principles of Internal Medicine*, pp. 2357–2372. McGraw-Hill, New York.

67 Mayhew, I.G. (1983) Seizure disorders. In: N. Robertson (ed), *Current Therapy in Equine Medicine*, pp. 344–349. WB Saunders, Philadelphia.

68 Duran, S.H., Ravis, W.R., Pedersoli, W.M. & Schumacher, J. (1987) Pharmacokinetics of phenobarbital in the horse. *American Journal of Veterinary Research*, **48**, 807–810.

69 Borris, D.J., Bertram, E.H. & Kapur, J. (2000) Ketamine controls prolonged status epilepticus. *Epilepsy Research*, **42**, 117–122.

70 Raidal, S.L. & Edwards, S. (2005) Pharmacokinetics of potassium bromide in adult horses. *Australian Veterinary Journal*, **83**, 425–430.

71 Baird-Heinz, H.E., Van Schoick, A.L., Pelsor, F.R., Ranivand, L. & Hungerford, L.L. (2012) A systematic review of the safety of potassium bromide in dogs. *Journal of the American Veterinary Medical Association*, **240**, 705–715.

72 Kowalczyk, D.F. & Beech, J. (1983) Pharmacokinetics of phenytoin (diphenylhydantoin) in horses. *Journal of Veterinary Pharmacology and Therapeutics*, **6**, 133–140.

73 Magdesian, K.G. (2006) Intensive care medicine. In: A.J. Higgins & J. Synder (eds), *The Equine Manual*, pp. 1255–1326. WB Saunders, Philadelphia.

74 Lunn, D.P., Cuddon, P.A., Shaftoe, S. & Archer, R.M. (1993) Familial occurrence of narcolepsy in miniature horses. *Equine Veterinary Journal*, **25**, 483–487.

75 Nau, R., Sorgel, F. & Eiffert, H. (2010) Penetration of drugs through the blood-cerebrospinal fluid/blood-brain barrier for treatment of central nervous system infections. *Clinical Microbiology Reviews*, **23**, 858–883.

76 Platt, H. (1973) Septicaemia in the foal. A review of 61 cases. *British Veterinary Journal*, **129**, 221–229.

77 Furr, M. (2008) Bacterial infections of the central nervous system. In: M. Furr & S. Reed (eds), *Equine Neurology*, pp. 187–196. Blackwell Publishing, Ames.

78 Giguere, S. (2006) Antimicrobial drug use in horses. In: S. Giguere, J.F. Prescott, J.D. Baggot *et al.* (eds), *Antimicrobial Therapy in Veterinary Medicine*, pp. 449–462. Blackwell Publishing, Ames.

79 Gardner, S.Y. & Papich, M.G. (2001) Comparison of cefepime pharmacokinetics in neonatal foals and adult dogs. *Journal of Veterinary Pharmacology and Therapeutics*, **24**, 187–192.

80 Gardner, S.Y., Sweeney, R.W. & Divers, T.J. (1993) Pharmacokinetics of cefotaxime in neonatal pony foals. *American Journal of Veterinary Research*, **54**, 576–579.

81 Ringger, N.C., Brown, M.P., Kohlepp, S.J., Gronwall, R.R. & Merritt, K. (1998) Pharmacokinetics of ceftriaxone in neonatal foals. *Equine Veterinary Journal*, **30**, 163–165.

82 Dowling, P.M. & Kruth, S. (2006) Antimicrobial therapy of selected organ systems. In: S. Giguere, J.F. Prescott, J.D. Baggot *et al.* (eds), *Antimicrobial Therapy in Veterinary Medicine*, pp. 357–379. Blackwell Publishing, Ames.

83 Brown, M.P., Kelly, R.H., Gronwall, R.R. & Stover, S.M. (1984) Chloramphenicol sodium succinate in the horse: Serum, synovial, peritoneal, and urine concentrations after single-dose intravenous administration. *American Journal of Veterinary Research*, **45**, 578–580.

84 Gronwall, R., Brown, M.P., Merritt, A.M. & Stone, H.W. (1986) Body fluid concentrations and pharmacokinetics of chloramphenicol given to mares intravenously or by repeated gavage. *American Journal of Veterinary Research*, **47**, 2591–2595.

85 Varma, K.J., Powers, T.E. & Powers, J.D. (1987) Single- and repeat-dose pharmacokinetic studies of chloramphenicol in horses: Values and limitations of pharmacokinetic studies in predicting dosage regimens. *American Journal of Veterinary Research*, **48**, 403–406.

86 Hart, K.A., Flaminio, M.J., LeRoy, B.E., Williams, C.O., Dietrich, U.M. & Barton, M.H. (2008) Successful resolution of cryptococcal meningitis and optic neuritis in an adult horse with oral fluconazole. *Journal of Veterinary Internal Medicine*, **22**, 1436–1440.

87 Steckel, R.R., Adams, S.B., Long, G.G. & Rebar, A.H. (1982) Antemortem diagnosis and treatment of cryptococcal meningitis in a horse. *Journal of the American Veterinary Medical Association*, **180**, 1085–1089.

88 Giguere, S. (2006) Antifungal chemotherapy. In: S. Giguere, J.F. Prescott, J.D. Baggot *et al.* (eds), *Antimicrobial Therapy in Veterinary Medicine*, pp. 301–322. Blackwell Publishing, Ames.

89 Prades, M., Brown, M.P., Gronwall, R. & Houston, A.E. (1989) Body fluid and endometrial concentrations of ketoconazole in mares after intravenous injection or repeated gavage. *Equine Veterinary Journal*, **21**, 211–214.

90 Davis, J.L., Salmon, J.H. & Papich, M.G. (2005) Pharmacokinetics and tissue distribution of itraconazole after oral and intravenous administration to horses. *American Journal of Veterinary Research*, **66**, 1694–1701.

91 Negroni, R. & Arechavala, A.I. (1993) Itraconazole: Pharmacokinetics and indications. *Archives of Medical Research*, **24**, 387–393.

92 Mootsikapun, P., Chetchotisakd, P., Anunnatsiri, S. & Choksawadphinyo, K. (2003) The efficacy of fluconazole 600 mg/day versus itraconazole 600 mg/day as consolidation therapy of cryptococcal meningitis in AIDS patients. *Journal of the Medical Association of Thailand*, **86**, 293–298.

93 Saag, M.S., Cloud, G.A., Graybill, J.R. *et al.* (1999) A comparison of itraconazole versus fluconazole as maintenance therapy for AIDS-associated cryptococcal meningitis. National Institute of Allergy and Infectious Diseases Mycoses Study Group. *Clinical Infectious Diseases*, **28**, 291–296.

94 Ball, M.A., Rebhun, W.C., Gaarder, J.E. & Patten, V. (1997) Evaluation of itraconazole-dimethyl sulfoxide ointment for treatment of keratomycosis in nine horses. *Journal of the American Veterinary Medical Association*, **211**, 199–203.

95 Korenek, N.L., Legendre, A.M., Andrews, F.M. *et al.* (1994) Treatment of mycotic rhinitis with itraconazole in three horses. *Journal of Veterinary Internal Medicine*, **8**, 224–227.

96 Latimer, F.G., Colitz, C.M., Campbell, N.B. & Papich, M.G. (2001) Pharmacokinetics of fluconazole following intravenous and oral administration and body fluid concentrations of fluconazole following repeated oral dosing in horses. *American Journal of Veterinary Research*, **62**, 1606–1611.

97 Davis, J.L., Salmon, J.H. & Papich, M.G. (2006) Pharmacokinetics of voriconazole after oral and intravenous administration to horses. *American Journal of Veterinary Research*, **67**, 1070–1075.

98 Colitz, C.M., Latimer, F.G., Cheng, H., Chan, K.K., Reed, S.M. & Pennick, G.J. (2007) Pharmacokinetics of voriconazole following intravenous and oral administration and body fluid concentrations of voriconazole following repeated oral administration in horses. *American Journal of Veterinary Research*, **68**, 1115–1121.

99 Vermes, A., Guchelaar, H.J. & Dankert, J. (2000) Flucytosine: A review of its pharmacology, clinical indications, pharmacokinetics, toxicity and drug interactions. *Journal of Antimicrobial Chemotherapy*, **46**, 171–179.

100 Magnarelli, L.A., Ijdo, J.W., Van Andel, A.E., Wu, C., Padula, S.J. & Fikrig, E. (2000) Serologic confirmation of Ehrlichia equi and Borrelia burgdorferi infections in horses from the northeastern United States. *Journal of the American Veterinary Medical Association*, **217**, 1045–1050.

101 James, F.M., Engiles, J.B. & Beech, J. (2010) Meningitis, cranial neuritis, and radiculoneuritis associated with Borrelia burgdorferi infection in a horse. *Journal of the American Veterinary Medical Association*, **237**, 1180–1185.

102 Imai, D.M., Barr, B.C., Daft, B. *et al.* (2011) Lyme neuroborreliosis in 2 horses. *Veterinary Pathology*, **48**, 1151–1157.

103 Divers, T.J. & Chang, Y. (2009) Lyme disease. In: N.E. Robinson & K.A. Sprayberry (eds), *Current Therapy in Equine Medicine*, pp. 143–144. Saunders Elsevier, St Louis.

104 Mervine, P. (2003) Treatment of neuroborreliosis. *Pediatric Infectious Disease Journal*, **22**, 671–672.

105 Hurcombe, S. (2008) Equine hepatic encephalopathy. In: M. Furr & S. Reed (eds), *Equine Neurology*, pp. 257–268. Blackwell Publishing, Ames.

106 Ahboucha, S. & Butterworth, R.F. (2004) Pathophysiology of hepatic encephalopathy: A new look at GABA from the molecular standpoint. *Metabolic Brain Disease*, **19**, 331–343.

107 Poh, Z. & Chang, P.E. (2012) A current review of the diagnostic and treatment strategies of hepatic encephalopathy. *International Journal of Hepatology*, **2012**, 480309.

108 Bismuth, M., Funakoshi, N., Cadranel, J.F. & Blanc, P. (2011) Hepatic encephalopathy: From pathophysiology to therapeutic management. *European Journal of Gastroenterology & Hepatology*, **23**, 8–22.

109 Wen, J., Liu, Q., Song, J., Tong, M., Peng, L. & Liang, H. (2013) Lactulose is highly potential in prophylaxis of hepatic encephalopathy in patients with cirrhosis and upper gastrointestinal bleeding: Results of a controlled randomized trial. *Digestion*, **87**, 132–138.

110 Goulenok, C., Bernard, B., Cadranel, J.F. *et al.* (2002) Flumazenil vs. placebo in hepatic encephalopathy in patients with cirrhosis: A meta-analysis. *Alimentary Pharmacology and Therapeutics*, **16**, 361–372.

111 Marsden, M.D. (2008) Stereotypic and other behavior problems. In: M. Furr & S. Reed (eds), *Equine Neurology*, pp. 373–402. Blackwell Publishing, Ames.

112 Dodman, N.H., Shuster, L., Court, M.H. & Dixon, R. (1987) Investigation into the use of narcotic antagonists in the treatment of a stereotypic behavior pattern (crib-biting) in the horse. *American Journal of Veterinary Research*, **48**, 311–319.

113 Kamerling, S.G., Hamra, J.G. & Bagwell, C.A. (1990) Naloxone-induced abdominal distress in the horse. *Equine Veterinary Journal*, **22**, 241–243.

114 Houpt, K.A. & McDonnell, S.M. (1993) Equine stereotypes. *Compendium on Continuing Education for the Equine Practice*, **15**, 1265–1272.

115 Baldessarini, R.J. & Tarazi, F.I. (2001) Drugs and the treatment of psychiatric disorders. In: J.G. Hardman, L.E. Limbird & A.G. Gilman (eds), *Goodman's and Gilman's Pharmacological Basis of Therapeutics*, pp. 485–520. McGraw-Hill, New York.

116 Baird, J.D., Arroyo, L.G., Vengust, M. *et al.* (2006) Adverse extrapyramidal effects in four horse given fluphenazine decanoate. *Journal of the American Veterinary Medical Association*, **229**, 104–110.

117 Brashier, M. (2006) Fluphenazine-induced extrapyramidal side effects in a horse. *Veterinary Clinics of North America: Equine Practice*, **22**, e37–e45.

118 Brewer, B.D., Hines, M.T., Stewart, J.T. & Langlois, J.F. (1990) Fluphenazine induced Parkinson-like syndrome in a horse. *Equine Veterinary Journal*, **22**, 136–137.

119 Kauffman, V.G., Soma, L., Divers, T.J. & Perkons, S.Z. (1989) Extrapyramidal side effects caused by fluphenazine decanoate in a horse. *Journal of the American Veterinary Medical Association*, **195**, 1128–1130.

120 Stitzel, R.E. (1976) The biological fate of reserpine. *Pharmacological Reviews*, **28**, 179–208.

121 Alper, M.H., Flacke, W. & Krayer, O. (1963) Pharmacology of reserpine and its implications for anesthesia. *Anesthesiology*, **24**, 524–542.

122 Memon, M.A., Usenik, E.A., Varner, D.D. & Meyers, P.J. (1988) Penile paralysis and paraphimosis associated with reserpine administration in a stallion. *Theriogenology*, **30**, 411–419.

CHAPTER 13

Clinical pharmacology of the equine musculoskeletal system

Bradford Bentz

Equine Medicine and Surgery, Bossier City, LA, USA

Nonsteroidal anti-inflammatory drugs

Introduction

Nonsteroidal anti-inflammatory drugs (NSAIDs) are commonly used in horses for the elimination and control of musculoskeletal pain and inflammation. NSAIDs block the cyclooxygenase (COX) enzyme, interrupting formation of thromboxane, prostacyclin, and the prostaglandins from arachidonic acid. This results in antipyretic action, pain relief, anti-inflammatory effects, and inhibition of platelet clumping. NSAIDs may also alter immune system responses and suppress inflammatory mediators other than the COX products. As a class, NSAIDs are associated with gastrointestinal ulceration and reduction in kidney perfusion. However, the NSAIDs used in horses do not all exhibit the same pharmacologic properties and toxicological profiles. Due to their potential for side effects, judicious NSAID use is always recommended. Negative side effects are observed more often when these agents are used at high doses or administered for prolonged periods of time or in the presence of exacerbating conditions, such as dehydration. Ensuring good patient hydration and considering coadministration of medications for the prophylaxis of gastrointestinal ulceration are advisable [1, 2]. There is minimal evidence of any clinical benefit to simultaneous administration or 2 or more NSAIDs. NSAIDs administered together will be additive in their toxic potential. A recent investigation also showed a lack of reduced toxicity when a COX-selective NSAID (firocoxib) was administered with a nonselective COX inhibitor (phenylbutazone (PBZ)) [3]. See Chapter 5 for a more detailed discussion on the general aspects of the pharmacology of NSAID.

Specific NSAIDs commonly used in horses
Aspirin

Aspirin is the weakest NSAID commonly used in horses, and for this reason, it is rarely used as a primary treatment for inflammatory conditions or pain management. Although most of the other NSAIDs reversibly inhibit activity on platelet COX, aspirin irreversibly binds to COX in platelets and therefore is associated with the greatest antiplatelet activity of the NSAID. This has made aspirin the NSAID of choice to decrease platelet aggregation and inhibit thrombus formation. The recommended dose for aspirin in the horse is partially dependent on its intended effect. Although it is a poor analgesic, it has been used for analgesia at doses of 25–50 mg/kg bwt every 12 h. For antiplatelet activity, aspirin may be administered at 10–20 mg/kg bwt every 24–48 h. Clinical applications for the use of aspirin as an inhibitor of platelet aggregation include the management of conditions that involve, or that may involve, damage to vascular endothelium and clot formation. These conditions include laminitis, thromboembolic colic, recurrent uveitis, and endotoxemia.

Aspirin administered to the horse is partially metabolized in the blood and liver to salicylic acid, which is rapidly excreted by the kidneys into the urine. As salicylic acid is a natural component of grass hay, horses

Equine Pharmacology, First Edition. Edited by Cynthia Cole, Bradford Bentz and Lara Maxwell.

consuming it will have low concentrations of the compound in their urine. Most medication control programs for equine athletes have adopted maximum permitted thresholds for salicylic acid in urine samples to account for this natural source [1, 2].

Phenylbutazone

PBZ is the most commonly used NSAID in horses, and it exhibits significant analgesic, anti-inflammatory, and antipyretic activity via inhibition of COX. It is available in formulations approved for oral (PO) and intravenous (IV) administrations. The injectable formulation can only be administered by careful IV administration, because it causes severe tissue damage if extravasated or if administered intramuscularly or subcutaneously. Following oral administration, PBZ is well absorbed, but the rate of absorption is delayed by the presence of food. In the blood, greater than 99% of the PBZ is carried bound to plasma proteins [4, 5]. In the liver, a portion of the PBZ is metabolized to oxyphenbutazone, a metabolite with activity similar to that of PBZ but with a slower rate of elimination. Because of the persistence of the metabolite, some of the therapeutic effects of PBZ will persist for more than 24 h after administration. The enzymatic capacity of the liver to metabolize PBZ becomes saturated following administration of relatively low dosages, which can dramatically decrease the rate of drug elimination. High doses of PBZ can therefore easily overwhelm the liver's ability to metabolize the drug, resulting in toxicity. PBZ and oxyphenbutazone will cross the placenta and are excreted in mare's milk, so cautious use or avoidance is warranted in nursing mares [1, 2, 4–9].

PBZ is used extensively in horses for a wide variety of musculoskeletal disorders; however, navicular disease, laminitis, and degenerative joint disease are among the most commonly treated disorders. Depending on the condition and severity of disease, PBZ may alleviate lameness or other pain for up to several days following its use. For severe musculoskeletal pain (e.g., laminitis), an initial dose of 4.4 mg/kg bwt q12 h is often administered. In order to avoid development of toxic effects, however, this dose should be rapidly tapered to a dose of 2.2 mg/kg bwt q12 h. If pain control is inadequate, concomitant therapy with a different class of analgesic, such as opioids, should be considered. For less severe pain and inflammation, an initial dose of 2.2 mg/kg bwt q12 h is appropriate. As soon as clinically possible, this

dose should also be decreased to 2.2 mg/kg bwt q24 h to minimize the risk of toxicity. In part due to drug accumulation associated with the slow excretion of oxyphenbutazone, PBZ is regarded as the NSAID with the greatest potential for toxicity in horses [1, 2, 8–12]. Clinical evidence of PBZ toxicity may occur in horses at any time during therapy. In particular, some horses appear to exhibit gastrointestinal discomfort or dysfunction with doses as low as 1 g per day and/or a duration of therapy of only a few days. Therefore, long-term use of PBZ for chronic conditions requires careful monitoring. When treatment extends beyond 5–7 days, the dosage interval should be extended to an every other day administration whenever clinically possible.

Ulcer prophylaxis should be considered to further minimize the risks of toxicity, particularly in horses that have exhibited sensitivity to the toxic effects of NSAID. Antiulcer therapy may also be warranted in horses receiving or expected to receive PBZ for more than 5–7 days. A commonly employed approach to ulcer prophylaxis is the administration of a proton pump inhibitor, such as omeprazole, or an H_2 antagonist, such as ranitidine.

Although toxicity to the gastrointestinal tract is the most prominent adverse effect of PBZ therapy in horses, other organ systems are also subject to toxicity. For example, PBZ also causes kidney damage from inhibiting the prostaglandins that maintain renal blood flow, and the nephrotoxic effect is significantly exacerbated by dehydration. In addition, PBZ competes for the same cellular binding sites as thyroid hormone. Treating horses for just 4 or 5 days causes significant decreases in both serum thyroxine T4 and free thyroxine concentrations [13, 14]. As a result, administration of PBZ to horses results in a greater than normal response to injection with thyroid-stimulating hormone [14]. Liver disease may impair elimination of PBZ, leading to higher concentrations of free PBZ in the blood and potentially toxicity.

Dipyrone

Although it has been used in horses for many years, the pharmacology of dipyrone has not been well investigated in this species. Dipyrone is thought to act similarly to other NSAIDs by inhibiting COX. Although FDA-approved formulations are no longer available, compounded formulations for IV, IM, or SC administration to horses can be obtained. Preparations of compounded products, however, are not regulated by the FDA, but rather, the pharmacies that produce them are regulated by state pharmacy boards with varying degrees of oversight. Therefore, the sterility, potency, and purity of these preparations may be suspect depending on the quality of the pharmacy formulating them.

Although not all equine veterinarians agree, dipyrone is reported to exhibit mild analgesic, antipyretic, and anti-inflammatory properties. Dipyrone also reportedly inhibits bradykinin-induced spasms of the gastrointestinal tract (e.g., spasmodic colic), but is not as efficacious as flunixin meglumine for visceral pain. High doses or chronic therapy with dipyrone may result in damage to the bone marrow as manifest by abnormal blood cell production. Other adverse reactions include gastrointestinal upset, pain at the injection site, skin reactions, hemolytic anemia, tremors, and anaphylactic reactions. Dipyrone should not be administered to horses with blood or bone marrow abnormalities [1, 2].

Flunixin meglumine

Flunixin meglumine is a potent inhibitor of COX that is available in injectable formulations, as well as pastes and granules for oral administration. Flunixin meglumine is rapidly absorbed following oral administration, and peak serum concentrations occur within 30 min of dosing. The onset of anti-inflammatory and analgesic action is within 2 h of administration, and the duration of action may extend to 36 h. As with other NSAIDs, flunixin is highly bound to serum proteins. Flunixin also accumulates in inflamed tissue and therefore its analgesic effects may persist longer than the drug is detectable in blood [1, 2, 11, 12]. It is primarily eliminated by the kidneys, as unchanged parent molecule in the urine.

Flunixin is used as an anti-inflammatory and analgesic agent in horses for a variety of conditions including colic, colitis, exertional rhabdomyolysis, endotoxemia, pleurodynia, laminitis, ocular inflammation and pain, and other musculoskeletal disorders. The recommended dose is 1.1 mg/kg bwt once daily, but higher doses and frequencies are often used initially for painful conditions, such as colic. Low-dose therapy with flunixin, at one-quarter the recommended dose, administered three to four times a day, exhibits antiendotoxic effects without masking signs of colic pain or causing toxicity. Although not universally accepted, some veterinarians believe that high doses of flunixin may mask signs of severe visceral pain and interfere with the clinician's ability to determine when surgical intervention is necessary. Flunixin causes similar adverse effects as PBZ but appears to have a wider safety margin. High doses can result in loss of appetite, depression, and gastrointestinal tract ulcers. IM injections of flunixin have been associated with fatal cases of clostridial myositis, so that route should be avoided even though it is a labeled route of administration.

Meclofenamic acid

Meclofenamic acid has been used for many years as an analgesic and an anti-inflammatory agent for musculoskeletal conditions in horses. As with most other NSAIDs, feeding prior to dosing may delay absorption of meclofenamic acid from the horse's stomach. Meclofenamic acid is typically administered orally to horses at a dose of 2.2 mg/kg bwt once a day. There is currently no FDA-approved product available in the USA, but it can be obtained from compounding pharmacies. Because the anti-inflammatory and analgesic action of meclofenamic acid can take 36–96 h to develop, it is often used, when permitted, in anticipation of joint inflammation or in preparation for a competition [1, 2, 15]. Consistent with its delayed onset of action, clinical efficacy can persist for days after therapy is discontinued. Repeated daily dosing does not result in drug accumulation, making it a useful drug for chronic inflammatory conditions, such as navicular disease or bone spavin. Many horses can be maintained comfortably with twice weekly administration without apparent side effects. Meclofenamic acid appears to have a wide safety margin as compared to most of the other NSAIDs. At typical therapeutic doses, however, some decrease in blood protein concentrations has been observed. Doses much higher than the those commonly recommended appear to be necessary to induce toxicity, which may include mouth ulcers, loss of appetite, depression, edema, and weight loss [1, 2, 15].

Ketoprofen

The propionic acid derivative ketoprofen, like other NSAIDs, concentrates in inflamed tissues and persists in those tissues for longer than it can be detected in the blood. Therefore, the anti-inflammatory effects of ketoprofen are not directly related to its concentration in the blood. Ketoprofen is rapidly eliminated from the blood, thereby reducing the chance of nephrotoxicity associated with drug accumulation. The anti-inflammatory effects of ketoprofen appear to peak at about 12 h after administration and last for approximately 24 h [1, 2, 16, 17]. In one study, the analgesia produced by ketoprofen administered at a dose of 3.63 mg/kg bwt was superior to that produced by a 4.4 mg/kg dose of PBZ [16]. Ketoprofen has been reported to have anti-inflammatory effects independent of COX inhibition, including inhibition of bradykinin and lipoxygenase pathways, although the antilipoxygenase effect has not been reliably substantiated to occur *in vivo* [1]. In addition, a cartilage-protective effect, reported in studies using cartilage cultures in the laboratory, has not been demonstrated in the horse.

Ketoprofen is recommended for musculoskeletal injuries, where a single dose may provide pain relief and anti-inflammatory activity for 24 h. Clinically in horses, ketoprofen does not appear to offer significant benefit over the use of flunixin meglumine, except it appears to be less likely to cause gastrointestinal ulcers than other NSAIDs. In a small toxicity study in horses, ketoprofen produced fewer gastrointestinal lesions than treatment with flunixin meglumine or PBZ [11]. At doses many times that recommended, clinical signs of ketoprofen toxicity are similar to those seen with other NSAIDs [1, 2, 12, 16, 17].

Firocoxib

Firocoxib is the first cyclooxygenase-1 (COX1)-sparing drug to be approved by the FDA for use in horses. *In vitro* studies have shown firocoxib to be highly selective for the cyclooxygenase-2 (COX2) isozyme, which is primarily responsible for the production of inflammatory mediators. It is concurrently very sparing of the COX1 isozyme, which is primarily involved in the production of prostaglandins for maintenance of physiologic functions, including gastric cytoprotection, renal homeostasis, and normal platelet function [1, 2, 18]. The recommended dose of firocoxib is 0.1 mg/kg bwt once daily, which corresponds to a 45.5 mg dose for a 1000 lb horse. Firocoxib is eliminated primarily in the urine as a decyclopropylmethylated metabolite. Although some of the COX2-selective NSAIDs are promoted as disease-modifying agents in the treatment of osteoarthritis (DMOAD), it is unclear if this characteristic is exhibited by firocoxib. Therefore, in the management of pain due to osteoarthritis, it remains important to focus on interventions that reduce and slow the progression of the osteoarthritis in addition to addressing pain relief with this or any other NSAID [1, 2, 18].

Topical diclofenac sodium

The phenylacetic acid derivative diclofenac is a nonselective COX and lipoxygenase inhibitor that is commonly used in human medicine. The safety profile of topical diclofenac has been clearly established in humans; its efficacy is equivalent or superior to that of other commonly used NSAIDs, whereas the risk for gastrointestinal irritation and renal toxicity is relatively low. Although there is not a diclofenac product approved for oral or parenteral administration in horses, the FDA has approved a 1% diclofenac liposomal cream formulation (Surpass® [1% diclofenac sodium] Topical Anti-Inflammatory Cream, IDEXX Pharmaceuticals, Portland, ME) for topical administration to horses for control of joint pain and inflammation associated with osteoarthritis. The product is recommended for administration to the horse by application of a five inch (5") ribbon of the cream twice daily over the affected joint for up to 10 days. Topical diclofenac may be effective for the control of joint pain and inflammation associated with osteoarthritis [2]. However, at least one study that investigated the anti-inflammatory efficacy of diclofenac diethylamine applied epicutaneously at a dose rate of 0.44 mg/kg bwt in a model of acute arthritis in horses did not find the drug to be efficacious [19]. Another study was performed to evaluate the urinary and serum concentrations of diclofenac after topical administration of 1% liposomal diclofenac cream for 10 days at the label dose, as well as at 2× and 4× the label dose. The results demonstrated the slow absorption and elimination of 1% liposomal diclofenac cream. Following 10 days of topical application of 1% diclofenac liposomal cream at 1×, 2×, and 4× the recommended label dose, diclofenac and 4-hydroxydiclofenac were present in all urine samples collected up to 72 h after the final application. The highest urine concentrations of diclofenac occurred 6 h after the final application of the cream. After administration of 1×, 2×, and 4× the label dose twice daily for 10 days, the decline in diclofenac and 4-hydroxydiclofenac concentrations occurred gradually over the next 3 days, with both the parent compound and the active metabolite present in concentrations above the limit of quantitation of the assay (4.0–8.0 ng/ml) 72 h after the last application of each dosage regimen [20].

Although the clinical efficacy of diclofenac has been questioned, recent work has suggested that the commercially available form of diclofenac for horses exhibits disease-modifying effects for therapy of osteoarthritis [21, 22]. Such claims have led to the use of the topical formulation of diclofenac in horses with a tendency toward swelling of the fetlock joints after hard work, as well as for routine management of horses with joint inflammation and/or disease. Treatment protocols for the therapy of synovitis and capsulitis focus on two endpoints: symptom-modifying effects and disease-modifying effects. Comparison of diclofenac sodium to PBZ in disease-modifying effects appears to favor diclofenac over PBZ [22]. In this comparison, the severity of cartilage lesions evaluated histologically was less severe in the diclofenac-treated group than the PBZ-treated group. In addition, fewer side effects are likely to be encountered with topical diclofenac usage as compared to the use of most systemically administered NSAID [2, 21, 22].

Etodolac

Etodolac is a slightly COX2-selective NSAID that is used infrequently in horses. In one study, the pharmacokinetics of etodolac administered at a dose of 20 mg/kg bwt IV and PO were determined in adult horses [23]. IV administration was associated with a mean plasma half-life of 2.67 h, whereas oral administration produced an average maximum plasma concentration of 32.57 μg/ml and had a bioavailability of 77%. In the same study, *in vitro* determination of the COX1 versus COX2 selectivity of etodolac demonstrated that it is only slightly selective for the COX2 enzyme in the horse [23]. Although an earlier investigation demonstrated the clinical efficacy of etodolac administered daily at a dose of 23 mg/kg bwt, PO, in horses with lameness due to navicular syndrome, it should not be viewed as a selective COX2 agent with the presumed improved safety profile often associated with these agents in veterinary species [24]. This same investigation also revealed that there was no additional clinical benefit when etodolac was administered at the same dose twice a day instead of once [24].

Carprofen

Carprofen is an NSAID of the 2-arylpropionate subclass that is available as a racemic solution for use in horses in some countries, but not in the USA [25]. In one study,

carprofen administered IV at doses of 0.7 and 4 mg/kg bwt was evaluated for the ability to suppress components of the inflammatory response [26]. While the lower dose resulted in moderate but transient inhibition of thromboxane production, it failed to affect prostaglandin, leukotriene B4, and β-glucuronidase concentrations in inflamed tissue. The higher dose produced greater and more persistent inhibition of serum thromboxane production and concurrently inhibited PGE2 synthesis and partially inhibited LTB4 and β-glucuronidase production in inflamed tissue [26]. The concentration–time profiles for the R(−) and S(+) enantiomers in plasma and fluids collected from inflamed and noninflamed tissues showed that the predominant enantiomer in all three was the R(−) form. Penetration of both enantiomers into inflamed tissues was slow and limited, and passage into noninflamed tissue was even lower. Although swelling was reduced by both doses, only the higher dose had an antipyretic effect. This study concluded that carprofen does not exhibit selective inhibition of the COX isozymes. The recommended clinical dose of carprofen is 0.7 mg/kg bwt. Because at this dose it demonstrated minimal inhibition of COX2, it has been suggested that its therapeutic effects may be derived partially through other inflammatory pathways, such as by weak inhibition of 5-lipoxygenase.

In clinical use, carprofen has exhibited a favorable margin of safety [26–28]. This might be explained by its weak COX inhibitory activity. When the drug was given PO at a dose rate of 0.7 mg/kg bwt for 14 consecutive days, there was no evidence of any accumulation of carprofen in plasma [27]. Carprofen was also well tolerated following IV and PO administration. IM administration, however, resulted in elevated levels of plasma creatine kinase, suggesting muscle cell damage. Carprofen has not been approved for use in horses in the USA, but has been used in clinical equine practice as an alternative NSAID.

Meloxicam

The pharmacokinetics of meloxicam in the horse have been evaluated after IV and PO administration in both fed and fasted horses [29]. A single dose of orally administered meloxicam was associated with high bioavailability that was not significantly different in fasted versus fed horses at 85.3 and 95.9%, respectively. However, the mean peak plasma concentrations were lower in fed horses at 1727 µg/l compared to 2577 µg/l in fasted horses [29]. Following oral administration of meloxicam at a dose of 0.6 mg/kg bwt once daily for 14 days, the terminal half-life was approximately 7.75 h and the bioavailability was about 97.5%. The drug was determined not to accumulate with repeated dosing. Urinary excretion of meloxicam was constant for 13 days and fell below the limit of detection of the analytical method used in the study 3 days after the final dose was administered [29].

The efficacy of meloxicam was evaluated in a study using a model of right carpal arthritis [30]. The results of this study indicated a median effective dose (ED_{50}) for clinical lameness of 0.265 mg/kg bwt. The calculated median effective plasma concentration for this lameness model was reported to be 195 ng/ml. The study concluded that meloxicam was a potent anti-inflammatory drug in horses. A daily dose of 0.6 mg/kg bwt was recommended for use [30]. Although meloxicam has been used clinically in horses to a limited extent, additional studies in horses to verify its efficacy and safety are needed.

Naproxen

A limited amount of objective information is available regarding the oral and parenteral use of naproxen in the horse. One pharmacokinetic investigation defined the disposition of naproxen following IV administration at a dose of 5 mg/kg bwt [31]. Ninety-seven percent of the circulating naproxen was bound to plasma proteins, and the appearance of free drug within the plasma was dose dependent. The peak synovial fluid concentration of naproxen occurred 6 h after administration. A large percentage of the dose administered was conjugated by the liver prior to elimination, and only a small amount was excreted as unconjugated drug by renal clearance. In one study, naproxen was still detectable in the urine 48 h after IV administration of a dose of 5 mg/kg bwt [31]. The reported bioavailability of naproxen in horses after oral administration varies from 50 to 87% [32]. The reported serum half-life of naproxen also varies from 4 to 7 h [32]. Recommended clinical doses range from 5 to 10 mg/kg bwt, PO, q12 h. Although there are no specific equine studies demonstrating the clinical efficacy of naproxen, anecdotal reports suggest it is an effective NSAID in horses. Several days of therapy may be required before the effects are clinically evident.

Deracoxib

One study has evaluated the pharmacokinetics of deracoxib administered orally to horses [33]. In this study, following oral administration of a dose of 2 mg/kg bwt, the terminal elimination half-life of deracoxib in horses was determined to be 12.5 h, and the mean maximum plasma concentration occurred 6.33 h after dosing. Evaluation of this drug *in vitro* suggested a slight COX2 selectivity with a COX1/COX2 ratio of approximately 26 for the IC_{50} and 22 for the IC_{80}. It was also stated that computer simulations indicated that following a dose of 2 mg/kg bwt, plasma concentrations would remain above the COX2 IC_{80} for 12 h and above the IC_{50} for 24 h [33].

Tramadol

Tramadol, a centrally acting synthetic analgesic, is commonly used in humans to treat conditions for which NSAIDs are also commonly prescribed, and so it will be discussed in this section. It is not an NSAID; however, it is a weak agonist of the µ opioid receptor, and it also increases serotonin release and inhibits reuptake of norepinephrine within the central nervous system (CNS). The pharmacokinetics of tramadol in the horse have been well defined, and it appears to be gaining popularity as an analgesic in performance horses [34–36]. Nevertheless, the results of pharmacokinetic and efficacy studies of tramadol in horses provide only tepid support for its use in this species. For example, the bioavailability of tramadol in the horse is extremely low at 3% and it has a short elimination half-life. In one investigation, tramadol was reported to be detectable in urine for between 1 and 24 h following its administration. In other studies that used thermal nociceptive analgesia models, tramadol administered at doses of 2 mg/kg bwt provided minimal analgesia [34–36]. Higher doses with relatively short dosing intervals may be necessary to achieve reliable analgesia in the horse. At this time, neither IV nor PO administered tramadol appears to produce significant analgesia in horses. There are no significant objective data to evaluate the use of tramadol in foals.

Pharmacological approaches for the treatment of navicular syndrome

The definition of navicular syndrome has evolved over the years from the simple reference to abnormalities of the navicular bone itself to the recognition and inclusion of pain in the caudal heel and the entire podotrochlear apparatus. The structures now considered to be part of and to contribute to the clinical manifestations of "navicular syndrome" include the collateral sesamoidean ligaments, the distal sesamoidean impar ligament, the navicular bursa, the deep digital flexor tendon, and the navicular bone [37–39]. Diagnostic evaluation of horses with navicular syndrome has expanded correspondingly to focus on all of these structures through the evolution of diagnostic imaging, including digital radiography, nuclear scintigraphy, advanced ultrasonography, and magnetic resonance imaging (MRI).

There are numerous theories behind the cause of navicular syndrome. Regardless of its cause, it is important to recognize that the term syndrome is often used to describe the clinical manifestations of these numerous proposed etiologies. Navicular syndrome is most appropriately diagnosed clinically. That is, clinical signs of pain localized to the podotrochlear apparatus and caudal heel are often termed navicular syndrome but are further substantiated by the documentation of pathological changes affecting the structures of the podotrochlear apparatus [37–39]. With the advent of the use of MRI for foot pain, many subtle pathologic changes are now detectable. The therapies for navicular syndrome are numerous and are frequently based on the proposed etiology. The proposed etiology may vary from one case to the next and from clinician to clinician. The primary theories for the cause of navicular syndrome are a vascular etiology with thrombosis and ischemia and a degenerative etiology. Other contributing factors include genetics, conformation, hoof trimming and shoeing, and chronic use injury [37–39].

Although isoxsuprine is commonly used to treat navicular disease, its use remains controversial. No consistent relationship between radiological evidence of navicular disease, severity of lameness, and response to isoxsuprine treatment has been shown [40–44]. While some investigations have indicated that horses treated with isoxsuprine exhibit positive responses with respect to clinical assessment scores, others showed no clinical benefit and have failed to elucidate any analgesic activity or mechanism of action for reports of clinical improvement. Isoxsuprine binds to beta adrenoreceptors, exhibiting both antagonistic and agonist activities. Its proposed clinical effects include vasodilation, uterine relaxation, as well as reductions in blood viscosity and platelet aggregation. The combined vasodilatory activity

and reduction in blood viscosity form the basis of its theoretical use to treat navicular disease, even though a firm understanding of the pathogenesis of navicular syndrome has not been determined. Following oral administration to horses, isoxsuprine was poorly absorbed, with a bioavailability of 2.2% and a high first-pass effect [42]. The reported elimination half-life in plasma of isoxsuprine was estimated to be less than 3 h and it also exhibited a high volume of distribution. Elimination of isoxsuprine is primarily by renal excretion. In an investigation evaluating equine digital and laminar flow in response to isoxsuprine administration, no increase in blood flow was found [43]. Despite the investigational evidence to the contrary, clinical benefit of isoxsuprine in the treatment of horses with navicular syndrome is anecdotally reported with a high frequency.

Pentoxifylline is another medication commonly used to treat navicular syndrome. Similar to isoxsuprine, pentoxifylline theoretically counteracts the vascular events associated with navicular syndrome. Pentoxifylline has been used in humans to treat disorders of microcirculation. Extrapolation from its activity in humans has led to its use as a rheologic agent in navicular syndrome in horses. Pentoxifylline has been proposed to increase red cell deformability, reduce blood viscosity, and facilitate the dissolution of thrombi, and together, these effects are theorized to improve perfusion and facilitate oxygen delivery to the tissue of the podotrochlear apparatus. Pentoxifylline, which is chemically related to theophylline and caffeine, is also a phosphodiesterase inhibitor and may produce some degree of concurrent vasodilation by this mechanism. Clinical trials of pentoxifylline administered orally at doses ranging from 4.5 to 7 mg/kg bwt q8 h have shown promise, but the use of this drug in the clinical setting is primarily based on its theoretical activities. A 2006 investigation of the pharmacokinetics of pentoxifylline in horses suggested that a dose of 10 mg/kg bwt, PO, q12 h will produce serum concentrations reported to be efficacious in humans [45]. It was also reported that serum concentrations in the horse decreased with repeat administrations, and therefore, the dose may need to be increased if clinical response diminishes with repeat administrations [45].

Warfarin has also been suggested as a potential treatment for navicular disease based on the presumption that decreased blood flow is a significant factor in the disease pathogenesis [37–39]. In one study, the dose of warfarin administered was adjusted until the one-stage prothrombin time (OSPT) was prolonged by 2–4 s [46]. The initial dose was 0.018 mg/kg bwt, PO, and that dose was increased, or in some cases decreased, by 20% until the desired prolongation of OSPT was produced. Final doses varied from 0.012 to 0.75 mg/kg bwt. Seventeen of 20 animals became sound and the remaining 3 showed a marked improvement in their gait. In this study, horses had been lame for an average of 9 months, and on average, horses responded to treatment in 7 weeks [46]. Due to a narrow therapeutic window, the use of warfarin requires close monitoring of coagulation and bleeding parameters. Because there is some evidence that warfarin and PBZ compete for protein binding sites in the blood, concurrent therapy with these two agents should be avoided [9, 10]. Warfarin use in the horse has been associated with numerous side effects including epistaxis, gastrointestinal bleeding, bleeding at venipuncture sites, and hematoma formation following trauma [47]. Its use in the horse for treatment of any disorder should be well justified, carefully considered, and well monitored.

Orgotein is a superoxide dismutase that has been used as an anti-inflammatory agent, and it has been the subject of limited research attention for the treatment of navicular disease and aseptic arthritis of traumatic origin [48, 49]. In one study on navicular syndrome, 3 of 7 horses treated with juxtabursal injections of orgotein were reported to have improved [49]. The current use of this agent for the treatment of these conditions appears to be limited as it has been replaced by newer therapies with significantly more supportive research.

Approved for use in the horse in the European Union (EU), tiludronic acid (TA) was specifically developed and marketed for the treatment of navicular syndrome [50]. The drug is a bisphosphonate that works by inhibiting osteoclastic activity. Although the EU product is labeled for IV administration, some practitioners administer TA by regional limb perfusion (RLP) to treat specifically localized lameness. This modality of administration, however, has not been evaluated for safety or efficacy. The proposed effect of tiludronate is to minimize remodeling and degeneration of bone in association with navicular syndrome [50]. Controlled clinical trials have demonstrated that TA is useful in the management of navicular disease, when administered at a dose of 1 mg/kg bwt [50]. Use of this medication is recommended in association with corrective shoeing.

Clinical improvement of horses with navicular syndrome is often seen with treatment of the distal interphalangeal joint with hyaluronan and/or corticosteroids. This approach has been evaluated using triamcinolone alone and in combination with hyaluronan [51]. The results of this study documented the diffusion of triamcinolone from the distal interphalangeal joint into the navicular bursa following intra-articular (IA) administration. The diffusion was determined to be occurring directly and not through systemic distribution. The addition of hyaluronan to the injection did not affect diffusion of the corticosteroid into the navicular bursa [51]. Based on the positive results observed in this study, IA therapy of the distal interphalangeal joint is a reasonable initial approach to managing well-selected cases of navicular syndrome. However, caution must be exercised in treating horses with signs of navicular syndrome without adequate diagnostic imaging. The need for repetitive and/or frequent injections should be a strong indication for aggressive diagnostic imaging in order to ascertain the complete spectrum of podotrochlear pathology and the potential consequences of repetitive injections.

Direct injection of the navicular bursa is a frequently offered intervention when medical therapy and shoeing changes alone fail to maintain soundness in the affected horse. The horses reported to be most responsive to intrathecal injection of the bursa were those with navicular bursitis that was not associated with other degenerative changes of the podotrochlear apparatus [52]. Triamcinolone is the corticosteroid most frequently used for this purpose. Despite a longer proposed duration of effect, the use of methylprednisolone should be avoided due to its perceived propensity to lead to soft tissue calcification and deep flexor tendon rupture. As with injection of the distal interphalangeal joint for treatment of navicular syndrome, complete diagnostic imaging should always be strongly considered in order to evaluate the complete spectrum of podotrochlear pathology, the likelihood of a positive clinical response, and the prognosis for future management and performance. Numerous other interventions have been found to be helpful in various instances of navicular syndrome. These may include extracorporeal shock wave therapy and various proposed corrective shoeing interventions. Long-term management of a horse with navicular syndrome frequently involves combinations of the aforementioned therapies [2].

Pharmacological approaches to the treatment of laminitis

The numerous proposed etiologies of laminitis and their potential concurrent interplay in its development underscore the need for the initial focus of the treatment to be targeted at any underlying diseases or conditions that have predisposed the horse to develop laminitis. Among others, these conditions include gastrointestinal disturbances, endocrinopathies, pneumonia or pleuropneumonia, septic metritis, severe lameness affecting weight bearing in another limb, acute uncontrolled ingestion of feed concentrates or lush green pasture, and toxin ingestion or exposure [53–57]. Because our understanding of the pathophysiology of laminitis is incomplete, a diverse array of treatments have been developed to address the local pathologic events in the laminae. In general, the emphasis is on breaking the self-perpetuating cycle of pain–hypertension–inflammation, which is believed to be critical in the progression of laminitis. The NSAID PBZ and flunixin meglumine are the drugs most commonly administered to provide pain relief and anti-inflammatory effects. See the earlier section in this chapter specific NSAIDS commonly used in horses for dosage recommendations.

Much of the data on the initiating events of laminitis point to the involvement of a vasoconstrictive event that ultimately leads to reduction in digital blood flow and laminar perfusion [57]. Some authors believe that the ischemic episode is more specifically associated with venoconstriction. Because of this, many of the treatments of laminitis focus on improving digital blood flow, Starling's forces of fluid movement, and laminar perfusion. The medications most commonly used for this purpose include acepromazine administered at a dose of 0.03–0.06 mg/kg bwt, IM, q6–8 h; isoxsuprine hydrochloride administered at a dose of 1.2 mg/kg bwt, PO, q12 h; and topically applied nitroglycerine gel administered at a dose of 2–4 mg/h [58, 59]. Though these therapies are used extensively in clinical practice, their efficacy is questionable due to the fact that none of these approaches have been shown to increase digital blood flow or laminar perfusion and because it is unclear to what extent vasoconstriction is actually responsible for the development of laminitis. In fact, for laminitis that is associated with a gastrointestinal disturbance and endotoxemia, it is theorized that vasodilation may not be appropriate as it may lead to increased exposure of

the digital vascular endothelium to the damaging effects of the toxin. Therefore, some practitioners employ methods to help induce vasoconstriction in the developmental or prodromal stages of laminitis. A commonly employed intervention is packing the feet in ice to induce vasoconstriction in response to the cold temperature. It is believed that to be efficacious continuous cold therapy is necessary throughout the developmental phase of laminitis [58, 59]. This can be logistically difficult to accomplish and rebound hyperemia may be a negative sequel to removal of the cold therapy. In human models of sepsis, IV lidocaine has been reported to reduce leukocyte adhesion and endothelial cell activation. Based on these findings, continuous rate infusions (CRI) of lidocaine have gained significant popularity in the management of acute laminitis. In addition to antiendotoxic effects, lidocaine infusions also provide significant analgesia. In a model of black walnut extract-induced laminitis, however, lidocaine CRI failed to produce detectable anti-inflammatory effects in equine skin and laminae [60]. Regardless of this finding, because there is a plethora of scientific literature documenting the anti-inflammatory effects of lidocaine in human and equine sepsis and ileus and because it is inexpensive, is relatively safe, and provides analgesia, lidocaine CRI will continue to be employed in the management of acute equine laminitis.

Another proposed contributing factor in the development of laminitis is microthrombosis with platelet activation and clumping occurring within the digital vessels. In an attempt to address this theoretical component of the development of laminitis, anticoagulation and platelet inactivation therapy has been proposed. For this purpose, SQ or IV heparin has been administered at a dose of 40 U/kg bwt q6–8 h. Aspirin has been also used at a dose of 10–20 mg/kg bwt, PO, q48 h. The clinical efficacy of both heparin and aspirin remains unclear.

Dimethyl sulfoxide (DMSO) has also been utilized extensively in the treatment of laminitis. The utilization of this compound has been based on its proposed anti-inflammatory and free-radical scavenging properties. This latter effect may be particularly helpful in combating the effects of ischemia–reperfusion injury. The dose of DMSO most commonly advocated for this use is 1 g/kg bwt, diluted in isotonic fluid to a concentration that does not exceed 20%. IV administration of concentrations higher than 20% has been associated with intravascular hemolysis. Most clinicians use this treatment every 8–12 h for the first several days of laminitis therapy. Some practitioners prefer to administer the same dose of the diluted solution by nasogastric intubation. DMSO is readily absorbed following intragastric administration, and the approach avoids any risk of intravascular hemolysis as well as the need to place an IV catheter.

A final important consideration in the management of laminitis is the need to provide foot support [58, 59]. This should begin with thick supportive bedding, with sand being ideal. Frog support is often helpful in the control of foot pain and the biomechanical forces that may tend to promote further inflammation and edema. Mechanical support may also be provided by using thick Styrofoam cut to the foot contours and taped into place on the bottom of the entire sole of the foot. In addition, there are many shoes or other support pads that are made commercially to be used for the provision of mechanical foot support in the laminitic horse. Over time, and after the resolution of the acute bout of laminitis, corrective shoeing and trimming will likely be necessary.

Some husbandry practices can decrease the risk initiating a laminitic episode. For example, uncontrolled access to lush pastures and overfeeding should be strictly avoided. Careful control of caloric intake and monitoring of any metabolic condition that predisposes to insulin resistance and a Cushingoid phenotype are also imperative. (see Chapter 15, for more in-depth discussion.)

Perineural and intra-articular anesthesia (diagnostic blocking for lameness exams)

Local anesthesia is primarily used for diagnostic purposes during lameness examinations, and it is accomplished by perineural injection and/or by IA injection of a short-acting local anesthetics. These agents produce anesthesia by blockade of the voltage-gated sodium channels in the neuronal membrane that serve to propagate the nerve impulse. A number of the local anesthetic agents, including procaine and mepivacaine, also induce vasodilation. The duration of effect of local anesthetics when administered perineurally can be increased by the concurrent administration of epinephrine, which will cause local vasoconstriction.

Lidocaine is commonly used for perineural anesthesia. The activity of lidocaine is characterized by rapid onset and an intermediate duration of effect. Mepivacaine has largely replaced lidocaine for IA anesthesia, because it appears to produce less joint inflammation postinjection. Lidocaine appears to be the most irritating of the routinely used blocking agents, and for this reason, many equine veterinarians routinely use mepivacaine for both IA and perineural diagnostic anesthesia [61].

Mepivacaine, which can be used for both perineural and IA anesthesia, has a reasonably rapid onset and medium duration of action. It is also reported to be less irritating to the joint tissue than lidocaine. Frequently, following diagnostic anesthesia of a joint, a therapeutic IA intervention is desired. Traditionally, it has been considered less than optimal to treat a joint on the same day that the joint has been anesthetized. This appears to be much less problematic to the joint when mepivacaine is utilized for joint anesthesia over lidocaine [61].

Like lidocaine and mepivacaine, bupivacaine is used in horses for perineural anesthesia. This agent is selected for use when the preferred duration of perineural anesthesia is much longer than that provided by other local anesthetics. Procaine is a local anesthetic of the amino-ester group. It is most frequently encountered in equine practice as an additive to penicillin G, where its presence helps minimize pain of IM injection. Otherwise, the use of procaine has largely been replaced by lidocaine due to its superior activity [61].

Morphine

Morphine is not a local anesthetic, but rather, it is an opioid narcotic analgesic agent that is most often administered to horses either parenterally (IV or IM) or epidurally. It can also be administered IA, however, to produce local analgesia in horses experiencing severe joint pain, although the specific dose, safety profile, and efficacy of this use have not been determined. At least one source, however, has recommended a dose of 0.1 mg/kg bwt. Some clinicians advocate its dilution with saline at 1 ml/10 kg bwt [62]. In a canine stifle arthrotomy model of analgesia, this dose provided analgesia for at least 6 h. Morphine can produce significant reductions in intestinal motility and intestinal transit times that increase the risk of colic in horses following its administration, although it is not clear if the dose used IA causes these effects.

Pharmacological management of osteoarthritis

The development and progression of osteoarthritis varies from primary degenerative conditions to secondary causes ranging from acute injury to low-intensity chronic joint trauma. Despite the various etiologies of osteoarthritis, the pathophysiology is constant. Inflammation of a joint leads to the initiation of capsulitis and synovitis. This inflammation is believed to result in a cascade of inflammatory mediators, initiated by IL-1 that can lead to the release of enzymes, including collagenase, stromelysin, serine proteinases, matrix metalloproteinase, and others, associated with cartilage degeneration. Osteoarthritis is a by-product of the daily trauma beginning with enzymatic release, followed by cartilage degradation, leaching of proteoglycan, and unwinding of the collagen due to the inflammatory mediators. Collagen molecules then appear to stimulate more inflammation, and a self-perpetuating cycle is initiated. Over time and without control, this enzymatic degradation leads to development of advanced osteoarthritis. The results are articular cartilage damage, synovial membrane thickening, and joint capsule fibrosis. Because of this, some of the most promising approaches to control and manage osteoarthritis are early interventions, when only capsulitis and synovitis are present, and before any long-term cartilage and joint damage has developed [2, 63–65].

Corticosteroid use in the management of osteoarthritis

Although corticosteroids have been used for many years in the management of equine osteoarthritis, recently, their use in managing osteoarthritis has received a great deal of negative attention. Some of the negative impressions of corticosteroids may have stemmed from their cavalier use and the subsequent adverse effects that developed in equine athletes. Chronic corticosteroid use in racehorses with arthritis was associated with ill-advised continued performance and subsequent injury of the treated joint. Concurrently, a body of research was produced that suggested that the use of corticosteroids in joints was associated with direct cartilaginous damage [2, 62–66]. Despite these impressions and reports, however, we now realize that the reality of appropriate corticosteroid use in the management of equine osteoarthritis is significantly

different than what these previous positions suggested. Most of the problems associated with IA corticosteroid administration can be attributed to poor injection technique, poor case selection, or less than ideal selection of the specific drug. Exceptionally high doses of corticosteroids and/or repeated injections are now regarded as strong indicators of the need for further diagnostics and consideration of other concurrent problems or disorders. At least a 6-month window between treatments was suggested to be prudent with a need for more frequent injections potentially indicating undiagnosed problems. When used judiciously, corticosteroids can be appropriate and cost-effective for the control and management of inflammatory joint disease. Through their anti-inflammatory actions and blocking of enzymes that are produced by inflamed joints, they are included in the class of medications considered to be DMOAD. Inflamed joint tissues do not produce joint fluid or hyaluronic acid (HA) in normal amounts or quality. IA corticosteroids can help to reestablish the ability of the joint to produce components that are critical to maintaining joint health. Clinical signs of joint disease, such as lameness, synovial effusion, and heat and pain on joint flexion, can usually be reduced more quickly and for a longer duration when IA corticosteroids are used in comparison to other IA monotherapies [2, 62–65].

Corticosteroids: Mechanism of action

Corticosteroids are proposed to exhibit disease-modifying activity primarily through their suppression of the two major mediators of cartilage degeneration: IL-1 and tumor necrosis factor (TNF). Corticosteroids also inhibit the movement of inflammatory cells to the site of inflammation and inhibit neutrophil function by impairing release of enzymes and decreasing phagocytosis. Corticosteroids inhibit the production of inflammatory mediators primarily through the induction of lipocortin, which inhibits phospholipase A_2 formation. The inhibition of phospholipase A_2 prevents the breakdown of membrane phospholipids to fatty acids, thereby preventing their subsequent oxygenation into inflammatory eicosanoids, such as prostaglandins and leukotrienes, by the COX and lipoxygenase pathways, respectively. In contrast to NSAIDs that only inhibit the COX enzymes, corticosteroids inhibit both eicosanoid pathways. In acute inflammation, corticosteroids also help maintain the integrity of the blood vessels, reduce edema formation, and limit the movement of white blood cells into injured tissues. Other less well-defined anti-inflammatory actions of corticosteroids include inhibition of metalloproteinases, inhibition of monocyte–macrophage complexes at the site of inflammation, and inhibition of plasminogen activator activity. The inhibition of cytokines and degradative enzymes involved in the pathogenesis of osteoarthritis is the probable mechanism for the exhibition of disease-modifying characteristics by corticosteroids. Studies have demonstrated that low doses of corticosteroids produce these cartilage-sparing effects without negatively affecting the chondrocyte [1, 2, 66].

Corticosteroid duration of action

Control of endogenous corticosteroid production is achieved through a negative feedback loop to the pituitary gland, with high concentrations of the endogenous corticosteroid cortisol inhibiting the release of adrenocorticotropic hormone (ACTH), which in turn inhibits further cortisol release. The administration of exogenous corticosteroids also inhibits ACTH release, and the duration of this inhibition has been used as an objective measure of the duration and potency of the various synthetic corticosteroids. Whether the duration of suppression of ACTH secretion is relevant to the duration of effect of a corticosteroid injected IA, however, is not clear. The reality is that estimating the clinical duration of action and the relative potency of corticosteroids administered IA is difficult and may vary depending on the parameters used. Most corticosteroids that are used clinically are prodrug ester formulations that must be hydrolyzed to become biologically active. In addition, some formulations of synthetic corticosteroids are mixtures of readily soluble and poorly soluble esters for both rapid and sustained actions [2, 66]. In the systemic circulation, the rate of corticosteroid prodrug hydrolysis can affect the onset and duration of action, as well as the perceived potency of the drug. However, in joints, most corticosteroids are rapidly converted to their active forms within synovial fluid. Table 13.1 compares the solubility and release rates of corticosteroid formulations commonly used for IA medication. The duration of IA corticosteroid activity has been associated with the continued presence of the drug in joint fluid, but clinically the anti-inflammatory effects of many IA corticosteroids appear to last well beyond the period in which they are detectable in joint fluid. When comparing the three corticosteroids commonly administered

Table 13.1 Comparison of solubility of corticosteroid esters and release rates.

Ester	Solubility	Release rate
Succinate	Very soluble	Rapid: minutes
Phosphate	Very soluble	Rapid: minutes
Acetate	Moderately soluble	Slow: 2–14 days
Acetonide	Poorly soluble	Very slow: weeks
Dipropionate	Poorly soluble	Very slow: weeks

IA to cortisol, methylprednisolone and betamethasone are generally considered to exhibit intermediate to long durations of action, while triamcinolone produces effects intermediate in duration. Regarding the potency of these three agents, betamethasone is considered the most potent and methylprednisolone the least [2, 66]. Table 13.2 compares the potency and duration of action of endogenous produced and exogenously administered corticosteroids [2, 66].

Specific corticosteroids
Triamcinolone acetonide

Triamcinolone is administered to horses systemically and IA. It is between three and five times more potent than cortisol and 1.25 times more potent than prednisolone [66]. Most veterinarians regard its duration of action as intermediate. Both IA and "remote site" administration of triamcinolone has been reported to be associated with disease-modifying effects in the management of osteoarthritis and osteochondral fragments in horses [2, 67]. Numerous studies have demonstrated that triamcinolone produces improvements in the degree of clinical lameness, synovial fluid composition and synovial membrane, and articular cartilage parameters [67]. Because the disease-modifying effects produced by triamcinolone are commonly considered to be superior to those produced by methylprednisolone, equine veterinarians generally prefer to use triamcinolone for IA treatment of high-motion joints and/or for use any time cartilage-sparing effects are desired. The recommended dose of triamcinolone acetonide is between 6 and 18 mg per horse. Most equine veterinarians advocate that the total dose should not exceed 18 mg, because anecdotally dosages exceeding 18 mg can lead to the development of acute laminitis. The perceived association between laminitis and corticosteroids

Table 13.2 Comparison of corticosteroid potency and duration of action.

Drug	Relative anti-inflammatory potency	Approximate duration of action based on adrenal suppression (h)	Duration of action
Cortisol (hydrocortisone)	1	<12	Short acting
Cortisone	0.8	<12	Short acting
Prednisolone	4	12–36	Intermediate
Prednisone	4	12–36	Intermediate
Methylprednisolone	5	12–36	Intermediate (often regarded as long acting in joint)
Triamcinolone	3–5	24–48	Intermediate
Isoflupredone	17–50	—	Long acting (often regarded as short to intermediate in joint)
Betamethasone	25–30	32 to >48	Long acting (short to intermediate in a joint)
Dexamethasone	25–30	32 to >48	Long acting
Flumethasone	30 to >120	>48	Long acting

Potency is relative to that of 1.0 for cortisol. Table reproduced with permission from Bentz BG, Revenaugh MS. (2010) Equine intra-articular injection. In: Jann HW, Fackelman GE, (eds.) *Rehabilitating the Athletic Horse*; Nova Science Publishers Inc, New York: pp. 87–115.

appears to be strongest for triamcinolone. Therefore, triamcinolone should be used with caution in horses with a history or a predisposition to laminitis; the latter would include ponies and horses with metabolic syndrome and equine pituitary pars intermedia dysfunction. Although methylprednisolone is generally considered more likely to produce osseous metaplasia, a dystrophic mineralization of soft tissue structures adjacent to the joint, it is also a risk with IA triamcinolone administrations. Despite these possible adverse events, when used appropriately, corticosteroids, particularly triamcinolone, may improve the health of the joint by its extensive and well-documented disease-modifying effects.

Methylprednisolone acetate

Methylprednisolone, when administered IA, is generally regarded as long acting with a potency that is approximately 5 times that of cortisol [66]. It is the corticosteroid most commonly administered IA to horses, and there are a plethora of studies examining its effects when administered via this route. In some instances, these studies provide conflicting results [68–73]. For example, several studies have reported detrimental effects of multiple doses of methylprednisolone acetate on cartilage metabolism, function, and repair in high-motion joints including the carpus, fetlock, and tarsocrural joints. IA use of methylprednisolone has also been

associated with negative effects on chondrocyte metabolism and OCD defect healing. At high concentrations, methylprednisolone has been reported to inhibit proteoglycan synthesis and to negatively affect the structural organization of collagen within the joint cartilage, while lower concentrations appear to produce these effects in a reversible manner. As the corticosteroid concentrations reported to adversely affect cartilage matrix synthesis appear to exceed those required to inhibit the synthesis of inflammatory and destructive mediators, lower doses are advocated to effectively control joint inflammation without causing detriment to articular cartilage. In contrast to these results, however, another investigation using equine cartilage explants showed no difference in the counteraction of the negative effects of IL-1 with either methylprednisolone or triamcinolone acetonide or their dose titration [73]. The relevance of this model to *in vivo* findings, however, is unclear. With bodies of evidence indicating the potential for both positive and negative effects on cartilage, it is generally assumed that methylprednisolone has a potential to cause negative effects on articular cartilage. Therefore, the total dose administered in any given treatment and the repeated use of methylprednisolone should be limited. The lowest effective dose is an empirical decision and may vary with the disease and the horse being treated. A commonly recommended dose is 120 mg for large joints, with a total dose range of

40–240 mg/horse. The duration of effect is reported to average from 3 to 4 weeks. IA injection of methylprednisolone has been associated with a local inflammatory response, commonly referred to as joint flare. Lower doses of methylprednisolone may be clinically effective and less likely to produce joint flare and detrimental effects on articular cartilage. Because of the potential for detrimental effects on articular cartilage, many equine practitioners avoid the use of methylprednisolone in high-motion joints but use it extensively in the distal tarsal joints and proximal interphalangeal joints [64, 65]. Anecdotally, IA administration of methylprednisolone appears to be associated with osseous metaplasia more commonly than other corticosteroids.

Betamethasone sodium phosphate/ betamethasone acetate

At 25–30 times the potency of cortisol, betamethasone is one of the more potent anti-inflammatory corticosteroids used for IA injection in horses [66]. Although the data is limited, there appear to be less documented detrimental effects of betamethasone on articular tissue in horses than other commonly used corticosteroids [74]. Anecdotal reports have also indicated that betamethasone may be less likely to produce joint flare than other corticosteroids. Although much of what is known regarding the effects of betamethasone is based on anecdotal reports and limited objective evaluations, many equine practitioners choose to use betamethasone in high-motion joints for its presumptive cartilage-sparing effects. Commercially available formulations of betamethasone are products approved for use in humans that often combine a rapid onset, short-acting water-soluble phosphate ester with a more lipid-soluble acetate ester for a more prolonged effect. A formulation that contains only the short-acting sodium phosphate ester is available as well. Depending on the size of the joint being treated, a dose range of 3–12 mg has been recommended for IA administration in humans.

Isoflupredone acetate

Isoflupredone is 17 times more potent than cortisol and 4 times more potent than prednisolone [66]. The usual intrasynovial dose for joint inflammation, tendinitis, or bursitis is 5–20 mg or more if treating a large joint. Isoflupredone acetate reportedly exerts an inhibitory influence on the mechanisms and the tissue changes associated with inflammation. Vascular permeability is decreased, exudation diminished, and migration of the inflammatory cells markedly inhibited [66]. That said, this drug is not as frequently used for IA therapy in horses. Anecdotal reports of temporary gastrointestinal upset resulting from higher dosages of isoflupredone exist. Combining isoflupredone with triamcinolone in the same syringe, which some have advocated in the past, may result in precipitation and is not a recommended combination.

Dexamethasone

Dexamethasone, which is 25 times more potent than cortisol, has been used for IA administration, although this practice is not common. When administered via this route, it has a rapid onset and short duration of action [66]. It is primarily administered systemically or orally in horses for the treatment of nonorthopedic inflammatory conditions.

Flumethasone

Chemically derived from prednisolone, flumethasone is significantly more potent and has a longer duration of effect than its parent molecule [66]. Flumethasone has been investigated as an IA medication, but its primary application at this time is as a systemically administered corticosteroid, a periarticular medication for treatment of sacroiliac and lumbosacral joint pain, and a component of other nonarticular therapies, such as mesotherapy [2]. Depending on the assay method used, flumethasone has been reported to be 700 times more potent than hydrocortisone and is significantly more potent than prednisolone or dexamethasone [66]. In the horse, flumethasone is primarily used for disorders of the musculoskeletal system in which permanent structural changes have not occurred and in the management of allergic reactions.

Other medications in the management of osteoarthritis
Hyaluronic acid

HA (also called hyaluronan or hyaluronate) is a nonsulfated glycosaminoglycan distributed widely throughout connective, epithelial, and neural tissues. It is produced by a membrane lining the joint capsule, released into the joint fluid, and then taken up by the joint cartilage. HA provides joint lubrication and protection of joint cartilage from the shear and compressive forces of joint motion. HA also reduces articular prostaglandin concentrations and scavenges free radicals. It is one of the chief components of the extracellular matrix and is a major component of the synovial fluid, increasing the viscosity of the fluid. Along with lubricin, it is one of the synovial fluid's main lubricating components. In articular cartilage, HA is present as a coat around each chondrocyte. Aggrecan monomers bind to hyaluronan in the presence of link protein and form large highly negatively charged aggregates. These aggregates hold water and are responsible for the resilience of cartilage.

HA is harvested from such sources as rooster comb and umbilical cord and is formulated for IA or IV administration. It is often used IA in conjunction with corticosteroids. HA has been reported to exhibit anti-inflammatory effects, pain relief, and improvement of joint mobility. Analgesic properties of this compound are believed to be due to its ability to reduce the sensitivity of articular nerve endings and its anti-inflammatory effects. Disease-modifying effects of HA have been postulated. For example, exogenous HA is proposed to potentiate the synthesis of endogenous HA by synovial cells and to promote proteoglycan synthesis. HA is also reported to protect cartilage from the effects of IL-1 and other inflammatory mediators. Cartilage-sparing effects are reported to occur following IA injection of HA by suppression of inflammatory cytokines and degradative proteinases [2, 75].

Research and anecdotal reports have suggested that using the highest molecular weight HA may be associated with the greatest benefit, particularly for IA administration. Table 13.3 presents the current FDA-approved HA products, their molecular weights, and recommended doses. It has been suggested that HA preparations with molecular weights exceeding 1×10^6 daltons produce superior benefits relative to those seen observed with lower molecular weight preparations. For example, cartilage-sparing effects of higher molecular weight preparations appear to be superior to lower molecular weight preparations in some models. Whether this can be directly correlated with superior clinical *in vivo* benefits, however, is less clear [2, 75]. Although the results of both human and equine clinical trials do suggest that utilizing higher molecular weight compounds is preferable, these study findings are not universally supported by other research models of synovial inflammation and joint disease. For this reason, the true ideal molecular weight of HA for clinical use remains unclear. Some current recommendations have proposed the use of HA with molecular weight in the range of $0.5-2.0 \times 10^6$d. Although these reports suggest that the highest molecular weights are most preferable, there appears to be a point where the benefit of high molecular weight is lost, and indeed, there is some evidence that molecular weights greater than $3-4 \times 10^6$d may lead to reduction of endogenous HA production [75]. Table 13.4 reviews some of the reported disease-modifying effects of HA in relation to molecular weight of the molecule.

IV formulations provide a convenient and less invasive route of HA administration relative to IA administration. When it is given IV, HA is presumed to disperse to all the joint capsules in the body. It is unclear if or how HA administered IV actually produces benefit to the joints. Indeed, it has been proposed that IV administered HA does not appear to penetrate the joints, but rather, it attaches to anti-inflammatory receptors on the joint capsule. Clinical benefit of HA may be exhibited through its potential to reduce nerve impulses and sensitivity to pain in the joint, through significant reduction of inflammatory mediators and matrix metalloproteinases, and by acting as a signaling molecule on cell surface receptors to regulate cellular proliferation, cell migration, and gene expression [75]. This activity

Table 13.3 FDA-approved HA products.

Brand name	Manufacturer	Molecular weight (daltons)*	Concentration (mg/ml)	Suggested dose (mg)†
Hyalovet®	Boehringer Ingelheim Vetmedica, Inc., St. Joseph, Missouri	$4-7 \times 10^5$	10	20
Hylartin V®	Zoetis Animal Health Kalamazoo, MI	3.5×10^6	10	20
Hyvisc®	Boehringer Ingelheim Vetmedica, Inc., St. Joseph, Missouri	2.1×10^6	11	20
Legend®	Bayer Corporation, Shawnee Mission, KS	3.0×10^5	10	40

*As stated by manufacturer.
†IA dosages are those recommended for small- to medium-sized joints. Some manufacturers recommend twice the dose for larger joints (e.g., tibiotarsal).

Table 13.4 Reported disease-modifying effects of hyaluronan relative to molecular weight.

Cell/tissue	Effect	Influence of MW (daltons)	Comments
Leukocytes	↓ Migration, chemotaxis, adhesion	>1×10^6 superior to <1×10^6	
	↓ Free-radical scavenging	>1×10^6 superior to <1×10^6	
Synovial fibroblasts	↑ Synthesis of HA	0.5×10^6 optimal	High concentrations of low MW
	↓ PGE2 release	2×10^6 superior to $0.2–1.0 \times 10^6$	↓synthesis as does MW >$3–4 \times 10^6$
Chondrocytes/ cartilage	↓ PGE2 release	2×10^6 superior to 0.5×10^6	Low MW inhibits synthesis
	↓ Proteoglycan release	$0.3 \times 10^6 = 2 \times 10^6$	1×10^6 less effective than
	↑ PG synthesis	0.8×10^6 superior to <0.3×10^6	$0.5–0.7 \times 10^6$
	↓ IL-1 induced, ↓PG and collagen synthesis	1×10^6 superior to <0.5×10^6	
	↓ chondrocyte apoptosis	$0.5–0.7 \times 10^6$ superior to <0.1×10^6	
	↑ TIMP-1 release	2×10^6 superior to 1×10^6 superior to 0.5×10^6	

may be more likely to be operative when directly administered into the joint; however, IV administered HA has been proposed to exhibit more potent anti-inflammatory activity than IA administered HA. If IV administered HA does not enter joints, there can be no lubrication effect. Horses treated with IV administered HA have been reported to exhibit a reduced degree of lameness compared to untreated horses. The anti-inflammatory effect of HA when given IV appears to be between 2 and 7 days [2].

Combination therapy with corticosteroids and hyaluronic acid

The use of a combination of a corticosteroid with HA for IA therapy is standard practice in equine medicine. It is believed that the concurrent administration of HA facilitates the efficacy of the corticosteroid, allowing a lower dose to be administered. The cartilage-sparing effect of HA is also potentially a benefit in this combination therapy [75]. Corticosteroid and HA combination therapy has been reported to be synergistic in human patients with osteoarthritis.

Polysulfated glycosaminoglycan (PSGAG)

Polysulfated glycosaminoglycan (PSGAG) is a semisynthetic preparation from bovine trachea that is comprised principally of chondroitin sulfate, a glycosaminoglycan found in the aggregating proteoglycan of cartilage. The compound is a large, sulfated, and charged molecule comprised of galactosamine, glucosamine, and hexuronic acid. After its administration, PSGAG binds to cartilage components. Although the mechanism of

action of PSGAG in joints is unclear, there are numerous human and animal studies that demonstrate beneficial effects in damaged joints. PSGAG has been purported to exhibit anti-inflammatory properties, to decrease the effect of destructive enzymes associated with joint inflammation and disease, and to stimulate normal production of HA and glycosaminoglycan. PSGAG was initially used in humans in the 1960s. It was reported to lead to reductions in the severity of clinical signs in human and equine arthritis patients. Clinical improvement is likely attributable to anti-inflammatory effects, including the inhibition of PGE2 synthesis and of cytokine release. Early reports suggested that PSGAG stimulates the synthesis of proteoglycans and collagen by chondrocytes, an effect that appeared to contribute to the healing of damaged cartilage. Subsequent studies have failed to specifically demonstrate any stimulation of proteoglycan synthesis. While PSGAG is considered by many to be an effective means of preventing cartilage degeneration in a joint, it does not appear to heal joint defects. The continued investigation of this compound has failed to show significant effects in the early healing of cartilage lesions. In fact, in one study, repair tissue in healing cartilage under the influence of this compound appeared to be inferior to that found in untreated animals [76]. Instead, PSGAG appears to help prevent cartilage degeneration. PSGAG works on the collagen fibers and intercollagenous tissues that comprise the matrix, or origination point, of joint cartilage. PSGAG appears in some reports to exhibit mild to moderate anticatabolic effects and capability of inhibiting the activity of a number of degradative enzymes known to be present in articular tissues. Various animal arthritis models have provided some support for a disease-modifying effect of PSGAG *in vivo*, and in most cases, beneficial effects were primarily attributed to inhibition of degradative enzymes. The end result would presumably be a healthier joint, more capable of resisting the wear and tear imposed by athletic use. Despite these findings, some clinicians do not believe that the drug can significantly protect cartilage. Regardless of these viewpoints, the use of this product may be more important for long-term joint health and maintenance and synovitis [2, 76].

FDA-approved formulations of PSGAG are available for IA and IM administration. PSGAG is marketed for preventive or therapeutic intervention of degenerative joint disease. The IA formulation is a higher concentration than the IM formulation in order to facilitate IA dosing of the compound into small joints. The IA administration of PSGAG was commonly used for many years but became less popular when it appeared to be associated with an increased incidence of joint infection and joint flare relative to that reported from IA corticosteroid administration. Following IA administration of PSGAG, it was suggested that the treated joint was more susceptible to *Staphylococcus* infections [77]. A subsequent study addressed this finding and concluded that administration of 125 mg of amikacin concurrently with the PSGAG would mitigate any increased risk of infection [78]. While it is likely to be safer, it is suggested that IM PSGAG produces less clinical benefit relative to IA PSGAG. When administering PSGAG IM, a 500 mg dose at 4-day intervals for seven total treatments is recommended by the manufacturer. The administered PSGAG complex is reported to remain in the cartilage for 4 days, where it facilitates cartilage and overall joint health. The frequency of PSGAG administration is usually based on the therapeutic response and its duration. There is considerable variability in the symptomatic relief with PSGAG treatment. Contrary to popular practices, the commercial PSGAG product should be stored at room temperature. A significant increase of injection site reactions has been reported when the product is stored at cooler temperatures.

Medical device formulations of PSGAG and hyaluronan

Because of the popularity of the FDA-approved formulations of PSGAG and HA, an ever-expanding number of products are being produced by many companies in order to compete for these markets. None of these products are FDA-approved drugs; rather, most are registered with the FDA as medical devices, and their label does not indicate that they can be used to treat osteoarthritis. Veterinarians need to understand that medical devices are not included in the Animal Medicinal Drug Use Clarification Act (AMDUCA), and therefore, the use of these products in an extralabel manner is not permitted as it is for FDA-approved drugs. This is an important point because should an adverse event occur following administration of one of these products in a manner that is not consistent with their label, a practitioner could be held liable for the injury. Therefore, veterinarians should discuss the use of these products with their insurance carrier to ascertain whether they would be covered in the event of an injury. In addition to the legal concerns of using these products, there are also questions regarding their efficacy and safety. For example, one investigation in 2004, which was funded by the manufacturer of an FDA-approved PSGAG product, the clinical efficacy of a chondroitin sulfate product marketed as a substitute for the approved product was evaluated using a model of equine carpal osteoarthritis [79]. The study concluded that the chondroitin sulfate product was markedly less effective than the FDA-approved PSGAG at improving the parameters of osteoarthritis evaluated in the model. It should also be remembered that as medical devices the manufacturer of these formulations do not have to meet the rigorous standards required of FDA-approved products. They do not have to demonstrate that they are safe and efficacious, nor are they necessarily manufactured under good manufacturing practices as are FDA-approved products. Nevertheless, there appears to be extensive use of these medical device products because they are more economical [2].

Interleukin-1 receptor antagonist protein

Interleukin-1 receptor antagonist protein (IRAP) is a newer therapeutic agent introduced into the arsenal of IA therapies. As its name implies, this protein works by blocking the IL-1 receptor. IL-1 is one of the major progenitors in the inflammatory cascade leading to synovitis and joint pain. By blocking this interaction, it is believed that pain and inflammation in the joint can be moderated or eliminated. It is reported to require a series of IA injections. First developed for use in humans, the product is derived from autologous harvest of the antagonist protein from the patient's own blood. The procedure has now been adapted for use in equine joints [80].

The commercially available product consists of a packet for harvesting the protein from whole blood. The process for obtaining IRAP is relatively easy but requires specific equipment, such as a centrifuge that accommodates 60 ml syringes and an incubator. The kit provides a 60 ml syringe containing glass beads to stimulate monocytic production of the antagonist protein and an anticoagulant. A jugular vein is aseptically prepared and 60 ml of blood is collected. The syringe is then incubated at 37°C for 24–29 h. The syringe is then centrifuged to separate the IRAP-rich plasma from the cellular components. The plasma is then harvested in 4 ml aliquots and frozen until use. Prior to injecting into a joint, the IRAP plasma is passed through a 0.2 μ millipore filter. Typically, 4 ml is injected once a week for three treatments [80]. In large-volume joints, such as the stifle, an 8 ml dose is commonly used. Depending on the condition being treated, the horse is often rested until it receives the second injection, and it is then permitted to gradually return to training. Associated articular soft tissue injuries are important to consider in treating any lameness, and therefore, as with other IA therapies, response to treatment is likely to be incomplete or of short duration, if such an injury exists. Joints affected with synovitis or mild degenerative joint disease are reported to have the best response to this therapy [80].

Despite some promising reports, the efficacy of IRAP therapy is still the subject of some debate. Much of the debate centers on case selection and which horses might benefit most from the procedure. For example, IRAP exhibits characteristics of DMOAD, and as such, it has been suggested to be helpful in horses to reduce or prevent inflammation from returning too quickly in joints treated with corticosteroids and HA. This approach was suggested to help minimize the need to repeat joint injections with HA and corticosteroids. IRAP has also been recommended for joints that have been previously treated with IA corticosteroids but that are now unresponsive to those medications [80]. IRAP has also been used as initial therapy for many horses; however, because the procedure is expensive, this approach will not be universally feasible for all horses and practices. Because corticosteroids are much less expensive, are effective, and also exhibit disease-modifying

characteristics, they are an excellent initial approach for many cases. IRAP is likely to be most economical and helpful if it is used when corticosteroids fail to produce the desired result and the owner is willing to accept the expense of this therapy.

Tiludronic acid

TA is a bisphosphonate that is approved for the treatment of navicular disease and osteoarthritis of the distal tarsus in the EU, but not currently in the USA [81]. With FDA permission, it can be imported into the USA, and equine clinicians in this country have expanded the use of this product well beyond the label applications [2, 82, 83]. As a drug class, bisphosphonates reduce bone resorption by inhibiting the activity of osteoclasts. In horses, TA has not been associated with a negative effect on bone formation or bone mineralization when used at the recommended dose. TA has also been reported to exhibit anti-inflammatory effects on arthritis, mediated by IL-1, through inhibition of cartilage-resorbing enzymes [2, 83, 84]. This property of TA may be beneficial in treating degenerative osteoarticular pathologies and suggests that the drug exhibits osteoarthritis disease-modifying properties. In addition to inhibition of the osteoclasts, TA inhibits the osteoblastic synthesis of interleukin-6 and its activation of osteoclasts. Intestinal absorption of calcium is also increased in a dose-dependent manner by TA, without increasing the excretion of calcium, and it facilitates the binding of calcium to bone by increasing the size of hydroxyapatite crystals being formed. Through these mechanisms, TA enhances calcium absorption, increases bone density, and acts as a regulator of bone remodeling. As a consequence of its various pharmacological properties, TA may be beneficial in the treatment of lameness where bone pathology is involved, in particular, where radiographs show that osteolysis and sclerosis are features of the pathology [2, 84].

TA is reported to be helpful in the treatment of lameness associated with navicular syndrome, osteoarthritis, bone spavin, and other osseous causes of lameness. It is reported to be most effective for cases with clinical signs of less than 6 months' duration. In a double-blind, placebo-controlled clinical trials of navicular disease, treatment with TA at a dose of 1 mg/kg bwt, IV, produced a significant improvement as demonstrated by long-term reduction in lameness and resumption of athletic activity [81]. A placebo-controlled clinical trial of TA involving the treatment of back pain associated with bony lesions of the vertebral column resulted in a significant improvement in back flexibility [82]. TA is recommended at a dose of 0.1 mg/kg bwt once daily for 10 days by slow IV injection. TA has also been administered at a dose of 1.0 mg/kg bwt, administered as a single bolus IV, diluted in at least 1 l of fluids. Anecdotal reports indicate a higher rate of side effects, particularly colic, when the entire 10-day dose of the medication is administered as a single bolus particularly if the drug is not fully dissolved in the IV fluids. Renal failure has also been sporadically reported in association with the administration of TA, and some of the cases have been severe and permanent.

TA has also been administered as an RLP. Using RLP has been hypothesized to increase drug delivery to the affected area(s) because of the high concentrations that can be achieved and to concurrently reduce the cost because smaller total volumes of the drug are administered. The use of TA via RLP is growing in popularity among performance horse veterinarians, but its efficacy is untested. The dose chosen for administration is empirical and dependent on the region and joint(s) being treated. Commonly, a single 50 mg vial is used for distal limb perfusion. Recently, the administration of TA IA has also been reported for the management of osteoarthritis, particularly in the stifle and vertebral articulations. Articular administration is reported in Europe, but has not yet gained wide acceptance as an IA therapy in the USA.

Pentosan polysulfate

Pentosan polysulfate has recently gained recognition and use in the USA for the treatment of equine osteoarthritis. There is an FDA-approved formulation of pentosan polysulfate that is administered orally to humans for the treatment of interstitial cystitis, but there is no FDA-approved equine formulation. In the USA, compounded preparations of pentosan polysulfate are available, as well as a formulation that is registered with the FDA as a medical device. As discussed in the earlier section on NSAIDs, veterinarians need to understand that compounded products are not formulated or produced under the same rigorous standards as FDA-approved products. There is no guarantee of their sterility, potency, purity, or stability. In a similar manner, as discussed in the section on Medical Device Formulations of PSGAG and Hyaluronan, medical devices are not manufactured under the same standards as FDA-approved products,

nor have they been shown to be safe and effective. Finally, there is no extralabel use permitted of medical devices under current FDA regulations.

Pentosan polysulfate is prepared from xylan, a hemicellulose extract of Beachwood. Structurally, it resembles glycosaminoglycans, and like other compounds in that class, it exhibits heparin-like anticoagulant activity [85]. In the joint, pentosan polysulfate reportedly stimulates chondrocyte metabolism and production of proteoglycans and increases synovial fibroblast production of high molecular weight hyaluronan. Pentosan also exhibits anti-inflammatory effects by inhibiting the formation of arachidonic acid mediators and the release of lysosomal enzymes, such as hyaluronidase, histamine, cathepsin B, and PMN elastase, that are implicated in the degradation of the cartilage matrix [2, 86–90]. Other activities of pentosan include stimulation of fibrinolysis and activation of plasminogen. Through these mechanisms, pentosan polysulfate promotes dissolution of thrombi and fibrin deposits in synovial tissues and in subchondral blood vessels. These effects may make pentosan polysulfate a useful drug in the stimulation of joint repair and healing, and this medication is classified as a DMOAD [2, 86–90]. Side effects in the horse have not been specifically investigated or reported; however, in humans, they include bleeding tendencies, hair loss, diarrhea, nausea, and headache. Contraindications to the use of pentosan in humans include clotting defects, traumatic or other hemorrhage, infections, renal or hepatic failure, and surgery within 48 h of administration. Most commonly, pentosan polysulfate is administered IM, but a recent report discusses direct IA administration [90]. For IM administration, pentosan polysulfate is administered at a dose of 3 mg/kg bwt or 1.5 g/500 kg horse. Treatment is currently advocated at 5–7-day intervals for four injections and then every 3–4 months thereafter, but variations of this dosing regimen are common.

Platelet-rich plasma

The use of platelet-rich plasma (PRP) for the treatment of musculoskeletal disorders has recently increased significantly. Both soft tissue and articular applications are now widely accepted [91–98]. To produce PRP, whole blood is collected from the horse and immediately centrifuged in order to concentrate platelets and circulating growth factors (TGF-β, IGF, EGF, TGF-α, PDGF, VEGF) that are believed to improve and speed healing. For soft tissue injuries, after resolution of the initial swelling, the PRP is separated from other blood components and injected into the soft tissue lesion using ultrasound guidance. For both soft tissue and IA therapies, multiple injections are often reported to be necessary at 2–4-week intervals in order to appreciate clinical improvement. IA PRP therapy is becoming more common, particularly when other therapies prove to be ineffective and/or if there is associated articular soft tissue injury [96, 97]. While IA applications of PRP are expanding, its use for tendon and ligamentous injury is now well established to help speed and facilitate healing and to improve the physiological quality of the healed tissue through the promotion of the formation of more normal tissue and reduced scarring. PRP is, by definition, a concentrate of platelets above that of whole blood, and there appears to be a minimal concentration of platelets necessary to produce clinical articular benefits. A platelet concentration that is 3 times that of blood is considered the minimum enrichment, while a concentration 5 times that of blood is considered optimal [97, 98]. Specialized centrifuges and techniques are necessary to produce the required platelet density in the PRP. Depending on the centrifugation system, a variable number of red and white cells are found within the PRP preparation, and it is unclear how these cellular components affect the therapeutic activity of PRP [91–94]. There is also evidence that concentrations greater than 8 times that of plasma may actually be detrimental to the healing process [97, 98]. There is some confusion over the need to activate PRP with thrombin, calcium chloride, or glass beads prior to its injection. It has been unclear if activation is necessary for internal application as it has been argued that there is likely enough endogenous tissue thromboplastin for platelet activation. Regardless of these points, PRP is believed to facilitate joint health, cartilage repair, and soft tissue healing through the expression of numerous growth factors and the potential facilitation of more rapid healing with less scar tissue formation. PRP is used most frequently in soft tissue therapy of tendon and ligament injury but is also gaining popularity as an IA therapy and for treatment of articular soft tissue injury involving the meniscus and ligaments of the stifle [61, 97].

Stem cells/bone marrow

In-depth reviews of stem cell therapies are provided elsewhere, but a brief overview will be provided here [99, 100]. Stem cells are immature cells that mature into the various body cell types. Stem cells can be harvested from embryonic tissue but also from other tissues including bone marrow, fat, and umbilical cord blood. In equine practice, stem cell therapy has focused primarily on stem cells that are capable of differentiating into musculoskeletal tissue [101–108]. A pluripotent stem cell represents a more primitive form of stem cell, often of embryonic origin, that is capable of differentiation into any of the cells of the major embryonic germ layers (endoderm, mesoderm, ectoderm). Such stem cells are identified by the ability to induce teratoma formation in test mice. By contrast, multipotent stem cells of mesenchymal origin are restricted in their differentiation to chondrocytes, osteoblasts, adipocytes, fibroblasts, and marrow stroma [103]. Current equine practice has focused on using these cells for regenerative therapy. Although autologous mesenchymal stem cells are easily harvested from bone marrow and fat, they comprise only a very small percentage of the nucleated cells in the harvest. For therapy that requires higher stem cell numbers, clonal expansion in the laboratory is necessary. Direct, unprocessed autogenic preparations of bone marrow aspirates have been used to treat musculoskeletal injuries with anecdotal reports of success. The beneficial effects of such a practice are unclear, but may not be attributable solely to the low number of stem cells in the aspirate. Other beneficial factors such as growth factors and fibronectin aid in cell migration and physiological healing and may help account for a clinical benefit. The use of autologous stem cells also minimizes the risk of tissue rejection. In addition to improved healing, stem cell therapy may also produce rapid improvement of clinical signs. Following harvest and concentration, stem cells and the marrow cofactors are injected into the damaged ligament or tendon, where the cells can eventually develop into normal, healthy tissue. The timing of the intervention is important. Ideally, stem cells and other factors are introduced into the damaged tissue after control of the acute inflammation. This often means, depending on the injury and the clinician, injection between 2 and 7 days or so after the injury. With stem cell injection, the inflammatory response is quieted and the response to the injury is propelled toward an expanded regenerative phase that produces less scar tissue. With the injection and reduced inflammation, clinical pain relief is often achieved. The continued wound healing and expanded regeneration at the site of injury perpetuates regeneration presumably toward replacement with more normal physiological tissue. The major advantage to stem cell therapy is the quality of this healing [102–108]. The ideal volume of injection and number of stem cells used for therapy are undefined and may vary with clinician preference, the lesion size and type, sites or structures treated, concentration of cells, and presence or absence of other regenerative factors in the injection.

In addition to bone marrow, fat is another source for the harvesting of stem cells [106]. In the horse, mesenchymal stem cells are often harvested from the tail head; however, they may be harvested from any fat on the body. Following surgical removal of the appropriate volume of fat, the harvested fat is sent to a commercial laboratory that extracts, cultures, and concentrates the stem cells from the fat sample. The concentrate is sent back, usually within 48 h, and this turnaround time makes the concentrated stem cells available for injection right about the time that an acute injury is capable of benefiting from their introduction into the wound. A number of investigations suggest excellent healing with adult mesenchymal stem cells as indicated by reduced inflammation, improved collagen fiber uniformity, and higher tendon healing scores.

A major portion of the reported clinical use of stem cell therapy is for the treatment of discrete core lesions of the digital flexor tendons and suspensory ligament. However, applications of stem cell therapy and other regenerative therapies are rapidly expanding. Other proposed stem cell therapy applications include injuries of the check, collateral, and cruciate ligaments and meniscal injuries of the stifle [2]. IA regenerative therapies and stem cell use are rapidly expanding in the horse. Such therapy has been employed for conditions such as osteochondrosis dissecans cysts involving various joints but is also being investigated and used for other articular diseases including degenerative joint disease and for disorders outside of the musculoskeletal system [108].

Urinary bladder matrix

Urinary bladder matrix (UBM) has been regarded as a simple inert biological scaffold, with its three-dimensional structure providing mere physical support [109]. However, the matrix harbors numerous growth factors and inhibitors, as well as an inherent ability to attract the body's own stem cells to an area of injury for healing and tissue restoration [2]. The A-Cell® product (ACell Inc., Columbia, MD), which is derived from pig urinary bladder, uses this extracellular matrix milieu to provide the framework for the coordination and signaling of tissue repair, regeneration, and replacement. For equine tendon and ligament injuries, the appealing characteristic of A-Cell® therapy is its simplicity for use. It is produced as a powder for reconstitution and thereby obviates the need to harvest tissue and isolate and concentrate stem cells before using it therapeutically [2, 110, 111].

A-Cell® has been successfully used for injuries of the suspensory ligament and suspensory branches, superficial and deep flexor tendons, and check ligaments [109]. A recent investigation in dogs with osteoarthritis of the hip joint found that IA injections of UBM may be helpful for that indication as well [110]. Clinical use of the commercial UBM product is likely being significantly driven by anecdotal reports of success, because the scientific literature supporting its use is fairly sparse. For example, a recent study, using a collagenase-induced model of superficial digital flexor tendonitis, failed to show any difference between UBM-treated and UBM-untreated control tendons [111]. Depending on the lesion, the recommended dose ranges from 0.2 to 0.4 g of UBM powder reconstituted with saline to a volume of 6–10 ml. As with other regenerative therapies, a complete evaluation of the lesion should be performed by ultrasonography before treatment in order to define the specific location and severity. Then after the initial inflammatory response has subsided in a few days to a week, the reconstituted product is directly injected under ultrasound guidance [2, 109, 111]. Injections of UBM have been reported to produce pain and swelling. This response is believed to occur due to an inflammatory response to the product. The expected postinjection inflammation should be clearly described to the client and may be controlled with anti-inflammatory therapy prior to or immediately following the procedure. Controlled exercise has also been reported to be helpful. The use of UBM has been estimated to reduce recovery time by about 30% with appropriate rehabilitation. Following therapy with UBM, the ultrasonographic evaluation of fiber patterns in treated tendons at 60 days has been reported to be similar to the ultrasonographic appearance of fiber patterns seen following stem cell therapy [2, 109]. The most difficult injuries to treat successfully have been reported to be those affecting the suspensory branches. The greatest success has been reported with treatment of proximal suspensory and superficial digital flexor injuries. A-Cell has also been reported to exhibit anti-bacterial activity, and there have been anecdotal reports that it has been used to treat tendon sheath sepsis with promising results.

Pain modulators

Pain modulators are occasionally used in horses with osteoarthritis to help control and break a potential pain–inflammatory cycle as well as the stress response to pain. Agents used as pain modulators include local anesthetic agents, when used for purposes other than diagnostic evaluation, and locally or systemically administered plant extracts that do not provide any other therapeutic activity. Pure pain modulation without addressing the underlying cause and pathology is dangerous to the horse. For this reason, surveillance for the use of pain modulators is a continued focus of regulatory bodies of all equestrian competitions. Furthermore, the use of some of these substances has been associated with severe tissue reaction and subsequent litigation for damages; therefore, they should be used with caution. Pain-modulating medications have been administered systemically, by local injection (e.g., perineural), by topical application and transdermal patches.

Capsaicin

Capsaicin is the active chemical in hot chili peppers. It acts by stimulating the release of substance P, one of the key chemicals responsible for transmitting the nervous signal for pain. Repeated application of capsaicin may act to deplete the nerve's stores of substance P and halt the transmission of the pain signal [2]. A number of products containing capsaicin have been developed and marketed for use in the horse. Because these products are not marketed as drugs, they are not required to prove their efficacy or safety to the FDA. Nevertheless, one report in 2003 concluded that topical application of capsaicin over the palmar digital nerves provided measurable pain relief for up to 4 h in horses with induced foot lameness [112]. If topical capsaicin is effective in alleviating pain, it must be remembered that it has no reported disease-modifying properties and its effects would be similar to those of a local anesthetic. While that might be appropriate in some medical situations, it could also facilitate severe damage induced by continued

use of a horse with an injury that requires management beyond simply pain modification. On initial application, capsaicin generally produces a mildly painful burning and tingling sensation of short duration and occasionally significant skin reactions. Testing for the use of topical capsaicin and related blocking agents is being successfully conducted at many equine competitions using thermography [2].

Pitcher plant extract

Pitcher plant, Sarraceniaceae, extract (Sarapin, High Chemical Company, Levittown, PA) is administered by injection either perineurally or by infiltrating specific sites. It can be used alone or in combination with other medications, such as corticosteroids, various homeopathic agents, and/or B vitamins. Pitcher plant extract injection has been placed in defined acupuncture points as part of a number of purported acupuncture therapies. Systemic administration of pitcher plant extract has also been anecdotally reported, but it is not approved for use by this mode of administration. A single equine investigation into the efficacy of anesthesia provided by such an extract applied in the region of the abaxial sesamoids failed to identify any significant nociceptive effects using a hoof withdrawal reflex heat latency model [113].

Nutraceuticals: Chondroitin sulfates/ glucosamines

Nutraceutical, a portmanteau of the words "nutrition" and "pharmaceutical," is a term applied to products derived from food sources that claim to provide extra health benefits, in addition to the basic nutritional value found in foods. In the USA, these products cannot claim to treat or cure any disease, because they would then be considered drugs and then subject to regulation by the FDA. Instead, they are generally labeled as products that support the function of a specific organ or organ system. Because they are not regulated as drugs, their purity, potency, and stability are not guaranteed. In addition, third-party analyses of nutraceuticals often find that the products to do contain what their labels claim they contain.

Products that claim to support joint health are some of the most commonly marketed nutraceuticals, and most of these contain combinations of chondroitin sulfate and glucosamines. Cartilage cells normally synthesize glucosamine from glucose and amino acids; however, they can also use externally supplied, preformed glucosamine. Regardless of the source, the chondrocytes use glucosamine to synthesize glycosaminoglycans and hyaluronan. Glucosamine also regulates cartilage synthesis of proteoglycans and collagen. Chondroitin sulfate is the principal glycosaminoglycan of aggregating proteoglycan, often called aggrecan. Chondroitin resembles PSGAG in structure, though less sulfated, and it has been reported to exhibit mechanisms of action that parallel those of PSGAG. There is evidence that these compounds may have some positive effects on joint health. In laboratory investigations, glucosamine increased proteoglycan synthesis by chondrocytes and reduced the synthesis of matrix metalloproteinases induced by inflammatory mediators. Importantly, these effects were reported to occur at concentrations of glucosamine approaching those achieved following oral administration. In chondrocyte culture experiments, the chondroprotective effects of chondroitin sulfate included stimulation of proteoglycan synthesis and inhibition of matrix-degrading enzymes. Chondroitin sulfate has been shown to have protective effects on proteoglycan loss in animal models of joint inflammation. Despite the results of studies that indicate they have some efficacy, to date, there is no significant evidence that indicates that these agents are absorbed as intact molecules from the equine intestinal tract.

Other substances have also been evaluated as nutraceuticals that support joint health. For example, a 2007 study demonstrated modest but significant benefits of an oral soy and avocado (ASU) supplement in an equine osteoarthritis model [114]. The benefits of oral ASU were reported to include disease-modifying effects, which were more significant than those seen with parenteral PSGAG and HA and oral HA products. Advocates of nutraceuticals believe that these compounds not only provide symptomatic relief of arthritis pain but also help to prevent the continued degeneration of articular cartilage. Though these effects are unverified, there appears to be significant anecdotal evidence of the benefits of these compounds from the equine industry. It has been suggested that the most likely benefit of the use of these compounds may be more in helping to slow the progression of osteoarthritis, rather than as a specific way of controlling the clinical manifestation of existing disease [2].

Other nutraceuticals: Dimethylglycine and methylsulfonylmethane

Dimethylglycine (DMG) is also a nutraceutical advocated for the improvement of stamina and endurance by increasing oxygen utilization and improving lactic acid metabolism. Like other nutraceuticals, despite favorable anecdotal reports, DMG has yet to be shown to produce these benefits in any well-controlled study [2].

Methylsulfonylmethane (MSM) is also a nutraceutical derived from DMSO, a known anti-inflammatory agent. It contains sulfur, which is a necessary component of several amino acids, and therefore, it is promoted as providing the building blocks for normal tissues. By transference, it is purported to produce clinical benefit in horses with degenerative joint disease, although there are no published scientific studies specifically documenting a beneficial effect from feeding MSM to horses [2].

Medications used for the treatment of epaxial and other muscle pain

Methocarbamol

Back pain, muscle spasticity, and muscle pain may be associated with numerous clinical conditions, including trauma, myositis, muscular and ligamentous sprains and strains, vertebral conditions, neurologic disorders, and exertional rhabdomyolysis. A thorough evaluation for each of these potential causes permits a targeted and specific therapeutic approach that maximizes the likelihood of a successful outcome.

Muscle spasms can be extremely painful. An increase in tonic stretch reflexes originates from the CNS with subsequent stimulation of descending neural tracts leading to hyperexcitability of the motor neurons. Muscle-relaxing agents can help alleviate muscle hyperexcitability and spasm by modifying the stretch reflex or by interfering with the excitation–contraction coupling mechanism in the muscle. Centrally acting muscle relaxants block the interneuronal pathways in the spinal cord and reticular activating system. As a result, these agents often produce mild sedation. Methocarbamol is a centrally acting muscle relaxant that has a chemical structure similar to guaifenesin. It diminishes skeletal muscle hyperactivity while maintaining normal muscle tone [2, 115]. Methocarbamol is frequently used to treat muscle spasms associated with back problems and exertional rhabdomyolysis at doses ranging from

25 to 75 mg/kg bwt, PO, q12 h or 15–25 mg/kg bwt, IV, q6–8 h. Methocarbamol can safely be administered concomitantly with NSAIDs or corticosteroids. An injectable formulation of methocarbamol is FDA approved for use in horses in the treatment of inflammatory and traumatic conditions of skeletal muscle in order to reduce muscle spasm and to promote muscle relaxation. The oral formulation of methocarbamol, which is a formulation approved for use in humans, is also commonly used in performance horse practice for the treatment and management of sore backs and muscle strain. It has also been prescribed preventively for horses prone to exertional rhabdomyolysis, although there is no evidence that it is effective for this purpose. As a centrally acting muscle relaxant, methocarbamol may produce sedation that can affect coordination and performance, and therefore, it should not be administered concomitantly with other drugs that depress the CNS. Overdosing of methocarbamol is primarily characterized by CNS depression, but salivation, weakness, and ataxia may also be observed.

Medications used to treat/prevent rhabdomyolysis

Dantrolene is a hydantoin derivative that is structurally and pharmacologically different from other skeletal muscle relaxants. Unlike methocarbamol, dantrolene has a direct action on muscle and is believed to interfere with the release of calcium from the sarcoplasmic reticulum. Dantrolene has no discernible effects on respiratory or cardiac function, but may cause dizziness and sedation. In veterinary medicine, dantrolene is recommended for the treatment of malignant hyperthermia in pigs but has been used in horses to treat postanesthetic myositis and exertional rhabdomyolysis. Dantrolene has also been used for the prevention of exertional rhabdomyolysis in performance horses prone to the condition or with confirmed recurrent exertional rhabdomyolysis (RER) [116–119]. It is administered at doses ranging from 2 to 4 mg/kg bwt, PO, q12 h or 800 mg/horse 1 h before exercise.

Phenytoin is another hydantoin derivative, primarily used as an anticonvulsant in humans. Phenytoin has been reported to be effective in some horses susceptible to exertional rhabdomyolysis. Some clinicians have also used this medication to help control the clinical signs of

stringhalt. Phenytoin appears to alter the function of neurotransmitters at the neuromuscular junction, the release of calcium from the sarcoplasmic reticulum, and the sodium flux at the sarcolemma. Dosages are adjusted to maintain serum concentrations of 5–10 µg/ml. Monitoring of serum concentrations is recommendable due to the highly variable nature of the kinetics of phenytoin in the horse. Reported doses have ranged between 1.4 and 2.7 mg/kg bwt, PO, q12 h. However, another recommendation suggested a starting dose of 6–8 mg/kg bwt, PO, q12 h for 3–5 days, followed by incremental increases of 1 mg/kg every 3–4 days as long as the horse continues to exhibit clinical signs of rhabdomyolysis and is not showing signs of sedation [116–119].

Dietary management and exercise are also important in the control of rhabdomyolysis secondary to muscle disorders such as polysaccharide storage myopathy and RER. These conditions can be diagnosed with appropriate testing that may include blood chemistry, electrolyte evaluations, vitamin E and selenium evaluations, exercise testing, muscle biopsy, and/or genetic testing. For management of muscle disorders that increase the frequency and likelihood of rhabdomyolysis, a reduction in the amount of starch fed and a relative increase in dietary fat intake are often coupled with a regular exercise program. Other practices such as mineral and vitamin supplementation may also be helpful [116–119].

Medications used in the prevention and management of hyperkalemic periodic paralysis

Hyperkalemic periodic paralysis (HYPP) is a disorder of genetic origin and is associated with a defect in skeletal muscle potassium channels. The disease occurs in Quarter Horses and horses of Quarter Horse lineage, such as paints. It is inherited as an autosomal dominant trait with incomplete penetrance. Affected horses exhibit episodes of muscle weakness and trembling in association with high blood potassium levels. Homozygous horses are more severely affected, and episodes may lead to dysphagia and recumbency [120, 121].

Long-term control of HYPP may be facilitated by dietary reduction of high-potassium feeds and forage. Regular administration of diuretics that facilitates potassium excretion may also be helpful. Acetazolamide, administered at a dose of 2–4 mg/kg bwt, PO, q8–12 h, has been recommended to help minimize the recurrence of clinical episodes of HYPP. Hydrochlorothiazide, administered at a dose of 0.5–1.0 mg/kg bwt, PO, q12 h, may also be helpful. Mild acute episodes are most often managed by administration of a grain feed and/or a low-potassium syrup, such as Karo corn syrup, and light exercise. More clinically severe episodes may require more intensive management with IV glucose administration in fluids with or without insulin. In addition to glucose, the slow administration of IV sodium bicarbonate or calcium gluconate to effect is also used to treat severe acute episodes of HYPP [120, 121].

Medications used to treat toxin-induced musculoskeletal disorders

Botulism
Botulism is a disease caused by elaboration of a toxin produced by *Clostridium botulinum* organisms. Although there are eight different toxins, most clinical cases of botulism appear to be caused by toxins B, C, and D. Vaccination and good husbandry interventions are the most important steps that can be taken to reduce the risk of botulism. Disease outbreaks may be associated with contaminated feed sources, such as hay or grain, or exposure to decaying animal or plant material. Horses are exquisitely sensitive to the effects of the botulism toxin. Diagnosis is based on elimination of other causes of weakness, trembling, loss of tail tone, loss of tongue tone, dysphagia, and/or recumbency. Diagnosis may also be supported by isolation of the toxin from a wound or stomach contents [122–124].

Treatment and management of botulism cases require intensive supportive care, and chances of recovery may be improved with administration of botulism antitoxin. Currently, a bivalent antitoxin A and B is commercially available, and a trivalent antitoxin A, B, and E has been investigated in humans. The volume of antitoxin necessary to treat botulism is unclear, but frequently more antitoxin is administered in a single dose than is necessary, because the amount of toxin circulating is generally very low. Clinical judgment should be used to determine initial doses, and response to therapy should be used as a gauge for the need for additional doses. Unfortunately, the cost of the antitoxin may itself limit repeat administrations. Administration of antitoxin is only effective for binding of unbound toxin and has no effect on toxin that has already bound to end-plate receptors. This toxin binding is irreversible and it requires generation of new receptors by the horse in order to recover from the effects of the toxin. Concurrent antimicrobial coverage for secondary infections, bladder catheterization, rectal evacuation, nutritional support, and, occasionally, mechanical ventilation and slinging are necessary to sustain treatment efforts and provide the opportunity for the horse or foal to recover [122–124].

Tetanus
Tetanus is caused by toxin(s) elaborated by *Clostridium tetani* organisms. The toxins liberated by the sporulating clostridial organisms include tetanospasmin and tetanolysin. Tetanospasmin produces the typical clinical signs of tetanus seen in animals, whereas tetanolysin damages the cytoplasmic membranes facilitating passage of other molecules, such as tetanospasmin, into the cell. Contrary to the clinical signs of botulism, tetanus is manifest as spastic paralysis. Clinically, this may appear as hypersensitivity to noise; a typical "sawhorse" stance; hyperreflexia; erect ears; stiff tail; stiff jaw, causing difficulty eating; sweating; and increases in heart and respiratory rates. The diagnosis is based on typical clinical signs, vaccination history, presence of a wound, identification of toxin in blood and/or culture, and identification of *C. tetani* [124].

Like botulism, tetanus is treated by administration of a tetanus antitoxin (TAT), which can be administered either IV or intrathecally, although IV administration is much more common. As is the case with botulism, prevention is far more rewarding than treating tetanus. Vaccination is simple, inexpensive, and effective and is a universal recommendation for all horses. In the early stages of tetanus, tranquilizers and/or barbiturate sedatives have been recommended in conjunction with administration of 300 000 IU of TAT twice a day. Doses of TAT, however, have varied from as high as 2.5 million IU once to 220 IU/kg bwt, IV, q12 h. One investigation reported better outcomes with 2500 IU administered SQ once a day for 3 days [125]. For intrathecal administration, either into the atlanto-occipital or lumbosacral space, positive results have been reported with the administration of 5–10 000 IU of TAT directly into the subarachnoid space. It is recommended that an equal volume of CSF be removed before injecting the

TAT. Another recommendation was the concurrent administration of 20–100 mg of prednisolone sodium succinate in order to help control meningeal inflammation. In addition, draining and cleaning of any wounds to minimize any anaerobic environment and, if secondary infections are of concern, administering either metronidazole, which is the antimicrobial of choice, penicillin, or a broad-spectrum antimicrobial with good activity against anaerobic organisms are also recommended. Affected horses should be placed in a quiet, dark box stall with elevated feed and water sources. A sling may be necessary for horses having difficulty standing or rising. Cavalier administration of equine TAT should be avoided. Acute hepatic necrosis has been associated with the administration of equine TAT, and it can occur up to several weeks following its administration [124].

Corynebacterium pseudotuberculosis infections (ulcerative lymphangitis, pigeon fever, pigeon breast)

The primary clinical manifestation of infection with *Corynebacterium pseudotuberculosis* organisms is abscessation or ulcerative lymphangitis. Abscess formation appears to occur more frequently in the Western states in the summer and fall. As it often affects the pectoral muscles, it has been given the colloquial term pigeon fever or pigeon breast, because the chest swells like that of a pigeon. Biting flies are believed to transmit the causative agent. Abscesses may occur either singularly or multifocally and recurrence is common. The abscesses typically drain thick, caseous pus, and the horses may present with edema, dermatitis, fever, and lethargy. Multiple horses on a farm may be affected and the disease may manifest as a perpetuating herd problem. The diagnosis is confirmed by culture. Initial therapy to manage these infections is to encourage the abscesses to open and drain, using surgical drainage if necessary. Internal abscessation may occur in chronic cases. If drainage is impossible, antimicrobial therapy may then be warranted. Penicillin is regarded as the drug of choice in most instances of *C. pseudotuberculosis* infections, and high doses of 50 000 IU/kg bwt are recommended to ensure antimicrobial distribution and penetration of the abscess(es) [126, 127].

Ulcerative lymphangitis, which is much less common than abscessation, occurs when the cutaneous lymphatics draining an abscess become infected. Hindlimbs may be more commonly affected, but infection of the forelimbs is possible. First, multiple hard nodules appear followed by abscessation, drainage, and ulceration. Although the individual lesions appear to resolve after draining, new lesions usually develop. The limb often becomes painful and exhibits swelling and/or pitting edema. Swelling often extends up the limb, and the lymphatic vessels become hardened. The diagnosis is presumptively made by the appearance of the limb with ulcerating abscessation. Definitive diagnosis is made by culture. Antimicrobial therapy is warranted and should be initiated as soon as possible. Abscesses may be incised and drained, but penicillin in high doses is necessary. Anti-inflammatory therapy is required to help control swelling and pain. Aggressive limb bandaging with pressure and hydrotherapy are often employed to help reduce swelling, although pain may be more severe with pressure bandaging. Severe cases may require much more intensive analgesia to help prevent complications, such as alternate limb laminitis. The positive outcomes of these cases depend on maintaining the normal physiology of the limb by prevention of fibrosis and permanent damage to the lymphatics [126, 127]. For cases unresponsive to penicillin, culture and sensitivity is strongly recommended [126].

Appendicular cellulitis

Appendicular cellulitis presents in a nearly identical manner as ulcerative lymphangitis. Because the causative organism(s) is not *C. pseudotuberculosis*, however, there is no abscessation. The limb becomes thickened and swollen with pitting edema presumably in response to wound infection with bacteria other than *C. pseudotuberculosis*. Diffuse subcutaneous infection appears to spread up the limb and may or may not involve the lymphatics. As with ulcerative lymphangitis, pain may be severe and the animal may refuse to bear weight during ambulation. Fever and lethargy are common. Pain management is imperative and adequate support of the opposite limb(s) is necessary to minimize the likelihood of laminitis. Culture and sensitivity may be warranted to target antimicrobial therapy, but many veterinarians approach this condition by administration of broad-spectrum antimicrobials such as penicillin/gentamicin, penicillin/enrofloxacin, or penicillin/third-generation cephalosporin combinations.

Organisms that have been reported to be associated with this condition include *Staphylococcus, Streptococcus, Pasteurella, Pseudomonas, Fusobacterium, Actinobacillus, Salmonella, and Nocardia*. In addition to antimicrobial therapy, treatment also often involves anti-inflammatory therapy with NSAIDs and/or corticosteroids, mild diuretic therapy often using trichlormethiazide/dexamethasone (i.e., Naquasone®, Merck Animal Health, Summit, NJ) or furosemide, pressure bandaging, hydrotherapy, and hand walking when possible. Treatment of appendicular cellulitis and similar conditions may be protracted. The goal is to maintain normal appendicular physiology by prevention of scarring and fibrosis [128–132].

Vasculitis and purpura hemorrhagica

Vasculitis is often an immune-mediated condition associated with systemic infection of a virus or bacterium. Inflammation of the blood vessels occurs with antigen–antibody, type III hypersensitivity, and reactions in the walls of the small vessels and capillaries, followed by vascular inflammation and necrosis. The result is edema, hemorrhage and thrombosis, and pain primarily of the distal limb(s). The condition may closely resemble a cellulitis of the affected limb(s) but often presents in more than one or all of the limbs. Organisms associated with vasculitis in the horse include *Streptococcus equi var equi*, often called purpura hemorrhagica, other streptococcal organisms, equine herpes virus, equine viral arteritis virus, equine infectious anemia virus, and equine granulocytic ehrlichiosis. A definitive diagnosis of vasculitis can be achieved by punch biopsy of the affected areas of the limb. Therapy involves treatment of the primary underlying condition, control of vascular inflammation, immunosuppression, supportive care, and pain management. This often involves the administration of antibiotics (e.g., penicillin for *S. equi var equi*), anti-inflammatory therapy with NSAID, immunosuppression with corticosteroids, and pain management as necessary. Dexamethasone is the most commonly used corticosteroid for treatment of vasculitis. Recommended doses range from 0.05 to 0.2 mg/kg bwt, IV or IM, q12–24 h. Horses with purpura hemorrhagica may require protracted therapy with corticosteroids for 4–6 weeks. Flumethasone administered at a dose of 0.005–0.011 mg/kg bwt or 2.5–5.0 mg/450 kg may be a reasonable corticosteroid to use in place of dexamethasone [132, 133].

Immune-mediated polymyositis

An immune-mediated polymyositis has been reported to occur in Quarter Horses and related bloodlines and a genetic basis has been suggested. The disease has been described on a much more limited basis in other breeds including the Thoroughbred and Icelandic pony. The clinical signs in affected horses are a rapid onset of muscle atrophy affecting the epaxial and gluteal muscle regions. Cervical muscle atrophy has also been reported. Generalized weakness may be a manifestation of significant muscle atrophy. In about 1/3 of the identified cases, an association with previous exposure to *S. equi* or other respiratory disease has been reported. Because hematologic abnormalities are minor in most affected horses, a diagnosis requires biopsy of the epaxial and gluteal muscles. Biopsy specimens reveal lymphocytic vasculitis, anguloid atrophy, lymphocytic myofiber infiltration, and fiber necrosis with macrophage infiltration and regeneration [134].

Treatment of affected horses involves administration of corticosteroids. Horses with concurrent evidence of streptococcal infection should be treated with antibiotics. Administration of corticosteroids is reported to help rapidly improve clinical signs and minimize further muscle atrophy. Dexamethasone has been recommended for initial therapy at a dose of 0.05 mg/kg bwt for 3 days, followed by prednisolone at a dose of 1 mg/kg bwt, PO, for 7–10 days, tapered by 100 mg/week over 1 month. Muscle mass can recover over two to three months. Horses that are not treated with corticosteroids may develop more severe muscle atrophy. Recurrence of myositis and associated atrophy is common and may require repeat therapy [134].

Bacteria-associated myositis/myonecrosis

The development of myositis in association with a *S. equi var equi* infection is relatively uncommon. Affected horses initially manifest clinical signs associated with "strangles" including submandibular lymphadenopathy and/or guttural pouch empyema but then develop myositis presenting with a stiff gait and firm, swollen, and painful epaxial and gluteal muscles. Myositis often progresses despite aggressive antimicrobial and anti-inflammatory therapies. Many cases become persistently recumbent and ultimately require euthanasia. Evaluation of blood parameters reveals findings indicative of a bacterial infection and myositis/rhabdomyolysis. A diagnosis of the condition requires concurrent evidence of infection with *S. equi var equi* and myositis. Unless recently vaccinated, titers to the M protein of *S. equi var equi* are reported to be low [134, 135].

One proposed explanation for the development of the myositis is the occurrence of a toxic-shock-like syndrome in affected horses. Alternatively, rhabdomyolysis may occur due to a bacteremia with local multiplication and production of exotoxins or proteases within the skeletal muscles. Although *S. equi var equi* has not been cultured in skeletal muscle from horses with rhabdomyolysis, the bacteria have been identified in affected muscle using immunofluorescent stains [134, 135].

A high mortality rate has been reported in horses receiving IV penicillin therapy after the appearance of clinical signs of strangles and myopathy. Although streptococcal species are usually susceptible to β-lactam antibiotics, the high mortality rate in penicillin-treated horses suggests that consideration of other antimicrobials may be warranted. An antimicrobial that inhibits protein synthesis, such as rifampin, combined with IV penicillin has been proposed as potentially beneficial in enhancing survival rates of horses with *S. equi var equi* rhabdomyolysis. Standard therapies for control and management of strangles should be concurrently implemented. NSAID and possibly high doses of short-acting corticosteroids may help control the inflammatory response. Pain management is a major part of therapy and may dictate the case progression and prognosis. Horses should be kept in a deeply bedded stall and, if recumbent, turned from side to side every 4 h or as frequently as possible. Persistent recumbency will add to muscle damage; therefore, when possible, horses may benefit from a sling if they will bear some weight.

Clostridial myositis/myonecrosis is often occurs following contamination of IM injection sites, and less often with other wounds. Horses typically present with localized pain, SC edema and/or crepitus. Abscessation is common in association with the injection site or wound. A high mortality rate may be associated with clostiridal myositis, at least partially depending on the isolate. Clostridial isolates seem to be most commonly *C. perfringens*. This isolate

is associated with the highest rate of survival. Other isolates include *C. septicum, C. ramosum, C. chauvoei*, and may be associated with higher mortality rates. Because of the severity of these infections, rapid and aggressive treatment and wound management is imperative. Clinical management is similar to infectious myositis of other bacterial causes. Aggressive surgical debridement allows for drainage of accumulated purulent or other fluid, and for oxygenation of the anaerobic environment. It is performed in conjunction with aggressive antimicrobial therapy, directed by culture and sensitivity. High doses of potassium penicillin (25–50 000 u/kg q 6 h) or another antimicrobial with good anaerobic activity, such as metronidazole (20–25 mg/kg q 6–8 h) are often utilized for these clostridial isolates. Other necessary therapies often necessary include those directed at systemic toxicity, laminitis prevention and good nursing care.

MRSA infections of the musculoskeletal system

There is increasing recognition in both human and veterinary medicines of the presence and transmission of methicillin-resistant and multidrug-resistant strains of *Staphylococcus aureus*. Wound infections with these strains are becoming more common, necessitating appropriate management and treatment by veterinarians and caretakers alike. Antimicrobial selection for the treatment of infections with MRSA should be guided by culture and sensitivity testing. This testing is also important for epidemiologic control. The common "first-line" antimicrobial agents utilized in humans for treatment of MRSA include doxycycline, trimethoprim–sulfamethoxazole, quinolone antimicrobial agents, and clindamycin [136, 137]. Fortunately, three of these compounds are commonly prescribed therapeutically and cost effectively in horses. Unfortunately, MRSA typically exhibits variable sensitivity to these medications in human patients, underscoring the importance of culture and sensitivity testing. Vancomycin has been used to treat multidrug-resistant forms of MRSA as a "last-line" drug, but resistance is emerging. At this time, most MRSA are sensitive to newer agents, such as linezolid or daptomycin. The oxazolidinone linezolid is a synthetic antimicrobial agent used for the treatment of serious infections caused by resistant Gram-positive organisms. It acts by inhibiting bacterial protein synthesis and it can be administered both IV and PO. It is probably cost prohibitive for use in the horse at this time. Daptomycin is a novel lipopeptide that is produced by the soil saprotroph *Streptomyces roseosporus*, and it is used to treat infections caused by multidrug-resistant bacteria, particularly Gram-positives, in humans, but has not been studied in the horse. Good hygiene and disinfection practices are critically important to prevent the spread of the resistant bacteria [136, 137].

Drugs used for regional administration and treatment of septic arthritis/osteomyelitis/physitis

Regional/local antimicrobial administration is commonly used to treat infections of the limbs, synovial structures, and body cavities. There are several methods of administration including direct injection, isolated limb retrograde venous injection using an Esmarch tourniquet, isolated limb infusion also with an Esmarch tourniquet, isolated limb intraosseous injection using a cannulated bone screw or other delivery system, continuous infusion using a balloon constant rate infusion system, and implantation of antimicrobial-impregnated sponges or beads [138–145]. The antimicrobial agents most commonly used for such administrations are the aminoglycosides. This is primarily because of their spectrum of activity, their concentration-dependent bactericidal action and a post antibiotic effect. One of the key advantages to the use of regional administration of antimicrobials is that very high concentrations at the site of infection can be achieved. In one study, administration of 1 g of gentamicin produced a C_{max} value in synovial fluid of 2.86 µg/ml [138]. In contrast, when 1 g of gentamicin was administered by isolated limb retrograde venous injection and by direct IA injection, C_{max} values of 589 and 64535 µg/ml, respectively, were obtained [138]. The C_{max} concentrations were 0.72 (IV administration), 147 (isolated limb retrograde venous infusion), and 16134 (direct articular injection) times greater than the reported MIC for the pathogen of interest (4 µg/ml) [138]. The C_{max} concentrations obtained appear to be at least partially dependent on the site of administration, with locations of administration closer to the site of infection or joint producing higher concentrations. Isolated limb intraosseous injections

have also been reported to be effective in obtaining high C_{max} concentrations, well in excess of the MIC of the offending pathogen [138].

Continuous infusion systems have been used for intrasynovial antimicrobial delivery and are available commercially [139–141]. In one study, a continuous delivery system using implantation of gentamicin-impregnated sponges was evaluated in tarsocrural joints [141]. Median peak synovial concentrations ranged from 115 to 332 µg/ml 3 h after implantation of a purified bovine collagen sponge impregnated with 130 mg of gentamicin into the plantarolateral pouch. Synovial fluid gentamicin concentrations fell to below 4 µg/ml by 48 h. Peak concentrations achieved were greater than 20 times that of the MIC of commonly isolated bacterial pathogens [141]. Importantly, this technique did not produce significant inflammation. Because such systems deliver antimicrobial agents continuously, they may also prove to be appropriate for use with time-dependent antimicrobial agents into synovial structures [141]. The system proved to be a useful adjunctive treatment to systemic antimicrobial therapy for the treatment of chronic and refractory cases of septic synovitis. Antimicrobial-impregnated polymethyl methacrylate and collagen sponges may also facilitate slow-release delivery of appropriate antimicrobial agents to local tissue in the treatment of septic arthritis.

Lyme disease

Lyme disease is caused by the spirochete *Borrelia burgdorferi*. Transmission to the horse occurs by a tick vector of the *Ixodes* genus. The putative clinical manifestations of Lyme disease in both humans and horses include signs relating to the skin and musculoskeletal and nervous systems. Lyme disease in humans is often manifest in its early stage by a rash (erythema migrans) and non-specific symptoms of fever, malaise, fatigue, headache, myalgia, and arthralgia. However, the indisputable clinical occurrence of Lyme disease in both horses and humans remains difficult to substantiate. Clinical cases are reported to peak during the summer months. According to the results of a questionnaire pertaining to equine Lyme borreliosis in Germany, the existence of the disease in the horse was reported to be confirmed by over half of the respondents [146]. The equine clinical manifestations of Lyme disease appear to be chronic poor performance and/or various orthopedic manifestations, the most common being shifting leg lameness. Neuroborreliosis has also been reported in the horse. A geographical distribution of equine Lyme disease cases is presumed to mirror human case distribution. The northeastern coast, areas of Wisconsin and Minnesota, and northwestern California are reportedly areas of the highest incidence of human cases [146–150].

The diagnosis of Lyme disease is made primarily by the combination of compatible clinical signs and supportive laboratory testing. The most common supportive test result in the diagnosis of Lyme disease is a positive serum antibody. Serological testing is available using an immunofluorescence assay (IFA), ELISA, and Western blot analysis. The IFA test was associated with the highest number of false-positive test results. The Western blot analysis was reported to be the most reliable of the three tests for the serological diagnosis of *B. burgdorferi* infection in horses. It is recommended that serological examination of horses should be initially performed using ELISA, followed by confirmation of positive ELISA test results using the Western blot test. Polymerase chain reaction (PCR) testing is available and primarily advocated for testing of synovial biopsy samples, synovial fluid, and cerebrospinal fluid. Less preferred samples for PCR include whole blood or urine [151–154]. A more recent approach to testing horses suspected to have Lyme disease involves evaluation of the serum for antibody to three specific outer surface proteins expressed by *B. burgdorferi*. This multiplex assay is proposed to help identify and distinguish vaccination antibody from antibody associated with early infection and from antibody associated with chronic infection [155].

Effective antibiotic therapy for Lyme disease is problematic. *B. burgdorferi* spirochetes use several mechanisms to resist antibiotic and immune destruction. *In vivo* antibiotic resistance is conferred by the ability to live intracellularly in fibroblasts, endothelial cells, glial cells, and others. Since some antibiotics, such as beta-lactams, are most effective against actively dividing organisms, the well-documented slow division of this spirochete potentiates its ability to evade antimicrobial activity. Some cultures of *B. burgdorferi* have taken up to 10.5 months to grow, and this finding could significantly impact the proposed length of treatment. L-forms of some bacteria have been shown to specifically impact the ability to produce chronic infection. L-forms of *B.* *burgdorferi* have also been identified and may further facilitate this characteristic of *B. burgdorferi*. These L-forms of *B. burgdorferi* also develop resistance by losing their cell wall and the ability to replicate. These characteristics render the spirochete much less susceptible to cell wall-acting antibiotics such as beta-lactams and to replication-dependent antibiotics. Considering these points in the therapeutic approach to Lyme disease, it may be realistic to use two antibiotics simultaneously, one antibiotic that acts on the surface of the organism and the other internally. Many horses diagnosed with Lyme disease, often due to the presence of fevers and/or lamenesses, are treated with IV oxytetracycline and/or oral doxycycline with reported positive clinical responses. Children under the age of eight are often treated with cefuroxime axetil and not doxycycline. Children over eight years of age are often managed with either doxycycline or amoxicillin with cefuroxime axetil. This combination, or a similar one, may be useful in younger, older, and/or immunosuppressed equine patients. In human patients, IV therapy may need to be followed by prolonged oral antimicrobial therapy, and treatment has been advocated for 2 months beyond the stabilization or past any recurrence of clinical signs of "Lyme symptoms." In one investigation, three groups of 4 ponies each were experimentally infected with *B. burgdorferi* by tick exposure. Each group was then treated with either doxycycline, ceftiofur, or tetracycline for 28 days [156]. While tetracycline treatment eliminated the infection, the responses to doxycycline and ceftiofur treatments were inconsistent. Following five months of antibiotic treatment, tissue necropsy specimens were culture positive in all of the ponies that exhibited increased antibody levels after antimicrobial treatment [156]. However, all four tetracycline-treated ponies were antibody and postmortem tissue culture negative. The prevention of Lyme disease may be a consideration in areas where the *Ixodes* ticks persist and where cases have been reported. A recombinant OspA (rOspA) vaccine was reported to be protective in a pony challenge model [157].

References

1 Dowling, P.M. (2011) *Myths and truths about controlling pain and inflammation in horses.* Alberta Agriculture and Rural Development, Alberta, CA, pp. 1–10. http://www1.agric.gov. ab.ca [accessed on May 5, 2014].

2 Bentz, B.G. & Revenaugh, M.S. (2010) Extra-articular therapies used in the management of lameness. In: H.W. Jann & G.E. Fackelman (eds), *Rehabilitating the Athletic Horse*, pp. 117–158. Nova Science Publishers Inc, New York.

3 Kivett, L., Taintor, J. & Wright, J. (2013) Evaluation of the safety of a combination of oral administration of phenylbutazone and firocoxib in horses. *Journal of Veterinary Pharmacology and Therapeutics*, doi:10.1111/jvp.12097.

4 Buur, J.L., Baynes, R.E., Smith, G.W. & Riviere, J.E. (2009) A physiologically based pharmacokinetic model linking plasma protein binding interactions with drug disposition. *Research in Veterinary Science*, **86** (2), 293–301.

5 Chan, T.Y. (1995) Adverse interactions between warfarin and nonsteroidal antiinflammatory drugs: Mechanisms, clinical significance, and avoidance. *Annals of Pharmacotherapy*, **29** (12), 1274–83.

6 Keegan, K.G., Messer, N.T., Reed, S.K., Wilson, D.A. & Kramer, J. (2008) Effectiveness of administration of phenylbutazone alone or concurrent administration of phenylbutazone and flunixin meglumine to alleviate lameness in horses. *American Journal of Veterinary Research*, **69** (2), 167–173.

7 Foreman, J. & Ruemmler, R. (2011) Phenylbutazone and flunixin meglumine used singly or in combination in experimental lameness in horses. *Proceedings 57th Annual Convention of the American Association of Equine Practitioners*. San Antonio, p. 83.

8 Clay, S., Woods, W.E., Nugent, T.E. *et al.* (1984) Population distributions of phenylbutazone and oxyphenbutazone after oral and i.v. dosing in horses. *Journal of Veterinary Pharmacology and Therapeutics*, **7** (4), 265–76.

9 Tobin, T., Chay, S., Kamerling, S. *et al.* (1986) Phenylbutazone in the horse: A review. *Journal of Veterinary Pharmacology and Therapeutics*, **9** (1), 1–25.

10 Gerring, E.L., Lees, P. & Taylor, J.B. (1981) Pharmacokinetics of phenylbutazone and its metabolites in the horse. *Equine Veterinary Journal*, **13** (3), 152–7.

11 Toutain, P.L., Autefage, A., Legrand, C. & Alvinerie, M. (1994) Plasma concentrations and therapeutic efficacy of phenylbutazone and flunixin meglumine in the horse: Pharmacokinetic/pharmacodynamic modelling. *Journal of Veterinary Pharmacology and Therapeutics*, **17** (6), 459–469.

12 MacAllister, C.G., Morgan, S.J., Borne, A.T. & Pollet, R.A. (1993) Comparison of adverse effects of phenylbutazone, flunixin meglumine and ketoprofen in horses. *Journal of the American Veterinary Medical Association*, **202** (1), 71–77.

13 Ramirez, S., Wolfsheimer, K.J., Moore, R.M., Mora, F., Bueno, A.C. & Mirza, T. (2008) Duration of effects of phenylbutazone on serum total thyroxine and free thyroxine concentrations in horses. *Journal of Veterinary Internal Medicine*, **11** (6), 371–374.

14 Morris, D.D. & Garcia, M. (1983) Thyroid-stimulating hormone: Response test in healthy horses and effect of phenylbutazone on equine thyroid hormones. *American Journal of Veterinary Research*, **44** (3), 503–507.

15 Snow, D.H., Baxter, P. & Whiting, B. (1981) The pharmacokinetics of meclofenamic acid in the horse. *Journal of Veterinary Pharmacology and Therapeutics*, **4** (2), 147–56.

16 Owens, J.G., Kamerling, S.G., Stanton, S.R. & Keowen, M.L. (1995) Effects of ketoprofen and phenylbutazone on chronic hoof pain and lameness in the horse. *Equine Veterinary Journal*, **27** (4), 296–300.

17 Landoni, M.F. & Lees, P. (1996) Pharmacokinetics and pharmacodynamics of ketoprofen enantiomers in the horse. *Journal of Veterinary Pharmacology and Therapeutics*, **19** (6), 466–74.

18 Kvaternick, V., Pollmeier, M., Fischer, J. & Hanson, P.D. (2007) Pharmacokinetics and metabolism of orally administered firocoxib, a novel second generation coxib, in horses. *Journal of Veterinary Pharmacology and Therapeutics*, **30** (3), 208–17.

19 Villarino, N.F., Vispo, T.J., Marcos, F. & Landoni, M.F. (2006) Inefficacy of topical diclofenac in arthritic horses. *American Journal of Animal and Veterinary Sciences*, **1** (1), 8–12.

20 Anderson, D., Kollias-Baker, C., Colahan, P., Keene, R.O., Lynn, R.C. & Hepler, D.I. (2005) Urinary and serum concentrations of diclofenac after topical application to horses. *Veterinary Therapeutics*, **6** (1), 57–66.

21 Bertone, J.J., Lynn, R.C., Vatistas, N.J., Kelch, W.J., Sifferman, R.L. & Hepler, D.I. (2002) Clinical field trial to evaluate the efficacy of topically applied diclofenac cream for the relief of joint lameness in horses. *Proceedings of the 48th Annual Convention of the American Association of Equine Practitioners*. Orlando, FL, pp. 190–193.

22 Frisbie, D.D., McIlwraith, C.W., Kawcak, C.E., Werpy, N.M. & Pearce, G.L. (2009) Evaluation of topically administered diclofenac liposomal cream for treatment of horses with experimentally induced osteoarthritis. *American Journal of Veterinary Research*, **70** (2), 210–215.

23 Davis, J.L., Papich, M.G., Morton, A.J., Gayle, J., Blikslager, A.T. & Campbell, N.B. (2007) Pharmacokinetics of etodolac in the horse following oral and intravenous administration. *Journal of Veterinary Pharmacology and Therapeutics*, **30** (1), 43–48.

24 Symonds, K.D., MacAllister, C.G., Erkert, R.S. & Payton, M.E. (2006) Use of force plate analysis to assess effects of etodolac in horses with navicular syndrome. *American Journal of Veterinary Research*, **67** (4), 557–561.

25 Davies, N.M. & Teng, X.W. (2003) Importance of chirality in drug therapy and pharmacy practice: Implications for psychiatry. *Advances in Pharmacy*, **1** (3), 242–252.

26 Lees, P. & Landoni, M.F. (2002) Pharmacodynamics and enantioselective pharmacokinetics of racemic carprofen in the horse. *Journal of Veterinary Pharmacology and Therapeutics*, **25** (6), 433–448.

27 McKellar, Q.A., Bogan, J.A., von Fellenberg, R.L., Ludwig, B. & Cawley, G.D. (1991) Pharmacokinetic, biochemical and tolerance studies on carprofen in the horse. *Equine Veterinary Journal*, **23** (4), 280–284.

28 Lees, P., McKellar, Q., May, S.A. & Ludwig, B. (1994) Pharmacodynamics and pharmacokinetics of carprofen in the horse. *Equine Veterinary Journal*, **26** (3), 206–208.

29 Committee for Veterinary Medicinal Products. (2002) *Meloxicam* (extension to horses) summary report. EMEA/

MRL/833/02-FINAL. European Agency for the Evaluation of Medicinal Products, Canary Warf.

30 Toutain, P.L. & Cester, C.C. (2004) Pharmacokinetic-pharmacodynamic relationships and dose response to meloxicam in horses with induced arthritis of the right carpal joint. *American Journal of Veterinary Research*, **65** (11), 1533–1541.

31 Soma, L.R., Uboh, C.E., Rudy, J.A. & Perkowski, S.Z. (1995) Plasma and synovial fluid kinetics, disposition, and urinary excretion of naproxen in horses. *American Journal of Veterinary Research*, **56** (8), 1075–1080.

32 Cagnardi, P., Gallo, M., Zonca, A., Carli, S. & Villa, R. (2011) Pharmacokinetics and effects of alkalization during oral and intravenous administration of naproxen in horses. *Journal of Equine Veterinary Science*, **31** (8), 456–462.

33 Davis, J.L., Marshall, J.F., Papich, M.G., Blikslager, A.T. & Campbell, N.B. (2011) The pharmacokinetics and in vitro cyclooxygenase selectivity of deracoxib in horses. *Journal of Veterinary Pharmacology and Therapeutics*, **34**, 12–16.

34 Shilo, Y., Britzi, M., Eytan, B., Lifschitz, T., Soback, S. & Steinman, A. (2008) Pharmacokinetics of tramadol in horses after intravenous, intramuscular and oral administration. *Journal of Veterinary Pharmacology and Therapeutics*, **31** (1), 60–65.

35 Dhanjal, J.K., Wilson, D.V., Robinson, E., Tobin, T.T. & Dirokulu, L. (2009) Intravenous tramadol: Effects, nociceptive properties, and pharmacokinetics in horses. *Veterinary Anaesthesia and Analgesia*, **36** (6), 581–590.

36 Cox, S., Villarino, N. & Doherty, T. (2010) Determination of oral tramadol pharmacokinetics in horses. *Research in Veterinary Science*, **89** (2), 236–241.

37 Dyson, S., Murray, R., Blunden, T. & Schramme, M. (2006) Current concepts of navicular disease. *Equine Veterinary Education*, **18** (1), 45–56.

38 Dyson, S. (2011) Radiological interpretation of the navicular bone. *Equine Veterinary Education*, **23** (2), 73–87.

39 Ceva Animal Health Ltd (2009) *Understanding Navicular Disease*. Ceva Animal Health Ltd, Chesham, Bucks.

40 Turner, A.S. & Tucker, C.M. (1989) The evaluation of isoxsuprine hydrochloride for the treatment of navicular disease: A double-blind study. *Equine Veterinary Journal*, **21** (5), 338–341.

41 Rose, R.J., Allen, J.R., Hodgson, D.R. & Kohnke, J.R. (1983) Studies on isoxsuprine hydrochloride for the treatment of navicular disease. *Equine Veterinary Journal*, **15** (3), 238–243.

42 Erkert, R.S. & MacAllister, C.G. (2002) Isoxsuprine hydrochloride in the horse: A review. *Journal of Veterinary Pharmacology and Therapeutics*, **25** (2), 81–87.

43 Ingle-Fehr, J.E. & Baxter, G.M. (1999) The effect of oral isoxsuprine and pentoxifylline on digital and laminar blood flow in healthy horses. *Veterinary Surgery*, **28** (3), 154–160.

44 Lizarraga, I., Castillo, F. & Valderrama, M.E. (2004) An analgesic evaluation of isoxsuprine in horses. *Journal of Veterinary Medicine A*, **51** (7–8), 370–374.

45 Liska, D.A., Akucewich, L.H., Marsella, R., Maxwell, L.K., Barbara, J.E. & Cole, C.A. (2006) Pharmacokinetics of pentoxifylline and its 5-hydroxyhexyl metabolite after oral and intravenous administration of pentoxifylline to healthy adult horses. *American Journal of Veterinary Research*, **67** (9), 1621–1627.

46 Colles, C.M. (1979) A preliminary report on the use of warfarin in the treatment of navicular disease. *Equine Veterinary Journal*, **11** (3), 187–190.

47 Vrins, A., Carlson, G. & Feldman, B. (1983) Warfarin: A review with emphasis on its use in the horse. *Canadian Veterinary Journal*, **24** (7), 211–213.

48 Coffman, J.R., Johnson, J.H., Trischler, L.G., Garner, H.E. & Scrutchfield, W.L. (1979) Orgotein in equine navicular disease: A double blind study. *Journal of the American Veterinary Medical Association*, **174** (3), 261–264.

49 Ahlengard, S., Tufvesson, G., Petterson, H. & Andersson, T. (1978) Treatment of traumatic arthritis in the horse with intra-articular orgotein (Palosein®). *Equine Veterinary Journal*, **10**, 122–124.

50 Denoix, J.M., Thibaud, D. & Ricco, B. (2003) Tiludronate as a new therapeutic agent in the treatment of navicular disease: A double-blind placebo-controlled clinical trial. *Equine Veterinary Journal*, **35** (4), 407–413.

51 Boyce, M., Malone, E.D., Anderson, L.B. *et al.* (2010) Evaluation of diffusion of triamcinolone acetonide from the distal interphalangeal joint into the navicular bursa in horses. *American Journal of Veterinary Research*, **71** (2), 169–175.

52 Bell, C.D., Howard, R.D., Taylor, D.S., Voss, E.D. & Werpy, N.M. (2009) Outcomes of podotrochlear (navicular) bursa injections for signs of foot pain in horses evaluated via magnetic resonance imaging: 23 cases (2005–2007). *Journal of the American Veterinary Medical Association*, **234** (7), 920–925.

53 Pollitt, C.C. (1999) Equine laminitis: A revised pathophysiology. *Proceedings 45th Annual Convention of the American Association of Equine Practitioners*. Albuquerque, NM.

54 Huntington, P., Pollitt, C. & McGowan, C. (2008) *Recent research into laminitis*. Proceedings of the Kentucky Equine Nutrition Conference: Facing Today's Nutritional Challenges, Advanced Management of Gastrointestinal and Metabolic Diseases, Lexington, KY, April 15–16, pp. 1–17.

55 Falerios, R.R., Nuovo, G.J. & Belnap, J.K. (2009) Calprotectin in myeloid and epithelial cells of laminae from horses with black walnut extract-induced laminitis. *Journal of Veterinary Internal Medicine*, **23**, 174–181.

56 White, N.A. (2005) Equine laminitis. *Proceedings Waltham Seminar*. Washington, DC.

57 Hood, D.M., Grosenbaugh, D.A., Mostafa, M.B., Morgan, S.J. & Thomas, B.C. (1993) Predisposition for venoconstriction in the equine laminar dermis in equine laminitis. *Journal of Veterinary Internal Medicine*, **7** (4), 228–234.

58 Pollitt, C.C. (2003) Laminitis. In: M.R. Ross & S.J. Dyson (eds), *Diagnosis and Management of Lameness in the Horse*, pp. 325–339. Saunders, St Louis, MO.

59 Stokes, A.M., Eades, S.C. & Moore, R.M. (2004) Pathophysiology and treatment of acute laminitis. In: S.M. Reed, W.M. Bayly & D.C. Sellon (eds), *Equine Internal Medicine*, pp. 522–531. Saunders, St. Louis, MO.

60 Williams, J.M., Lin, Y.J., Loftus, J.P. *et al.* (2010) Effect of intravenous lidocaine administration on laminar inflammation in the black walnut extract model of laminitis. *Equine Veterinary Journal*, **42** (3), 261–269.

61 Bentz, B.G. & Revenaugh, M.S. (2010) Equine intra-articular injection. In: H.W. Jann & G.E. Fackelman (eds), *Rehabilitating the Athletic Horse*, pp. 87–115. Nova Science Publishers Inc, New York.

62 Bentz, B.G. (2012) Pain management in the wounded/injured horse. *Proceedings of the North American Veterinary Conference*. Orlando, FL.

63 McIlwraith, C.W. (2010) Management of joint disease in the sport horse. *Proceedings of the 17th Kentucky Equine Research Nutrition Conference*; Lexington. pp. 61–81.

64 Carter, J., Carter, G.K., Easter, J.L., Frisbie, D., McClure, S. & Mitchell, R.D. (2007) Managing equine joint inflammation: A roundtable discussion on diagnostic and treatment options. Supplement to *Compendium on Continuing Education for the Practicing Veterinaria Equine Edition*, **2** (3A), 1–16.

65 Caron JP. (2006) Therapy for equine joint disease. Large *Animal Veterinary Rounds*, **6** (7), 1–6. www.canadian veterinarians.net/larounds [accessed on May 5, 2014].

66 US Pharmacopeial Convention (2004) *Corticosteroid-Glucocorticoid Effects (Veterinary—Systemic)*, pp. 1–67. The United States Pharmacopeial Convention, Rockville, MD.

67 Frisbie, D.D., Kawcak, C.E., Trotter, G.W., Powers, B.E., Walton, R.M. & McIlwraith, C.W. (1997) Effects of triamcinolone acetonide on an in vivo equine osteochondral fragment exercise model. *Equine Veterinary Journal*, **29**, 349–359.

68 Murray, R.C., DeBowes, R.M., Gaughan, E.M., Zhu, C.F. & Athanasiou, K.A. (1998) The effects of intra-articular methylprednisolone and exercise on the mechanical properties of cartilage in the horse. *Osteoarthritis Cartilage*, **6** (2), 106–114.

69 Frisbie, D.D., Kawcak, C.E., Baxter, G.M. *et al.* (1998) Effects of 6alpha-methylprednisolone acetate on an equine osteochondral fragment exercise model. *American Journal of Veterinary Research*, **59** (12), 1619–1628.

70 Carter, B.G., Bertone, A.L., Weisbrode, S.E., Bailey, S.Q., Andrews, J.M. & Palmer, J.L. (1996) Influence of methylprednisolone acetate on osteochondral healing in exercised tarsocrural joints of horses. *American Journal of Veterinary Research*, **57** (6), 914–922.

71 Shoemaker, R.S., Bertone, A.L., Martin, G.S. *et al.* (1992) Effects of intra-articular administration of methylprednisolone acetate on normal articular cartilage and healing of experimentally induced osteochondral defects in horses. *American Journal of Veterinary Research*, **53** (8), 1446–1453.

72 Murray, R.C., Znaor, N., Tanner, K.E., DeBowes, R.M., Gaughan, E.D. & Goodship, A.E. (2002) The effect of intra-articular methylprednisolone acetate and exercise on equine carpal subchondral and cancellous bone microhardness. *Equine Veterinary Journal*, **34** (3), 306–310.

73 Dechant, J.E., Baxter, G.M., Frisbie, D.D., Trotter, G.W. & McIlwraith, C.W. (2003) Effects of dose titration of methylprednisolone acetate and triamcinolone acetonide on interleukin-1 conditioned equine articular cartilage explants in vitro. *Equine Veterinary Journal*, **35** (5), 444–450.

74 Foland, J.W., McIlwraith, C.W., Trotter, G.W., Powers, B.E. & Lamar, C.H. (1994) Effect of betamethasone and exercise on equine carpal joints with osteochondral fragments. *Veterinary Surgery*, **23** (5), 369–376.

75 Necas, J., Bartosikova, L., Brauner, P. & Kolar, J. (2008) Hyaluronic acid (hyaluronan): A review. *Veterinarni Medicina*, **53** (8), 397–411.

76 Todhunter, R.J., Minor, R.R., Wootton, J.A., Krook, L., Burton-Wurster, N. & Lust, G. (1993) Effects of exercise and polysulfated glycosaminoglycan on repair of articular cartilage defects in the equine carpus. *Journal of Orthopaedic Research*, **11** (6), 782–795.

77 Gustafson, S.B., McIlwraith, C.W. & Jones, R.L. (1989) Comparison of the effect of polysulfated glycosaminoglycan, corticosteroids, and sodium hyaluronate in the potentiation of a subinfective dose of Staphylococcus aureus in the midcarpal joint of horses. *American Journal of Veterinary Research*, **50** (12), 2014–2017.

78 Gustafson, S.B., McIlwraith, C.W., Jones, R.L. & Dixon-White, H.E. (1989) Further investigations into the potentiation of infection by intra-articular injection of polysulfated glycosaminoglycan and the effect of filtration and intra-articular injection of amikacin. *American Journal of Veterinary Research*, **50** (12), 2018–2022.

79 White, G.W., Stites, T., Jones, W. & Jordan, S. (2004) Efficacy of intramuscular chondroitin sulfate and compounded acetyl-d-glucosamine in a positive controlled study of equine carpitis. *Proceedings 50th Annual Convention of the American Association of Equine Practitioners*. Denver.

80 Hague, B.A. (2005) Clinical impression of Orthokine (IRAP) treating joint disease in the performance horse. *Proceedings ACVS Diplomate Resort Meeting*. Bretton Woods, NH, p. 45.

81 CEVA Sante Animale (2008) *Tildren 500 mg Infusion. Marketing Brochure*, pp. 1–10. Animal Health LTD, Chesham.

82 Coudry, V., Thibaud, D., Riccio, B., Audigié, F., Didierlaurent, D. & Denoix, J.M. (2007) Efficacy of tiludronate in the treatment of horses with signs of pain associated with osteoarthritic lesions of the thoracolumbar vertebral column. *American Journal of Veterinary Research*, **68** (3), 329–337.

83 Delguste, C., Amory, H., Piccot-Crézollet, C. *et al* (2007) Pharmacological effects of tiludronate in horses after long term immobilization. *Bone*, **41** (3), 414–421.

84 Kamm, L., McIlwraith, W. & Kawcak, C. (2008) A review of the efficacy of tiludronate in the horse. *Journal of Equine Veterinary Science*, **28** (4), 209–214.

85 Dart, A., Perkins, N., Dowling, B.T., Livingston, C. & Hodgson, D. (2001) The effect of three different doses of

sodium pentosan polysulfate on haematological and hae-mostatic variables in adult horses. *Australian Veterinary Journal*, **79** (9), 624–627.

86 Fuller, C.J., Ghosh, P. & Barr, A.R. (2002) Plasma and syno-vial fluid concentrations of calcium pentosan polysulphate achieved in the horse after intramuscular injection. *Equine Veterinary Journal*, **34** (1), 61–64.

87 Little, C. & Ghosh, P. (1996) Potential use of pentosan poly-sulfate for the treatment of equine joint disease. In: C.W. McIlwraith & G.W. Trotter (eds), *Joint disease in the horse*, pp. 281–292. WB Saunders Co, Philadelphia, PA.

88 McIlwraith, C.W., Dart, A.J., Hughes, F.E., McInnes, R. & Teitzel, R. (2011) *The Role of Pentosan Polysulfate in Multimodal Treatment Plans: A Roundtable Discussion*. International Veterinary Supplies, Kembla Grange.

89 McIlwraith, C.W., Frisbie, D.D. & Kawcak, C.E. (2012) Evaluation of intramuscularly administered pentosan polysulfate for treatment of experimentally induced osteoar-thritis in horses. *American Journal of Veterinary Research*, **73** (5), 628–633.

90 Kwan, C., Bell, R., Koenig, T. *et al.* (2012) Effects of intra-articular sodium pentosan polysulfate and glucosamine on the cytology, total protein concentration and viscosity of synovial fluid in horses. *Australian Veterinary Journal*, **90** (8), 315–320.

91 Sutter, W. (2007) *PRP: Platelet-rich plasma*. Vet-Stem, Poway, CA. www.vet-stem.com/pdfs/sutter.pdf [accessed on May 5, 2014].

92 Waselau, M., Sutter, W.W., Genovese, R.L. & Bertone, A.L. (2008) Intralesional injection of platelet-rich plasma fol-lowed by controlled exercise for treatment of midbody suspensory ligament desmitis in Standardbred racehorses. *Journal of the American Veterinary Medical Association*, **232** (10), 1515–1520.

93 Kaneps, A.J. (2008) *Platelet-Rich Plasma: A New Treatment for Tendon and Ligament Injuries in Horses*, pp. 1–4. New England Equine Medical and Surgical Center, Dover, NH.

94 Texor, J. (2011) Platelet-rich plasma: Improving treatment for tendon and ligament injuries. *CEH Horse Report*, **29** (1), 1–6.

95 Texor, J. (2011) *Platelet-rich plasma: The rest of the story*. Ontario. www.lakeimmunogenics.com/downloads/LI-PRP.pdf [accessed on May 5, 2014].

96 Carmona, J.U., Argüelles, D., Climent, F., *et al.* (2005) Autologous platelet-rich plasma injected intraarticularly diminished synovial effusion and degree of lameness in horses affected with severe joint disease. *Proceedings 14th Annual Scientific Meeting European College Veterinary Surgeons*. Lyon.

97 Sutter, W.W. (2011) PRP: Indications for intra-articular use. *Proceedings ACVS Veterinary Symposium*. Chicago, IL, pp. 104–107.

98 Weibrich, G., Hansen, T., Kleis, W., Buch, R. & Hitzler, W.E. (2004) Effect of platelet concentration in platelet-rich plasma on peri-implant bone regeneration. *Bone*, **34**, 655–671.

99 Fortier, L.A. & Smith, R.K.W. (2008) Regenerative Medicine for Tendinous and Ligamentous Injuries of Sport Horses. *Veterinary Clinics of North America. Equine Practice*, **24**, 191–201.

100 Koch, T.G., Berg, L.C. & Betts, D.H. (2009) Current and future regenerative medicine- Principles, concepts and therapeutic use of stem cell therapy and tissue engi-neering in equine medicine. *Canadian Veterinary Journal*, **50** (2), 155–165.

101 Herthel, D.J. (2001) Enhanced suspensory ligament healing in 100 horses by stem cells and other bone marrow components. *Proceedings for the 47th. Annual American Association of Equine Practitioners*, **47**, 319–321.

102 Pacini, S., Spinabella, S., Trombi, L. *et al.* (2007) Suspension of bone marrow derived undifferentiated mesenchymal stromal cells for repair of superficial digital flexor tendon in race horses. *Tissue Engineering*, **13**, 2949–2955.

103 Taylor, S.E., Smith, R.K. & Clegg, P.D. (2007) Mesenchymal stem cell therapy in equine musculoskeletal disease: Science, fact or clinical fiction? *Equine Veterinary Journal*, **39** (2), 172–180.

104 Smith, R.K.W. (2008) Mesenchymal stem cell therapy for equine tendinopathy. *Disability and Rehabilitation;*, **30** (20–22), 1752–1758.

105 Wilkie, M.M., Nydam, D.V. & Nixon, A.J. (2007) Enhanced early chondrogenesis in articular defects following arthroscopic mesenchymal stem cell implan-tation in an equine model. *Journal Orthopaedic Research*, **25** (7), 913–925.

106 Vidal, M.A., Kilroy, G.E., Lopez, M.J., Johnson, J.R., Moore, R.M. & Gimble, J.M. (2007) Characterization of equine adipose tissue-derived stromal cells: Adipogenic and osteogenic capacity and comparison with bone marrow-derived mesenchymal stromal cells. *Veterinary Surgery*, **36** (7), 613–622.

107 Vidal, M.A. & Lopez, M.J. (2011) Adipogenic differentia-tion of adult equine mesenchymal stromal cells. *Methods in Molecular Biology*, **702**, 61–75.

108 Reiners, S. (2012) The current status of regenerative medicine (stem cell therapy). *Proceedings North American Veterinary Conference*. Orlando, FL.

109 Mitchell, R.D. (2006) Treatment of tendon and ligament injuries with UBM powder. In: A. Linder (ed.) *Proceedings Conference on Equine Sports Medicine and Science; Management of Lameness Causes in Sport Horses*. Wageningen Academic Publishers, Cambridge, pp. 213–217.

110 Rose, W., Wood, J.D., Simmons-Byrd, A. & Spievack, A.R. (2009) Effect of a xenogeneic urinary bladder injectable bioscaffold on lameness in dogs with osteoarthritis of the coxofemoral joint (Hip): A randomized, double blinded controlled trial. *International Journal of Applied Research in Veterinary Medicine*, **7** (1), 13–22.

111 Wallis, T.W., Baxter, G.M., Werpy, N.M., Mason, G.L., Frisbie, D.D. & Jarloev, N. (2010) Acellular urinary bladder matrix in a collagenase model of superficial digital flexor tendonitis in horses. *Journal of Equine Veterinary Science*, **30** (7), 365–370.

112 Seino, K.K., Foreman, J.H., Greene, S.A., Goetz, T.E. & Benson, G.J. (2003) Effects of topical perineural capsaicin in a reversible model of equine foot lameness. *Journal of Veterinary Internal Medicine*, **17** (4), 563–566.

113 Harkins, J.D., Mundy, G.D., Stanley, S.D., Sams, R.A. & Tobin, T. (2003) Lack of local anesthetic efficacy of Sarapin in the abaxial sesamoid block model. *Journal of Veterinary Pharmacology and Therapeutics*, **20** (3), 229–232.

114 Kawcak, C.E., Frisbie, D.D., McIlwraith, C.W., Werpy, N.M. & Park, R.D. (2007) Evaluation of avocado and soybean unsaponifiable extracts for treatment of horses with experimentally induced osteoarthritis. *American Journal of Veterinary Research*, **68** (6), 598–604.

115 Muir, W.W., Sams, R.A. & Ashcraft, S. (1984) Pharmacologic and pharmacokinetic properties of methocarbamol in the horse. *American Journal of Veterinary Research*, **45** (11), 2256–2260.

116 McKenzie, E.C., Valberg, S.J., Godden, S.M., Finno, C.J. & Murphy, M.J. (2004) Effect of oral administration of dantrolene sodium on serum creatine kinase activity after exercise in horses with recurrent exertional rhabdomyolysis. *American Journal of Veterinary Research*, **65** (1), 74–79.

117 Valberg, S.J. (2006) Exertional rhabdomyolysis. *Proceedings Of the 52nd Annual Convention of the American Association of Equine Practitioners*. San Antonio, TX, pp. 365–372.

118 Valberg, S.J. (2010) Management of tying-up in sport horses: Challenges and successes. *Proceedings of the 17th Kentucky Equine Research Nutrition Conference*. Lexington, KY, pp. 82–93.

119 Valberg, S.J. (2010) Review of muscle diseases in sport horses. *Proceedings Veterinary Sport Horse Symposium*. Lexington, KY, pp. 107–120.

120 Reynolds, J.A. (2004) *Equine Hyperkalemic Periodic Paralysis (HYPP) Overview and Management Strategies. Technical Edge*. ADM Alliance Nutrition, Quincy IL.

121 Zeilmann, M. (1993) HYPP—hyperkalemic periodic paralysis in horses. *Tierärztliche Praxis*, **21** (6), 524–527.

122 Sanofi Pasteur Limited (2005) *Botulism Antitoxin Bivalent (Equine) Types A and B*. Package Insert R2-0705 USA. Sanofi Pasteur Limited, Toronto, ON.

123 Sprayberry, K.A., Carlson, G.P. (1997) *Review of botulism*. Proceedings of the 43rd Annual Convention of the AAEP, Phoenix, AZ, December 7–10, **43**, pp. 379–381.

124 Furr, M. (2008) Clostridial neurotoxins: Botulism and tetanus. In: R. Furr (ed), *Equine Neurology*, pp. 221–229. Blackwell Publishing, Ames, IA.

125 Green, S.L., Little, S.B., Baird, J.D., Tremblay, R.R.M. & Smith-Maxie, L.L. (1994) Tetanus in the horse: A review of 20 cases (1970–1990). *Journal Veterinary Internal Medicine*, **8** (2), 128–132.

126 MacLeay, J.M. (2004) Diseases of the musculoskeletal system: Suppurative myositis: Abscessation. In: S.M. Reed, W.M. Bayly & D.C. Sellon (eds), *Equine Internal Medicine*, 2nd edn, pp. 514–515. Saunders, St Louis, MO.

127 Rees, C.A. (2004) Disorders of the skin. In: S.M. Reed, W.M. Bayly & D.C. Sellon (eds), *Equine Internal Medicine*, 2nd edn, p. 693. Saunders, St Louis, MO.

128 Adam, E.N. & Southwood, L.L. (2007) Primary and secondary limb cellulitis in horses: 44 cases (2000–2006). *Journal of the American Veterinary Medical Association*, **231**, 1696–1703.

129 Fjordbakk, C.T., Arroyo, L.G. & Hewson, J. (2008) Retrospective study of the clinical features of limb cellulitis in 63 horses. *Veterinary Record*, **162**, 233–236.

130 Eckhoff, A. & Davis, E.G. (2007) Septic cellulitis. *Compendium on Continuing Education for the Practising Veterinarian Equine Edition*, **2** (1), 32–39.

131 Getman, L.M. (2011) Alternative therapies for cellulitis. *Proceedings ACVS Veterinary Symposium, the Surgical Summit*. Chicago, IL, pp. 585–587.

132 Dyson, S.J. (2003) The swollen limb. In: M.R. Ross & S.J. Dyson (eds), *Diagnosis and Management of Lameness in the Horse*, pp. 150–152. Saunders, St Louis, MO.

133 Sellon, D.C. (2004) Disorders of the hematopoietic system: Acquired disorders of hemostasis; Vasculitis. In: S.M. Reed, W.M. Bayly & D.C. Sellon (eds), *Equine Internal Medicine*, pp. 752–755. Saunders, St. Louis, MO.

134 Valberg, S.J. (2006) Immune-mediated myopathies. *Proceedings of the 52nd Annual Convention of the American Association of Equine Practitioners*. San Antonio, TX, pp. 354–358.

135 Rees, C.A. (2004) Disorders of the skin: Vasculitis and purpura hemorrhagica. In: S.M. Reed, W.M. Bayly & D.C. Sellon (eds), *Equine Internal Medicine*, pp. 712–713. Saunders, St. Louis, MO.

136 Orsini, J.A., Snooks-Parsons, C., Stine, L. *et al.* (2005) Vancomycin for the treatment of methicillin-resistant staphylococcal and enterococcal infections in 15 horses. *Canadian Journal of Veterinary Research*, **69** (4), 278–286.

137 Institute for International Cooperation in Animal Biologics. (2011) *Methicillin resistant staphylococcus aureus (MRSA) technical fact sheet*. Iowa State University, College of Veterinary Medicine, Ames, IA. http://www.cfsph.iastate.edu/Factsheets/pdfs/mrsa.pdf [accessed on May 5, 2014].

138 Errico, J.A., Trumble, T.N., Bueno, A.C., Davis, J.L. & Brown, M.P. (2008) Comparison of two indirect techniques for local delivery of a high dose of an antimicrobial in the distal portion of forelimbs of horses. *American Journal of Veterinary Research*, **69** (3), 334–342.

139 Meagher, D.T., Latimer, F.G., Sutter, W.W. & Saville, W.J. (2006) Evaluation of a balloon constant rate infusion system for treatment of septic arthritis, septic tenosynovitis, and contaminated synovial wounds: 23 cases (2002–2005). *Journal of the American Veterinary Medical Association*, **228** (12), 1930–1934.

140 Lescun, T.B., Vasey, J.R., Ward, M.P. & Adams, S.B. (2006) Treatment with continuous intrasynovial antimicrobial infusion for septic synovitis in horses: 31 cases (2000–2003). *Journal of the American Veterinary Medical Association*, **228** (12), 1922–1929.

141 Ivester, K.M., Adams, S.B., Moore, G.E., VanSickle, D.C. & Lescun, T.B. (2006) Gentamicin concentrations in synovial fluid obtained from the tarsocrural joints of horses after implantation of gentamicin-impregnated collagen sponges. *American Journal of Veterinary Research*, **67** (9), 1519–26.

142 Kettner, N.U., Parker, J.E. & Watrous, B.J. (2003) Intraosseous regional perfusion for treatment of septic physitis in a two-week-old foal. *Journal of the American Veterinary Medical Association*, **222** (3), 346–350.

143 Haerdi-Landerer, M.C., Habermacher, J., Wenger, B., Sutter, M.M. & Steiner, A. (2010) Slow release antibiotics for treatment of septic arthritis in large animals. *Veterinary Journal*, **184** (1), 14–20.

144 Carstanjen, B., Boehart, S. & Cislakova, M. (2010) Septic arthritis in adult horses. *Polish Journal of Veterinary Sciences*, **13** (1), 201–12.

145 Morton, A.J. (2005) Diagnosis and treatment of septic arthritis. *Veterinary Clinics of North America: Equine Practice*, **21** (3), 627–649.

146 Gall, Y. & Pfister, K. (2006) Survey on the subject of equine Lyme borreliosis. *International Journal of Medical Microbiology*, **296** (Suppl 40), 274–279.

147 Imai, D.M., Barr, B.C., Daft, B. *et al.* (2011) Lyme neuroborreliosis in two horses. *Veterinary Pathology*, **48**, 1151–1157.

148 James, F.M., Engiles, J.B. & Beech, J. (2010) Meningitis, cranial neuritis, and radiculoneuritis associated with Borrelia burgdorferi infection in a horse. *Journal of the American Veterinary Medical Association*, **237** (10), 1180–1185.

149 Butler, C.M., Houwers, D.J., Jongejan, F. & van der Kolk, J.H. (2005) Borrelia burgdorferi infections with special reference to horses. A review. *Veterinary Quarterly*, **27** (4), 146–156.

150 Cohen, D., Bosler, E.M., Bernard, W., Meirs, D., Eisner, R. & Schulze, T.L. (1988) Epidemiologic studies of Lyme disease in horses and their public health significance. *Annals of the New York Academy of Sciences*, **539**, 244–257.

151 Tara, B., Manion, T.B., Khan, M.I., Dinger, J. & Bushmich, S.L. (1998) Viable Borrelia burgdorferi in the urine of two clinically normal horses. *Journal of Veterinary Diagnostic Investigation*, **10**, 196–199.

152 Dzierzecka, M. & Kita, J. (2002) The use of chosen serological diagnostic methods in Lyme disease in horses. Part II. Western blot. *Polish Journal of Veterinary Sciences*, **5** (2), 79–84.

153 Dzierzecka, M. & Kita, J. (2002) The use of chosen serological diagnostic methods in Lyme disease in horses. Part I. Indirect immunofluorescence and enzyme-linked immunosorbent assay (ELISA). *Polish Journal of Veterinary Sciences*, **5** (2), 71–77.

154 Straubinger, R.K. (2000) PCR-based quantification of Borrelia burgdorferi organisms in canine tissues over a 500-day postinfection period. *Journal Clinical Microbiology*, **38** (6), 2191–2199.

155 Anonymous. (2012) *Multiplex lyme assay for horses.* Animal Health Diagnostic Center, Cornell University, Ithaca, NY. https://ahdc.vet.cornell.edu/docs/Lyme_Disease_Multiplex_Testing_for_Horses.pdf

156 Chang, Y.F., Ku, Y.W., Chang, C.F. *et al.* (2005) Antibiotic treatment of experimentally Borrelia burgdorferi-infected ponies. *Veterinary Microbiology*, **107** (3–4), 285–294.

157 Chang, Y.F., McDonough, S.P., Chang, C.F., Shin, K.S., Yen, W. & Thomas, D.T. (2000) Human granulocytic ehrlichiosis agent infection in a pony vaccinated with a Borrelia burgdorferi recombinant OspA vaccine and challenged by exposure to naturally infected ticks. *Clinical and Diagnostic Laboratory Immunology*, **7** (1), 68–71.

CHAPTER 14

Therapy of the eye

Amber Labelle

Veterinary Teaching Hospital, University of Illinois Urbana-Champaign, Urbana, IL, USA

Ocular anatomy, routes of ocular drug administration, and barriers to drug penetration

Ocular anatomy impacts the delivery of drugs to the ocular surface and intraocular tissues. What is unique about ocular pharmacology is not the specific agents used in therapy, but the unique mechanisms of drug delivery dictated by ocular anatomy and the barriers to drug penetration it presents. Understanding this anatomy will improve the clinician's ability to effectively treat ocular disease.

Eyelids

The eyelids should be considered similar to skin elsewhere on the body. The most unique feature of the eyelids from a drug delivery standpoint is their proximity to the ocular surface. Care must be taken when administering topical medications to the eyelids to ensure that the drug formulation is compatible with the ocular surface or else to carefully avoid contaminating the ocular surface with the formulation.

The vascular nature of the eyelids makes treatment with systemic rather than topical medications ideal. For drugs with high potential for systemic toxicity, local application of an ointment, suspension, or emulsion is an alternative. When using a topical formulation, careful consideration should be given to its compatibility with the ocular surface. For example, many chemotherapeutic agents may be safe for use in the periocular skin but are highly toxic to the corneal epithelium. When using a preparation with known or suspected ocular surface toxicity, it is advisable to avoid the eyelid margin and to exercise great care in the application of the preparation to the periocular skin.

The ocular surface: Cornea, sclera, and conjunctiva

The ocular surface is covered by the precorneal tear film, which in the horse has a volume of approximately 230 µl (compared to ~8–10 µl in man). The normal equine tear flow rate is approximately 30 µl/min, and the tear film is completely replaced every 7 min [1]. The precorneal tear film is drained from the ocular surface via the nasolacrimal duct. It is important to remember that tear flow may be higher in horses with painful ocular disease, and that can significantly influence the pharmacokinetics of drugs applied to the ocular surface.

The cornea consists of five layers: the precorneal tear film, corneal epithelium, collagenous stroma, Descemet's membrane, and corneal endothelium. The juxtaposition of the hydrophobic corneal epithelium and hydrophilic stroma presents a significant barrier to drug penetration. The corneal epithelium is continuous with the conjunctival epithelium, making this hydrophobic barrier continuous over the ocular surface. While the cornea is conventionally considered to lack lymphatics, the conjunctiva and eyelids are rich in lymphatic vessels.

Efficacious drug concentrations can readily be achieved in the highly vascular conjunctiva via systemic or topical administration. The conjunctiva may also act as a drug repository, binding drugs and slowly releasing them into the precorneal tear film. As described in the previous section, the hydrophobic conjunctival epithelium is poorly permeable to hydrophilic preparations. Subconjunctival injections can be used to bypass the conjunctival barrier. Conversely, the conjunctival vasculature is a major site of drug absorption into the systemic circulation, and this absorption can decrease regional drug concentrations, shortening the duration

---

Equine Pharmacology, First Edition. Edited by Cynthia Cole, Bradford Bentz and Lara Maxwell.
© 2015 John Wiley & Sons, Inc. Published 2015 by John Wiley & Sons, Inc.

of effect after topical administration. It is important to remember that any topically administered drug can theoretically have a systemic effect. However, for most compounds, the amount of drug absorbed through the conjunctiva is clinically irrelevant for the average 450 kg horse. Though in smaller patients, such as foals and miniature horses, the effects of systemic absorption may be clinically significant and should be considered when designing treatment regimens.

Treating disease of the cornea is one of the most common ocular challenges for the equine practitioner. Systemic administration of medication is not useful for treating the avascular cornea as this mode of administration does not achieve therapeutic drug concentrations in the precorneal tear film or in the corneal tissue itself. Therefore, topical drug application is most frequently used for treating corneal disease. Topical administration has several advantages: (i) it is relatively easy to accomplish, (ii) it produces high drug concentrations on the corneal surface, and (iii) the total amount of drug administered can easily be altered by varying the dose and/or frequency of administration.

Unfortunately, properties of the precorneal tear film can also limit the effectiveness of topically applied medications. Peak drug concentrations occur immediately after a drug is administered to the ocular surface, followed by a rapid decline as the drug is diluted in the precorneal tear film. Drug concentrations further decline as the precorneal tear film is cleared from the ocular surface via the nasolacrimal drainage system. Because the amount of drug that penetrates the cornea (and anterior chamber) is directly correlated to the amount of drug in the precorneal tear film, most of the absorption of topically administered drugs occurs in the first 10–20 min after administration. The rate of elimination of a drug from the precorneal tear film may be increased in painful, inflamed eyes due to increased lacrimation and thus increased drug dilution. The precorneal tear film also contains enzymes that may contribute to the degradation or metabolism of drugs, further decreasing drug concentrations and therefore the amount of drug absorbed.

Penetration of a given drug into and through the cornea is limited by the size and polarity of the drug molecule. The ideal drug would be one of relatively small molecular size that could change its polarity from lipophilic (to facilitate passage through the epithelium/endothelium) to hydrophilic (to facilitate passage through the stroma). Lack of significant corneal penetration does not imply a drug is not useful for treating corneal disease, only that it is more suited for treating superficial disease. To be effective in the treatment of deep corneal diseases, such as infectious keratitis and stromal abscesses, adequate corneal penetration is essential.

Multiple approaches can be used to improve drug penetration of the cornea. Firstly, altering the formulation of the drug can increase its penetration. For example, some drugs are formulated as inactive lipophilic compounds, which facilitate their penetration through the corneal epithelium. Once in the anterior chamber, they are metabolized to the active drug form. Secondly, utilizing an ointment rather than a solution or including a gel-forming polymer in the formulation can increase contact time between the cornea and drug, thereby increasing the time available for absorption. Some commercially available antiglaucoma medications, such as timolol hydrochloride, utilize this gel-forming technology to increase corneal contact time. Such gel-forming polymers are currently not widely available but may become more common in the future. Thirdly, increasing the frequency of administration or administering a higher concentration of the drug will increase the precorneal tear film concentration and thus the corneal concentration. Fourthly, removing the epithelial barrier by physical debridement will decrease the barrier to corneal penetration for all drugs. Finally, adding preservatives to drug formulations can improve their corneal penetration. Many preservatives, such as benzalkonium chloride, also act to increase the size of the spaces between epithelial cells in order to improve the passage of a drug through the epithelial barrier.

Subconjunctival administration of medication is another avenue for reaching the cornea, and it can be used as an alternative or in combination with topical administration. This route of administration is more invasive than topical, cannot be performed frequently, and cannot be performed by an owner, all of which limit its clinical utility for most diseases. A notable exception is the use of repository drug formulations, such as triamcinolone acetate, that slowly release the drug over time.

Anterior segment: Anterior/posterior chamber, iris, ciliary body, and lens

The anterior segment consists of all the structures posterior to the cornea back to and including the lens. The anterior chamber is the fluid-filled space between the cornea and iris, while the posterior chamber is the small fluid-filled space between the posterior iris face and the anterior surface of the lens. The posterior chamber is easily confused with the vitreous, which is the large space posterior to the lens that is filled with the vitreous humor. The uveal tract includes the iris, ciliary body, and choroid. The iris and ciliary body comprise the anterior uvea, while the choroid is considered the posterior uvea.

The uveal tract is vascular tunic of the eye and is the anatomic location of the blood–aqueous barrier (BAB). The BAB is similar to the blood–brain barrier in that it acts as an obstacle to intraocular drug penetration. In the iris, melanocytes may act as a repository for drugs, such as clenbuterol and atropine, that possess a high affinity for melanin. The anterior uveal tract is bathed in aqueous humor, a low-protein fluid with a density similar to that of water and with a relatively high turnover rate. Drugs in the aqueous humor, whether they are injected intracamerally (into the anterior chamber) or diffuse through the cornea, are removed relatively rapidly. The lens is surrounded by both the aqueous and vitreous humors and has no direct access to the uveal vasculature.

Treatment of the anterior segment can be accomplished via a number of routes of administration, including systemic, topical, subconjunctival, episcleral/suprachoroidal, and intracameral. Each route of administration has advantages and disadvantages and must overcome its own barriers to intraocular penetration. For example, the major barrier to intraocular drug penetration of systemically administered drugs is the BAB, and only a limited number of medications can penetrate it. However, many intraocular diseases, particularly inflammatory conditions, compromise the BAB, resulting in an increase in its permeability that allows systemically administered medications to reach clinically significant concentrations in the anterior segment. Topical administration is frequently utilized to treat intraocular diseases, but the cornea, conjunctiva, and sclera represent major barriers to drug absorption (see Section "Ocular Surface"). Subconjunctival administration bypasses the corneal/conjunctival barrier, but as previously discussed, its clinical utility is somewhat limited. Episcleral or suprachoroidal injections or implantation of devices effectively accesses intraocular structures, but both require specialized equipment and expertise to perform safely. The most common suprachoroidal drug administration is surgical implantation

of a cyclosporine A implant device for treatment of equine recurrent uveitis (ERU). Because of the rapid turnover of aqueous humor, intracameral injections into the anterior chamber are only useful for administration of medications that do not require extended residence times. For example, tissue plasminogen activator (TPA), a potent fibrinolytic, can be injected intracamerally because it has an extremely rapid mechanism of action that requires only minutes to produce substantial efficacy. Intracameral injection, however, requires expertise and is not suitable for repeated use or for an owner to perform. Although the lens is bathed in aqueous humor and touches the anterior vitreous face, achieving therapeutic concentrations in these ocular fluids does not necessarily imply that similar intralenticular concentrations have been attained.

In summary, selection of a route of drug administration for the treatment of diseases of the anterior segment is dictated by the disease process as well as patient and owner factors (including willingness/ability of the owner to carry out the prescribed treatment). To accomplish the treatment goal, multiple routes of administration are frequently used.

Posterior segment: Vitreous humor, retina, optic nerve, and choroid

The posterior segment of the eye consists of the vitreous humor, retina, optic nerve, and choroid. The choroid is part of the uveal tract and is also termed the posterior uvea.

Routes of administration of drugs for treatment of diseases of the vitreous, retina, and optic nerve are limited compared to those used to treat the anterior segment of the eye. For example, the majority of topically administered drugs will not penetrate to the vitreous/retina sufficiently to achieve therapeutic concentrations. Although newer-generation pharmaceuticals, such as some nonsteroidal anti-inflammatory drugs (NSAIDs), may allow this depth of penetration, it should generally be assumed that topical drug administration is not effective for vitreoretinal disease unless the specific drug formulation indicates otherwise. Intravitreal or systemic administration is required for therapy of these posterior ocular structures. The retina is also protected by the blood–retinal barrier (BRB) that limits the penetration of systemically administered medications to this delicate intraocular tissue.

Orbit

The orbit is comprised of highly vascular muscle, fat, connective tissue, and bone. Its major function is to protect the globe and control ocular movement. The vascular nature of the orbit makes systemic administration the ideal route of administration for treatment of ocular disease. Topically administered medications do not sufficiently penetrate through the ocular surface barriers (such as the conjunctiva) to achieve therapeutic concentrations in the orbit. The orbit may be a site of direct injection, especially local anesthetics for the purposes of surgical anesthesia or postoperative analgesia. Great care must be taken when performing a retrobulbar (behind the globe) injection into the orbit to avoid inadvertent penetration of the globe.

Ophthalmic drug formulation

Ophthalmic drug formulations are specifically designed for the unique ocular microenvironment. For example, all FDA-approved ophthalmic formulations are sterile at the time of production. In addition, ophthalmic solutions are formulated so their pH and osmolarity are similar to that of precorneal tear film, that is, pH=7.4 and osmolarity=290 mOsm. Solutions with a pH or osmolarity different from that of tears can be irritating and induce lacrimation, which as previously discussed dilutes the drug concentration in the tear film. Equine patients may quickly become intolerant of medications delivered to the ocular surface that are irritating. One of the problems with using compounded ocular medications is that their sterility, pH, and osmolarity are unknown. Therefore, the use of compounded medications should be limited to situations where FDA-approved products are not available.

Many ophthalmic pharmaceuticals also contain preservatives to minimize growth of any microbial contaminants. These preservatives can be irritating to the corneal epithelium and may be associated with transient or persistent hypersensitivity, particularly with repeated use. While preservative-free formulas are available, they are often more expensive, have a considerably shorter shelf life, and possess an increased risk of contamination once opened.

Ophthalmic ointment formulations are more commonly used in the horse than solutions because they are easier to instill into the eye. Interestingly, they are used less frequently in human medicine because they cause significant blurring of vision by distorting the precorneal tear film. Ophthalmic ointments have several advantages over solutions. For example, ointments have a longer contact time, thus improving the ophthalmic bioavailability of a given drug. Ointments melt after they are instilled onto the ocular surface, and their viscous nature and petroleum base decrease their rate of drainage into the nasolacrimal duct and therefore their systemic absorption. Ointments may also feel more soothing to the patient and therefore be better tolerated. It is important to remember, however, that the petroleum ointment base induces significant granulomatous inflammation if it enters the anterior chamber; thus, the use of ointments should be avoided in any eye at risk of corneal rupture.

Methods of ocular drug delivery

The majority of drugs delivered to the eye are instilled topically onto the ocular surface in ointment or solution form. Ophthalmic ointments should be instilled in 1/4–1/2″ strips directly to the ocular surface. Alternately, the ointment can be applied to a clean or gloved finger and applied gently to the everted palpebral conjunctival surface of the lower eyelid. Solutions are more challenging to apply, as the equine ocular surface is parallel to the natural gravity-following trajectory of a drop of solution released from a bottle. While application of ocular solutions is possible in a compliant patient, placement of a subpalpebral lavage (SPL) system greatly facilitates administration of solutions. SPLs are useful when the horse is difficult to treat, the desired medication is a solution, the treatment will be long term, the lids and/or cornea is very fragile, and the frequency of treatment is high. It is important to ensure the SPL is correctly placed or inadvertent corneal trauma may occur. Commercially available kits include all the necessary equipment for placement of an SPL (Mila International, Erlanger, KY, USA).

For placement of an SPL, the horse should first be heavily sedated and well restrained, with most horses benefiting from placement of a twitch prior to SPL insertion. Auriculopalpebral and frontal nerve blocks should be performed, and then 1–2 ml of 2% lidocaine should be infiltrated subcutaneously where the SPL needle will exit the skin. The skin and ocular surface should be prepared with povidone–iodine solution, and then a topical anesthetic should be applied to the ocular surface. Once the horse is prepared, the dorsal conjunctival fornix should be palpated with a clean or gloved finger. The trochar should be guarded using a fingertip and then passed into the conjunctival fornix and through the eyelid. Every attempt should be made to pass the trochar as close to the dorsal orbital rim as possible. This ensures that the footplate of the SPL will be seated in the dorsal-most recess of the conjunctival fornix, which minimizes the potential for inadvertent movement of the footplate and thus corneal trauma. The SPL is then pulled completely through the lid until the footplate is seated in the conjunctival fornix. The tip of a finger is used to palpate and confirm correct positioning of the footplate. Alternatively, the SPL may also be placed in the inferior conjunctival fornix, which has also been associated with good treatment success [2]. The SPL should be secured to the horse's head using medical tape adhered to the tubing and sutured to the horse or other fixation system. A protective mask with a hard plastic cup is recommended to decrease trauma to the SPL at its insertion site (Eye Saver Mask, Jorgensen Labs, Loveland, CO, USA).

Although no peer-reviewed studies have compared the efficacy of various regimens for the administration of medications through an SPL, several guidelines are commonly accepted in practice. Firstly, given that the volume of the equine precorneal tear film is approximately 230 µl, administration of medication volumes greater than this will result in loss of medication through the nasolacrimal duct or onto the face as the precorneal tear film overflows the palpebral fissure. Therefore, recommended solution volumes are 0.1–0.2 ml. Secondly, after the volume of medication is injected into the SPL, 1.0 ml of air should be slowly injected behind it to push the solution through the length of the SPL tubing. Finally, a minimum interval of 5 min between each drug administration allows for absorption of each drug prior to administration of the next. This technique of administering each medication individually eliminates any potential for drug interactions that may decrease the local absorption or potency of the drugs.

Although topical is the most common route of administration of ocular drugs, other routes are also used. For example, subconjunctival injection of solutions is one method of bypassing the conjunctival barrier to intraocular drug penetration. Typically performed using a 27–25 g needle in a sedated and restrained patient after the application of topical anesthesia, the needle tip is carefully advanced under the conjunctiva, and the desired solution is injected. The injected volume should not exceed 1 ml, and great care should be taken to avoid inadvertent penetration of the sclera. It should be expected that some drug will leak out of the needle track and be absorbed as if it had been administered topically. Following a subconjunctival injection, aqueous solutions are generally completely absorbed within 8–12 h. Subconjunctival injections of ophthalmic solutions do not replace the need for topical therapy, particularly in cases of bacterial or fungal keratitis, but should be viewed as an adjunctive approach to increase intraocular drug concentrations.

Injection of a solution directly into the anterior chamber, referred to as intracameral administration, is indicated when it is not possible to achieve intraocular therapeutic concentrations by any other route of administration. For example, TPA can only be administered by intracameral injection. It can be performed using a 25–30 g needle inserted at the limbus into the anterior chamber in a sedated, restrained patient after the administration of topical anesthesia. The advantage of intracameral injection is the direct delivery of drug to the target tissue and the ability to rapidly obtain therapeutic concentrations. Nevertheless, transient intraocular inflammation (uveitis) can be expected as a result of an intracameral injection, and it also carries the risk of iris and/or lens laceration, intraocular hemorrhage, and septic endophthalmitis. The risk of septic endophthalmitis can be reduced by preparation of the ocular surface using a dilute povidone–iodine solution (see Section "Antiseptics"). The potential benefit of any drug injected into the anterior chamber must be weighed against the risk of intraocular toxicity. Toxicity to the corneal endothelium and lens is of particular concern. For example, TPA, a potent fibrinolytic that is useful in dissolving fibrin associated with intraocular inflammation, is toxic to the corneal endothelium at high doses.

Injection of drugs directly into the vitreous humor, referred to as intravitreal injection, can achieve high drug concentrations in that fluid. The primary indication for this route of administration is for treatment of diseases of the posterior segment, such as endophthalmitis or retinal disease, although repositol injections of corticosteroids are occasionally used for the treatment of chronic ERU. Intravitreal injection is performed using a 25–27 g needle inserted 10 mm posterior to the dorso-lateral limbus in a sedated, restrained patient after the administration of topical anesthesia. Fluid turnover in the vitreous is much slower than the aqueous, and therefore, therapeutic concentrations can be sustained for hours to weeks following an intravitreal injection, depending on the drug and its formulation. Intravitreal injection does carry the risks of inadvertent lens lacera-tion with subsequent phacoclastic uveitis, subretinal hemorrhage, retinal detachment, and septic endo-phthalmitis. The risk of septic endophthalmitis can be reduced by preparation of the ocular surface using a dilute povidone–iodine solution (see Section "Antiseptics").

Systemic administration of drugs can be very effective when the desired ocular target is a vascular structure. For example, the eyelids, conjunctiva, and orbit are an ideal target tissue for systemically administered medications because they are highly vascular. However, therapeutic concentrations of systemically administered medications are not achieved in avascular structures such as the pre-corneal tear film, cornea, and lens. Therapeutic drug concentrations may be achieved in the uveal tract and retina, following systemic administration, particularly if the integrity of the BAB or BRB has been compromised, which increases the intraocular penetration of most drugs.

Slow-release devices are a relatively novel drug delivery method. For example, bioerodible disks con-taining cyclosporine A surgically implanted in the suprachoroidal space have become the most successful reported treatment for ERU. Intravitreally implanted devices, however, have been less successful. Drug delivery devices are an area of intense research and development in human ophthalmology and more may eventually become available for veterinary applications.

Drug therapy for examination and diagnostic testing

Chemical restraint greatly facilitates examination of the painful equine eye. Alpha-2 agonists are the class of drug used most frequently for ocular examinations. These inexpensive agents, which include xylazine and detomidine, have a fairly short duration of action, a wide margin of safety, and minimal effects on ocular tissues that may adversely affect ocular examination parameters. A notable exception is assessment of aqueous tear production; in other species, alpha-2 ago-nists significantly decrease reflex tear production as accessed via the Schirmer tear test (STT). While xylazine has been reported to have no effect on equine STT values, there are no reports of the effects of romifidine or detomidine [3]. Therefore, ideally, STT should be per-formed prior to the administration of any alpha-2 agonist to minimize the possibility of confounding the results of the test. Xylazine has also been shown to cause a statistically significant decrease in intraocular pressure (IOP), although no studies have evaluated the effects of other alpha-2 agonists on IOP [4, 5]. This find-ing does not suggest that alpha-2 agonists should not be used to facilitate tonometry (the measurement of IOP) only that the practitioner should be consistent in the measurement technique, including using the same sedative at the same dose, in order to decrease vari-ability between measurements.

Opioids are generally not used for ophthalmic examination as they may be associated with increased spontaneous head movement in some horses. Please refer to Chapter 5, Anesthesia and Sedation in the Field, for more information on sedatives and their mecha-nisms of action.

Topical anesthetics

Topical anesthetics are useful to facilitate examination of a painful eye, tonometry, ocular ultrasound, obtain-ing diagnostic samples, and performing surgery on the ocular surface. Topical anesthetics approved for use in the eye are proparacaine hydrochloride 0.5% solution, tetracaine hydrochloride 0.5% solution, and tetracaine hydrochloride 1% solution. All three formulations are safe and effective for use in the horse. The duration of effect of a single drop of proparacaine is approximately 25 min, with the maximum anesthetic effect occurring 5 min postadministration [6]. A single drop of tetracaine has a somewhat longer duration of effect, but the maximum anesthetic effect also occurs 5 min postad-ministration [7]. Using two different local anesthetics increases the time to maximum anesthetic effect for both drugs. In humans, proparacaine is associated with less ocular discomfort on administration than tetracaine [8]. No such comparison has been made in the horse, however, and investigators noted no adverse ocular effects or signs of ocular discomfort with the use of 0.5 and 1% tetracaine [9]. Both proparacaine and tetra-caine appear suitable for use in the horse.

Mydriatics/cycloplegics

Mydriasis refers to dilation of the pupil, while cycloplegia is paralysis of the ciliary body. Equine practitioners must keep in mind that most cycloplegic drugs are also mydriatics, but not all mydriatics have cycloplegic properties. It is important to know which drugs have mydriatic or cycloplegic properties to allow for the selection of the appropriate drug. A drug that has only mydriatic properties is most appropriate to facilitate an ocular examination but would be inappropriate for the treatment of uveitis, where relief of ciliary body muscle spasm via cycloplegia provides analgesia to the patient.

Tropicamide 1% solution is the most common short-acting mydriatic used to facilitate diagnostic procedures. It is a parasympatholytic agent that blocks muscarinic acetylcholine receptors on the ciliary body and iris constrictor muscle, allowing the iris dilator muscle to act unopposed. It has short-acting mydriatic and cycloplegic effects, so its use is inappropriate where long-term cycloplegia is required, as in the treatment of uveitis. Maximal dilation occurs 30–60 min after administration and lasts for approximately 12 h. Rare individuals may remain dilated for up to 24 h after administration.

Phenylephrine 10% solution, a sympathomimetic agent that stimulates alpha-1 adrenoreceptors, has been shown to be ineffective as a mydriatic in horses when used as a sole agent. Phenylephrine is a potent vasoconstrictor, and when corneal vascularization is present, it can minimize conjunctival or corneal hemorrhage during diagnostic procedures, such as biopsy or obtaining samples for cytology. It also reduces chemosis (edema of the conjunctiva) to facilitate visualization of the ocular surface. Phenylephrine hydrochloride 2.5% solution is the formulation most commonly used to produce these effects.

Atropine sulfate 1% solution or ointment is a long-acting mydriatic/cycloplegic. It is a parasympatholytic agent that blocks muscarinic acetylcholine receptors in the iris and ciliary body. A single dose of atropine administered to a normal horse may induce mydriasis for more than 14 days. For this reason, use of atropine in diagnostic examinations is not recommended; tropicamide is more appropriate due to its shorter duration of action. Atropine is most commonly used to produce mydriasis and cycloplegia in the treatment of uveitis and keratitis. Although topical administration of atropine to the eye has experimentally been associated with decreased gastrointestinal motility in horses, clinical experience does not support this finding [10]. Horses treated with atropine should be monitored to detect early signs of colic; however, atropine is not contraindicated for use in horses and is a useful drug in the management of keratitis and uveitis.

Antiseptics

Povidone–iodine, an iodophor solution, is the most commonly used antiseptic for disinfection of periocular tissues and the ocular surface. The commercially available form of povidone–iodine is free aqueous iodine bound to a carrier molecule (polyvinylpyrrolidone). The role of the carrier molecule is to facilitate transfer of the free iodine to the target cell wall. A broad range of concentrations from 0.005 to 10% are reported to have antimicrobial activity. Somewhat counterintuitively, lower concentrations of povidone–iodine have been shown to have more rapid antimicrobial effects. Concentrations of 1–5% are recommended for preparation of periocular tissues, while 0.05–0.5% solutions are recommended for preparation of the ocular surface. All detergent-containing antiseptics, including povidone–iodine scrub, should be avoided for ocular and periocular use as severe ocular surface toxicity, including corneal ulceration, corneal edema, and chemosis, may result from their use [11].

Drug therapy for keratitis

Simple ulcerative keratitis

Selection of the appropriate drug therapy for a horse with a corneal ulcer is based primarily on the type of corneal ulcer present. Corneal ulcers can be divided into two major categories: simple and complicated. Simple ulcers are those in which (i) there has only been loss of epithelium with no loss of the underlying stroma, (ii) there is no evidence of infection (including cellular infiltrate in the stroma or keratomalacia, which is necrosis of cornea), and (iii) there are no underlying factors that may complicate ulcer healing, such as facial nerve paresis or an eyelid laceration or infection. Simple ulcers can be expected to heal by epithelialization within 5–10 days, depending on the size of the ulcer. Drug therapy for a simple ulcer consists of three components: preventing infection, controlling secondary uveitis, and providing analgesia to the patient.

Preventing infection

The avascular, warm, and moist cornea is an ideal environment for the growth of microorganisms. When the epithelial barrier has been breached, opportunistic pathogens including the normal ocular bacterial flora may colonize and invade the corneal surface. Normal equine ocular floras are primarily Gram-positive bacteria, with fewer Gram-negative bacteria and rare fungal organisms. Therefore, to prevent bacterial infections in simple ulcers, use of an antimicrobial with activity against both Gram-positive and Gram-negative organisms is recommended. Since simple ulcers do not involve the underlying stroma, the ability of the antimicrobial to penetrate into the deeper stromal layers is not an important selection factor. An antimicrobial ointment is generally selected as a first-line formulation in the treatment of a simple ulcer, as this is the easiest preparation for a handler to safely and effectively instill into the eye. Unfortunately, the commercial availability of antimicrobial ophthalmic ointments is quite limited, so it essential that the practitioner understand the advantages and limitations of the available formulations (Table 14.1).

Triple-antibiotic preparations (neomycin–polymyxin–bacitracin available as an ointment and neomycin–polymyxin–gramicidin available as a solution) are ideal antibiotic combinations for the prevention of infection in simple ulcers. Their broad spectrums of activity make them well suited for use in superficial corneal ulcerations. Although they do not penetrate into the cornea, as previously discussed, this is not a concern with simple ulcerations. Another antimicrobial choice is the commercially available ophthalmic preparation of oxytetracycline–polymyxin B (Terramycin, Pfizer Animal Health). The disadvantages of this combination are that the tetracyclines are bacteriostatic, not bactericidal, and the spectrum of activity of polymyxin B is primarily Gram-negative. Aminoglycoside ophthalmic formulations, such as gentamicin and tobramycin, are bactericidal but have a similar narrow spectrum of activity of primarily Gram-negative organisms and *Staphylococcus* spp. Aminoglycosides are best reserved for use when the results of culture and sensitivity testing indicate the presence of susceptible organisms. Chloramphenicol, which is highly lipophilic and thereby has excellent corneal penetration, is available in ophthalmic preparations, but it is only bacteriostatic and it has minimal activity against Gram-negative *Pseudomonas* organisms, which are highly pathogenic. Finally, the fluoroquinolone ciprofloxacin ophthalmic ointment is bactericidal with a broad spectrum of activity and excellent stromal penetration. Ciprofloxacin, however, is not recommended for use in cases of simple ulcerative keratitis because of growing concerns regarding the development of antimicrobial resistance. It should be reserved for cases of complicated ulcerative keratitis.

Given the limited availability of ophthalmic ointment preparations, triple-antibiotic formulations remain the only preparations that combine bactericidal effects with broad spectrums of activity. In addition, the availability of a triple-antibiotic solution allows its use through an SPL system where necessary. Regardless of the drug formulation (ointment or solution) or method of administration (direct instillation or SPL), treatment should be administered q6–8 h until uptake of fluorescein stain by the cornea is no longer observed and the patient is comfortable with no blepharospasm.

Controlling secondary uveitis and pain

The epithelium and superficial stroma of the cornea are densely innervated by the ophthalmic branch of cranial nerve V (trigeminal nerve), and as a result, simple corneal ulcers are extremely painful. To decrease pain and

Table 14.1 Commercially available ointment preparations.

Drug	Bactericidal/ bacteriostatic	Spectrum
Triple antibiotic (neomycin–polymyxin–bacitracin)	Bactericidal	G+ and G−
Erythromycin 0.5%	Bacteriostatic (bactericidal at high concentrations)	Primarily G+
Gentamicin 0.3%	Bactericidal	Primarily G−
Tobramycin 0.3%	Bactericidal	Primarily G−
Chloramphenicol 1%	Bacteriostatic	G+ and G− but *Pseudomonas spp.* usually resistant
Oxytetracycline–polymyxin B	Bacteriostatic/ bactericidal	G−, less G+
Ciprofloxacin 0.3%	Bactericidal	G+ and G−

inflammation, NSAIDs should be administered, either parenterally or orally (PO), until reepithelialization occurs. Flunixin meglumine has long been clinically held as the most effective NSAID for the treatment of intra-ocular inflammation, although peer-reviewed studies documenting its superiority are lacking. Initial doses of 1 mg/kg q12 h are recommended, decreasing to 0.5 mg/kg q12–24 h as the patient shows clinical improvement as evidenced by decreased blepharospasm and ocular discharge. Topical NSAIDs are generally not recommended for patients with simple corneal ulcers as administration of these drugs is associated with temporary, but significant, ocular pain and very rarely keratomalacia.

Ulcerative keratitis also stimulates branches of the trigeminal nerve that innervate the anterior uveal tract (including the iris and ciliary body), creating reflex uveitis; the more severe the keratitis, the more severe the uveitis. Stimulation of the trigeminal nerve causes secondary spasm of the ciliary body musculature and is a significant source of ocular pain in patients with ulcerative keratitis. Therefore, all patients with ulcerative keratitis should be treated for reflex uveitis.

Administration of topical atropine 1% ointment is useful for the relief of spasm of the ciliary body associated with reflex uveitis. Atropine also causes mydriasis, which can decrease the formation of posterior synechiae (adhesions between the iris and anterior lens capsule that deform the pupil and decrease its normal range of motion). In most patients with a simple corneal ulcer, a single administration of atropine is likely to be sufficient to cause cycloplegia and mydriasis. However, some patients, particularly those with wide corneal lesions, may require atropine administration q24 h until reepithelialization occurs in order to provide the adequate analgesia.

Complicated keratitis
Bacterial keratitis
Bacterial keratitis, which is very common in the horse, appears clinically as white to yellow to tan infiltrates in the stroma that may be associated with keratomalacia or loss of stroma (deep ulcer). The results of the clinical examination as well as cytology and culture and sensitivity testing are the keys to establishing an appropriate and rational treatment plan. Cytology can be utilized to direct initial treatment, but culture results are essential to confirm the diagnosis and refine the therapeutic plan. If no organisms are observed on cytology, broad-spectrum antimicrobial therapy should

still be instituted until culture/sensitivity results are received. However, as false-negative results from cytology and culture and sensitivity testing occur regularly with bacterial keratitis, if bacterial keratitis is strongly suspected, broad-spectrum antimicrobial therapy is indicated, even if cytology or culture and sensitivity testing does not confirm the diagnosis. Results of a complete ophthalmic examination (including the presence of infiltrate in the stroma) are as important to establishing a diagnosis of infectious keratitis as diagnostic testing (such as cytology).

Treatment of bacterial keratitis is often complex and prolonged. It is important to remember that when treating a bacterial infection in the corneal stroma, an antibiotic with good corneal penetration is required (Table 14.1). Triple-antibiotic combinations, while broad spectrum, have limited corneal penetration and are generally not the ideal choice for treating bacterial keratitis that involves the deeper stroma. A fluoroquinolone antibiotic, such as ciprofloxacin or ofloxacin that has superior corneal penetration, will be significantly more efficacious.

Although administration of antimicrobial ointments is an option, the use of an SPL to facilitate administration of ocular medications is recommended for most cases of bacterial keratitis because it will significantly extend the antimicrobial treatment options (Table 14.2). Commercially available and compounded preparations are routinely used in SPL systems. The compounded solutions listed in Table 14.2 can be prepared by diluting the intravenous (IV) preparations in sterile saline, water, or

Table 14.2 Ophthalmic antibacterial solutions.

Drug	Bactericidal/ bacteriostatic	Spectrum
Triple antibiotic (neomycin–polymyxin–gramicidin)	Bactericidal	G+ and G−
Gentamicin 0.3%	Bactericidal	Primarily G−
Tobramycin 0.3%	Bactericidal	Primarily G−
Ciprofloxacin 0.3%	Bactericidal	G+ and G−
Ofloxacin 0.3%	Bactericidal	G+ and G−
Moxifloxacin 0.5%	Bactericidal	G+ and G−
Compounded ophthalmic solutions		
Cefazolin 3.3–5.5%	Bactericidal	Primarily G+
Amikacin 1%	Bactericidal	Primarily G−

artificial tears. While the osmolarity and pH of these solutions are unknown, clinical experience has shown this approach to produce solutions that are generally effective and well tolerated. It should be kept in mind that the administration of two antimicrobial ophthalmic solutions may be necessary to provide the appropriate broad-spectrum activity required when treating bacterial keratitis.

Frequency of therapy depends on the severity of the disease. A maximum dosing interval of q6 h is recommended, and in severe cases, treatment as frequently as q2 h may be required. Treatment must continue until reepithelialization is complete.

Fungal keratitis

The clinical appearance of fungal keratitis is more variable than that of bacterial keratitis. Lesions range from superficial, white-gray, and lacy to reticulated subepithelial lesions associated with multifocal erosions of epithelium to large areas of stromal infiltrate associated with stromal loss and keratomalacia. Discoloration or brunescence of the stroma may also occasionally be observed. Cytology is more likely to recover organisms when the lesion is superficial, and serial sampling may be necessary to obtain the diagnosis. If a positive fungal culture is obtained, antifungal sensitivity testing can be performed. Although it does not have the same widely accepted standards as similar antimicrobial testing and thus the results may vary by laboratory, it can provide useful information to aid in the selection of an antifungal agent. Confirmation of the presence of a fungal infection can also be achieved using polymerase chain reaction (PCR) technology for the 16S ribosomal subunit of the fungal organism. PCR, however, does not allow for antifungal sensitivity testing. Selection of appropriate topical medication is further complicated by the geographic variability in sensitivity of fungal pathogens to antifungal agents. Therefore, knowledge of regional drug sensitivities is essential for appropriate antifungal selection. For this reason, a review of the current literature and consultation with local or regional ophthalmologists can be very helpful in establishing rational, regionally appropriate therapy (Table 14.3).

The only FDA-approved, commercially available antifungal ophthalmic preparation is natamycin (Natacyn, Alcon Laboratories, Inc.). All other preparations must be compounded. Commonly utilized solutions are easily

Table 14.3 Ophthalmic antifungal solutions.

Drug	Notes
Polyenes	
Natamycin 5%	Limited epithelial penetration
Triazoles	
Fluconazole 0.2%	Least potent of the triazoles
Itraconazole 1% in 30% DMSO	Can be compounded as an ointment
Voriconazole 1%	Most potent of the triazoles
Imidazoles	
Ketoconazole 1%	Low potency, rarely used
Miconazole 1%	Can be compounded as an ointment
Other	
Silver sulfadiazine 1%	Can be compounded as an ointment

prepared in the clinical setting from commercially available IV preparations. Solutions are considerably less challenging to compound than ointments, and the prolonged duration of treatment for fungal keratitis makes administration of a solution via SPL highly desirable. If an antifungal ointment is required, it should be formulated at reputable compounding pharmacy with experience in ophthalmic preparations.

The dosing interval for antifungal agents should initially be q6 h, and then after the first 24–36 h, it should be decreased to q2–4 h. This dosing regime is designed to initially induce a "slow" death of fungal organisms in order to avoid a sudden influx of inflammatory cells that may lead to catastrophic keratomalacia, followed by increasing concentrations of antifungal agents to promote complete elimination of the fungal pathogen. The duration of treatment is often prolonged, particularly in the case of deep stromal involvement. Surgical intervention is often required, but frequently, it does not alleviate the need for topical antifungal therapy. Treatment should continue until reepithelialization occurs and all cellular infiltrate resolves and for a minimum of 4 weeks total after initial diagnosis in order to minimize recurrence.

Keratomalacia

Keratomalacia results from the enzymatic activity of collagenases and proteases on the collagen fibers of the corneal stroma. Inhibition of collagenase and protease

Table 14.4 Agents for inhibition of collagenases/proteases.

Drug	Formulation	Dose
EDTA 0.2%	Solution	
Autologous serum	Solution	
Doxycycline	Tablet	20 mg/kg PO q24h, 10 mg/kg PO BID
Oxytetracycline–polymyxin B	Ointment	
N-acetylcysteine 5–10%	Solution	
Ilomastat 0.1%	Solution	

activity is an essential component of treating bacterial and fungal ulcerative keratitis in horses. Even when overt keratomalacia is not present, prophylactic therapy is indicated when treating these diseases.

Although there are a number of agents available to treat or prevent keratomalacia (Table 14.4), of the available anticollagenase/antiprotease agents, autologous serum has the broadest activity against the numerous destructive enzymes. In addition, autologous serum is readily obtained, inexpensive, and easy to administer. Anticollagenase/antiprotease agents should be administered frequently in cases of active keratomalacia and hourly in severe cases and can be tapered as the clinical picture improves. Combination therapy with other agents listed in Table 14.4 is also indicated in severely affected cases for maximum enzymatic inhibition.

Stromal abscess

Stromal abscesses appear clinically as focal areas of yellow/white infiltrate in the stroma that are associated with significant ocular pain and secondary uveitis. The presence of corneal vascularization is variable depending on the duration of the lesion. Ulceration of the overlying epithelium is likewise variable. When the epithelium is intact or when the abscess is located in the posterior 50% of the cornea, obtaining an etiologic diagnosis in most cases of stromal abscess is challenging. Empiric therapy, including antibiotic and antifungal therapy, is recommended due to increasing reports in the peer-reviewed literature identifying fungal organisms as major pathogens in this disease syndrome [12, 13].

Because the overlying epithelium is intact in many stromal abscess cases, the selection of antimicrobial and antifungal agents with adequate penetration is key to successful treatment. In addition, repeated debridement of the corneal epithelium may help to improve drug penetration. Even with surgical intervention, prolonged therapy is generally required in most cases, and therefore, use of an SPL and ophthalmic solutions is highly recommended.

Drug therapy for noninfectious keratitis

Immune-mediated keratitis

Immune-mediated keratitis (IMMK) is a syndrome of keratopathies with diverse clinical appearances [14]. Superficial, midstromal, and endothelial forms have been described, and empiric treatments have been proposed varying with the clinical appearance of the lesion. In general, the deeper the lesion, the more difficult it is to treat. Empiric therapies have included topical corticosteroids (prednisolone acetate, dexamethasone), topical calcineurin inhibitors (cyclosporine A, tacrolimus), potent topical NSAIDs (bromfenac), systemic steroids, systemic calcineurin inhibitors, and systemic tetracyclines [14, 15]. Objective comparisons between therapies are challenging because some cases may spontaneously resolve. Referral to a veterinary ophthalmologist is prudent in cases of IMMK.

Eosinophilic keratitis

Eosinophilic keratitis is an unusual keratopathy that appears clinically as white, chalky plaques associated with dense corneal vascularization in the perilimbal cornea [16]. An immune-mediated component is strongly suspected but not yet proven. A seasonal prevalence is noted, and horses that live in pasture are overrepresented in the afflicted population. Concurrent ulceration or secondary infection may also be noted. Cytology is diagnostic in most cases and reveals sheets of eosinophils with variable numbers of other inflammatory cells. Therapeutic options include topical corticosteroids, topical NSAIDs, topical immunomodulatory agents like cyclosporine A or tacrolimus, systemic corticosteroids, topical mast cell stabilizers such as lodoxamide tromethamine, and systemic antihistamines. Treatment often needs to be prolonged as resolution of the lesion is slow to occur. Topical corticosteroids are contraindicated when a secondary infection or ulceration is present. Referral to or consultation with a veterinary ophthalmologist may be indicated as these cases are often challenging to manage.

Drug therapy for uveitis

Acute uveitis

The goals of treating acute uveitis are to limit the side effects of inflammation until it can be completely eliminated and to reestablish the BAB. A combination of topical and systemic therapy is indicated for the majority of cases.

Systemic NSAIDs are indicated for most cases of uveitis. Although clinical studies comparing the efficacy of the various systemic NSAIDs are lacking, many clinicians recommend flunixin meglumine as the NSAID of choice for uveitis. The duration of NSAID treatment will depend upon the response to treatment. Generally, systemic NSAID therapy should be continued until no significant uveitis is apparent on clinical examination. Since systemic therapy may be prolonged, appropriate monitoring for the side effects of NSAIDs is indicated (see Chapter 5, Pharmacology of nonsteroidal anti-inflammatory drugs for side effects of NSAIDs).

Systemic corticosteroids may be incorporated into the treatment plan where use of NSAIDs is contraindicated (history of renal insufficiency or ulcerative gastrointestinal disease) or where inflammation is particularly severe. Corticosteroids are potent anti-inflammatories, but are not without their own unique risks and side effects. Systemic corticosteroids should be reserved for refractory cases of uveitis and then used only with caution and careful monitoring of the patient's systemic health. Oral dexamethasone at 0.04–0.08 mg/kg q24 h is well tolerated in most patients and can be slowly tapered over the course of 2–3 weeks (Table 14.5).

Topical administration of anti-inflammatory agents, either NSAIDs or corticosteroids, can be used as an alternative to systemic administration. The primary advantage of topical therapy is a decreased risk of side effects compared to systemic administration of NSAIDs and corticosteroids. Selection of a topical NSAID versus

Table 14.5 Topical anti-inflammatory drugs.

Drug	Formulation
Nonsteroidal anti-inflammatories	
Bromfenac 0.09%	Solution
Diclofenac 0.1%	Solution
Flurbiprofen 0.03%	Solution
Indomethacin 1%	Suspension
Ketorolac 0.4%	Solution
Nepafenac 0.1%	Solution
Corticosteroid anti-inflammatories	
Dexamethasone 0.1%	Solution
Loteprednol etabonate 0.5%	Suspension/ointment
Neomycin–polymyxin–bacitracin Dexamethasone	Ointment/solution
Prednisolone acetate 1%	Suspension

a corticosteroid depends on a number of patient factors. Concurrent ocular diseases and route of administration also influence the choice of what type of topical anti-inflammatory to select. Firstly, topical corticosteroids should never be administered when corneal ulceration is present. Even topical NSAIDs should be used with caution when corneal ulceration is present as they are rarely associated with acute and dramatic keratomalacia. Secondly, topical NSAIDs are not commercially available in ointment formulation, which makes their application more challenging. Finally, when inflammation is severe, topical NSAIDs and corticosteroids can be used concurrently. The major disadvantage to the use of topical corticosteroids is suppression of the ocular immune system, which leaves the cornea vulnerable to opportunistic pathogens should a corneal abrasion occur. Administration of topical corticosteroids is a well-known risk factor for the development of fungal keratitis. When selecting a topical corticosteroid, ensure that the selected drug is of appropriate potency with ability to penetrate the cornea. For example, hydrocortisone is a poor choice for the treatment of uveitis because it does not penetrate the cornea and does not achieve therapeutic concentrations in the anterior segment.

Frequency of treatment for acute uveitis is determined by severity of inflammation, with the most severe cases requiring treatment q2–4 h. Treatment is tapered as the inflammation resolves. It is important to remember that inflammation may be present even when the eye appears clinically normal. Persistent ocular hypotension and resistance to mydriasis are signs that subclinical uveitis is present. Topical treatment should be continued well past clinical resolution of inflammation.

Subconjunctival and intravitreal injections of reposital steroid formulations are effective for long-term (2–6 weeks) delivery of intraocular corticosteroids and can be extremely efficacious in controlling uveitis. In a study evaluating a number of commonly used corticosteroids, triamcinolone acetate was determined to be the least toxic to intraocular structures [17]. Reported doses of triamcinolone range from 1 to 40 mg, although most practitioners utilize doses of 1–2 mg. Methylprednisolone should not be administered subconjunctivally as it is rarely associated with formation of painful subconjunctival granulomas [18].

Great care must be taken when administering intravitreal corticosteroid injections to avoid secondary bacterial endophthalmitis. Appropriate preparation of the ocular surface, including use of povidone–iodine solution, and administration of topical antibiotics pre- and postinjection can help minimize the risk of this complication. Secondary bacterial or fungal infections of the cornea may also occur after intravitreal or subconjunctival corticosteroid injections. Because the immune system of the eye is suppressed, these patients must be closely monitored for any evidence of corneal abrasions or ulcerative keratitis and treated aggressively at the first sign of any breach in the ocular surface.

Drug therapy for controlling the side effects of uveitis

Uveitis also causes spasm of the ciliary body musculature, which is extremely painful. Therefore, administration of a topical cycloplegic agent, such as atropine 1%, to eliminate the spasm is recommended. Atropine also causes mydriasis, which decreases the risk of formation of posterior synechiae and stabilizes the BAB, though the mechanism by which it produces this latter effect is not well understood. When treating uveitis, atropine should be administered to effect q6–24 h. This rate of application is higher than for that of a simple ulcer because of the increased stimulus for miosis and ciliary body spasm in cases of uveitis. If full mydriasis is not observed within 48 h of the first application, inflammatory mediators, such as prostaglandins, may be responsible for the persistent miosis. In these cases,

increasing the dose of anti-inflammatory agents (either topical or systemic) may be helpful. Posterior synechiae may also cause a decreased response to atropine administration. It should be remembered that tropicamide 1% should not be used in cases of uveitis as it has only short-acting cycloplegic properties. In a similar manner, phenylephrine 2.5–10% solution is not an effective mydriatic when used as a sole agent in the horse, but may be used in some cases as an adjunctive therapy to augment mydriasis.

Acute and/or severe uveitis is also associated with intraocular fibrin formation. Fibrin promotes the formation of posterior synechiae, which may lead to visual impairment. TPA at a dose of 25 μg can be administered to lyse the fibrin, but it must be administered by intracameral injection, because the cornea is impermeable to it. Although TPA is unstable once reconstituted, it can be frozen at −80°C until use.

Active uveitis also causes diffuse corneal edema. This edema occurs secondary to transient endothelial dysfunction associated with inflammatory-induced alterations in the composition of aqueous humor. In these cases, because the edema is expected to be self-limiting as the intraocular inflammation improves, the application of topical hyperosmotics to reduce corneal edema is not recommended.

Equine recurrent uveitis

ERU is a form of autoimmune uveitis unique to the horse. The triggering stimulus that initiates the ERU cascade is controversial and poorly understood. Previous exposure to *Leptospira* spp., persistent leptospirosis, previous trauma, and a variety of other infectious organisms have all been implicated. Regardless of the underlying etiology, ERU results in chronic, self-perpetuating intraocular inflammation and is the most common cause of blindness in the horse. Active and quiescent phases of the disease are observed, as are both anterior and posterior segment manifestations. Active inflammatory episodes are treated similarly to acute uveitis as described previously. Unfortunately, the side effects of long-term topical and systemic anti-inflammatory therapy may lead to complications that are as vision threatening as the disease itself (e.g., fungal keratitis in patients treated with chronic topical corticosteroids). The need for a safe, chronic therapy for ERU led to the development of a suprachoroidal cyclosporine A (CSA) implant. CSA is a calcineurin inhibitor that decreases the activation of autoaggressive T cells. The CSA-impregnated bioerodible disk is surgically implanted beneath a partial-thickness scleral flap in the dorsotemporal quadrant of the globe. Once implanted, CSA is released into the suprachoroidal space with direct access to the uveal vasculature, allowing therapeutic concentrations of CSA to be achieved intraocularly. This unique surgical approach for a pharmacologic intervention was necessary because CSA has exceptionally poor corneal penetration, making topical administration useless for the treatment of intraocular disease. The goal of a CSA implant placement is to reduce the number, frequency, and severity of ERU episodes, and it has a reported long-term success rate of approximately 80% [19]. Unfortunately, the surgery is difficult and must be performed by someone skilled in microsurgical techniques.

Drug therapy for glaucoma

Equine glaucoma is a vision-threatening disease that is underdiagnosed and poorly understood in the horse. Primary glaucoma is a hereditary form of glaucoma recognized in humans and dogs where the aqueous humor pathway tract becomes dysfunctional in middle age. Secondary glaucoma is caused by an acquired dysfunction of the aqueous humor outflow pathway. ERU is the most commonly documented cause of secondary glaucoma in the horse [20, 21]. Primary glaucoma, where the aqueous drainage system is dysfunctional, is much less frequently reported in the horse. The goal of treating glaucoma is to preserve function of the optic nerve and retina. Reduction of IOP to a normal range is essential for optimizing optic nerve and retinal function. Treatment of glaucoma is often very frustrating and owners should be warned of the guarded long-term prognosis. Medical therapy for glaucoma can be divided into drugs that decrease the production of aqueous humor and those that increase the outflow of aqueous humor.

Drug therapy that decreases the production of aqueous humor

Carbonic anhydrase inhibitors (CAIs) inhibit the enzyme carbonic anhydrase, which is essential for the production of aqueous humor in the ciliary body. Available CAIs include brinzolamide 1% and dorzolamide 2%. While both have been demonstrated to reduce IOP in clinically normal horses, the reduction caused by brinzolamide was greater [22, 23]. Nevertheless, the widespread availability of affordable, generic dorzolamide has made it the most commonly used treatment for equine glaucoma. Topical CAIs should be administered q8–12 h. Peer-reviewed studies evaluating the effects of PO administered CAI acetazolamide on equine IOP are lacking. Nevertheless, anecdotal reports suggest that doses of 2–3 mg/kg PO q12 h are safe for use in adult horses with normal renal function.

Beta adrenergic receptor antagonists, known as beta-blockers, also decrease the production of aqueous humor via inhibition of cAMP activity in the ciliary body. The beta-blocker timolol maleate 0.5% has been demonstrated to reduce IOP in clinically normal horses [24]. Timolol and dorzolamide are available as a combination product for ease of administration. Beta-blockers, whether dosed with a CAI or as single agents, should be administered q8–12 h.

Drug therapy that increases the outflow of aqueous humor

Prostaglandin analogs such as latanoprost 0.005% and travoprost 0.004% cause dramatic increases in IOP outflow in other species, but have not been demonstrated to produce this effect consistently in the horse. Study results conflict on their ability to reduce IOP and also report a high rate of complications, including increased ocular pain [25, 26]. As prostaglandin analogs mimic the inflammatory effects of endogenous prostaglandins, this drug class should be used with great caution in horses with glaucoma associated with ERU.

Atropine 1% does not consistently reduce IOP in normal horses and can be associated with significant elevations in IOP in rare cases [27, 28]. Therefore, atropine is not recommended for the treatment of equine glaucoma.

Other drug therapy for glaucoma

Because equine glaucoma occurs most often secondary to ERU, control of intraocular inflammation is essential for adequate treatment of glaucoma. Given the association between ERU and glaucoma, it is prudent to carefully examine a glaucoma patient for any evidence of active inflammation, and liberal use of anti-inflammatory agents is warranted in cases of equine glaucoma. It should be noted that there is also an unusual, but poorly documented, phenomenon in the horse termed hypertensive iridocyclitis where transient increases in IOP are reduced with anti-inflammatory therapy alone.

References

1 Chen, T. & Ward, D.A. (2010) Tear volume, turnover rate, and flow rate in ophthalmologically normal horses. *American Journal of Veterinary Research*, **71**, 671–676.

2 Giuliano, E.A., Maggs, D.J., Moore, C.P., Boland, L.A., Champagne, E.S. & Galle, L.E. (2000) Inferomedial placement of a single-entry subpalpebral lavage tube for treatment of equine eye disease. *Veterinary Ophthalmology*, **3**, 153–156.

3 Brightman, A.H., 2nd, Manning, J.P., Benson, G.J. & Musselman, E.E. (1983) Decreased tear production associated with general anesthesia in the horse. *Journal of the American Veterinary Medical Association*, **182**, 243–244.

4 Trim, C.M., Colbern, G.T. & Martin, C.L. (1985) Effect of xylazine and ketamine on intraocular pressure in horses. *Veterinary Record*, **117**, 442–443.

5 van der Woerdt, A., Gilger, B.C., Wilkie, D.A. & Strauch, S.M. (1995) Effect of auriculopalpebral nerve block and intravenous administration of xylazine on intraocular pressure and corneal thickness in horses. *American Journal of Veterinary Research*, **56**, 155–158.

6 Kalf, K.L., Utter, M.E. & Wotman, K.L. (2008) Evaluation of duration of corneal anesthesia induced with ophthalmic 0.5% proparacaine hydrochloride by use of a Cochet-Bonnet aesthesiometer in clinically normal horses. *American Journal of Veterinary Research*, **69**, 1655–1658.

7 Monclin, S.J., Farnir, F. & Grauwels, M. (2011) Duration of corneal anaesthesia following multiple doses and two concentrations of tetracaine hydrochloride eyedrops on the normal equine cornea. *Equine Veterinary Journal*, **43**, 69–73.

8 Bartfield, J.M., Holmes, T.J. & Raccio-Robak, N. (1994) A comparison of proparacaine and tetracaine eye anesthetics. *Academic Emergency Medicine*, **1**, 364–367.

9 Monclin, S.J., Farnir, F. & Grauwels, M. (2011) Determination of tear break-up time reference values and ocular tolerance of tetracaine hydrochloride eyedops in healthy horses. *Equine Veterinary Journal*, **43**, 74–77.

10 Williams, M.M., Spiess, B.M., Pascoe, P.J. & O'Grady, M. (2000) Systemic effects of topical and subconjunctival ophthalmic atropine in the horse. *Veterinary Ophthalmology*, **3**, 193–199.

11 Mac Rae, S.M., Brown, B. & Edelhauser, H.F. (1984) The corneal toxicity of presurgical skin antiseptics. *American Journal of Ophthalmology*, **97**, 221–232.

12 Andrew, S.E., Brooks, D.E., Biros, D.J., Denis, H.M., Cutler, T.J. & Gelatt, K.N. (2000) Posterior lamellar keratoplasty for treatment of deep stromal abscesses in nine horses. *Veterinary Ophthalmology*, **3**, 99–103.

13 Plummer, C.E., Kallberg, M.E., Ollivier, F.J., Barrie, K.P. & Brooks, D.E. (2008) Deep lamellar endothelial keratoplasty in 10 horses. *Veterinary Ophthalmology*, **11** (Suppl 1), 35–43.

14 Matthews, A. & Gilger, B.C. (2009) Equine immune-mediated keratopathies. *Veterinary Ophthalmology*, **12** (Suppl 1), 10–16.

15 Gilger, B.C., Michau, T.M. & Salmon, J.H. (2005) Immune-mediated keratitis in horses: 19 cases (1998–2004). *Veterinary Ophthalmology*, **8**, 233–239.

16 Yamagata, M., Wilkie, D.A. & Gilger, B.C. (1996) Eosinophilic keratoconjunctivitis in seven horses. *Journal of the American Veterinary Medical Association*, **209**, 1283–1286.

17 Yi, N.Y., Davis, J.L., Salmon, J.H. & Gilger, B.C. (2008) Ocular distribution and toxicity of intravitreal injection of triamcinolone acetonide in normal equine eyes. *Veterinary Ophthalmology*, **11** (Suppl 1), 15–19.

18 Fischer, C.A. (1979) Granuloma formation associated with subconjunctival injection of a corticosteroid in dogs. *Journal of the American Veterinary Medical Association*, **174**, 1086–1088.

19 Gilger, B.C., Wilkie, D.A., Clode, A.B. et al. (2010) Long-term outcome after implantation of a suprachoroidal cyclosporine drug delivery device in horses with recurrent uveitis. *Veterinary Ophthalmology*, **13**, 294–300.

20 Annear, M.J., Wilkie, D.A. & Gemensky-Metzler, A.J. (2010) Semiconductor diode laser transscleral cyclophotocoagulation for the treatment of glaucoma in horses: A retrospective study of 42 eyes. *Veterinary Ophthalmology*, **13**, 204–209.

21 Miller, T.R., Brooks, D.E., Smith, P.J. & Sapienza, J.S. (1995) Equine glaucoma: Clinical findings and response to treatment in 14 horses. *Veterinary and Comparative Ophthalmology*, **5**, 170–182.

22 Germann, S.E., Matheis, F.L., Rampazzo, A., Burger, D., Roos, M. & Spiess, B.M. (2008) Effects of topical administration of 1% brinzolamide on intraocular pressure in clinically normal horses. *Equine Veterinary Journal*, **40**, 662–665.

23 Willis, A.M., Robbin, T.E., Hoshaw-Woodard, S., Wilkie, D.A. & Schmall, M.L. (2001) Effect of topical administration of 2% dorzlamide hydrochloride or 2% dorzlamide hydrochloride-0.5% timolol maleate on intraocular pressure in clinically normal horses. *American Journal of Veterinary Research*, **62**, 709–713.

24 Van Der Woerdt, A., Wilkie, D.A., Gilger, B.C., Strauch, S.M. & Orczeck, S.M. (2000) Effect of single- and multiple-dose 0.5% timolol maleate on intraocular pressure and pupil size in female horses. *Veterinary Ophthalmology*, **3**, 165–168.

25 Davidson, H.J., Pinard, C.L., Keil, S.M., Brightman, A.H. & Sargeant, J.M. (2002) Effect of topical ophthalmic latanoprost on intraocular pressure in normal horses. *Veterinary Therapeutics*, **3**, 72–80.

26 Willis, A.M., Diehl, K.A., Hoshaw-Woodard, S., Kobayashi, I., Vitucci, M.P. & Schmall, L.M. (2001) Effects of topical administration of 0.005% latanoprost solution on eyes of clinically normal horses. *American Journal of Veterinary Research*, **62**, 1945–1951.

27 Herring, I.P., Pickett, J.P., Champagne, E.S., Troy, G.C. & Marini, M. (2000) Effect of topical 1% atropine sulfate on intraocular pressure in normal horses. *Veterinary Ophthalmology*, **3**, 139–143.

28 Mughannam, A.J., Buyukmihci, N.C. & Kass, P.H. (1999) Effect of topical atropine on intraocular pressure and pupil diameter in the normal horse eye. *Veterinary Ophthalmology*, **2**, 213–215.

CHAPTER 15

Pharmacological treatment of equine endocrine diseases

Dianne McFarlane

Oklahoma State University, Stillwater, OK, USA

Introduction

In the adult horse, there are two endocrinopathic conditions that are amenable to pharmacological intervention, equine metabolic syndrome (EMS) and equine pituitary pars intermedia dysfunction (PPID). Early and accurate recognition and treatment of endocrine disease are recommended in horses to minimize the risk of development of life-threatening disease sequelae including laminitis and immunosuppression. Together, EMS and PPID are responsible for the majority of all equine laminitis cases, and treatment of the primary disease is an essential component of management of laminitis of all etiologies [1]. Unfortunately, currently available diagnostic tests for both EMS and PPID are plagued by false negatives early in disease. Therefore, therapeutic decision making must take into account the likelihood that early testing may not provide a definitive diagnosis.

Equine metabolic syndrome (EMS)

EMS is the name given to a collection of risk factors in horses that predict laminitis, including adiposity, hyperinsulinemia, insulin resistance, and thriftiness. This syndrome was once thought to be the consequence of hypothyroidism, and treatment with levothyroxine was the mainstay of therapy. The realization that the syndrome of obesity-associated laminitis in the horse is mechanistically more similar to metabolic syndrome in people and linked to insulin dysregulation was first suggested by Johnson in 2002 [2]. Further work in the field led to development of a 2010 consensus statement characterizing EMS as a phenotype that includes obesity, insulin resistance (or hyperinsulinemia), and a predisposition for laminitis [3]. Additional factors identified as part the syndrome included dyslipidemia, hyperleptinemia, and altered reproductive cycling. In addition to laminitis, other clinical sequelae of EMS of concern include exercise intolerance and infertility. Since the 2010 consensus statement was written, a great deal of additional data have been collected that have helped to clarify our understanding of EMS and endocrinopathic laminitis.

One of the most noteworthy recent findings is that it is serum insulin concentration, not tissue insulin resistance *per se*, that appears to trigger laminitis. In a series of experiments, it was shown that normal ponies and horses exposed to 48–72 h of continuous intravenous administration of insulin develop clinical and histological signs of laminitis [4, 5]. These data clearly support recent epidemiological studies showing a strong correlation between fasting serum insulin concentration and naturally occurring laminitis [6–12]. Further work has implicated insulin-mediated activation of the insulin-like growth factor 1 receptors in the hoof in the pathogenesis of laminitis through promotion of proliferation and elongation of the secondary lamellae [13]. The enhanced understanding of the underlying mechanisms of endocrinopathic laminitis will undoubtedly lead to exploration of novel drugs in the treatment and prevention of this devastating disease.

Treatment of EMS focuses around two major goals, reducing body weight (bwt) and decreasing serum the insulin concentration. These two goals overlap as a reduction in bwt will often result in an improvement in insulin sensitivity. Diet and exercise management are

Equine Pharmacology, First Edition. Edited by Cynthia Cole, Bradford Bentz and Lara Maxwell.
© 2015 John Wiley & Sons, Inc. Published 2015 by John Wiley & Sons, Inc.

the cornerstones of EMS treatment; pharmacological management is typically reserved for those horses that are resistant to management changes alone. Careful dietary management, with a strict reduction of soluble sugars, has been shown to be an effective means of controlling both bwt and insulin sensitivity in horses [14]. Exercise serves to both utilize calories and directly enhance tissue insulin sensitivity, and a regulated exercise program is strongly recommended in horses without orthopedic restrictions such as active laminitis. As one might expect, however, owner compliance is often problematic when rigorous dietary and exercise management is required.

Levothyroxine sodium

Thyroid hormone supplementation using levothyroxine sodium is perhaps one of the most overprescribed treatments in equine medicine. It has been prescribed for the treatment of EMS, laminitis, anhidrosis, fescue toxicosis, infertility, allergies, exertional rhabdomyolysis, lethargy, poor performance, and a plethora of other generally nonspecific clinical maladies [15–18]. Often, the diagnosis of hypothyroidism in these cases is based on either vague clinical signs alone or clinical signs and low resting thyroid hormones, thyroxine (T4) and triiodothyroxine (T3) [15–18]. Functional thyroid testing is rarely performed. When dynamic thyroid testing has been performed to assess the role of thyroid hormones in these conditions, hypothyroidism has not been a factor [15–18].

The use of short-duration, high-dose levothyroxine sodium to promote weight loss and improve insulin sensitivity in horses has been investigated [19–21]. The therapeutic goal is to induce mild hyperthyroidism, thereby accelerating metabolism and causing weight reduction. Thus, the dose currently recommended is higher than the previously suggested dose when the underlying cause of endocrinopathic laminitis was believed to be hypothyroidism. Dietary restriction and exercise must be initiated at the same time as levothyroxine, as a potential effect of high-dose levothyroxine is increased appetite. When levothyroxine was administered at a dose of 48 mg/day for 16–48 weeks, normal horses lost from 25 to 49 kg and demonstrated a 2-fold increase their insulin sensitivity [19–21]. When the same dose of levothyroxine was administered for 6 months to horses suffering from EMS, they did not lose any more weight than the untreated control group [22]. When the dose was increased to 72 mg/day for an additional

3 months, however, the levothyroxine-treated horses lost approximately 30 kg of bwt, which was significantly more than the weight lost by the untreated horses [22]. Both the 48 and 72 mg/kg dose groups had significant increases in the circulating T4 hormone and suppression of thyroid hormone release following TRH stimulation [21]. The effect of levothyroxine on metabolic rates has not been directly tested.

In people, adverse effects of high doses of levothyroxine include cardiac arrhythmias, left ventricular hypertrophy, and excitation. Levothyroxine actually has a black box label mandated by the FDA warning that it should not be used for weight loss, because the high dose required to produce that effect is associated with serious or life-threatening manifestations of toxicity. Nevertheless, in a 48-week study administering levothyroxine to six healthy mares, no adverse health effects were observed [20]. Variables monitored in that study included hematology, serum chemistry, cardiac troponin I, and echocardiographic measurements [20]. Although lifelong levothyroxine administration was previously recommended for treatment of EMS in horses, the current scientific literature indicates that no further benefits can be anticipated after 6–9 months of therapy. Therefore, once weight loss has been achieved, horses should be gradually weaned off levothyroxine to prevent iatrogenic hypothyroidism. The dose can be reduced by half every 2 weeks until the dose is 12.5 mg/day or lower [23]. After 2 weeks at that dose, the drug can be discontinued.

Metformin

Metformin is a biguanide drug that has been widely used as an oral antihyperglycemic agent in human medicine for more than 50 years [24]. It is recognized to have several potential antidiabetic mechanisms of action including reducing hepatic glucose production, enhancing tissue sensitivity to insulin, and increasing translocation of glucose type 4 (GLUT4) transporters to cell membranes in insulin-sensitive tissues [25]. These actions are thought to be produced by metformin-induced AMP kinase activation [26]. A second line of evidence suggests metformin may decrease oral absorption of glucose by altering gut flora to decrease dietary glucose availability and by sequestering glucose in the mucosa of the gastrointestinal tract [25, 27].

In humans, metformin had an absolute oral bioavailability of 40–60%, and an inverse relationship was observed between the dose ingested and the relative absorption, suggesting the involvement of an active, saturable absorption process. Metformin is rapidly distributed following absorption and does not bind to plasma proteins. No metabolites or conjugates of metformin have been identified, indicating a lack of hepatic metabolism. The drug is eliminated unchanged by renal secretion and is considered contraindicated in people with renal impairment [28]. The most commonly reported adverse event associated with metformin therapy in people is lactic acidosis, a relatively rare complication, which is fatal in 25% of the people affected [29].

Two studies have been performed analyzing metformin pharmacokinetics in horses. In the first, metformin was administered orally (PO) and IV at approximately 12 mg/kg bwt [30]. In this study, the bioavailability of PO administered metformin was only 7% in fasted horses and less than 4% in horses in a postprandial state. In addition, the elimination half-life was very short in horses, less than 30 min, compared to 6 h in humans. However, in a second pharmacokinetic study in horses, the elimination half-life was determined to be approximately 12 h following an oral dose of 30 mg/kg bwt. Although the bioavailability was not determined in the second study, mean steady-state serum concentration determined in four ponies receiving 15 mg/kg bwt q12 h for 20 days was low at 122 ng/ml, compared to the therapeutic target range in humans of 500–1000 ng/ml [31, 32].

Several efficacy studies have also been performed evaluating the effect of metformin on insulin dynamics, but unfortunately, they have produced conflicting results. For example, Vick and colleagues found transient improvement in insulin sensitivity using a hyperinsulinemic–euglycemic clamping technique in obese mares receiving 3 mg/kg bwt of metformin q12 h, but not when higher doses of 6 and 9 mg/kg bwt q12 h were administered [33]. In contrast, Tinworth and group, using the frequently sampled IV glucose tolerance test, did not find an effect of metformin administered at a dose of 15 mg/kg bwt to nonobese ponies [34]. In another study that used the same testing methods, again, no effect of metformin was noted when the dose was increased to 30 mg/kg bwt [35]. In contrast to these studies, Durham and coworkers showed an improvement in proxies of insulin sensitivity in obese, laminitic horses treated with metformin at a dose of 15 mg/kg bwt q12 h for 2 weeks [36]. The lack of concordance in these studies was attributed to differences in

dose, insulin sensitivity testing methods, and/or subject selection [37]. Interesting new data from Rendle et al. may provide some insight into the earlier discrepancies [38]. When 30 mg/kg of metformin was administered to normal horses or horses made insulin resistant through glucocorticoid administration, the response to an oral glucose challenge was markedly reduced [38]. These results suggest that it was the testing method that was responsible for the discrepancies and that the mechanism of action of metformin in horses is through inhibition of glucose absorption from the small intestine rather than enhancement of insulin sensitivity at the level of the tissue. Therefore, metformin, administered at a dose of 30 mg/kg bwt, may have a place in treatment of EMS and prevention of laminitis by preventing glucose-stimulated insulin release.

In people with diabetes, glipizides have a complementary action when administered concurrently with metformin. Glipizides selectively bind sulfonylurea receptors on the surface of the pancreatic beta cells and enhance insulin release. Therefore, in horses with EMS that already have excessive insulin secretion, treatment with glipizides is contraindicated.

Nutraceuticals

Numerous supplements have been suggested to improve insulin sensitivity in horses and ponies with insulin dysregulation, although peer-reviewed data supporting these claims are sparse. One study evaluated the efficacy of a magnesium chromium supplement in EMS horses using the frequently sampled IV glucose tolerance test and resting insulin and glucose concentrations as measures of insulin sensitivity. No improvement was observed after 16 weeks at the manufacturer's recommended daily dose [22]. Respondek et al. found that short-chain fructo-oligosaccharides improved insulin sensitivity in obese Arabian mares fed ad libitum; however, in obese horses with dietary carbohydrate restriction, short-chain fructo-oligosaccharides had no effect beyond that of diet alone [14, 39].

Pituitary pars intermedia dysfunction (PPID)

PPID is the most common endocrinopathy of aged horses, affecting 15–25% of horses 15–20 years or older [40–42]. Clinical signs of the disease include an abnormal hair coat, which may manifest as absent, incomplete, or late shedding, or lightening of coat color. Additional clinical signs include muscle atrophy, immunosuppression, mentation changes, polydipsia, polyuria, thermoregulatory dysfunction, and infertility. Laminitis also occurs in approximately 30% of PPID-affected horses, and conversely, 40–50% of horses with laminitis of unknown origin have biochemical or clinical evidence of PPID or EMS [12, 40–42].

Equine PPID results from a loss of hypothalamic-derived dopaminergic inhibition of the intermediate lobe of the pituitary, resulting in unchecked replication of intermediate lobe melanotropes and excessive secretion of proopiomelanocortin (POMC)-derived peptides, such as α-melanocyte-stimulating hormone, adrenocorticotropin, β-endorphin, and corticotropin-like intermediate lobe peptide. Damage to the dopaminergic neurons that innervate the intermediate lobe of the pituitary is associated with oxidative stress, accumulation of misfolded proteins, and failure of autophagic clearance and likely occurs early in the disease process [43]. Targeting these pathological processes in high-risk animals or those with early disease may prove beneficial and represent a future therapeutic strategy.

The treatment of PPID has several important components. Horses with PPID benefit from the provision of an optimized geriatric health management program, as well as pharmaceutical treatment of disease. Similar to other aged horses, PPID-affected animals require aggressive preventative health care to maximize their well-being and health status. In addition, vigilant monitoring of indicators of PPID-associated health concerns is required. Early identification and resolution of secondary complications, including laminitis, weight loss, and infections, can be instrumental in improving quality of life and longevity in PPID horses. When well cared for, horses with PPID can live into their 30s and even 40s.

Clinical signs and hormonal profiles differ among horses with PPID, suggesting that there may be multiple etiologies and syndromes of pars intermedia dysfunction. For example, hyperinsulinemia and/or insulin resistance occurs in approximately 40% of horses with PPID, and hyperinsulinemia is considered a risk factor for the development of laminitis in horses with endocrine disease [6–12, 44]. McGowan *et al.* reported hyperinsulinemia in more than 90% of laminitic horses with confirmed PPID, but the study group was small, only 11 horses,

and dynamic testing to evaluate insulin glucose regulation was not performed [11]. At this time, it remains unclear if laminitis only occurs in those PPID horses with insulin dysregulation. It is also unknown if insulin dysregulation is a cause, consequence, or unrelated secondary condition in horses with PPID. Furthermore, as several pituitary hormones have anti-inflammatory and analgesic properties, it is not clear if laminitis is more or less severe when PPID is present. Although irrefutable evidence from controlled studies is lacking, ample anecdotal evidence supports a predisposition of horses with EMS for later development of PPID. Understanding the different clinical syndromes may improve our ability to customize treatment of PPID to avoid unnecessary drug treatments while still lowering risk of development of PPID-associated secondary complications.

Dopaminergic agonist treatment

The use of dopaminergic agonists has been the mainstay of PPID treatment for more than 30 years. In the 1980s, Orth and group showed that administration of bromocriptine at a dose of 100 mg, PO or SQ, or pergolide mesylate at a dose of 5 mg, PO, caused a rapid decrease in plasma immunoreactive POMC-derived peptides in two horses with overt PPID [45]. Following publication of these results, pergolide mesylate was used to treat clinical cases of PPID at a dose of 3–5 mg/horse [46]. It was later shown that a lower, more economical dose of 1–2 mg/horse, which is equivalent to a dose of approximately 0.075 µg/kg bwt, PO, q24 h, also controlled clinical signs, and use of pergolide became widespread in equine practice [47].

Pergolide mesylate

Pergolide mesylate is an ergot-derived drug that was used in humans for the treatment of Parkinson's disease, a dopaminergic neurodegenerative disease that causes motor dysfunction. Pergolide is a dopamine receptor agonist with greater affinity for D2 than D1 receptors and a minor affinity for the serotonin 5HT-2A and 5HT-2A receptors as well as α-1 and α-2 adrenergic receptors [48, 49]. It functions in PPID by activating D2 receptors, the inhibitory Gi subtype of G protein-coupled dopaminergic receptors that are abundant on the melanotropes of the PI.

Limited information exists on the pharmacokinetics of pergolide in horses. Plasma drug concentrations were reported to be 4–10 times greater in horses than in humans administered the same dose of 10 µg/kg bwt, PO, suggesting greater bioavailability in horses [50]. Based on this data, the authors concluded that the current recommended starting dose of 1–2 µg/kg bwt, equivalent to 0.5–1 mg/horse, q24 h was sufficient to produce plasma concentrations equivalent to therapeutic drug concentrations targeted in people with pituitary dysfunction. In addition, the results of this study demonstrated that plasma pergolide concentrations decline rapidly following oral dosing, and therefore, twice-daily administration may be more appropriate in order to maintain therapeutic concentrations. However, this recommendation is based on the kinetics following administration of a single dose to healthy young horses and does not account for drug accumulation at steady state, alterations in target receptors that would occur with chronic drug exposure, or the effect of age and PPID on drug disposition. Additional studies are underway to assess pharmacokinetic properties in PPID horses after prolonged pergolide administration.

The principal adverse effect associated with pergolide in horses is anorexia, which is typically mild and occurs at onset of treatment [51]. Anorexia can usually be resolved by discontinuing treatment for a few days and then resuming it at a lower dose with a slow dose escalation over 7–14 days until the desired dose is reached. In some horses, splitting the dose into a twice-daily treatment improves appetite. In people, reports of valvular endocardiosis and regurgitation in Parkinson's disease patients chronically treated with pergolide led to the voluntary market withdrawal of pergolide mesylate (Permax™, Eli Lilly, Indianapolis, IN) from the market [52–55]. There is no evidence of similar valvular lesions occurring in horses treated with pergolide [51]. Although pregnant mares have been treated with the drug, safety of pergolide use during pregnancy and lactation has not been studied in equids.

After the withdrawal of Permax from the market, compounding pharmacies became the sole source of pergolide mesylate for the treatment of equine PPID. Therefore, the FDA-CVM released a statement that they would be "exercising enforcement discretion as appropriate over the pharmacy compounding of pergolide for use in animals" [56]. Unfortunately, pergolide is a particularly difficult drug to compound, because it is unstable in aqueous suspensions and degrades rapidly when exposed to light [57]. Analyses of pergolide

products from several compounding pharmacies revealed considerable degradation and a lot of variation of the actual drug concentrations in the marketed products from the strengths indicated on their labels [57, 58]. These variations in pergolide content have also been shown in different scoops of the same container of a compounded granular formulation and even from capsules derived from the same batch of raw drug [58]. In 2011, a veterinary-approved pharmaceutical pergolide mesylate (Prascend™, Boehringer Ingelheim, St Joseph, MO) was introduced for the treatment of PPID in horses and ponies, and the FDA-CVM issued a retraction of the exemption of extralabel regulations for pharmacies compounding pergolide stating, "the conditions under which the Agency was exercising enforcement discretion no longer exist" [56].

Several studies have demonstrated the efficacy of pergolide mesylate at improving both clinical signs and hormonal dysregulation in horses with PPID [51, 59–61]. In the largest of these studies, the field clinical efficacy trial conducted for FDA approval of Prascend, 76% of the 113 horses who completed the study were considered treatment successes [51]. In other smaller studies, pergolide was better than cyproheptadine at improving both clinical signs and the ACTH concentration in horses suffering from PPID [59–61]. In addition to decreasing secretion of pars intermedia hormones, another potential goal of therapy is to decrease the size of the pituitary, thus minimizing the effect of compression on adjacent pituitary and neural structures. The ability of pergolide to reduce pituitary gland size was investigated using computed tomography (CT) in a group of horses before and after 6 months of pergolide treatment [62]. No decrease in pituitary gland size was found; however, this study was potentially confounded by the effect of season, as the posttreatment CT scans were performed in the fall when pars intermedia and total pituitary gland size naturally increase [63].

Once pergolide therapy has been initiated, routine follow-up examinations are recommended. Ideally, both clinical response and endocrine testing should be monitored every 6–12 months. Some, but not all, horses will require periodic changes in dose for optimal hormonal regulation. Typically, in horses with a poor or incomplete response, the pergolide dose is increased by 1–2 µg/kg bwt, and the response is reassessed a month later.

As discussed earlier, early treatment of horses with PPID is considered optimal to prevent or limit development of life-threatening complications such as laminitis. However, early diagnosis of PPID is often difficult. Therefore, an important, as of yet unanswered, clinical question is whether to treat horses that test negative for PPID but that have nonspecific indicators (e.g., weight loss or infertility) or risk factors (e.g., age or EMS) of PPID. More research will be needed to answer this question.

Cyproheptadine

Cyproheptadine has been suggested as a second-line drug, best used in combination with pergolide mesylate when maximal tolerated doses of pergolide alone are insufficient to resolve clinical signs. Cyproheptadine is a serotonin antagonist with additional antihistamine, antimuscarinic, and calcium channel-blocking actions. Several small studies have shown a limited efficacy of cyproheptadine for resolving or improving clinical signs of PPID when used as a monotherapy at doses of 0.25–0.5 mg/kg bwt, PO, q24 h [59–61]. Cyproheptadine has been shown to lower the seizure threshold in mice, and therefore, the use of cyproheptadine in horses with a history of seizures or central neurologic disease is not advised. In addition, the drug should be discontinued in horses that develop neurologic signs while on treatment [64].

Trilostane

Trilostane is a competitive inhibitor of the enzyme 3-beta hydroxysteroid dehydrogenase, which functions in the synthesis of cortisol from cholesterol. The efficacy of trilostane was evaluated in 20 horses with clinical signs of PPID and laminitis [65]. After 30 days of treatment with trilostane at an average dose of 0.6 mg/kg bwt, PO, clinical signs of laminitis improved, but dexamethasone suppression test results remained abnormal in the majority of cases. Unfortunately, the results of this study were complicated by the absence of an untreated control group, which was not included in the study due to humane concerns. It is reasonable to assume that trilostane may improve clinical signs of the 20–40% of horses with PPID that have significant adrenal gland hyperplasia and hypercortisolemia [66–68]. However, the finding that it is insulin, and not cortisol, concentration that correlates with the risk of laminitis has made the value of trilostane treatment questionable, and no further research has been done to assess the utility of trilostane for PPID or endocrinopathic laminitis in the horse.

Supplements and nutraceuticals

Many nutraceuticals and natural remedies have been suggested as treatments for PPID. One of the more popular natural remedies is *Vitex agnus-castus* extract, also known as chasteberry extract. In a study of 14 horses with PPID, however, a commercial chasteberry extract failed to resolve clinical signs or improve diagnostic test results [69]. In fact, several animals deteriorated while on the Vitex, and use of the extract was discontinued prior to completion of the study. When these same horses were subsequently treated with pergolide, eight of nine improved. The results of this single study support the use of pergolide rather than chasteberry extract in the treatment of horses with PPID.

References

1 Tadros, E.M. & Frank, N. (2013) Endocrine disorders and laminitis. *Equine Veterinary Education*, **25**, 152–162.
2 Johnson, P.J. (2002) The equine metabolic syndrome peripheral Cushing's syndrome. *Veterinary Clinics of North America Equine Practice*, **18**, 271–293.
3 Frank, N., Geor, R.J., Bailey, S.R., Durham, A.E. & Johnson, P.J. (2010) Equine metabolic syndrome. *Journal of Veterinary Internal Medicine*, **24**, 467–475.
4 Asplin, K.E., Sillence, M.N., Pollitt, C.C. & McGowan, C.M. (2007) Induction of laminitis by prolonged hyperinsulinaemia in clinically normal ponies. *Veterinary Journal*, **174**, 530–535.
5 de Laat, M.A., McGowan, C.M., Sillence, M.N. & Pollitt, C.C. (2010) Equine laminitis: Induced by 48 h hyperinsulinaemia in Standardbred horses. *Equine Veterinary Journal*, **42**, 129–135.
6 Carter, R.A., Treiber, K.H., Geor, R.J., Douglass, L. & Harris, P.A. (2009) Prediction of incipient pasture-associated laminitis from hyperinsulinaemia, hyperleptinaemia and generalised and localised obesity in a cohort of ponies. *Equine Veterinary Journal*, **41**, 171–178.
7 Treiber, K., Carter, R., Gay, L., Williams, C. & Geor, R. (2009) Inflammatory and redox status of ponies with a history of pasture-associated laminitis. *Veterinary Immunology and Immunopathology*, **129**, 216–220.
8 McGowan, C.M., Frost, R., Pfeiffer, D.U. & Neiger, R. (2004) Serum insulin concentrations in horses with equine Cushing's syndrome: Response to a cortisol inhibitor and prognostic value. *Equine Veterinary Journal*, **36**, 295–298.
9 McGowan, C.M. (2008) The role of insulin in endocrinopathic laminitis. *Journal of Equine Veterinary Science*, **28**, 603–607.
10 Walsh, D.M., McGowan, C.M., McGowan, T., Lamb, S.V., Schanbacher, B.J. & Place, N.J. (2009) Correlation of plasma

insulin concentration with laminitis score in a field study of equine Cushing's disease and equine metabolic syndrome. *Journal of Equine Veterinary Science*, **29**, 87–94.

11 Karikoski, N.P., Horn, I., McGowan, T.W. & McGowan, C.M. (2011) The prevalence of endocrinopathic laminitis among horses presented for laminitis at a first-opinion/referral equine hospital. *Domestic Animal Endocrinology*, **41**, 111–117.

12 Donaldson, M.T., Jorgensen, A.J. & Beech, J. (2004) Evaluation of suspected pituitary pars intermedia dysfunction in horses with laminitis. *Journal of the American Veterinary Medical Association*, **224**, 1123–1127.

13 de Laat, M.A., Pollitt, C.C., Kyaw-Tanner, M.T., McGowan, C.M. & Sillence, M.N. (2013) A potential role for lamellar insulin-like growth factor-1 receptor in the pathogenesis of hyperinsulinaemic laminitis. *Veterinary Journal*, **197**, 302–306.

14 McGowan, C.M., Dugdale, A.H., Pinchbeck, G.L. & Argo, C.M. (2013) Dietary restriction in combination with a nutraceutical supplement for the management of equine metabolic syndrome in horses. *Veterinary Journal*, **196**, 153–159.

15 Breuhaus, B.A. (2009) Thyroid function in anhidrotic horses. *Journal of Veterinary Internal Medicine*, **23**, 168–173.

16 Breuhaus, B.A. (2003) Thyroid function in mature horses ingesting endophyte-infected fescue seed. *Journal of the American Veterinary Medical Association*, **223**, 340–345.

17 Breuhaus, B.A. (2011) Disorders of the equine thyroid gland. *Veterinary Clinics of North America*, **27**, 115–128.

18 Meredith, T.B. & Dobrinski, I. (2004) Thyroid function and pregnancy status in broodmares. *Journal of the American Veterinary Medical Association*, **224**, 892–894.

19 Frank, N., Elliott, S.B. & Boston, R.C. (2008) Effects of long-term oral administration of levothyroxine sodium on glucose dynamics in healthy adult horses. *American Journal of Veterinary Research*, **69**, 76–81.

20 Frank, N., Buchanan, B.R. & Elliott, S.B. (2008) Effects of long-term oral administration of levothyroxine sodium on serum thyroid hormone concentrations, clinicopathologic variables, and echocardiographic measurements in healthy adult horses. *American Journal of Veterinary Research*, **69**, 68–75.

21 Sommardahl, C.S., Frank, N., Elliott, S.B. *et al.* (2005) Effects of oral administration of levothyroxine sodium on serum concentrations of thyroid gland hormones and responses to injections of thyrotropin-releasing hormone in healthy adult mares. *American Journal of Veterinary Research*, **66**, 1025–1031.

22 Chameroy, K.A. (2010) *Diagnosis and management of horses with equine metabolic syndrome (EMS)*. PhD Dissertation, University of Tennessee, Knoxville. http://trace.tennessee.edu/utk_graddiss/871 [accessed on May 5, 2014].

23 Frank, N. (2009) Equine metabolic syndrome. In: B.P. Smith (ed), *Large Animal Internal Medicine*, 4th edn, pp. 1352–1355. Mosby, St Louis.

24 Rena, G., Pearson, E.R. & Sakamoto, K. (2013) Molecular mechanism of action of metformin: Old or new insights? *Diabetologia*, **56**, 1898–1906.

25 Lee, J.O., Lee, S.K., Kim, J.H. *et al.* (2012) Metformin regulates glucose transporter 4 (GLUT4) translocation through AMP-activated protein kinase (AMPK)-mediated Cbl/CAP signaling in 3T3-L1 preadipocyte cells. *Journal of Biological Chemistry*, **287**, 44121–44129.

26 Bailey, C.J., Wilcock, D. & Scarpello, J.H.B. (2008) Metformin and the intestines. *Diabetologia*, **51**, 1552–1553.

27 Zhou, G., Myers, R., Li, Y. *et al.* (2001) Role of AMP-activated protein kinase in mechanism of metformin action. *Journal of Clinical Investigation*, **108**, 1167–1174.

28 Duong, J.K., Kumar, S.S., Kirkpatrick, C.M. *et al.* (2013) Population pharmacokinetics of metformin in healthy subjects and patients with type 2 diabetes mellitus: Simulation of doses according to renal function. *Clinical Pharmacokinetics*, **52**, 373–384.

29 Renda, F., Mura, P., Finco, G., Ferrazin, F., Pani, L. & Landoni, G. (2013) Metformin-associated lactic acidosis requiring hospitalization. A national 10 year survey and a systematic literature review. *European Review for Medical and Pharmacological Sciences*, **17**, 45–49.

30 Hustace, J.L., Firshman, A.M. & Mata, J.E. (2009) Pharmacokinetics and bioavailability of metformin in horses. *American Journal of Veterinary Research*, **70**, 665–668.

31 Tinworth, K.D., Edwards, S., Noble, G.K., Harris, P.A., Sillence, M.N. & Hackett, L.P. (2010) Pharmacokinetics of metformin after enteral administration in insulin-resistant ponies. *American Journal of Veterinary Research*, **71**, 1201–1206.

32 Scheen, A.J. (1996) Clinical pharmacokinetics of metformin. *Clinical Pharmacokinetics*, **30**, 359–371.

33 Vick, M.M., Sessions, D.R., Murphy, B.A., Kennedy, E.L., Reedy, S.E. & Fitzgerald, B.P. (2006) Obesity is associated with altered metabolic and reproductive activity in the mare: Effects of metformin on insulin sensitivity and reproductive cyclicity. *Reproduction, Fertility and Development*, **18**, 609–617.

34 Chameroy, K., Frank, N. & Elliott, S.B. (2010) Effects of metformin hydrochloride on glucose dynamics during transition to grass paddocks in insulin-resistant horses [abstract]. *Journal of Veterinary Internal Medicine*, **24**, 690.

35 Durham, A.E., Rendle, D.I. & Newton, J.E. (2008) The effect of metformin on measurements of insulin sensitivity and beta cell response in 18 horses and ponies with insulin resistance. *Equine Veterinary Journal*, **40**, 493–500.

36 Tinworth, K.D., Boston, R.C., Harris, P.A., Sillence, M.N., Raidal, S.L. & Noble, G.K. (2012) The effect of oral metformin on insulin sensitivity in insulin-resistant ponies. *Veterinary Journal*, **191**, 79–84.

37 Durham, A.E. (2012) Metformin in equine metabolic syndrome: An enigma or a dead duck? *Veterinary Journal*, **191**, 17–18.

38 Rendle, D.I., Rutledge, F., Hughes, K.J., Heller, J. & Durham, A.E. (2013) Effects of metformin hydrochloride on blood glucose and insulin responses to oral dextrose in horses. *Equine Veterinary Journal*, **45**, 751–754.

39 Respondek, F., Myers, K., Smith, T.L., Wagner, A. & Geor, R.J. (2011) Dietary supplementation with short-chain fructo-oligosaccharides improves insulin sensitivity in obese horses. *Journal of Animal Science*, **89**, 77–83.

40 Brosnahan, M.M. & Paradis, M.R. (2003) Assessment of clinical characteristics, management practices, and activities of geriatric horses. *Journal of the American Veterinary Medical Association*, **223**, 99–103.

41 Ireland, J.L., Clegg, P.D., McGowan, C.M., McKane, S.A., Chandler, K.J. & Pinchbeck, G.L. (2012) Disease prevalence in geriatric horses in the United Kingdom: Veterinary clinical assessment of 200 cases. *Equine Veterinary Journal*, **44**, 101–106.

42 McGowan, T.W., Pinchbeck, G.P. & McGowan, C.M. (2012) Prevalence, risk factors and clinical signs predictive for equine pituitary pars intermedia dysfunction in aged horses. *Equine Veterinary Journal*, **45**, 74–79.

43 McFarlane, D., Dybdal, N., Donaldson, M.T., Miller, L. & Cribb, A.E. (2005) Nitration and increased alpha-synuclein expression associated with dopaminergic neurodegeneration in equine pituitary pars intermedia dysfunction. *Journal of Neuroendocrinology*, **17**, 73–80.

44 McGowan, T.W. (2010) *Aged horse health, management and welfare*. PhD Dissertation, University of Queensland, Brisbane. http://espace.library.uq.edu.au/view/UQ:180103 [accessed on May 5, 2014].

45 Orth, D.N., Holscher, M.A., Wilson, M.G., Nicholson, W.E., Plue, R.E. & Mount, C.D. (1982) Equine Cushing's disease: Plasma immunoreactive proopiolipomelanocortin peptide and cortisol levels basally and in response to diagnostic tests. *Endocrinology*, **110**, 1430–1441.

46 Beech, J. & Garcia, M.C. (1991) Diseases of the endocrine system. In: P.T. Colahan, I.G. Mayhew, A.M. Merritt & J.N. Moore (eds), *Equine Medicine and Surgery*, 4th edn, pp. 1737–1751. American Veterinary Publications, Goleta.

47 Peters, D.F., Erfle, J.B. & Slobojan, G.T. (1995) Low-dose pergolide mesylate treatment for equine hypophyseal adenomas (Cushing's syndrome). *Proceedings of the 41st Annual Convention of the American Association of Equine Practitioner*. AAEP, Lexington, pp. 154–155.

48 Kvernmo, T., Hartter, S. & Burger, E. (2006) A review of the receptor-binding and pharmacokinetic properties of dopamine agonists. *Clinical Therapeutics*, **28**, 1065–1078.

49 Perez-Lloret, S. & Rascol, O. (2010) Dopamine receptor agonists for the treatment of early or advanced Parkinson's disease. *CNS Drugs*, **24**, 941–968.

50 Gehring, R., Beard, L., Wright, A., Coetzee, J., Havel, J. & Apley, M. (2010) Single-dose oral pharmacokinetics of pergolide mesylate in healthy adult mares. *Veterinary Therapeutics*, **11**, E1–E8.

51 FDA (2011) *Freedom of information summary*. http://www.fda.gov/downloads/AnimalVeterinary/Products/ApprovedAnimalDrugProducts/FOIADrugSummaries/UCM280354.pdf [accessed on December 24, 2013].

52 Pritchett, A.M., Morrison, J.F., Edwards, W.D., Schaff, H.V., Connolly, H.M. & Espinosa, R.E. (2002) Valvular heart disease in patients taking pergolide. *Mayo Clinic Proceedings*, **77**, 1280–1286.

53 Corvol, J.C., Anzouan-Kacou, J.B., Fauveau, E. *et al.* (2007) Heart valve regurgitation, pergolide use, and parkinson disease: An observational study and meta-analysis. *Archives of Neurology*, **64**, 1721–1726.

54 Zanettini, R., Antonini, A., Gatto, G., Gentile, R., Tesei, S. & Pezzoli, G. (2007) Valvular heart disease and the use of dopamine agonists for Parkinson's disease. *New England Journal of Medicine*, **356**, 39–46.

55 Steiger, M., Jost, W., Grandas, F. & Van Camp, G. (2009) Risk of valvular heart disease associated with the use of dopamine agonists in Parkinson's disease: A systematic review. *Journal of Neural Transmission*, **116**, 179–191.

56 FDA (2012) *FDA statement on the compounding of pergolide products for animal use*. http://www.fda.gov/AnimalVeterinary/NewsEvents/CVMUpdates/ucm296371.htm [accessed on May 5, 2014].

57 Davis, J.L., Kirk, L.M., Davidson, G.S. & Papich, M.G. (2009) Effects of compounding and storage conditions on stability of pergolide mesylate. *Journal of the American Veterinary Medical Association*, **234**, 385–389.

58 Stanley, S.D. & Knych, H.D. (2011) Comparison of pharmaceutical equivalence for compounded preparations of pergolide mesylate. *Proceedings of the 56th Annual Convention of the American Association of Equine Practitioners*. AAEP, Lexington, pp. 274–276.

59 Donaldson, M.T., LaMonte, B.H., Morresey, P., Smith, G. & Beech, J. (2002) Treatment with pergolide or cyproheptadine of pituitary pars intermedia dysfunction (equine Cushing's disease). *Journal of Veterinary Internal Medicine*, **16**, 742–746.

60 Perkins, G.A., Lamb, S., Erb, H.N., Schanbacher, B., Nydam, D.V. & Divers, T.J. (2002) Plasma adrenocorticotropin (ACTH) concentrations and clinical response in horses treated for equine Cushing's disease with cyproheptadine or pergolide. *Equine Veterinary Journal*, **34**, 679–685.

61 Schott, H.C. (2002) Pituitary pars intermedia dysfunction: Equine Cushing's disease. *Veterinary Clinics of North America Equine Practice*, **18**, 237–270.

62 Pease, A.P., Schott, H.C., Howey, E.B. & Patterson, J.S. (2011) Computed tomographic findings in the pituitary gland and brain of horses with pituitary pars intermedia dysfunction. *Journal of Veterinary Internal Medicine*, **25**, 1144–1151.

63 Cordero, M., McFarlane, D., Breshears, M., Miller, L., Miller, M. & Duckett, W. (2012) The effect of season on histologic and histomorphometric appearance of the equine

pituitary gland. *Journal of Equine Veterinary Science*, **32**, 75–79.

64 Singh, D. & Goel, R.K. (2010) Proconvulsant potential of cyproheptadine in experimental animal models. *Fundamental & Clinical Pharmacology*, **24**, 451–455.

65 McGowan, C.M. & Neiger, R. (2003) Efficacy of trilostane for the treatment of equine Cushing's syndrome. *Equine Veterinary Journal*, **35**, 414–418.

66 Glover, C.M., Miller, L.M., Dybdal, N.O., Lopez, A., Duckett, W.M. & McFarlane, D. (2009) Extrapituitary and pituitary pathological findings in horses with pituitary pars intermedia dysfunction: A retrospective study. *Journal of Equine Veterinary Science.*, **29**, 146–153.

67 Boujon, C.E., Bestetti, G.E., Meier, H.P., Straub, R., Junker, U. & Rossi, G.L. (1993) Equine pituitary adenoma: A functional and morphological study. *Journal of Comparative Pathology*, **109**, 163–178.

68 Heinrichs, M., Baumgartner, W. & Capen, C.C. (1990) Immunocytochemical demonstration of proopiomelano-cortin-derived peptides in pituitary adenomas of the pars intermedia in horses. *Veterinary Pathology*, **27**, 419–425.

69 Beech, J. (2002) Comparison of Vitex agnus castus extract and pergolide in treatment of equine Cushing's syndrome. *Proceedings of the 48th Annual Convention of the American Association of Equine Practitioners*. AAEP, Lexington, pp. 175–177.

CHAPTER 16

Equine cardiovascular clinical pharmacology

Meg Sleeper

School of Veterinary Medicine, University of Pennsylvania, Philadelphia, PA, USA

Both in the acute phase and long term, horses are being treated for heart disease more and more commonly. Many therapies are empirical and based on data from other species; however, more data are becoming available regarding the efficacy of many of agents in the horse. It is important to remember, however, that most agents used for therapy of heart disease are not specifically approved for use in horses. In addition, the data available are often from studies that included only a small number of horses, making it impossible to predict idiosyncratic adverse effects. Moreover, many studies use healthy horses, making extrapolation to horses with heart disease tenuous at best. Finally, for many drugs administered to horses, oral bioavailability can be very poor, which limits dosing options [1].

Congestive heart failure

Congestive heart failure (CHF) occurs most frequently in the horse secondary to mitral and/or aortic regurgitation. However, heart failure has also been reported to occur secondary to congenital heart disease, pericardial disease, and myocardial disease in the horse [2]. The goals of medical therapy regardless of the underlying cause of CHF are to improve cardiac output, promote diuresis of excessive body fluid, and normalize tissue perfusion and oxygenation. There are four primary cardiovascular determinants of cardiac output that can be altered by drugs: preload, afterload, myocardial contractility (inotropy), and heart rate.

Acute management of CHF

Reduction of cardiac filling pressure or preload is one of the mainstays of heart failure treatment in all species, and the most commonly used medication is the diuretic furosemide (Table 16.1). Furosemide inhibits $Na+$, $K+$, and $Cl-$ resorption in the ascending loop of Henle, leading to increased excretion of water, $Na+$, $Cl-$, $K+$, $Ca++$, $Mg++$, $H+$, HCO_3-, and PO_4-. Furosemide should be administered intravenously or intramuscularly at a dose of 1–2 mg/kg bwt every 6–12 h to control pulmonary edema (Table 16.3). Subsequent dosing can be adjusted according to the patient's response. Intravenously administered furosemide (1 mg/kg) results in a diuretic effect within 5–10 min with a peak effect 15–30 min after injection. A rapid decline in the diuretic effect follows, which appears to be due to rapid elimination of the drug [3]. Intramuscular administration resulted in a more prolonged effect with excretion of about 50% more urine [3]. These results suggest IM administration is likely to be more effective than IV in the horse with CHF. The response may be suboptimal in horses with low cardiac output and poor renal perfusion. Additionally, aggressive therapy with furosemide can lead to significant dehydration and electrolyte disturbances, and these patients should be monitored closely. Monitoring is particularly critical in patients receiving concurrent digoxin, as dehydration and azotemia, hypokalemia, and hypomagnesemia predispose to cardiac glycoside toxicity.

Table 16.1 Classification of drugs used to treat CHF.

Effect	Drug
Preload reducers	Diuretics: furosemide
Afterload reducers	Hydralazine, ACEI
Positive inotropes	Digoxin, sympathomimetics, phosphodiesterase inhibitors (PDI)

Equine Pharmacology, First Edition. Edited by Cynthia Cole, Bradford Bentz and Lara Maxwell.
© 2015 John Wiley & Sons, Inc. Published 2015 by John Wiley & Sons, Inc.

Constant rate infusion (CRI) of furosemide has been reported in human and canine patients to increase urine volume and sodium excretion and possibly reduce fluctuations in electrolyte and fluid balance compared to bolus administration [4, 5]. One study compared furosemide CRI (0.12 mg/kg/h) to IV dosing of 1 mg/kg bwt furosemide every 8 h in five normal horses. The CRI of furosemide followed administration of a loading dose (0.12 mg/kg bwt IV). Four of the five horses produced more urine after CRI compared to bolus administration of furosemide over 24 h; however, the mean difference was not statistically significant. However, efficacy of CRI diuresis was markedly enhanced over the first 8 h, suggesting the administration method may be useful acutely in cases that require profound diuresis [6].

Bumetanide (2.2 µg/kg bwt IV) is a more potent loop diuretic than furosemide, which has been suggested to be useful in treating severely affected equine patients [7, 8]. In humans, it has more predictable absorption, and therefore response, than furosemide. The potential side effects and drug interactions, however, would be similar to those seen with furosemide. At this time, the preponderance of experience using furosemide in horses compared to bumetanide makes furosemide the preferred first choice diuretic.

Afterload reduction with arteriodilators is an important focus of CHF therapy in other species (Table 16.1). These drugs increase forward stroke volume and cardiac output and decrease the regurgitant fraction when left heart valve disease is present. However, there is limited data to substantiate the use of vasodilator therapy in the treatment of heart failure in horses. Hydralazine is an arterial vasodilator that has minimal effects on the venous system. It is available in an injectable and an oral formulation. Results from one study suggest the drug may have a direct, positive inotropic effect independent of afterload reduction [7]. In horses, hydralazine has been shown to result in vasodilation when administered at a dose of 0.5 mg/kg bwt IV [9]. In that study, cardiac output and heart rate increased for 260 min following the single dose, while mean arterial and central venous blood pressures did not change from baseline values. For long-term therapy, a dose of 0.5–1.5 mg/kg bwt, orally (PO), q12 h has been suggested, but efficacy by this route has not been tested [7, 10].

Diltiazem is a calcium channel blocker that is used in humans and dogs for management of supraventricular arrhythmias, and it leads to reduced systemic blood pressure in humans [11]. In a study designed to ascertain an effective dose and monitor the hemodynamic effects of diltiazem in the horse, intravenous (IV) diltiazem decreased systemic blood pressure and systolic function in normal horses [12]. In a later study, the same group demonstrated that the equine response to diltiazem is variable and its use requires careful monitoring of hemodynamic parameters [13]. In summary, diltiazem should only be used with extreme caution in horses affected with CHF unless additional studies suggest otherwise. Moreover, its efficacy when administered PO is uncertain. Nitrovasodilators and promazine have not been evaluated in horses.

Sympathomimetic agents are the drugs used most commonly in equine patients with myocardial failure (systolic failure) to increase cardiac inotropy (contractility) during the acute management of CHF (Table 16.1). These agents are short acting and must be administered by a CRI. Dobutamine (1–10 µg/kg/min IV) is the synthetic catecholamine that is used most frequently in the horse because it appears to be the least arrhythmogenic in this species. Dobutamine acts on cardiac B1 adrenoceptors to increase contractility, resulting in increased cardiac output and arterial pressure with minimal effect on peripheral vascular resistance, but does not significantly affect the heart rate [8]. In contrast, dopamine acts on variable receptors depending on its administration rate. At a low administration rate (<3 µg/kg/min IV), dopamine acts on dopamine receptors to increase blood flow in the renal and mesenteric vascular beds. At higher administration rates, it also acts on B1 adrenoceptors, resulting in increased cardiac output. However, at higher rates, dopamine also acts on peripheral α adrenoreceptors to cause vasoconstriction. For this reason and because dobutamine is less arrhythmogenic and improves cardiac output more than dopamine, dobutamine is generally preferred over dopamine in equine cases of cardiac failure [8].

Phosphodiesterase III inhibitors (PDEIII-I) have become an important part of heart failure management in small animal cardiac patients. These drugs result in increased cardiac contractility and vasodilation and are therefore often referred to as "inodilators." Pimobendan is a PDEIII-I, which also sensitizes the mechanical apparatus of the cardiomyocyte to calcium, thereby increasing contractility by another mechanism as well. In the dog, it is very fast acting and can be used in acute phase control of CHF, as well as long-term management

[14]. However, there are only anecdotal reports of the use of this agent in horses with CHF, and it is likely to remain cost prohibitive for the near future. In addition, pharmacokinetic/pharmacodynamic studies have not been performed in the horse to date. Milrinone is another PDEIII-I that is used in human patients for short-term treatment of severe myocardial failure. Milrinone has been shown to produce beneficial hemodynamic effects in halothane-anesthetized horses, although at this time it is likely to be cost prohibitive for most equine patients [15]. Although digoxin is available in an injectable form, the sympathomimetics are generally preferred because of the ease with which IV digoxin can lead to toxicosis. If deemed necessary, however, digitalization using the maintenance dose administered IV is less likely to cause toxicosis than loading doses, and a clinical response is generally observed within 48 h of the initial dose [16]. Monitoring of serum digoxin concentrations is important due to the variable disposition of the drug among different horses [16].

Arrhythmia management is discussed in a separate section of this chapter, but it is important to remember that significant bradycardia (<20 bpm) and tachycardia (>90 bpm) will decrease cardiac output. Therefore, optimizing the heart rate is an important part of therapy for the CHF patient.

Chronic management of CHF

Furosemide is the most commonly used preload reducer in the acute as well as chronic stages of heart failure. Once an animal has developed CHF, it is rare that medications can ever be stopped, and furosemide therapy is expected to continue for the remainder of the horse's life. Exceptions to this rule would be those cases in which cardiac function improves (i.e., CHF is secondary to a rapid tachyarrhythmia, myocarditis, etc. that respond to medical management). For the vast majority of cases, however, long-term therapy with furosemide is necessary (0.25–2 mg/kg bwt every 8–12 h IM or IV). Unfortunately, although furosemide is effective after administration PO in other species, systemic availability was poor and variable in a study evaluating oral furosemide administration in normal horses, and the drug is not recommended to be administered by this route in this species [6].

Angiotensin-converting enzyme inhibitors (ACEI) are a mainstay of chronic CHF therapy in other species. ACEI inhibit the conversion of angiotensin I to angiotensin II. Angiotensin II is a potent vasoconstrictor leading to increased systemic blood pressure, myocardial work, and myocardial oxygen demand. Angiotensin II has also been linked to deleterious myocardial remodeling. ACEI are the most commonly used afterload reducers in veterinary cardiology. However, although enaprilat, the active metabolite of enalapril, has been shown to cause arterial dilation in anesthetized horses, two other studies suggest that the prodrug administered PO to horses is not effective [17]. Following a single oral dose enalapril (0.5 mg/kg bwt), there was no demonstrable pharmacodynamic effect or suppression of ACE activity [18]. Similarly, following 2 months of oral administration in normal ponies, ACE activity was unchanged compared to controls [19]. Therefore, systemic availability of enalapril appears to be poor when administered PO in the horse either because it is poorly absorbed or because it is inadequately converted to its active form. Some clinicians believe they have seen a positive clinical response in horses with heart disease treated with enalapril. However, it is difficult to recommend it for use in horses unless further studies demonstrate an effective dose or formulation. Two reports exist in the literature suggesting alternative ACEI may be more effective in horses. A case report describes the beneficial use of ramipril (50 µg/kg bwt once daily) in a horse with CHF [20]. In another report, 20 horses with mitral valve disease were treated with quinapril (120 mg/horse/day for 8 weeks) [21]. In that study, the horses had improved stroke volume and cardiac output; however, the study was unblinded and there was no control group. Clearly, additional efficacy studies using ACEI in horses with heart disease are warranted.

Angiotensin receptor blockers have not been evaluated in the horse to date. However, hydralazine (see acute CHF section) has been recommended as an effective afterload reducer in the horse at a dose of 0.5–1.5 mg/kg bwt, PO, q12 h [7, 10].

The most commonly used positive inotropic agent in the horse for chronic therapy is digoxin. Digoxin blocks the myocardial Na+/K+ pump resulting in elevated intracellular Na+ concentrations, which are then exchanged for Ca++. The results are increased intracellular calcium concentrations and increased inotropy. Digoxin also increases parasympathetic activity and slows atrioventricular (AV) nodal conduction (see section on treating cardiac arrhythmias). The recommended dose is 2.2 μg/kg bwt, IV, q12 h or 11 μg/kg bwt, PO, q12 h [16, 22]. If it is deemed clinically important to rapidly digitalize a horse, a loading dose of 11 μg/kg bwt IV can be administered slowly or divided into two doses the first day, followed by oral maintenance dosing [10] (Table 16.3). The clinician must remember, however, that rapid digitalization significantly increases the risk of the development of toxic serum concentrations, and therefore, there are very few cases in which this approach is warranted. Because there is wide variability in the response to digoxin among horses, therapeutic drug monitoring is recommended. Trough and peak (~2 h post drug administration) concentrations of digoxin should be between 0.5 and 2.0 ng/ml [16]. When therapeutic drug monitoring is not possible, the electrocardiogram should be reviewed for signs of digoxin toxicity, including sinus bradycardia, PR prolongation, and ST interval and T wave changes [8]. Additional signs of digoxin toxicity include depression, anorexia, and constipation. Hypokalemia, hypoproteinemia, renal failure, and dehydration predispose to digoxin toxicity by increasing plasma concentrations of the active drug [8]. Acute digoxin toxicity can be treated by discontinuing digoxin administration and promoting diuresis. In addition, digoxin antibodies are available, but they are generally cost prohibitive in large animals. Digoxin should be administered with caution in horses with reduced renal function and is contraindicated in cases of suspected ionophore (i.e., monensin) or cardiac glycoside (i.e., *oleander* spp.) toxicosis. Pimobendan (see acute CHF section) is a more efficacious positive inotrope; however, as mentioned previously, it is expensive and there is no pharmacokinetic or pharmacodynamic data from horses.

Theophylline and aminophylline are xanthine derivatives and bronchodilators that have positive inotropic and chronotropic effects [23]. They are also PDEIII-I but they are rarely used for their inotropic effect, although they are useful in some cases of bradycardia (see the treatment of bradycardia section).

Medical management of cardiac arrhythmias

The treatment of cardiac arrhythmias should always include consideration of possible underlying disease processes and correction of acid–base and/or electrolyte imbalances. Some arrhythmias secondary to myocarditis will respond to corticosteroid therapy. Many antiarrhythmic agents, in particular the ventricular antiarrhythmics, have proarrhythmic potential and may actually predispose the patient to fatal arrhythmias. Therefore, therapy is only recommended if clinical signs are associated with the presence of the rhythm disturbance or if a rapid ventricular tachycardia (VT) is present.

Supraventricular arrhythmias

Atrial fibrillation (AF) is by far the most important dysrhythmia in horses. It is the most common cardiovascular cause of poor performance in the equine athlete [24]. An important factor in the formation of this arrhythmia is atrial size, which explains why horses are particularly predisposed. AF frequently occurs in horses with no evidence of underlying cardiac disease (lone AF); however, the longer the arrhythmia is present, the more likely electrical remodeling will occur, which results in increased stability of the arrhythmia [25–27]. Therefore, the longer the AF has been present, the more difficult it is to convert the horse to a sinus rhythm. Similarly, in horses with AF and underlying heart disease (underlying cardiomegaly increases the risk of AF development in this population), conversion is more difficult and recurrence of AF is more common [27].

Traditionally, oral quinidine sulfate has been the treatment of choice for horses with AF. Quinidine is a class IA sodium channel blocker, which increases the myocardial refractory period and prolongs the QRS and QT intervals (Table 16.2). It also has vagolytic and peripheral vasodilatory effects. Horses with recent onset AF (<2 months) may be treated effectively with IV quinidine (quinidine gluconate) [28]. The recommended dosing frequency is 1.1–2.2 mg/kg bwt every 10 min to a total dose of 9–11 mg/kg bwt (or until conversion or signs of toxicity develop) [7] (Table 16.3). If unsuccessful or if AF has been present for longer than 2 months, oral quinidine (quinidine sulfate) using a dosing regimen of 22 mg/kg bwt administered via nasogastric tube every 2 h to a total dose of 88–132 mg/kg bwt (or until conversion or signs of toxicity develop) is the standard protocol [28]. If neither conversion nor signs of toxicity occur, therapy can be continued at a dosing rate of 22 mg/kg bwt administered via nasogastric tube every 6 h. Therapeutic drug monitoring of quinidine serum concentrations is very helpful to avoid toxicity and is particularly critical in horses that are treated beyond the first day with quinidine. The maximum plasma concentration range is 2–5 µg/ml. When this range is exceeded, toxic signs are common and conversion to sinus rhythm is unlikely [28]. If quinidine plasma concentrations cannot be obtained promptly, a total dose of 88 mg/kg bwt q2 h should not

be exceeded [22]. Quinidine is contraindicated in horses with AF and concurrent heart failure. These horses should be treated as described above for CHF and with digoxin in order to control the ventricular response rate.

In horses without underlying heart disease, quinidine's efficacy ranges from 62 to 92% [29, 26]. However, the prognosis for successful conversion decreases and the likelihood of recurrence increases the longer the duration of the disease. Therefore, it is critical that a complete heart exam is performed prior to attempting conversion. Also, therapy with quinidine can result in potentially serious consequences including diarrhea, colic, and sudden death [29]. Other common adverse signs include systemic hypotension, upper respiratory tract edema, and depression [8]. Horses undergoing treatment should be kept in quiet surroundings, and the electrocardiogram should be monitored. It is important to monitor the ventricular response rate and to evaluate the ECG for other changes associated with quinidine toxicity including QRS prolongation or development of new cardiac arrhythmias. QRS prolongation greater than 125% should prompt discontinuation of quinidine therapy [8]. Similarly, rapid supraventricular or ventricular arrhythmias

Table 16.2 Classification of antiarrhythmic drugs.

Class	Drug
I	Sodium channel blockers
IA	Quinidine, procainamide
IB	Lidocaine, mexiletine, tocainide, phenytoin
IC	Flecainide, propafenone
II	Beta adrenergic receptor blockers Propranolol, sotalol
III	Potassium channel blockers Amiodarone, sotalol, bretylium
IV	Calcium channel blockers Diltiazem

Table 16.3 Drugs commonly used to treat cardiovascular disease.

Drug	Dose
Quinidine	Oral: 22 mg/kg bwt quinidine sulfate by nasogastric tube every 2 h (see text) IV: 1.1–2.2 mg/kg bwt q10 min up to total dose of 9–11 mg/kg bwt
Procainamide	Oral: 25–35 mg/kg bwt q8 h IV: 1 mg/kg/minute up to a total dose of 20 mg/kg bwt
Magnesium	IV: 1 g/min to effect up to a maximum of 25 g/450 kg horse
Lidocaine	IV: 0.1–0.25 mg/kg bwt slowly up to a total dose of 0.5 mg/kg bwt
Propranolol	IV: 0.05–0.16 mg/kg q12 h (administer over 1 min)
Digoxin	Oral: loading 34–70 µg/kg bwt, maintenance 11–35 µg/kg q12 h (use lower dose with tablets and higher dose with elixir) IV: loading 11–14 µg/kg bwt, maintenance 2.2–7 µg/kg bwt once a day (IV administration and/or loading dose protocols are not usually recommended due to the narrow therapeutic window (see text))
Furosemide	IV or IM: 0.25–2.0 mg/kg bwt as needed to control pulmonary edema; CRI, 0.12 mg/kg loading dose followed by 0.12 mg/kg/h
Hydralazine	Oral: 0.5–1.5 mg/kg bwt q12 h IV: 0.5 mg/kg bwt q12 h

(>100 bpm) should prompt discontinuation of quinidine and initiation of specific antiarrhythmic therapy. In man, high serum quinidine concentrations have abortogenic and teratogenic effects; however, in the one case report describing its use in a pregnant mare with AF, no ill effects were recognized [30].

Accelerated AV conduction occurs in up to half of horses treated with quinidine because of the drug's vagolytic effect [28]. For this reason, digitalization has historically been recommended prior to initiating quinidine therapy in horses with elevated heart rates. The addition of digoxin is also warranted if conversion to sinus has not occurred after 2 days of quinidine therapy. Quinidine decreases renal clearance of digoxin and can increase serum digoxin concentrations [31]. Therefore, therapeutic monitoring of digoxin serum concentrations is indicated for horses receiving both drugs. Diltiazem, administered IV, has also been evaluated as a way to control accelerated AV conduction. However, two of eight horses developed severe hypotension and sinus arrest during diltiazem administration [12]. The study concluded that IV diltiazem administration in healthy horses is reasonably safe but requires careful monitoring. It was hypothesized that if the frequency dependence of the diltiazem that has been demonstrated in other species occurs in horses, lower dosages in horses with tachycardia may be efficacious, thereby minimizing adverse effects. To test this hypothesis, the effect of diltiazem on AV conduction with IV coadministration of quinidine in horses was determined. The results of that study showed that diltiazem's effect on AV nodal conduction was rate dependent. During rapid electrical stimulation to model atrial tachycardia, diltiazem administration controlled the ventricular response rate when administered at a dose of 0.125–1.125 mg/kg bwt, although this dose did not slow the heart rate of normal horses [13]. Therefore, although IV diltiazem may be effective for rapid supraventricular rhythms, it should be used with careful hemodynamic monitoring, particularly in horses with cardiac dysfunction.

Beta-blockers such as propranolol (0.05–0.16 mg/kg bwt IV) can also be used to address the development of rapid supraventricular tachycardia during quinidine administration [7]. The pharmacologic effect achieved will depend on the degree of sympathetic tone present. Propranolol is available in oral and injectable formulations, but bioavailability is very low when administered

PO to horses [23]. Ventricular arrhythmias should be addressed with magnesium sulfate, lidocaine, or propranolol. (See further discussion of these agents under ventricular antiarrhythmic therapy.) Mineral oil or activated charcoal may be administered to limit further drug absorption, and IV fluid therapy is recommended in cases of hypotension and for cardiovascular support. Intravenous sodium bicarbonate (1 mEq/kg bwt) is useful to increase protein binding of free quinidine, which will decrease the circulating free or active drug [28]. Finally, phenylephrine (0.01–0.02 mg/kg bwt IV) can be administered in cases of intractable hypotension.

AF conversion with quinidine has been an established protocol with reasonable efficacy and low cost for years [24, 32]. However, because of the risks associated with quinidine therapy and the fact that it is not always effective, other alternatives for conversion of AF to sinus rhythm continue to be evaluated. Electrical cardioversion is routinely used in humans for restoration of sinus rhythm, and transvenous electrical cardioversion has proven to be effective in the treatment of equine lone AF as well [32–34]. The procedure appears to be well tolerated for the short term and is an excellent option for AF patients when available [35]. However, the procedure requires specialized equipment that is not widely available, and therefore, medical management of AF will continue to be widely used for equine AF patients. In addition, medical conversion approaches, other than quinidine, have also been evaluated, but it is important to keep in mind that at this time, quinidine remains the best choice for medical conversion of AF.

Procainamide is a class IA antiarrhythmic, similar to quinidine; however, it is less effective in treating supraventricular arrhythmias [8] (Table 16.2). The direct hemodynamic effects of procainamide are the same as quinidine, but they are less pronounced. For example, procainamide rarely results in significant hypotension. Its active metabolite, N-acetyl procainamide, blocks potassium channels in myocardial cells, prolonging the action potential. The recommended IV administration regime for procainamide in the horse is 1 mg/kg/min up to a total dose of 20 mg/kg bwt. The oral recommended dose is 25–35 mg/kg bwt, PO, q8 h [7] (Table 16.3).

Amiodarone is a class III antiarrhythmic, which has also been used in the treatment of horses with AF (Table 16.3). Because of extremely poor bioavailability and expense, oral amiodarone therapy has too many limitations to be useful in the horse [36]. However, in a pharmacokinetic and pharmacodynamic study of a single IV amiodarone administration in seven normal ponies, 5–7 mg/kg bwt over 3–5 min was well tolerated and no side effects were noted [37]. Cardiac effects of the drug included an increase in heart rate, changes in the T waves, and prolongation of the QT interval, when corrected for the increased heart rate. These ECG changes occurred at times when plasma amiodarone concentrations were in the therapeutic range (1.0–2.5 mg/l). In a clinical trial, six horses with chronic AF were treated with a protocol of IV amiodarone (5 mg/kg/h IV over 1 h followed by 0.83 mg/kg/h IV for 23 h and then 1.9 mg/kg/h IV for the following 30 h), and 4 were successfully converted to sinus rhythm [38]. Side effects in this small group of horses were mild and transient. In a second study, the same group used a different two-phase protocol of amiodarone administration to treat six horses with chronic AF. In the first phase, horses received an infusion of 6.52 mg/kg/h for 1 h followed by 1.1 mg/kg/h for 47 h. The second phase, which immediately followed completion of the first phase, consisted of a second loading dose of 3.74 mg/kg/h for 1 h, followed by 1.31 mg/kg/h for 47 h. Three of the six horses converted to sinus rhythm without side effects; however, the other 3 did not convert and all 3 had adverse signs associated with the administration [39]. Adverse signs only appeared in horses that received the drug for more than 36 h. The authors speculated that phospholipidosis may be a mechanism for amiodarone toxicity and that antioxidants, such as oral vitamin E, which reduce phospholipidosis, may be protective; however, this hypothesis has not been tested. From the small amount of data currently available, amiodarone may be an effective antiarrhythmic in the horse; however, caution should be exercised in using the drug for prolonged infusions.

Flecainide is a class IC sodium channel blocker, which has been effective for treating various supraventricular and ventricular arrhythmias in humans (Table 16.2). Ohmura et al. performed a dosing study and found that IV flecainide (1–3 mg/kg bwt IV administered at a rate of 0.2 mg/kg/min) effectively converted 6 of six horses with experimentally induced AF [40]. Two horses with naturally occurring AF were also successfully treated using 0.88–1.28 mg/kg bwt administered at a rate of 0.2 mg/kg/min. The drug was well tolerated in all of the horses. From their results, they suggest the effective equine flecainide dose is up to 2 mg/kg bwt administered

at 0.2 mg/kg/min. In a different study, however, evaluating IV flecainide for conversion in horses with chronic AF, only one of nine horses was successfully returned to sinus rhythm, and this horse had an AF duration of only 12 days [27]. In this study, flecainide was administered at a dose of 2 mg/kg bwt IV and at a rate of 0.2 mg/kg/ min for 10 min. In 3 of the horses, this regimen was followed by another dose of 1 mg/kg bwt at a rate of 0.05–0.10 mg/kg/min for 10–20 min. Horses that failed to convert were treated with the traditional quinidine protocol. Two horses developed ventricular dysrhythmias during the first 15 min of flecainide therapy, which necessitated discontinuing the drug. In contrast, quinidine sulfate given PO restored sinus rhythm in eight of the nine horses uneventfully [27].

In a study that evaluated PO administered flecainide, plasma concentrations of flecainide that were effective for treating AF in the Ohmura et al. study were obtained with doses of 4–6 mg/kg bwt of flecainide [41]. However, the purpose of the study was for pharmacokinetic analysis of oral flecainide in horses; efficacy was not evaluated. One published case report described successful conversion from AF using five doses of oral flecainide (4.1 mg/kg bwt, total dose 2.2 g); however, the horse exhibited signs of colic during the 17 h conversion [42]. These data collectively suggest that although flecainide might be effective in acute cases of AF, it is unlikely to be useful in cases of chronic AF and may cause significant adverse effects.

Sotalol (class III drug with additional β adrenergic blocking effects) and propafenone (class IC antiarrhythmic) have also been used in trials to investigate their use in equine AF cases; however, neither appears particularly effective in this population [43] (Table 16.3). Sotalol was administered as an IV infusion at a dose rate of 0.75–1.25 mg/kg bwt over 15 min, whereas propafenone was administered at a dose of 2 mg/kg bwt over 15 min followed 20 min later by a CRI of 7 μg/kg/min for 120 min. The six horses receiving propafenone had therapeutic concentrations of 20–500 ng/ml, but none of them converted to sinus rhythm. On the other hand, subsequent quinidine therapy resulted in conversion in all six. None of the three horses treated with sotalol converted to sinus rhythm either. Therefore, at this time, quinidine continues to be the first-line option for medical conversion of AF. However, ranolazine is an antianginal drug, which inhibits abnormal late Na+ channel currents. Oral ranolazine has shown efficacy in conversion of human AF, and it is possible future studies will show that it is effective in equines as well [44].

Although much less common than AF, atrial arrhythmias such as supraventricular tachycardia and/or frequent atrial premature contractions (APCs) have also been recognized as a cause of clinical signs in the horse. Intermittent APCs rarely result in symptoms or require specific therapy. In horses that are otherwise normal, atrial tachycardia rarely results in elevated resting heart rates because the high resting vagal tone in this species leads to physiologic AV block. However, with exercise or an underlying cause of vagal inhibition, significant tachycardias can develop. Many of the drugs listed in the AF section are reasonable options to control any supraventricular tachycardia, and conversion of atrial tachycardia can be attempted medically or by electrical cardioversion. Alternatively, digoxin can be used to slow AV nodal conduction and the ventricular response rate.

Ventricular arrhythmias

Antiarrhythmic agents are warranted if ectopy is severe enough to cause signs of low cardiac output, which occurs most often when the heart rate is >100 bpm. Based on extrapolation from human studies, in the presence of other risk factors (e.g., multiform complexes, and R on T phenomenon), it is also of benefit to suppress the ectopy. In addition, persistent tachycardia may result in secondary heart failure within days to weeks [7]. Lidocaine, magnesium sulfate, quinidine gluconate, propranolol, procainamide, phenytoin, and propafenone all have been advocated for the treatment of VT in the horse. In several horses with presumed myocarditis, corticosteroid administration resulted in successful conversion to sinus rhythm; however, its use would be contraindicated in the presence of an active infection [45].

Lidocaine is a local anesthetic and a class IB sodium channel blocker (Table 16.2). The recommended dosing regimen is 0.1–0.25 mg/kg bwt IV slowly every 5 min up to a total dose of 0.5 mg/kg bwt [22] (Table 16.3). The most significant side effects are neurologic (e.g., excitement, ataxia, muscle fasciculations, and seizures) secondary to central nervous system stimulation. Diazepam (0.05–0.4 mg/kg bwt IV) has been used to prevent or control lidocaine-induced seizures. Lidocaine is fast acting with a short duration of action and minimal cardiovascular effects. However, the equine nervous and/or musculoskeletal system is more sensitive than

the cardiovascular system [46]. In one study, a loading dose of 1.3 mg/kg bwt over 15 min followed by a CRI of 50 µg/kg/min resulted in one of six horses exhibiting signs of toxicosis, including tremors and collapse [47]. The target plasma concentration range of lidocaine is 1–2 µg/ml with toxic effects occurring in the 1.9–4.5 µg/ml range [47]. These authors concluded that a lower lidocaine infusion rate is better for long-term lidocaine infusions and that coadministration of highly protein-bound drugs could increase risk of lidocaine toxicity. One case report describes signs of toxicity in a horse that received a 1.3 mg/kg bwt loading dose of lidocaine followed by a CRI of 0.05 mg/kg/min [48]. Signs of toxicity, including muscle fasciculations and supraventricular tachycardia, in that horse developed after 1.5 h. Clinical signs, including the arrhythmia, resolved approximately 2 h after discontinuation of the lidocaine CRI.

Phenytoin sodium has similar actions to lidocaine but is generally less effective for the treatment of ventricular arrhythmias. However, phenytoin has been used in horses for controlling myotonia, rhabdomyolysis, and digitalis-induced cardiac arrhythmias [49, 50]. It was also successfully used to treat ventricular ectopy in seven horses that had not responded to lidocaine or procainamide [51]. The recommended protocol is 20 mg/kg bwt of phenytoin PO BID for 2 days and then reduced to 10–15 mg/kg bwt PO BID. There is also an IV dose recommendation of 5–10 mg/kg bwtfollowed by 1–5 mg/kg bwt IM BID or 10–15 mg/kg bwt PO BID, but it may be irritating to surrounding tissue because of its alkalinity. If possible, plasma concentrations should be determined regularly until a plateau concentration between 5 and 10 mg/l is achieved. Signs of sedation should be interpreted as excessively high serum concentrations and the dosage should be reduced. Additional adverse effects include muscle fasciculations.

Magnesium sulfate is a physiologic calcium channel blocker (Table 16.3). Magnesium decreases ventricular arrhythmias due to its ability to enhance homogeneity in repolarization [52]. Magnesium sulfate is slower acting than lidocaine and has no significant cardiovascular effects. Magnesium solutions containing calcium should not be used for this purpose. The most commonly recommended dosing regimen is 1 g/min to effect up to a maximum of 25 g [22].

Quinidine gluconate (1.1–2.2 mg/kg bwt IV boluses every 10 min up to a total dose of 9–11 mg/kg bwt) can also be used to treat VT [22, 45]. As stated previously, its propensity to cause hypotension and to produce negative inotropic effects may be undesirable, and hemodynamic monitoring is important. Quinidine should be avoided in horses with systolic dysfunction. When it must be used in animals with compromised cardiovascular function, concurrent IV administration of a balanced electrolyte solution at the rate of 3–4 ml/kg/h has been recommended [22].

Procainamide has similar actions to quinidine but with fewer cardiovascular side effects (see Section "Atrial Fibrillation"). Recommended dosing regimens include 1 mg/kg/min given IV up to a total dose of 20 mg/kg bwt or 25–35 mg/kg bwt given PO every 8 h [22].

Propafenone blocks fast sodium channels (class I antiarrhythmic) and also has weak B adrenoceptor antagonistic properties and mild class III and class IV activity [53] (Table 16.2). Human clinical studies have shown it to be useful for supraventricular arrhythmias and ventricular arrhythmias. The drug has rapid distribution in the body after IV administration, but there is large interindividual variability [53]. Dosing regimens are 0.5–1 mg/kg bwt IV (slowly) in 5% dextrose or 2 mg/kg bwt, PO, q8 h.

Amiodarone (see AF section) is an alternative antiarrhythmic, which was successfully used to treat a horse with refractory VT after therapy with magnesium, lidocaine, and propafenone was unsuccessful [38]. In this case, after conversion to sinus rhythm, therapy was switched to phenytoin; however, VT recurred and IV amiodarone was reinstituted. The VT again responded to amiodarone and a tapering protocol was initiated (5 mg amiodarone/kg/h for 1 h followed by 0.83 mg/kg/h for the next 23 h). Amiodarone was then tapered daily by 0.20 mg/kg/h over the next 5 days. On the 6th and 7th day, the horse received amiodarone 5 mg/kg IV over 10 min. Amiodarone was continued PO following the week of IV administration at 10 mg/kg bwt PO once daily for 1 week; then at 7.5 mg/kg bwt PO once daily for 2 weeks; then 5 mg/kg once daily for 2 weeks; and finally 2.5 mg/kg once PO for 2 weeks. Amiodarone was then discontinued, and 8 months postconversion, the horse remained in sinus rhythm. Although adverse effects with short-term amiodarone therapy in humans are reasonably rare, adverse effects with chronic therapy including thyroid, pulmonary, hepatic, gastrointestinal, ocular, and dermatologic disorders are more common. Therefore, the drug is probably best reserved for use in refractory VT cases.

Propranolol is a nonselective B adrenoceptor antagonist. It exerts its antiarrhythmic action by inhibiting the effects of catecholamines on myocardial function. It is infrequently used to treat supraventricular and ventricular arrhythmias in horses [8]. Because it is a competitive inhibitor, the degree of sympathetic tone present influences its efficacy. Dose rates range from 0.05 to 0.16 mg/kg bwt IV [8, 22]. Therapeutic concentrations of propranolol reduce myocardial contractility and slow the heart rate, effects that may be undesirable. The oral form of propranolol is not effective in the horse [8].

Pharmacologic treatment of ventricular fibrillation is rarely successful in horses. Lidocaine and bretylium have been suggested [7]. Bretylium (0.5–5 mg/kg IV) blocks potassium channels in myocardial cells.

Bradyarrhythmias

Sinus bradycardia, advanced AV block, and third-degree AV block require treatment if the heart rate is slow enough to negatively impact cardiac output, which is usually less than 24 bpm. The anticholinergic drugs atropine (0.01–0.02 mg/kg bwt IV) and glycopyrrolate (5–10 µg/kg bwt IV) can be used to treat pathologic bradyarrhythmias. These drugs are postganglionic muscarinic cholinergic receptor antagonists and increase heart rate by decreasing vagal tone. Side effects include decreased gastrointestinal motility and secretions, which can lead to signs of colic, increased respiratory dead space, and mydriasis [8]. These drugs are primarily used to treat transient bradyarrhythmias during anesthesia.

Some anesthesia-associated bradyarrhythmias do not respond to anticholinergics, and sympathomimetics, such as dobutamine or dopamine, may be effective. It is important to monitor the patient for metabolic disturbances, which can lead to bradycardia. For example, hyperkalemia can cause severe bradycardia, and occasionally, immune-mediated myocarditis can lead to complete heart block. Addressing the hyperkalemia with insulin and dextrose or calcium gluconate often results in an improved heart rate, and corticosteroid therapy may lead to resolution of complete heart block. However, if severe bradycardia persists and is not responsive to medical management, a temporary and/or permanent pacemaker is indicated [54–57].

As already stated, theophylline and aminophylline are xanthine derivatives with positive inotropic and chronotropic effects [23]. Side effects include excitement, cardiac arrhythmias, and tachycardia [8]. Aminophylline is recommended at 2–7 mg/kg bwt IV q6–12 h or 5 mg/kg bwt PO aminophylline tablets. It should not be administered IM because it can cause discomfort by this route [10]. The sustained-release formulation of theophylline should be administered at 5–15 mg/kg bwt PO q12–24 h [10, 23]. Both drugs should be dosed on lean body mass.

Acknowledgment

I would like to acknowledge Dr. Mary Durando for her help proofreading this chapter.

References

1 Bertone, J.J. (2007) Evidence-based drug use in equine medicine and surgery. *Veterinary Clinics of North America: Equine Practice*, **23**, 201–213.

2 Nout, Y.S., Hinchcliff, K.W., Bonagura, J.D., Meurs, K.M. & Papenfuss, T.L. (2003) Cardiac amyloidosis in a horse. *Journal of Veterinary Internal Medicine*, **17**, 588–592.

3 Tobin, T., Roberts, B.L., Swerczek, T.W. & Crisman, M. (1978) The pharmacology of furosemide in the horse. III Dose and time response relationships, effects of repeated dosing, and performance effects. *Journal of Equine Medicine and Surgery*, **2**, 216–226.

4 Adin, D.B., Taylor, A.W., Hill, R.C., Scott, K.C. & Martin, F.G. (2003) Intermittent bolus injection versus continuous infusion of furosemide in normal adult greyhound dogs. *Journal of Veterinary Internal Medicine*, **17**, 632–636.

5 Lahav, M., Regev, A., Ra'anani, P. & Theodor, E. (1992) Intermittent administration of furosemide vs continuous infusion preceded by a loading dose for congestive heart failure. *Chest*, **102**, 725–731.

6 Johansson, A.M., Gardner, S.Y., Levine, J.F. *et al.* (2004) Pharmacokinetics and pharmacodynamics of furosemide after oral administration to horses. *Journal of Veterinary Internal Medicine*, **18**, 739–743.

7 Mogg, T.D. (1999) Equine cardiac disease. Clinical pharmacology and therapeutics. *Veterinary Clinics of North America: Equine Practice*, **15**, 523–534, vii.

8 Muir, W.W., 3rd & McGuirk, S. (1987) Cardiovascular drugs. Their pharmacology and use in horses. *Veterinary Clinics of North America: Equine Practice*, **3**, 37–57.

9 Bertone, J.J. (1988) Cardiovascular effects of hydralazine HCl administration in horses. *American Journal of Veterinary Research*, **49**, 618–621.

10 Plumb, D.C. (2002) *Veterinary Drug Handbook.* Iowa State Press, White Bear Lake, MN.

11 Opie, L.H. (2009) Calcium channel blockers (calcium antagonists). In: L.H. Opie & B.J. Gersh (eds), *Drugs for the Heart*, pp. 59–87. Saunders Elsevier, Philadelphia, PA.

12 Schwarzwald, C.C., Bonagura, J.D. & Luis-Fuentes, V. (2005) Effects of diltiazem on hemodynamic variables and ventricular function in healthy horses. *Journal of Veterinary Internal Medicine*, **19**, 703–711.

13 Schwarzwald, C.C., Hamlin, R.L., Bonagura, J.D., Nishijima, Y., Meadows, C. & Carnes, C.A. (2007) Atrial, SA nodal, and AVnodal electrophysiology in standing horses: Normal findings andelectrophysiologic effects of quinidine and diltiazem. *Journal of Veterinary Internal Medicine*, **21**, 166–175.

14 Gordon, S.G., Miller, M.W. & Saunders, A.B. (2006) Pimobendan in heart failure therapy—a silver bullet? *Journal of the American Animal Hospital Association*, **42**, 90–93.

15 Muir, W.W. (1995) The haemodynamic effects of milrinone HCl in halothane anaesthetised horses. *Equine Veterinary Journal Supplement*, 108–113.

16 Sweeney, R.W., Reef, V.B. & Reimer, J.M. (1993) Pharmacokinetics of digoxin administered to horses with congestive heart failure. *American Journal of Veterinary Research*, **54**, 1108–1111.

17 Muir, W.W., 3rd, Sams, R.A., Hubbell, J.A., Hinchcliff, K.W. & Gadawski, J. (2001) Effects of enalaprilat on cardiorespiratory, hemodynamic, and hematologic variables in exercising horses. *American Journal of Veterinary Research*, **62**, 1008–1013.

18 Gardner, S.Y., Atkins, C.E., Sams, R.A. *et al.* (2004) Characterization of the pharmacokinetic and pharmacodynamic properties of the angiotensin-converting enzyme inhibitor, enalapril, in horses. *Journal of Veterinary Internal Medicine*, **18**, 231–237.

19 Sleeper, M.M., McDonnell, S.M., Ely, J.J. & Reef, V.B. (2008) Chronic oral therapy with enalapril innormal ponies. *Journal of Veterinary Cardiology*, **10**, 111–115.

20 Guglielmini, C., Giuliani, A., Testoni, S., Corletto, F. & Bernardini, D. (2002) Use of ACE inhibitor (ramipril) in a horse with congestive heart failure. *Equine Veterinary Education*, **14**, 297–306.

21 Gehlen, H., Vieht, J.C. & Stadler, P. (2003) Effects of the ACE inhibitor quinapril on echocardiographic variables in horses with mitral valve insufficiency. *Journal of Veterinary Medicine A*, **50**, 460–465.

22 Reef, V.B. & McGuirk, S.M. (2009) Diseases of the cardiovascular system. In: B.P. Smith (ed), *Large Animal Internal Medicine*, pp. 453–489. Mosby Elsevier, St. Louis, MO.

23 Baggot, J.D. (1995) The pharmacological basis of cardiac drug selection for use in horses. *Equine Veterinary Journal Supplement*, 97–100.

24 Young, L.E. & Van Loon, G. (2005) Editorial: Atrial fibrillation in horses: new treatmentchoices for the new millennium? *Journal of Veterinary Internal Medicine*, **19**, 631–632.

25 De Clercq, D., Van Loon, G., Tavernier, R., Duchateau, L. & Deprez, P. (2008) Atrial and ventricular electrical and contractile remodeling and reverse remodeling owing to short-term pacing- induced atrial fibrillation in horses. *Journal of Veterinary Internal Medicine*, **22**, 1353–1359.

26 Reef, V.B., Levitan, C.W. & Spencer, P.A. (1988) Factors affecting prognosis and conversion in equine atrial fibrillation. *Journal of Veterinary Internal Medicine*, **2**, 1–6.

27 Van Loon, G., Blissitt, K.J., Keen, J.A. & Young, L.E. (2004) Use of intravenous flecainide in horses with naturally-occurring atrial fibrillation. *Equine Veterinary Journal*, **36**, 609–614.

28 Reef, V.B., Reimer, J.M. & Spencer, P.A. (1995) Treatment of atrial fibrillation in horses: New perspectives. *Journal of Veterinary Internal Medicine*, **9**, 57–67.

29 Morris, D.D. & Fregin, G.F. (1982) Atrial fibrillation in horses: Factors associated with response to quinidine sulfate in 77 clinical cases. *Cornell Veterinarian*, **72**, 339–349.

30 Bertone, J.J., Traub-Dargatz, J.L. & Wingfield, W.E. (1987) Atrial fibrillation in a pregnant mare: Treatment with quinidine sulfate. *Journal of the American Veterinary Medical Association*, **190**, 1565–1566.

31 Parraga, M.E., Kittleson, M.D. & Drake, C.M. (1995) Quinidine administration increases steady state serum digoxin concentration in horses. *Equine Veterinary Journal Supplement*, 114–119.

32 McGuirk, S.M., Muir, W.W. & Sams, R.A. (1981) Pharmacokinetic analysis of intravenously and orally administered quinidine in horses. *American Journal of Veterinary Research*, **42**, 938–942.

33 Levy, S., Lauribe, P., Dolla, E. *et al.* (1992) A randomized comparison of external and internal cardioversion of chronic atrial fibrillation. *Circulation*, **86**, 1415–1420.

34 McGurrin, M.K., Physick-Sheard, P.W. & Kenney, D.G. (2008) Transvenous electricalcardioversion of equine atrial fibrillation: Patient factors and clinical results in 72 treatment episodes. *Journal of Veterinary Internal Medicine*, **22**, 609–615.

35 Bellei, M.H., Kerr, C., McGurrin, M.K., Kenney, D.G. & Physick-Sheard, P. (2007) Management and complications of anesthesia for transvenous electrical cardioversion of atrial fibrillation in horses: 62 cases (2002–2006). *Journal of the American Veterinary Medical Association*, **231**, 1225–1230.

36 DeClercq, D., Van Loon, G., Baert, K. *et al.* (2006) Intravenous amiodarone treatment in horses with chronic atrial fibrillation. *Veterinary Journal*, **172**, 129–134.

37 Trachsel, D., Tschudi, P., Portier, C.J. *et al.* (2004) Pharmacokinetics and pharmacodynamic effects of amiodarone in plasma of ponies after single intravenous administration. *Toxicology and Applied Pharmacology*, **195**, 113–125.

38 De Clercq, D., Van Loon, G., Baert, K., De Backer, P. & Deprez, P. (2007) Treatment with amiodarone of refractory ventricular tachycardia in a horse. *Journal of Veterinary Internal Medicine*, **21**, 878–880.

39 De Clercq, D., Van Loon, G., Baert, K. *et al.* (2007) Effects of an adapted intravenous amiodarone treatment protocol in horses with atrial fibrillation. *Equine Veterinary Journal*, **39**, 344–349.

40 Ohmura, H., Nukada, T., Mizuno, Y., Yamaya, Y., Nakayama, T. & Amada, A. (2000) Safe and efficacious dosage of flecainide acetate for treating equine atrial fibrillation. *Journal of Veterinary Medical Science*, **62**, 711–715.

41 Ohmura, H., Hiraga, A., Aida, H., Takahashi, T. & Nukada, T. (2001) Determination of oral dosage and pharmacokinetic analysis of flecainide in horses. *Journal of Veterinary Medical Science*, **63**, 511–514.

42 Risberg, A.I. & McGuirk, S.M. (2006) Successful conversion of equine atrial fibrillation using oral flecainide. *Journal of Veterinary Internal Medicine*, **20**, 207–209.

43 De Clercq, D., Van Loon, G., Tavernier, R., Verbesselt, R. & Deprez, P. (2009) Use of propafenone for conversion of chronic atrial fibrillation in horses. *American Journal of Veterinary Research*, **70**, 223–227.

44 Murdock, D.K., Kersten, M., Kaliebe, J. & Larrain, G. (2009) The use of oral ranolazine to convert new or paroxysmal atrial fibrillation: A review of experience with implications for possible "pill in the pocket" approach to atrial fibrillation. *Indian Pacing and Electrophysiology Journal*, **9**, 260–267.

45 Reimer, J.M., Reef, V.B. & Sweeney, R.W. (1992) Ventricular arrhythmias in horses: 21 cases(1984–1989). *Journal of the American Veterinary Medical Association*, **201**, 1237–1243.

46 Meyer, G.A., Lin, H.C., Hanson, R.R. & Hayes, T.L. (2001) Effects of intravenous lidocaine overdose on cardiac electrical activity and blood pressure in the horse. *Equine Veterinary Journal*, **33**, 434–437.

47 Milligan, M., Kukanich, B., Beard, W. & Waxman, S. (2006) The disposition of lidocaine during a 12-hour intravenous infusion to postoperative horses. *Journal of Veterinary Pharmacology and Therapeutics*, **29**, 495–499.

48 Mullen, K.R., Gelzer, A.R., Kraus, M.S., Mitchell, K. & Divers, T.J. (2009) ECG of the month. Cardiac arrhythmias in a horse after lidocaine administration. *Journal of the American Veterinary Medical Association*, **235**, 1156–1158.

49 Smith, P.A., Aldridge, B.M. & Kittleson, M.D. (2003) Oleander toxicosis in a donkey. *Journal of Veterinary Internal Medicine*, **17**, 111–114.

50 Wijnberg, I.D., van der Kolk, J.H. & Hiddink, E.G. (1999) Use of phenytoin to treatdigitalis-induced cardiac arrhythmias in a miniature Shetland pony. *Veterinary Record*, **144**, 259–261.

51 Wijnberg, I.D. & Ververs, F.F. (2004) Phenytoin sodium as a treatment for ventricular dysrhythmia in horses. *Journal of Veterinary Internal Medicine*, **18**, 350–353.

52 Parikka, H.J. & Toivonen, L.K. (1999) Acute effects of intravenous magnesium on ventricular refractoriness and monophasic action potential duration in humans. *Scandinavian Cardiovascular Journal*, **33**, 300–305.

53 Puigdemont, A., Riu, J.L., Guitart, R. & Arboix, M. (1990) Propafenone kinetics in the horse. Comparative analysis of

compartmental and noncompartmental models. *Journal of Pharmacological Methods*, **23**, 79–85.

54 Fennell, L., Church, S., Tyrell, D. *et al.* (2009) Double-outlet right ventricle in a 10-month-old Friesian filly. *Australian Veterinary Journal*, **87**, 204–209.

55 Reef, V.B., Clark, E.S., Oliver, J.A. & Donawick, W.J. (1986) Implantation of a permanent transvenous pacing catheter in a horse with complete heart block and syncope. *Journal of the American Veterinary Medical Association*, **189**, 449–452.

56 Taylor, D.H. & Mero, M.A. (1967) The use of an internal pacemaker in a horse with Adams-Stokes syndrome. *Journal of the American Veterinary Medical Association*, **151**, 1172–1176.

57 Van Loon, G., Fonteyne, W., Rottiers, H., Tavernier, R. & Deprez, P. (2002) Implantation of a dual-chamber, rate-adaptive pacemaker in a horse with suspected sick sinus syndrome. *Veterinary Record*, **151**, 541–545.

CHAPTER 17

Clinical pharmacology of diseases of the equine urinary system

Nora Nogradi[1] and Balazs Toth[2]

[1] Dubai Equine Hospital, Dubai, United Arab Emirates
[2] Equine Department and Clinic, Szent István University, Dora-Major, Hungary

Acute renal failure

Acute renal failure (ARF), also termed as acute kidney injury (AKI), is a syndrome characterized by rapid loss of urinary excretory function with or without evidence of structural changes in the renal parenchyma. ARF failure is a medical emergency. The sudden decline of glomerular filtration rate (GFR) results in rapid accumulation of nitrogenous and nonnitrogenous waste products along with disturbances in electrolyte and metabolic homeostasis. ARF is one of the major complications of human patients hospitalized for critical illness [1]. There are no direct data on the prevalence of ARF in horses, but anecdotal reports estimate that 0.5–1% of hospitalized horses have evidence of renal dysfunction. Horses at greater risk to develop such complications include those suffering from severe systemic inflammatory diseases that result in hypovolemia and cardiovascular compromise, those suffering from diseases that result in pigmenturia of any type, and horses that are treated with potentially nephrotoxic medications. A large proportion of the functional renal mass (about 75%) has to be damaged before any biochemical evidence of renal dysfunction is appreciated. Therefore, it is always recommended to monitor renal function in patients at risk, as early detection and management are essential for a favorable outcome.

The definition of ARF is traditionally based on alterations in clinical and clinicopathologic characteristics. According to a definition adapted from the human literature, ARF is suspected if serum creatinine levels increase by 50% when compared to baseline values during hospitalization or if there is a reduction in urine output resulting in oliguria of less than 0.5 ml/kg/h for more than 6 h [2]. While these guidelines can be difficult to apply in equine patients, they further emphasize the importance of monitoring renal function in hospitalized horses and suggest that a rise in serum creatinine concentration in an otherwise well-hydrated equine patient can be an alarming sign of impaired renal function. In most cases, however, the equine practitioner diagnoses renal failure in more advanced stages of the disease, evaluating horses with high serum creatinine and BUN concentrations and severe electrolyte disturbances.

Causes of ARF

ARF can be divided into three categories.

1 Prerenal failure (prerenal azotemia): reduced GFR is caused by decreased renal perfusion that is a result of hypotension, caused by anesthesia, sepsis, endotoxemia, or decreased cardiac output (i.e., severe arrhythmias or congestive heart failure), and/or hypovolemia, caused by decreased circulating blood volume secondary to acute blood or fluid losses (i.e., diarrhea, gastric reflux, or sweating). Temporary episodes of decreased renal perfusion will result in decreased urine output, but if perfusion is restored in a timely manner, persistent detrimental effects may not occur. On the other hand, prolonged episodes of decreased renal perfusion will result in hypoxic–ischemic injury to the renal parenchyma, eventually leading to intrinsic renal failure.

Equine Pharmacology, First Edition. Edited by Cynthia Cole, Bradford Bentz and Lara Maxwell.

2 Intrinsic renal failure (renal azotemia): the reduced GFR is caused by damage to some portion of the nephron (i.e., glomeruli, tubules, or interstitium). The specific parts of the nephron affected depend on the etiology. In horses, acute tubular necrosis (ATN), secondary to ischemia following prolonged renal hypoperfusion, is the most common cause of nephron damage. Other causes of ATN include administration of nephrotoxic medications, such as nonsteroidal anti-inflammatory drugs (NSAID), aminoglycosides, tetracyclines, polymyxin B, amphotericin B, and/or vitamin D products; pigment nephropathy due to rhabdomyolysis or intravascular hemolysis; and ingestion of heavy metals, such as Hg, Cd, Zn, As, or Pb, or toxic agents, such as acorns, cantharidin, pyrrolizidine, and alkaloid-containing plants. Glomerular damage as a cause of ARF is rare in horses but does occur. Diseases associated with damage to the glomerulus include immune-mediated glomerulopathies, such as purpura hemorrhagica, which occurs secondary to viral or bacterial infections, such as *Streptococcus equi* spp. *equi* infection. Interstitial nephritis in horses is rare and most commonly associated with infection by *Leptospira* species.

3 Postrenal failure (postrenal azotemia): this occurs when an obstruction of the urinary tract prevents the emptying of urine from the kidneys. Obstruction will result in a rapid rise in the serum creatinine concentration due to the inability of the kidneys to excrete it; if urine flow can be restored quickly, however, the azotemia should resolve spontaneously. A prolonged obstruction, however, can cause pressure necrosis of the tubules and renal interstitium, resulting in intrinsic renal failure with more detrimental consequences.

Management of ARF

When managing horses with ARF, it is very important to identify and correct the causative factors, although the overall goal of therapy is supportive. This includes administration of intravenous fluids to restore renal perfusion in order to preserve as much functional capacity as possible. When the exact nature of the underlying disease process responsible for intrinsic renal disease is not known at the time of diagnosis, treatment and further diagnostic testing should be carried out simultaneously. Following a thorough clinical examination and clinicopathologic evaluation, the hydration status and rate of urine production, if any, need to be determined. Before developing a fluid plan for the horse with ARF, it is important to classify the disease as anuric, oliguric, or nonoliguric renal failure.

Therapy for anuric or oliguric renal failure

ARF, characterized by decreased or a total lack of urine production, is a medical emergency that requires hospitalization and critical monitoring of the patient, so that interventions to increase diuresis can be made in a timely manner. The longer the anuric or oliguric state persists, the less likely it is that the condition can be fully reversed. Urine production in a healthy, adult horse is around 1–2 ml/kg/h; however, it is greatly affected by hydration status. Adapting the guidelines from human medicine to use in equine patients, oliguric renal failure can be suspected in azotemic horses that produce less than 0.5 ml/kg/h while receiving maintenance IV fluid therapy, while anuria is defined as a lack of urine production despite IV fluid therapy [2].

A thorough evaluation of the horse in ARF should include assessment of perfusion parameters, urinalysis, complete blood count, plasma lactate, and chemistry panel as well as measurement of central venous pressure (CVP) and indirect blood pressure when available. If there are no signs of fluid overload (weight gain, subcutaneous (SC) edema, or evidence of pulmonary edema) and CVP is not increased (adults < 12–15 cmH$_2$O, neonates < 10–12 cmH$_2$O), the fluid challenge method of fluid administration should be followed [3] (Figure 17.1). IV administration of a 20 ml/kg bwt (i.e., ~10 l for adult horses, 1 l for neonatal foals) bolus of isotonic crystalloid solution is followed by subsequent reevaluation of perfusion parameters and CVP. The type of fluid chosen for correction of dehydration should be based on the patient's electrolyte balance. If hyponatremia (i.e., Na < 125 mEq/l) is marked, fluid therapy can be initiated with 0.9% NaCl, which has a sodium content of 154 mEq/l. Normosol-R®, Plasma-Lyte A®, and lactated Ringer's solution all have lower sodium concentrations of 130–140 mEq/l and are, therefore, better options in horses with sodium concentrations in the normal range. If no increase in urine production occurs following the fluid bolus and clinical and clinicopathologic parameters show no evidence of fluid overload, subsequent boluses can be administered with repeated evaluation of the patient between boluses. Animals that remain anuric may become volume overloaded by excessive fluid

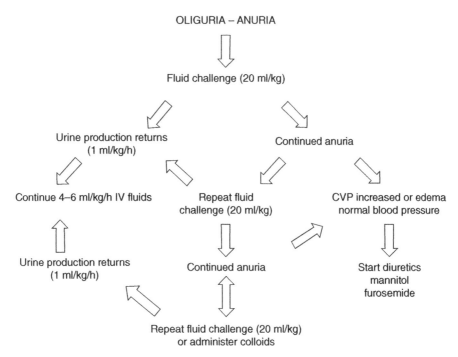

OLIGURIA – ANURIA

Fluid challenge (20 ml/kg)

Urine production returns
(1 ml/kg/h)

Continued anuria

Continue 4–6 ml/kg/h IV fluids

Repeat fluid
challenge (20 ml/kg)

CVP increased or edema
normal blood pressure

Urine production returns
(1 ml/kg/h)

Continued anuria

Start diuretics
mannitol
furosemide

Repeat fluid challenge (20 ml/kg)
or administer colloids

Figure 17.1 Algorithm for the management of oliguric renal failure in horses.

infusion. In such cases, measurements of CVP can be used to determine the endpoint of fluid administration, as it is a sensitive marker of fluid overload. The rise in CVP will precede clinical signs, such as pulmonary or SC edema formation. Measurement of CVP requires placement of a central venous catheter into the cranial vena cava or right atrium. If CVP measurements are not feasible, serial weight measurements of the patient can also be informative; however, this method is far less sensitive and accurate in detecting fluid overload. If clinical signs of hypoperfusion are still present when the limit of fluid therapy is reached, direct or indirect blood pressure measurements should be taken. Hypotension due to systemic illness commonly contributes to decreased renal perfusion in critically ill neonatal foals; however, it occurs less commonly in adult horses. If hypotension is present after fluid replacement therapy, colloid administration should be considered, while inotrope and vasopressor therapy remains the ultimate option for the reestablishment of normal renal blood flow in hypotensive or hypoperfused patients (see Chapter 15). If there is no evidence of hypotension, but no urine production occurs with the administration of multiple fluid boluses, diuretic therapy should be initiated.

Furosemide, a loop diuretic, administered IV, is the diuretic of choice in cases of anuric or oliguric renal failure, as it can increase the rate of urine flow and enhance potassium excretion. It also produces an increase in GFR and a redistribution of blood from the renal medulla to the cortex. Response to furosemide treatment is variable in horses with oliguric and anuric renal failure. Horses with tubular debris or pigment accumulation have decreased delivery of furosemide to the active site at the lumen of the thick ascending limb of the loop of Henle, resulting in a less pronounced or even the absence of a diuretic effect. The duration of effect of furosemide is between 2 and 3 h, although the elimination half-life greatly depends on renal function. Continuous rate infusion (CRI) of furosemide has been shown to be superior to a single-dose administration in producing greater urine volume in the first 8 h of administration [4]. A loading dose of 0.12 mg/kg bwt furosemide given intravenously should be followed by a CRI at a rate of 0.12 mg/kg/h. If CRI administration is not an option, a single dose of furosemide at a dose of 1 mg/kg bwt, IV, should be administered. If no urine production occurs within 60 min, other diuretic agents should be considered. Mannitol, an osmotic diuretic, would be a logical next step. Mannitol is also freely filtered by the glomeruli and is not substantially secreted, reabsorbed, or metabolized. It acts by diffusing from the bloodstream into the renal interstitium, creating an osmotic gradient, thereby increasing medullary blood flow. The increased perfusion washes out the medullary osmotic gradient and results in increased urine volume. A bolus of 0.25–0.5 g/kg bwt administered as a 20% solution, IV, can be repeated twice, 30 min apart. Adverse effects of mannitol therapy include development of fluid overload that can result in acute pulmonary edema. Therefore, a dose of 1 g/kg bwt should not be exceeded at any given time regardless of the response.

No improvement in anuria or oliguria despite aggressive diuretic therapy suggests irreversible pathological changes in the renal parenchyma and carries a poor to grave prognosis. Dopamine had been used in the past to reverse oliguria in patients with ARF, but due to the lack of efficacy and occurrence of side effects, it is no longer recommended for oliguric renal failure, except to support blood pressure [5]. Additional options for these patients include hemodialysis and peritoneal dialysis. While hemodialysis is a commonly used therapeutic option for ARF in small animal medicine, there is only limited information available regarding hemodialysis in horses. A more widely available technique is peritoneal dialysis that allows removal of toxic waste products, including creatinine and BUN, by the administration of large amounts of dialysate solution into the peritoneal cavity. The solute exchange occurs by way of diffusion, as waste products at higher concentration in the blood will diffuse across the peritoneum into the dialysis fluid and be removed with the fluid exchange. Contraindications for peritoneal dialysis include peritonitis, severe clotting disorders, and severe hypoalbuminemia. Both intermittent and continuous dialysis techniques have been described in horses with ARF [6, 7]. For **intermittent peritoneal dialysis**, the horse is equipped with an indwelling peritoneal catheter or drain (28–32 Fr size) at the most dependent part of the abdomen. Placement of the catheter can be performed with the horse standing, under sedation and local anesthesia. Then, peritoneal lavage is performed with 10–15 l of dialysate solution. After infusion of the fluid, the catheter is occluded and the horse is walked for about 30 min to maximize contact time between the lavage fluid and the peritoneal lining, and then the fluid is

allowed to drain out. The procedure can be repeated daily; however, it is important to monitor the amount of fluid that is recovered, as fluid retention has been described as the most common complication of intermittent peritoneal dialysis. If there is no improvement with intermittent dialysis or there are complications associated with the procedure, **continuous peritoneal dialysis** can be attempted. This procedure requires the placement of an inflow catheter in the left flank and an outflow drain at the most dependent part of the abdomen. Continuous infusion of the dialysate solution is performed at a rate of 4–6 ml/kg/h. The details of the procedure have been described elsewhere [8]. In previous reports, continuous peritoneal dialysis was used for 3–4 days without complications and resulted in partial resolution of the azotemia. Regarding the dialysate solution, it has been recommended to use balanced polyionic solutions (Normosol-R, Plasma-Lyte A, lactated Ringer's solution, Hartmann's solution) with dextrose and other additions depending on the patient's metabolic status. Normal saline solution can only be used for short-term dialysis, as it has been shown to predispose patients to adhesion formation with long-term use. The addition of dextrose creates hypertonicity, which is crucial to achieve ultrafiltration and removal of excess water. The exact dextrose concentration to be used depends on the patient's hydration status. In an otherwise normovolemic patient, a 1.5% dextrose solution is adequate, while a dialysate solution with up to 4.25% dextrose concentration has been described for patients with severe fluid overload [9]. The dialysate solution should be warmed to body temperature prior to infusion. It is not the goal of peritoneal dialysis to achieve full replacement of renal function, but to remove enough solutes and control electrolyte and acid–base balance to temporarily maintain homeostasis until renal function returns. Once renal blood flow is restored, the remaining functional nephrons will determine the ultimate recovery of GFR. If there is no improvement in the azotemia or urine production with the implementation of peritoneal dialysis, the prognosis is grave. If urine production returns, guidelines for therapy should follow recommendations for nonoliguric renal failure.

Therapy for nonoliguric renal failure

A subset of horses with ARF presents with clinical signs of polyuria (PU) and polydipsia (PD). The goal of fluid therapy in these cases is to increase diuresis, in order to remove uremic toxins, while the electrolyte and metabolic homeostasis is maintained. If we consider maintenance fluid requirement for an adult horse under normal circumstances to be 2 ml/kg/h, then the goal is to achieve diuresis by providing two to three times the maintenance rate in ARF. While these are good guidelines to start with, it is always important to monitor urine output closely and tailor the fluid rate to the needs of the individual horse. In a horse with excessive PU, fluid rate may need to be increased significantly to match the losses.

The type of IV fluid used for diuresis depends on the electrolyte status of the horse. In horses with ARF that do not have significant electrolyte abnormalities, a balanced polyionic solution (Normosol-R, Plasma-Lyte A, lactated Ringer's solution) is the ideal choice. These crystalloids have similar electrolyte composition to equine plasma and therefore can serve as replacement fluids and can also be used for diuresis in patients with renal failure, if no major electrolyte disturbances need to be corrected. Please refer to Chapter 8, for more information on the composition of these fluids. As a general rule, once fluid therapy is initiated, it is recommended that it be continued for a minimum of 72 h, as diuresis may not result in immediate changes in serum creatinine and BUN concentrations. If there is no change in the levels of uremic toxins in the blood after 3 days of fluid therapy, the damage to the kidneys is likely permanent, and the diagnosis of chronic renal failure (CRF) can be made. As long as these horses continue to produce adequate urine volume, fluid therapy can be discontinued, and management of CRF can be attempted.

If uremic toxin levels decrease in response to fluid therapy, diuresis should be continued until there is no additional change in values over a 24 h period. Initially, there may be a more substantial decrease in the plasma BUN and creatinine concentrations, as fluid therapy will lead to hemodilution and a proportionate decrease of these compounds. Depending on the success of reversal of the acute component of the renal disease, a low-level chronic impairment can be still present. Tapering of the fluid support should be performed very slowly in any patient where long-standing fluid therapy is implemented but is particularly important in horses with renal disease. Weaning the horse off of IV fluid support over a 3–4-day period, by decreasing the amount of fluid given by 25% every 24 h, is generally recommended.

If the urine output diminishes by a corresponding degree and azotemia does not return, tapering of the fluid volume can be continued. If urine output does not diminish as the volume of fluid administered decreases, then the kidneys are unable to regulate fluid balance, and further reduction of IV fluid support will result in dehydration. In such cases, diuresis should be continued and tapering can be attempted in a few days at a slower rate (10% per day). Once IV fluid therapy is successfully discontinued, creatinine and BUN levels as well as water consumption should be monitored daily for 2–3 days. When the horse is discharged from the hospital, management recommendations include avoiding of nephrotoxic medications and activities that can result in episodes of temporary dehydration, such as strenuous exercise, for a couple of months postdischarge.

Special considerations in the management of ARF
Monitoring
Horses hospitalized for ARF require intensive care and monitoring. The reversal of anuric renal failure is a challenging therapeutic goal, and the importance of close monitoring and timely intervention cannot be overemphasized. It is especially important in the first 2–3 days of therapy and should include serial physical examinations, weight measurements, and blood work evaluations (electrolytes, acid–base balance, hydration parameters, and uremic toxins). Measurement of urine output via an indwelling urinary catheter facilitates fine-tuning of fluid therapy. Whereas measurement of urine output is not practical in adult patients, it should be performed in recumbent neonates. Once urine production returns, the level of care and monitoring can be decreased, but it is important to continue monitoring hydration parameters and record serial weight measurements to guide proper fluid therapy during diuresis.

Hyperkalemia
Hyperkalemia is a common feature of ARF and is most likely to be encountered in severely oliguric or anuric patients. It is often corrected with the restoration of renal perfusion and subsequent urine production. However, in cases of prolonged hyperkalemia (>6 mEq/l), medical management should focus on correction to prevent life-threatening complications associated with cardiac arrhythmias. In these cases, hyperkalemia can be temporarily managed by volume expansion with 0.9%

NaCl. If 0.9% NaCl is not available, fluid therapy with potassium-containing fluids (Normosol-R, Plasma-Lyte A, lactated Ringer's solution) will also decrease hyperkalemia by improving renal perfusion and enhancing potassium excretion by the kidneys, although the volume expansion effect will not be as pronounced. Additional therapeutic options for hyperkalemia include the IV administration of calcium, sodium bicarbonate, and glucose infusions, with or without concurrent administration of insulin. These therapeutics help to direct the excess potassium from the extracellular to the intracellular space. Serial electrocardiographic monitoring is recommended during stabilization. Arrhythmias should resolve within minutes after correction of hyperkalemia. These therapeutic options, however, only provide temporary relief from effects of hyperkalemia. Therefore, once potassium levels are normalized, focus should shift back to reversal of anuric renal failure and resumption of urine flow.

Complications

Complications encountered during the treatment course of ARF include anorexia, gastric ulceration, diarrhea, anemia, catheter site issues, and the development of neurologic signs. Minimizing azotemia is the key to minimizing most of these complications. In addition, treatment with gastroprotectants can improve appetite, and providing highly palatable and easily digestible feed will encourage horses with ARF to eat. Parenteral nutrition should be considered if anorexia persists for longer than 3 days of therapy. Antimicrobial therapy is indicated when the underlying disease process is infectious in nature, when multiple urinary catheterization procedures are undertaken, or when peritoneal dialysis is performed. An antimicrobial agent with broad-spectrum coverage and activity in the urine should be selected. For guidelines to antimicrobial selection, see the section discussing bacterial urinary tract infections (UTI). Careful aseptic care of the IV catheter can minimize the risk of catheter site complications.

Management of acute leptospirosis

Leptospirosis is considered a sporadic cause of acute tubulointerstitial nephritis that can lead to ARF, as well as placentitis, abortion, and premature births in horses. *Leptospira interrogans* serovars *bratislava*, *pomona*, *kennewicki*, *grippotyphosa*, and *hardjo* have been reported in horses [9]. While there are only a few reports of leptospirosis as a cause of ARF, anecdotally, it appears to be more common and should be considered in horses that present with acute-onset depression, fever, and azotemia. Laboratory abnormalities in horses with leptospirosis include leukocytosis, hyperfibrinogenemia, azotemia, and isosthenuric urine. Ultrasound examination typically reveals enlarged, swollen kidneys, and a renal biopsy generally demonstrates tubulointerstitial nephritis. A microscopic agglutination test (MAT) on serum is often normal titer (<1:200) because acutely infected animals have not seroconverted. Evaluation of convalescent titers in 10–14 days will generally show a substantial increase, confirming the presumptive diagnosis. *Leptospira* organisms may also be detected in urine by the fluorescent antibody test (FAT), silver staining, dark-field microscopy, or PCR. Since the bacteria shed intermittently, it is recommended to collect three to five urine samples over a 24–48 h period and pool them together for testing. Another option is to administer furosemide at a dose of 1 mg/kg bwt, IV, once and use the second urine stream for sample collection, as this technique has been shown to increase urinary shedding of the organism.

Appropriate treatment for leptospirosis varies depending on the severity and duration of clinical signs. Antimicrobial therapy is always indicated and the regimen and drug selection should be based on *in vitro* susceptibility testing and anecdotal treatment response. As horses with clinical leptospirosis can be azotemic, it is important to consider the potential for nephrotoxicity when selecting the specific antimicrobial. Although the effects of antimicrobial therapy on outcome and duration of clinical illness have been variable, therapy has been shown to prevent leptospiruria or at least reduce its duration in most cases [10]. The most widely used antimicrobials for the treatment of leptospirosis in human medicine include penicillins, cephalosporins, and doxycycline. While there is no direct data on the efficacy of these agents on leptospirosis in horses, they are recommended in this species as well. While oxytetracycline is effective against *Leptospira* organisms *in vitro*, it is not ideal for the treatment of leptospirosis in horses, as the active metabolites of tetracyclines are not present in the equine urinary system at high enough concentrations to be effective [11]. In addition, the documented nephrotoxic effect of oxytetracycline makes it a less favorable choice in the azotemic patient. Nephrotoxicity has not been reported as a consequence of doxycycline administration to horses. This drug is eliminated unchanged through the gastrointestinal tract and urine, and it has been shown that oral administration to foals results in high urinary concentrations [5, 12]. Therefore, the use of sodium or potassium penicillin at a dose 22 000 U/kg bwt, IV or IM, q6 h; ceftiofur at a dose of 2.2 mg/kg bwt, IV, q12 h; doxycycline at a dose of 10 mg/kg bwt, orally (PO), q12 h; or enrofloxacin at a dose of 7.5 mg/kg bwt, IV, q12 h has been recommended for the treatment of equine leptospirosis [13]. Controlled studies are needed to provide scientific data on additional antimicrobial recommendations, as well the duration of treatment. Supportive therapy in these cases should focus on the management of ARF. In addition, isolation of suspect or confirmed cases leptospirosis is highly recommended to prevent disease spread to other horses. Additionally, it is important to consider the zoonotic risk, which necessitates protective clothing for individuals taking care of affected horses. About 10% of infected humans will show systemic clinical signs with mortality reaching as high as 10% in the clinically affected individuals [10].

Chronic renal failure

CRF is a syndrome of progressive loss of renal function over time. It is caused by decline in GFR, which leads to a loss of urine-concentrating ability, retention of water-soluble nitrogenous waste products, alterations in electrolyte and acid–base status, and dysfunction of several hormonal and homeostatic regulatory mechanisms. There are multiple causes of renal disease in horses that affect distinct sites within the nephron. For example, glomerular disease can be further categorized into glomerulonephritis, nonspecific glomerulopathy, renal glomerular hypoplasia, or amyloidosis, while tubulointerstitial disease can be caused by tubular necrosis, pyelonephritis, nephrolithiasis, hydronephrosis, renal dysplasia, and papillary necrosis. Regardless of the initiating cause, the progressive nature of chronic renal disease will ultimately lead to the destruction of the entire nephron. Histopathologic changes in the kidneys are usually not disease specific; hence, a biopsy is not typically helpful in determining the etiology of the renal disease.

Clinical features of CRF

Unlike ARF, CRF develops over a period of weeks, months, or years. The loss of functional nephrons results in a decreased GFR, which leads to increased plasma concentrations of substances normally eliminated via renal excretion and the clinical manifestation of uremic syndrome. Horses with CRF usually present with anorexia, chronic weight loss, lethargy, rough hair coat, and tartar buildup and may exhibit PU/PD. In addition to excreting metabolic waste products and maintaining electrolyte and fluid balance, the kidneys also play a pivotal role in endocrine function. CRF therefore can manifest in decreased production of the peptide hormone erythropoietin, resulting in the development of a nonregenerative anemia [14].

Diagnosis of CRF is based on historical information, clinical signs, and clinicopathologic findings, including azotemia that is unresponsive to diuresis with IV fluids, electrolyte disturbances, and persistent isosthenuria (i.e., urine specific gravity of 1.007–1.012). Renal ultrasonography can provide information on the morphology of the kidneys and has been recently identified as a valuable diagnostic modality to predict prognosis in horses with CRF [15].

Management of CRF

CRF is due to irreversible pathological changes in the renal parenchyma, and as a result, progression of disease is expected over time. Depending on the severity of renal damage and the accompanying uremic syndrome, the short-term prognosis of CRF can be good, while long-term outcome is always poor. Corrective treatment for CRF, such as renal transplantation, is not available in horses. Therefore, the goal of therapy is to focus on ameliorating the clinical signs and enhance the quality of life of the patient by managing the clinical signs such as anorexia, weight loss, and anemia and hindering the progression of the disease. It is difficult to determine the speed at which a particular patient's disease will progress. In a recent report, no clinical or clinicopathologic findings were found to be associated with long-term survival in horses with CRF that were discharged from the hospital [15]. This finding emphasizes the importance of long-term management and dietary changes in these cases postdiagnosis. Based on empirical data, horses that maintain a fair to good appetite and a good body condition score carry the best long-term prognosis.

Special considerations for management of CRF

Water and electrolyte balance

Due to the decrease in urine-concentrating ability, PU and compensatory PD are common in horses with CRF. Therefore, it is critical to ensure that horses with CRF always have free access to adequate fresh water. Episodes of temporary dehydration, caused by lack of access to water, gastrointestinal complications such as diarrhea or reflux, or sweating due to strenuous exercise or hot weather, can result in rapid and severe decline in renal function and exacerbation of the renal disease (ARF or CRF). In these cases, the amount of fluid that needs to be replaced depends on the level of hypovolemia and dehydration, as well as the ongoing fluid loss requirements. If continuous fluid therapy is needed, the clinician should include the increased fluid requirements secondary to PD, along with other losses and maintenance needs. Once fluid therapy can be discontinued, a slow tapering schedule should be followed. Please refer to the guidelines outlined in the Section "Acute Renal Failure". It is important to note that horses with CRF have altered water and electrolyte homeostasis. As a consequence, the rapid administration of IV fluids that would otherwise be tolerated by a horse with normal renal function can result in edema formation in the horse with CRF. The type of fluid should be tailored to the electrolyte needs of the patients. Horses with CRF can exhibit hyponatremia and hypochloremia, in which case 0.9% NaCl solution may be adequate to replace fluid and electrolyte losses. In cases where no apparent electrolyte disturbances are evident but dehydration necessitates fluid therapy, a balanced polyionic solution (Normosol-R, Plasma-Lyte A, lactated Ringer's solution) can be used. In the past, oral salt supplementation was recommended in the management of CRF to maintain water intake and increase urine production. Recent recommendations, however, caution against excessive salt supplementation in the absence of hyponatremia and hypochloremia, as maintenance of sodium excretion in animals with CRF represents an adaptation of individual nephrons to the altered electrolyte state and the high-dietary-sodium intake can have negative consequences on this balance [16].

The decreased GFR in patients with CRF results in decreased excretion of hydrogen ion and increased loss of bicarbonate via the urine. Additionally, dietary changes beneficial in the management of CRF include avoiding excess protein intake, which in turn results in a further decreased acid excretion due to the decreased ammonia production. In cases where metabolic acidosis is apparent (i.e., plasma bicarbonate <20 mEq/l), supplementation with sodium bicarbonate at a dose of 50–150 g/day should be initiated. It is important to tailor the dose to the needs of the individual patient, as the increased sodium intake can result in edema formation. Decrease or discontinuation of supplementation may be feasible once target metabolic status is reached.

Nutrition

Reduction of dietary protein intake is the cornerstone of CRF management in dogs and cats. While there is no scientific data to support the beneficial effects of decreased protein intake in horses with CRF, it has been recommended to maintain the total dietary crude protein intake between 10 and 12% of body weight [17]. Further reduction of protein intake can result in decreases in body weight, muscle mass, and serum albumin concentration. Generally, it is recommended to limit the consumption of high-protein and high-calcium forage sources, such as alfalfa and oat hay, and provide good quality grass hay or pasture to meet the roughage requirements of the horse. However, it is important to keep in mind that energy needs supersede those of protein synthesis. Consequently, sufficient caloric intake is necessary to prevent catabolism of endogenous proteins that can result in weight loss and further exacerbation of the renal disease. Feeding good quality, low-protein concentrates or oats and increasing the fat intake with the addition of corn oil (i.e., 8–16 oz/day) or rice bran can help to meet energy requirements. Providing a highly palatable diet is just as important as the constitution of the diet. Horses with CRF are lethargic and anorexic due to the increased circulating levels of uremic toxins, while the presence of gingivitis, in addition to oral and gastric ulceration, further exacerbates anorexia. Feeding small amounts of highly palatable feeds, such as concentrates, frequently throughout the day and keeping these horses on pasture will help maintain body condition. Additionally, gastroprotectants can be administered to diminish anorexia associated with gastric discomfort (see Chapter 12). The horse with CRF and chronic wasting may benefit from judicious administration of anabolic steroids, such as nandrolone or boldenone, to improve appetite and metabolic status; however, the risks and benefits of administration need to be evaluated in each individual case.

Supportive therapy

Since CRF presents as the clinical manifestation of diffuse inflammatory and degenerative processes in the kidneys, there is a good pathophysiologic rationale behind using antioxidants in these cases, as inflammation will lead to the increased generation of free oxygen radicals. The beneficial effects of antioxidants have been suggested in small animal patients with CRF [18]. Vitamin E is a cofactor of the glutathione peroxidase enzyme, which is one of the key antioxidant systems in the body, whereas ascorbic acid is a cofactor of multiple redox enzymes. There are currently no scientific data to support the use of antioxidant therapy in horses with CRF, but the potential beneficial effects combined with the unlikely harmful effects make the use of both ascorbic acid and vitamin E appealing. Vitamin E can be administered at a dose of 5000 IU/day as an oral suspension, whereas ascorbic acid can be given PO at a dose of 10–20 g daily. The beneficial effects of omega-3 polyunsaturated fatty acid (PUFA) supplementation have been recently postulated in many chronic diseases, including CRF both in people and small animals. The biological mechanism behind the purported effects of omega-3 PUFAs (α-linolenic acid [ALA], eicosapentaenoic acid [EPA], or docosahexaenoic acid [DHA]) is the skewed synthesis toward the anti-inflammatory eicosanoids, rather than the proinflammatory eicosanoids, during an inflammatory process. The direct effects of omega-3 PUFA supplementation in horses with CRF have not been evaluated, but based on experiences from other species, they may decelerate the progression of renal disease [19, 20]. There are numerous commercially marketed supplements available for horses, but the optimal dose remains unknown. Based on recommendations in small animals, an omega-3/omega-6 ratio of 1:5–10 seems to be beneficial. This would equal to about 10–50 g of omega-3 PUFA supplemented daily based on a diet containing 2–4% fat.

Therapeutic approaches to urinary incontinence and retention

Urinary incontinence is the inability to control micturition and results in intermittent or continuous urine leakage. Disorders of micturition include problems with urine storage (incontinence) and bladder emptying (urine retention). It is a frustrating problem in horses, as a definitive diagnosis is often difficult to establish, and therefore, treatment modalities are limited, while the amount of nursing care required from clients to keep an incontinent horse comfortable is substantial. Causes of incontinence and urine retention may be nonneurogenic or neurogenic in origin [21]. Congenital and acquired disorders of the lower urinary tract or altered detrusor and sphincter tone innervations should also be considered. Secondary cystitis (sabulous cystitis) is a characteristic feature of micturition disorders, while primary bacterial cystitis is considered rare in horses. Thus, cystitis without any predisposing cause should also raise a suspicion of urinary incontinence.

Etiology

Nonneurogenic incontinence has been linked to uni- or bilateral ectopic ureter, urolithiasis, cystitis, urethritis, and neoplasia of the lower urinary tract. In broodmares, incontinence has been occasionally noted after trauma to the external urethral sphincter from breeding accidents, dystocia, or poor vulvar conformation. Iatrogenic trauma from accidental insertion of a vaginal speculum into the bladder has been also described as a cause of incontinence [22]. In contrast to ovariectomized female dogs, estrogen-responsive incontinence resulting from low urethral sphincter tone has been seldom reported in mares and is considered a rare phenomenon.

In older geldings and stallions, a myogenic bladder paralysis has been described without apparent neurologic deficits. The end result is accumulation of large amounts of crystallized sediment in the bladder, termed sabulous cystitis, which leads to overstretching and consequent atony of the detrusor muscle. The etiology of incomplete bladder evacuation in these cases is speculative. However, difficulty in attaining normal urination posture secondary to chronic spondylitis, lumbosacral pain, or sacroiliac pain has been proposed [23].

Neurogenic incontinence is defined as the dysfunction of the neural pathways associated with normal micturition. This reflex involves sacral parasympathetic (pelvic nerve, S2–S4), somatic (pudendal nerve), and lumbar sympathetic (hypogastric nerve L1–L4) branches. These nerves are under the central control of the brainstem and cerebral cortex. Depending on the location of a lesion, neurogenic incontinence can be further divided into upper motor neuron (UMN) and lower motor neuron (LMN) deficits:

- LMN deficits—overflow bladder

  Damage to the sacral spinal cord segments or to the pelvic nerves will result in urethral sphincter and detrusor atony with subsequent urinary retention and overflow incontinence. Rectal examination in these cases reveals a large, flaccid bladder that is easily expressed. Equine herpesvirus 1 myeloencephalopathy (EHM), equine protozoal myeloencephalitis (EPM), lumbosacral vertebral trauma, cauda equina neuritis, equine motor neuron disease (EMND), or neoplasia can lead to an LMN bladder. Epidural administration of alcohol has also been anecdotally reported to result in iatrogenic bladder paralysis.

- UMN deficits—autonomic bladder

  Injury to the spinal cord cranial to the sacral segments will lead to increased urethral sphincter tone and disorders of micturition. Rectal examination in these cases reveals a spastic bladder that can be small, normal sized, or distended and is difficult to express. Incontinence resulting from UMN dysfunction is rare in horses but may be associated with meningitis, EHM, EPM, neoplasia, trauma, or an idiopathic origin [24].

The characterization of the bladder dysfunction is helpful for neuroanatomical localization. However, it is important to recognize that horses with UMN bladder signs will develop an overflow bladder (LMN bladder) over time, due to the accumulation of urine sediment as a result of incomplete emptying. Therefore, it is possible to diagnose overflow bladder (LMN bladder) in neurologic horses, without evidence of sacral spinal cord segment involvement.

A unique form of neurogenic bladder has been anecdotally reported in newborn foals with no causative or etiologic agent identified. It is speculated that this phenomenon may be part of the neonatal maladjustment syndrome (NMS), but foals may not display any other characteristic signs of NMS, such as lack of suckle, aimless wondering, vocalizing. These foals typically have a distended and spastic bladder (UMN signs) and exhibit stranguria. It is crucial to recognize and address the neurogenic bladder in foals, as it can lead to reopening of the urachus or even bladder rupture.

Clinical signs

Chronic, prolonged contact of urine with the skin leads to scalding and dermatitis around the perineum and medial aspect of the hindlimbs. Acute-onset neurogenic

incontinence may be accompanied by other neurologic deficits in adult horses. With LMN dysfunction, urine dribbling is usually continuous (flaccid, paralytic bladder), and other signs, including loss of anal and tail tone, fecal retention, perineal sensory deficits, and hindlimb weakness, are common. UMN dysfunction manifests as intermittent urine leakage, and spinal ataxia can be apparent as well. In these cases, bladder rupture can occur as a result of exaggerated sphincter tone. Dysuria or stranguria along with an abnormal or absent urine flow is suggestive of obstructive uropathy (urolithiasis, urethritis, and neoplasia). Neonatal foals with neurogenic bladder will exhibit stranguria, while there may not be any other clinical signs present.

Diagnosis

The diagnosis of urinary incontinence is based on history, clinical signs, and the results of diagnostic procedures. Neurologic evaluation, rectal palpation, urinalysis, hematology, serum chemistry, transrectal and transabdominal ultrasonography, and endoscopy of the lower urinary tract may be indicated. Evaluation of intravesicular and urethral pressures via cystometrography and urethral pressure profilometry has been described, but is not practical or feasible in most situations. Scintigraphy may also aid in diagnosis if vertebral spinal trauma or other degenerative changes exist [25]. Computed tomography and magnetic resonance imaging can be utilized in foals and miniature breeds, when other diagnostic approaches fail to provide a diagnosis. Pertinent information from history includes trauma, previous lumbosacral pain, breeding accidents, ongoing neurological disease, and dystocia. Incontinence since birth raises the suspicion of congenital malformation of the lower urinary tract (ectopic ureter), whereas stranguria/pollakiuria in a foal is suggestive of a transient neurogenic bladder. Urinary tract infection is a common sequel to micturition disorders, and therefore, urinalysis and routine urine culture should be performed in all cases.

Management

Treatment of **nonneurogenic incontinence** depends on the underlying cause and includes approaches aimed at ameliorating the primary problem (ectopic ureter, uroliths). A Caslick's procedure can be performed in mares with poor pelvic conformation. In certain instances, the underlying problem cannot be resolved, as in the case of infiltrative neoplasia and some congenital abnormalities.

In cases of **neurogenic incontinence**, diagnosis and treatment of the primary neurologic problem are important, while in the meantime, evacuation of the bladder and maintenance of an indwelling urinary catheter can help to prevent development of sabulous cystitis and further loss of detrusor muscle function. Some authors that have followed recovery of horses long-term after EHM have suggested that continuing bladder dysfunction may be due to the common practice of only emptying the bladder twice daily and that more frequent bladder evacuation may be indicated for treatment of the neurogenic bladder. If crystalline sediment is already present, it can be lavaged with large volumes of isotonic fluids through the urinary catheter. In cases of chronic incontinence, this procedure may need to be repeated on a regular basis, as accumulation of the sabulous material in the bladder due to incomplete evacuation can lead to exacerbation of the clinical signs. Pharmacologic intervention can be attempted in all cases of micturition disorders; however, success is usually limited to cases where the acute onset is followed by timely intervention, as a chronically distended urinary bladder is less likely to regain function due to the excessive neurologic and myogenic damage.

If some detrusor activity is detectable, treatment with bethanechol chloride (0.02–0.08 mg/kg bwt, SQ, q8 h or 0.3–0.5 mg/kg bwt, PO, q8 h) stimulates bladder contraction and may be helpful for LMN dysfunction [26]. Horses unresponsive to parasympathomimetics are poor candidates for long-term management. It is recommended to use the smallest effective dose, as this drug will exert gastrointestinal side effects through its widespread cholinergic actions in the body. If the bladder is of normal or small size and urethral tone is inadequate (as determined by urethral pressure measurements or more practically by observing continuous voiding without stranguria), phenylpropanolamine (PPA) can be administered at a dose of 1 mg/kg bwt, PO, q12 h). PPA is a sympathomimetic, α adrenergic stimulant and should be administered with caution as it has been reported to cause excitement, panting, or anorexia in small animals. PPA is thought to stimulate α adrenergic receptors directly and stimulate both α1 adrenergic and β adrenergic receptors indirectly by causing the release of norepinephrine. Other pharmacologic effects of PPA include vasoconstriction, mild CNS stimulation, and appetite suppression. Since there are no pharmacokinetic or scientific data available on the effect of PPA in horses, the use of the drug is presently anecdotal.

Some mares with sphincter atony respond positively to estradiol cypionate administered at a dose of 5–10 µg/kg bwt, IM, every other day [27]. The therapeutic rationale for the administration of estrogens is based on a proposed enhanced norepinephrine response on α adrenoceptors, which stimulates the smooth muscles of the urethral sphincter.

Conversely, urethral sphincter tone can be decreased, and urine voiding improved by the addition of the α adrenergic blocker phenoxybenzamine administered at a dose of 0.7 mg/kg bwt, PO, q6 h in cases of UMN bladder disorders. Phenoxybenzamine has a slow onset of action, and the effective dose is usually increased gradually over 3- to 4-day intervals in small animals, whereas data in horses is scarce. The quality of the urine stream is often used to gauge phenoxybenzamine effectiveness. If the stream is weak but continuous and of normal diameter, bethanechol may be used to increase detrusor contractility; however, it must not be used until the functional urethral obstruction is relieved. Hypotension is a major adverse effect of phenoxybenzamine in small animals, and the dose is routinely decreased if the animal shows any indication of weakness or disorientation. The dose should only be increased if a favorable response is not observed after 3 or 4 days, and rapid dose changes should be avoided. Glaucoma is a rare complication of phenoxybenzamine treatment in people; it is unknown if this occurs in horses.

Diazepam administered at a dose of 0.02–0.1 mg/kg bwt, slow IV, can also be used for UMN bladder disorders while the patient is hospitalized, as it decreases external urethral sphincter tone through its relaxant effect on skeletal muscles. However, this relaxant effect is short lasting (1–2 h). Acepromazine administered at a dose of 0.01–0.05 mg/kg bwt, IM, q8 h also has α adrenergic antagonist activity in addition to its tranquilizing effect and may be useful in some UMN cases.

To prevent urine scalding, the affected areas should be cleaned once or twice daily followed by topical applications of petroleum jelly or zinc oxide. Foals with neurogenic bladder will require long-term urinary catheterization for 3–10 days in addition to broad-spectrum antimicrobials. Serial urine culture and sensitivity (C&S) evaluations are recommended to monitor the accompanying cystitis and tailor the antimicrobial therapy.

In general, incontinence caused by neurogenic origin carries a poor prognosis for recovery except for transient, potentially treatable or maintainable neurologic diseases (EPM, EHM, or neurogenic bladder in neonatal

Table 17.1 Names, indications, and doses of the drugs most commonly in neurogenic incontinence.

Drug	Indication	Dose
Bethanechol	LMN—decreased detrusor activity	0.02–0.08 mg/kg SQ q8 h 0.3–0.5 mg/kg PO q8 h
Diazepam	UMN—increased sphincter tone	0.02–0.1 mg/kg IV
Acepromazine	UMN—increased sphincter tone	0.01–0.05 mg/kg IV, IM, SQ q8 h
Phenoxybenzamine	UMN—increased sphincter tone	0.7 mg/kg PO q6 h
PPA	LMN—decreased sphincter tone	1 mg/kg PO q12 h
Estradiol cypionate	LMN—decreased sphincter tone	5–10 μg/kg IM EOD

foals) [28]. In other cases, incontinence presents as a chronic problem accompanied with sabulous cystitis. Management in these cases can be attempted with periodic lavages of the urinary bladder and certain pharmacological agents (Table 17.1) [29].

Treatment of urinary tract infections

Bacterial UTIs are uncommon in horses [30]. While there is no direct data on the incidence of UTI in horses, it is most frequently diagnosed as an ascending infection secondary to urolithiasis or functional impairment of the bladder, such as incontinence or urine retention, that interfere with normal urine flow. As with other infections, environmental, host, and infectious agent interaction plays a role in the development of disease. Host protective factors include production of secretory IgA and defensins on the surface of the uroepithelium, as well as innate and acquired immune responses. Classification of UTI is based on the presence of detectable abnormalities in host defense mechanisms that allow colonization of pathogenic bacteria within the urinary tract. In cases of uncomplicated UTI, there are no underlying structural, neurologic, or functional abnormalities of the urinary tract identified. In these cases, colonization is likely due to a transient defect in the patient's defense mechanisms. In general, uncomplicated UTI requires a shorter treatment course and carries a better prognosis for recovery in comparison to complicated UTI. In cases of complicated UTI, colonization of the urinary tract is secondary to a structural, neurologic, or functional abnormality, and resolution of the infection requires correction of the primary cause. The majority of the horses diagnosed with bacterial UTI have an underlying disease process. Contributing factors to the development of UTI in these cases include obstruction of normal urine flow by masses, uroliths, or strictures; disruption of the uroepithelium by trauma or neoplasia; or reduction of normal urogenital flora.

Long-term urinary catheterization is rarely performed in equids except for recumbent neonatal foals or horses with neurogenic bladder. Prolonged catheterization favors biofilm formation and bacterial adhesion with subsequent colonization. Additionally, urinary catheters enable bacteria to ascend from the distal urethra or external genitalia to the bladder. A further complicating factor is that maintenance of an indwelling urinary catheter is not feasible to the same extent as in humans. These circumstances allow colonization of pathogenic agents in the urinary tract; thus, horses with indwelling urinary catheters will predictably develop UTI.

Escherichia coli is one of the most commonly isolated organisms from urine in clinically healthy horses as well as those with UTI. Uropathogenic strains of *E. coli* selectively emerge from the fecal flora and possess virulence factors that play a critical role in their predominance. These factors include fimbriae that attach to the uroepithelium, lipopolysaccharides (LPS) that promote interleukin production and neutrophil chemotaxis, and alpha hemolysin that generates inflammation through complex and diverse pathways [31]. Other commonly isolated organisms from ascending UTI include *Proteus*, *Klebsiella*, *Enterobacter*, *Streptococcus*, *Staphylococcus*, *Corynebacterium*, and *Pseudomonas* species. Most of these bacteria are part of the normal urogenital flora; however, in the presence of predisposing factors, the more pathogenic flora can overgrow. Rarely, hematogenous spread of pathogenic organisms to the urinary tract can occur in neonatal foals with bacterial sepsis.

Diagnosis

Differentiation of uncomplicated from complicated UTI is crucial for a successful recovery and often requires extensive diagnostic testing. Urinalysis is the most useful test in the diagnosis of bacterial UTI. Visualization of more than 20 microorganisms and more than 10 white blood cells (WBC) per high-power field during examination of the urine sediment is highly suggestive of UTI [32]. History and physical examination may aid in localizing the disease within the urinary tract (nephritis, ureteritis, cystitis, or urethritis). Nonetheless, extensive diagnostic testing may be required to identify the underlying cause. A complete blood count may be unremarkable or can reveal mature neutrophilia or left shift. Plasma fibrinogen concentration can be elevated in cases of pyelonephritis or cases where abscess formation within the urinary tract is present. Urine C&S testing is highly recommended prior to treatment with antimicrobials. More than 10 000 colony-forming units (CFU) of bacteria per milliliter of urine have been considered diagnostic for UTI. It must be noted that urine samples collected from female horses and those collected via free-catch sampling have higher CFU counts [33]. Endoscopy of the urinary tract, to look for the presence of strictures, adhesions, uroliths, neoplasias, or mucosal defects, is considered a standard diagnostic tool in the workup of UTI. It may also aid in the evaluation of ureters (hematuria, decreased or no flow) and provide the opportunity to collect samples from the left and right ureters separately. Ultrasonography, both percutaneous and transrectal, of the urinary tract is recommended to evaluate the kidneys and ureters for urolithiasis and abscesses.

Antimicrobial drugs used to treat infections in the renal tract

The use of antimicrobial drugs remains the cornerstone of UTI management in equids. However, as mentioned earlier, UTI is almost always a secondary problem (i.e., complicated UTI). Therefore, it is critical to resolve the primary issue before or parallel to the initiation of antimicrobial treatment. Bacterial susceptibility, urinary excretion of the drug, and convenience of administration are the primary considerations for antimicrobial selection. For cases of uncomplicated UTI, 1–2 weeks of antimicrobial therapy is recommended. Complicated UTI or recurrent cases may require treatment for up to 6–8 weeks, whereas complete resolution of renal abscesses may require 2–6 months of therapy. Clinical signs, clinicopathologic findings, and microbial culture results must be considered before cessation of treatment.

Specific antimicrobial drugs

The selection of antimicrobials is based upon empirical information until C&S is available. Oral sulfonamides in cases of uncomplicated UTI in adult horses are often the first-line therapy, while complicated UTI cases and foals are treated with IV antimicrobials, including cephalosporins alone or in combination with an aminoglycoside in nonazotemic patients. More details on the pharmacology of the antimicrobial agents discussed in this chapter can be found in Chapter 2.

Potentiated sulfonamides (trimethoprim–sulfonamide)

Sulfonamides are excreted by glomerular filtration and active tubular secretion. These antimicrobials reach high concentrations in the urine and are good choices for treatment of UTI. Dihydropyrimidines, such as trimethoprim, and the sulfonamides are bacteriostatic alone, but in combination therapy, they often have a synergistic bactericidal effect. Trimethoprim–sulfamethoxazole (TMS) has broad-spectrum activity, a reasonable price, and the convenience of oral administration, which make it an excellent choice for UTI prophylaxis in cases of incontinence or urolithiasis or for the treatment of uncomplicated UTI. Many uropathogenic bacteria, including *Streptococcus* species, *Staphylococcus* species, and *E. coli*, are sensitive to TMS. Uncommonly reported complications associated with TMS use include crystalluria, interstitial nephritis, and hematuria in other species. The dose range is 15–30 mg/kg bwt, PO, q12 h.

β–lactam antimicrobials

Penicillins are also commonly used to treat UTIs in horses. They are often the primary drugs of choice as penicillins reach high concentrations in urine. However, the need for parenteral administration of penicillin in horses limits their utility when prolonged treatment is needed. Since penicillin G has primarily Gram-positive, anaerobic, and only a limited Gram-negative spectrum of activity, both the long-acting procaine ester formulation (PPG) administered at a dose of 22 000 U/kg bwt, IM, q12 h and the potassium salt formulation administered at a dose of 22 000 U/kg bwt, IV, q6 h should be concomitantly administered with aminoglycosides or a fluoroquinolone to enhance activity against Gram-negative uropathogens.

Aminopenicillins in the form of ampicillin administered at a dose of 20–40 mg/kg bwt, IV, q8–12 h may be used either alone or in combination with aminoglycosides to provide broad-spectrum coverage. Because they penetrate the LPS layer of Gram-negative bacteria better than penicillin, they have improved activity against these pathogens. Ampicillin is commonly used in neonatal foals and to lesser extent in adults due to its cost.

Imipenem was developed to combat β-lactamase-associated antimicrobial resistance. This antimicrobial has a broad spectrum of activity and is highly concentrated in urine when combined with cilastatin. The use of imipenem is almost always cost prohibitive in adult horses but can be used in miniature horses and foals but only when the presence of a multiresistant organism is confirmed by C&S testing. Pharmacokinetic data suggests a dose of 10–20 mg/kg bwt, IV, q6 h would be appropriate.

Cephalosporins are also excellent choices for treatment of UTI in horses. Ceftiofur is a third-generation cephalosporin that is effective against a wide range of Gram-positive and Gram-negative organisms. Some Gram-negative bacteria, however, may be resistant to ceftiofur at the commonly recommended dose of 2.2 mg/kg bwt, IV or IM, q12 h, and therefore, its use combined with other antimicrobials is occasionally recommended based on the results of C&S testing. Other third-generation cephalosporins, including cefotaxime administered at a dose of 25–40 mg/kg bwt, IV, q6 h and ceftazidime administered at a dose of 40 mg/kg bwt, IV, q6 h, are commonly used in neonatal foals, but should not be considered for initial treatment of UTI unless C&S testing supports their use. Their cost and complications, such as antimicrobial-induced colitis, associated with their use limit their use in adult horses.

Aminoglycosides

Aminoglycosides are bactericidal antimicrobials that are eliminated via glomerular filtration, leading to high concentrations of active drug in urine and renal tubular epithelial cells. Despite their high concentrations in urine, aminoglycosides are not used for initial treatment of UTI because they are potentially nephrotoxic and because they have limited activity in urine due to the low oxygen tension and alkaline pH. Their potential therapeutic advantage is in treating aerobic Gram-negative bacteria causing ascending or hematogenous pyelonephritis. The dosage of gentamicin is 6.6 mg/kg bwt, IV, q24 h, and the dosage of amikacin is 21–25 mg/kg bwt, IV, q24 h. Amikacin is usually cost prohibitive in adult horses and is reserved to treat microbes resistant to gentamicin (i.e., resistant *Enterococcus sp.*). Gentamicin, however, has better activity than amikacin against *Streptococcus sp.* and nonenteric Gram-negative organisms, including most *Klebsiella* and *Pseudomonas sp.*

Fluoroquinolones

Enrofloxacin has been used for the treatment of UTI in adult horses. It has great efficacy against *Staphylococcus sp.* and Gram-negative bacteria and penetrates well into abscesses. Although its use is highly discouraged in immature horses due to its cartilage-damaging effects, there may be situations where enrofloxacin is the best option for therapy. In these cases, some clinicians believe that concomitant administration of hyaluronic acid and/or polysulfated glycosaminoglycans can decrease the severity of the cartilage damage, although there are no scientific studies supporting this theory. Oral compounded formulations are widely available, but the clinician needs to remember that the quality and stability of compounded formulations cannot be assumed. Enrofloxacin should only be used when C&S results indicate the presence of organisms resistant to other antimicrobials typically considered for initial therapy, such as potentiated sulfonamides. The recommended dose of enrofloxacin is 5 mg/kg bwt, IV, q24 h or 7.5 mg/kg bwt, PO, q24 h.

Supportive therapy

Supportive therapy including administration of IV fluids and NSAIDs may be indicated in individual cases. Phenazopyridine, a urinary analgesic and local anesthetic, has been used with success in both foals and adult horses at a dose of 4 mg/kg bwt, PO, q8–12 h to alleviate signs associated with urinary discomfort. Phenazopyridine is an azo dye compound that acts to confer relief from irritation or spasm of the urinary tract mucosa via local anesthetic activity. It will stain the urine, skin, and any material that inadvertently come into contact with it. In humans with urinary tract inflammation, the agent alleviates symptoms of dysuria, frequency, burning, and the sensation of urgency. Side effects include aggravation of oxidative stress and development of methemoglobinemia, and therefore, long-term administration (i.e., >7 days) is not recommended.

Management of renal abscesses

Rarely, cases of equine infectious nephritis and renal abscessation occur as sequelae to primary bacterial sepsis from *Rhodococcus equi*, *Corynebacterium pseudotuberculosis*, or *S. equi* spp. *equi* infections. Regardless of the cause, prolonged antimicrobial therapy from 1 to 6 months with a drug that can penetrate the abscess capsule is indicated. After initial stabilization of the horse, an additional consideration in these cases is to find a drug that can be administered PO and long term. These criteria are met by chloramphenicol administered at a dose of 50 mg/kg bwt, PO, q8 h, enrofloxacin, and doxycycline. Another alternative would be rifampin administered at a dose of 5 mg/kg bwt, PO, q12 h in combination with another antimicrobial, because resistance to rifampin develops quickly when it is used as a sole agent. Rifampin is highly lipophilic and has excellent penetration into tissues, cells, and abscesses [11]. Administration of multiple antimicrobials PO increases the risk of development of colitis, and therefore, close monitoring of these horses is recommended. Ultrasound-guided drainage and lavage of large abscesses can be attempted in cases that are accessible via a percutaneous approach. In cases of pyelonephritis or renal abscessation that is refractory to treatment, unilateral nephrectomy may be an option, if the other kidney is functional.

Parasitic infections

Parasitic lesions associated with the nematodes *Strongylus vulgaris*, *Halicephalobus deletrix*, and *Dioctophyme renale* in equine kidneys should be also considered in cases unresponsive to antimicrobial drugs [32]. Aberrant larval migration of *S. vulgaris* in the renal artery and parenchyma has been described but usually is an incidental finding during postmortem examinations. Passage through the renal parenchyma may result in infarctions or hemorrhage. In cases of suspected larval migration, anthelmintic therapy with fenbendazole administered at a dose of 10 mg/kg bwt, PO, q24 for 5 days is recommended.

Therapeutic options for urolithiasis

Urolithiasis is an uncommon disease in horses, with the prevalence reported in a study from California to be around 0.11% over a 20-year period [34]. Prevalence, however, likely varies in the different regions of the USA, due to the changes in pasture and soil composition. While calculus formation can occur anywhere in the urinary tract, the bladder remains the most common site, followed by the kidneys, and calculi can also be found lodged in the urethra or ureters. There is no documented age, breed, or sex predilection associated with urolith formation. However, it appears to be a more common problem in males, due to their relatively narrow and long urethra. Factors contributing to mineral formation in the urinary tract include supersaturation of the urine, urine retention, a genetic tendency to excrete large amounts of calcium and uric acid in the urine, and lack of inhibitors of crystal growth [35]. In addition, UTIs, invasive procedures, and any damage to the renal parenchyma, such as papillary crest necrosis, all increase the risk for secondary mineral formation. The most common type of calculus in the equine urinary tract is calcium carbonate, while struvite and oxalate stones are a far less common.

Diagnosis

Horses with urolithiasis can present with variable clinical signs, depending on the location of the calculi. Horses with calculi in the upper urinary tract can present with clinical signs of renal failure, whereas uroliths in the bladder or in the urethra can result in hematuria, stranguria, or pain, often interpreted as colic. In a recent retrospective study, 69% of the horses diagnosed with CRF had some type of mineral buildup in the upper or lower urinary tract [15]. Urinary calculi can also be an incidental finding during routine diagnostic evaluation, with no evidence of pathology at the time of evaluation. Urinary calculi in the kidneys can be detected with percutaneous ultrasound examination, while stones lodged in the ureters can be visualized with transrectal ultrasound examination. Urinary calculi in the lower urinary tract can grow quite large and can be palpated during rectal examination in most cases; however, transrectal ultrasound examination can be helpful in questionable cases. It is recommended to evaluate renal function by serum biochemistry panels in horses with urolithiasis, as well as test for a concurrent UTI by obtaining a sterile urine sample for urinalysis and culture.

Management of urinary calculi

Multiple surgical techniques have been described for the removal of urinary calculi, including laparocystotomy, perineal urethrotomy, and laparoscopic cystotomy, while more recently introduced techniques, such as laser lithotripsy and shock wave therapy, aim at stone disruption and removal without major surgical intervention. Details on these procedures can be found elsewhere [36].

In all cases that undergo surgical resolution of urolithiasis, therapy to support renal function should be initiated. Once urine flow is established, diuresis with 4–6 ml/kg/h polyionic crystalloid fluids can be initiated. This will allow flushing of the cellular and mineral debris caused by the procedure. In cases where renal damage is apparent, the aforementioned recommendations for the *Management of ARF* can be followed. As horses with urolithiasis often have accompanying UTI, it is always necessary to initiate antimicrobial therapy, preferably before the surgical procedure. See the guidelines outlined in Section "Antimicrobial Drugs Used to Treat Infections in the Renal Tract".

Once the obstruction is resolved, management changes can be attempted to prevent reoccurrence of the problem. For example, dietary changes to limit calcium intake are recommended. Horses in general consume a high-calcium diet and as a result excrete large quantities of calcium in the urine. Acidification of the urine of horses with recurrent urolithiasis can also be an option, as calcium crystals are readily soluble in urine with a pH below 6. Effective acidification of equine urine, however, is not easily accomplished. Feeding a diet with a low dietary cation–anion difference (DCAD) is useful in the long-term management of these cases, as it influences systemic pH and urinary excretion of minerals. A DCAD value of less than 100 mEq/kg of dry feed decreases urine pH and enhances excretion of minerals, especially calcium [37]. It is recommended that owners have their commercial feed products and hay analyzed for DCAD values.

Urinary acidifiers can also be used; however, the amount of supplement required to effectively decrease urine pH is unpalatable for most horses. Both ammonium chloride and ammonium sulfate have been described for the management of urolithiasis in horses. The ammonium of PO supplemented ammonium chloride is converted by the liver to urea, freeing hydrogen ions and decreasing bicarbonate concentration. Therefore, efficacy depends on hepatic conversion of ammonium chloride, which requires normal liver function. Ammonium chloride administered at a dose of 330 mg/kg bwt, PO, q24 h has been shown to decrease

urine pH into the acidic range [38], but this high dose is usually unpalatable for the horse, and administration may require daily nasogastric intubation. In another report, ammonium sulfate administered at a dose of 175 mg/kg bwt, PO, q12 h was used successfully to decrease urine pH and limit the recurrence of uroliths in a horse [39]. Ammonium sulfate is thought to be more palatable, and horses may eat it mixed in pellets or grain. Oral administration of ascorbic acid has been proven to decrease the urinary pH below 6; however, the dose of 1–2 g/kg bwt, PO, q24 h is extremely high and may not be practical [38]. Administration of urinary acidifiers is only recommended in patients with normal renal function, as altering metabolic homeostasis can be harmful to kidneys with an already compromised function.

References

1 Odutayo, A., Adhikari, N.K., Barton, J. *et al.* (2012) Epidemiolo of acute kidney injury in Canadian critical care units: A prospective cohort study. *Canadian Journal of Anesthesia*, **59** (10), 934–942.

2 Mehta, R.L., Kellum, J.A., Shah, S.V. *et al.* (2007) Acute Kidney Injury Network: Report of an initiative to improve outcomes in acute kidney injury. *Critical Care*, **11**, R31.

3 Fielding, C.L. & Magdesian, K.G. (2009) Fluid therapy for renal failure. In: B.P. Smith (ed), *Large Animal Internal Medicine*, pp. 1495–1496. Mosby, St. Louis.

4 Johansson, A.M., Gardner, S.Y., Levine, J.F. *et al.* (2003) Furosemide continuous rate infusion in the horse: Evaluation of enhanced efficacy and reduced side effects. *Journal of Veterinary Internal Medicine*, **17**, 887–895.

5 Womble, A., Giguère, S. & Lee, E.A. (2007) Pharmacokinetics of oral doxycycline and concentrations in body fluids and bronchoalveolar cells of foals. *Journal of Veterinary Pharmacology and Therapeutics*, **30**, 187–193.

6 Han, J.H. & McKenzie, H.C. (2008) Intermittent peritoneal dialysis for the treatment of acute renal failure in two horses. *Equine Veterinary Education*, **20**, 256–264.

7 Gallatin, L.L., Couëtil, L.L. & Ash, S.R. (2005) Use of continuous-flow peritoneal dialysis for the treatment of acute renal failure in an adult horse. *Journal of the American Veterinary Medical Association*, **226**, 756–759, 732.

8 Reuss, S.M., Franklin, R.P., Peloso, J.G. & Gallatin, L.L. (2006) How to perform continuous peritoneal dialysis in an adult horse. *American Association of Equine Practitioners*, **52**, 96–100.

9 Bersenas, A.M. (2011) A clinical review of peritoneal dialysis. *Journal of Veterinary Emergency and Critical Care*, **21**, 605–617.

10 Hines, M.T. (2007) Leptospirosis. In: D.C. Sellon & M.T. Long (eds), *Equine Infectious Diseases*, pp. 301–309. WB Saunders, St. Louis.

11 Haggett, E.F. & Wilson, W.D. (2008) Overview of the use of antimicrobials for the treatment of bacterial infections in horses. *Equine Veterinary Journal*, **20**, 443–448.

12 Agwuh, K.N. & MacGowan, A. (2006) Pharmacokinetics and pharmacodynamics of the tetracyclines including glycylcyclines. *Journal of Antimicrobial Chemotherapy*, **58**, 256–265.

13 Kim, D., Kordick, D., Divers, T. & Chang, Y.F. (2006) In vitro susceptibilities of Leptospira spp. and Borrelia burgdorferi isolates to amoxicillin, tilmicosin, and enrofloxacin. *Journal of Veterinary Science*, **7**, 355–359.

14 Schott, H.C. (2009) Chronic renal failure. In: S. Reed, W. Bayley & D. Sellon (eds), *Equine Internal Medicine*, 3rd edn, pp. 1231–1252. WB Saunders, St. Louis.

15 Nogradi, N., Toth, B., Whitcomb, M., Riley, R., Pusterla, N. & William, R. (2012) Factors associated with short term and long term outcome in horses with chronic renal failure. ACVIM Forum Research Abstracts Program, Presented at the Annual Meeting of the American College of Veterinary Internal Medicine, New Orleans, LA, May 30–June 2.

16 Grauer, G.F. (2003) Renal failure. In: R.W. Nelson & C.G. Couto (eds), *Small Animal Internal Medicine*, 3rd edn, pp. 608–623. Mosby, St. Louis.

17 Jarvis, N.G. (2009) Nutrition of the aged horse. *Veterinary Clinics of North America Equine Practice*, **25**, 155–166, viii.

18 Brown, S.A. (2008) Oxidative stress and chronic kidney disease. *Veterinary Clinics of North America Small Animal Practice*, **38**, 157–166, vi.

19 Friedman, A.N. (2010) Omega-3 fatty acid supplementation in advanced kidney disease. *Seminars in Dialysis*, **23**, 396–400.

20 Brown, S.A., Brown, C.A., Crowell, W.A. *et al.* (2000) Effects of dietary polyunsaturated fatty acid supplementation in early renal insufficiency in dogs. *Journal of Laboratory and Clinical Medicine*, **135**, 275–286.

21 Sponseller, B.E. (2003) Urinary incontinence. In: N.E. Robinson (ed), *Current Therapy in Equine Medicine*, 5th edn, pp. 824–826. Mosby, St. Louis.

22 Gehlen, H. & Klug, E. (2001) Urinary incontinence in the mare due to iatrogenic trauma. *Equine Veterinary Education*, **13**, 183–186.

23 Couëtil, L.L., Hoffman, A.M., Hodgson, J. *et al.* (2007) Inflammatory airway disease of horses. *Journal of Veterinary Internal Medicine*, **21**, 356–361.

24 Scarrat, W.K., Buechner-Maxwell, V.A. & Karzenski, S. (1999) Urinary incontinence and incoordination in three horses associated with equine protozoal myeloencephalitis. *Journal of Equine Veterinary Science*, **19**, 642–645.

25 Kay, A.D. & Lavoie, J.P. (1987) Urethral pressure profilometry in mares. *Journal of the American Veterinary Medical Association*, **191**, 212–216.

26 Booth, T.M., Howes, D.A. & Edwards, G.B. (2000) Bethanechol-responsive bladder atony in a colt foal after cystorrhaphy for cystorrhexis. *Veterinary Record*, **147**, 306–308.

27 Watson, E.D., McGorum, B.C. & Keeling, N. (1997) Oestrogen-responsive urinary incontinence in two mares. *Equine Veterinary Education*, **9**, 81–84.

28 Carr, E.A. (2009) Urinary incontinence. In: B.P. Smith (ed), *Large Animal Internal Medicine*, pp. 935–937. Mosby, St. Louis.

29 Rendle, D.I., Durham, A.E., Hughes, K.J., Lloyd, D. & Summerhays, G.E. (2008) Long-term management of sabulous cystitis in five horses. *Veterinary Record*, **162**, 783–787.

30 Schott, H. (2003) Urinary tract infection and bladder displacement. In: N.E. Robinson (ed), *Current Therapy in Equine Medicine*, pp. 837–839. Mosby, St. Louis.

31 Frye, M.A. (2006) Pathophysiology, diagnosis, and management of urinary tract infection in horses. *Veterinary Clinics of North America Equine Practice*, **22**, 497–517, x.

32 Schott, H. (2009) Urinary tract infections. In: S. Reed, W. Bayly & D. Sellon (eds), *Equine Internal Medicine*, 3rd edn, pp. 1254–1258. WB Saunders, St. Louis.

33 MacLeay, J.M. & Kohn, C.W. (1998) Results of quantitative cultures of urine by free catch and catheterization from healthy adult horses. *Journal of Veterinary Internal Medicine*, **12**, 76–78.

34 Laverty, S., Pascoe, J.R., Ling, G.V., Lavoie, J.P. & Ruby, A.L. (1992) Urolithiasis in 68 horses. *Veterinary Surgery*, **21**, 56–62.

35 Jose-Cunilleras, E. & Hinchcliff, K.W. (1999) Renal pharmacology. *Veterinary Clinics of North America Equine Practice*, **15**, 647–664, ix.

36 Duesterdieck-Zellmer, K.F. (2007) Equine urolithiasis. *Veterinary Clinics of North America Equine Practice*, **23**, 613–629, iv.

37 Wall, D.L., Topliff, D.R., Freeman, D.W., Breazile, J.E., Wagner, D.G. & Stutz, W.A. (1993) *The effect of dietary cation–anion balance on mineral balance in the anaerobically exercised horse*. Proceedings of the 13th Equine Nutrition and Physiology Society, University of Florida, Gainesville, FL, 21–23 January 1993, 504, pp. 50–53.

38 Wood, T., Weckman, T.J., Henry, P.A., Chang, S.L., Blake, J.W. & Tobin, T. (1990) Equine urine pH: Normal population distributions and methods of acidification. *Equine Veterinary Journal*, **22**, 118–121.

39 Remillard, R.L., Modransky, P.D., Welker, F.H. & Thatcher, C.D. (1992) *Dietary management of cystic calculi in a horse. Journal of Equine Veterinary Science*, **12**, 359–363.

Index

Equine Pharmacology, First Edition. Edited by Cynthia Cole, Bradford Bentz and Lara Maxwell.
© 2015 John Wiley & Sons, Inc. Published 2015 by John Wiley & Sons, Inc.

Printed and bound by CPI Group (UK) Ltd, Croydon, CR0 4YY

16/04/2025

14658461-0006